D1401911

Anaesthesia
of the
CAT

Anaesthesia of the CAT

edited by

L.W. Hall

and

P.M. Taylor

University of Cambridge
Cambridge, UK

Baillière Tindall

LONDON PHILADELPHIA TORONTO SYDNEY TOKYO

Baillière Tindall   24–28 Oval Road
W.B. Saunders   London NW1 7DX, UK
Company Ltd
　　　　　　　The Curtis Center
　　　　　　　Independence Square West
　　　　　　　Philadelphia, PA 19106–3399, USA

　　　　　　　55 Horner Avenue
　　　　　　　Toronto, Ontario M8Z 4X6, Canada

　　　　　　　Harcourt Brace & Company
　　　　　　　(Australia) Pty Ltd
　　　　　　　30–52 Smidmore Street
　　　　　　　Marrickville, NSW 2204, Australia

　　　　　　　Harcourt Brace Japan
　　　　　　　Ichibancho Central Building
　　　　　　　22-1 Ichibancho
　　　　　　　Chiyoda-ku, Tokyo 102, Japan

© 1994 Baillière Tindall

All rights reserved. No part of this publication may be
reproduced, stored in a retrieval system or transmitted, in
any form or by any means, electronic, mechanical,
photocopying or otherwise, without the prior permission
of Baillière Tindall,
24–28 Oval Road, London NW1 7DX, UK

A catalogue record for this book is available from the
British Library

ISBN 0–7020–1665–9

This book is printed on acid-free paper

Typeset by J&L Composition Ltd, Filey, North Yorkshire
Printed and bound in Great Britain by The Bath Press, Avon

Contents

Contributors

J. Aldrich University of California Veterinary Medical Teaching Hospital, Davis, CA 95616, USA

J.C. Brearley, Anaesthesia Unit, Animal Health Trust, PO Box 5, Newmarket, Suffolk CB8 7DW, UK.

D.H. Dyson, University of Guelph, Ontario Veterinary College, Guelph, Ontario N1G 2W1, Canada.

R.J. Evans, University of Cambridge, Dept of Clinical Veterinary Medicine, Madingley Road, Cambridge CB3 0ES, UK.

P.A. Flecknell, Comparative Biology Centre, The Medical Centre, University of Newcastle upon Tyne, Newcastle, UK.

L.W. Hall, University of Cambridge, Dept of Clinical Veterinary Medicine, Madingley Road, Cambridge CB3 0ES, UK.

S.C. Haskins, University of California, Dept of Surgery and Radiological Sciences, School of Veterinary Medicine, Davis, CA 95616, USA.

J.E. Ilkiw, University of California, Dept of Surgical and Radiological Sciences, School of Veterinary Medicine, Davis, CA 95616, USA.

A.R. Jefferies, Animal Pathology Division, University of Cambridge, Dept of Clinical Veterinary Medicine, Madingley Road, Cambridge CB3 0ES, UK.

J.C.M. Lewis, International Zoo Veterinary Group, Keighley Business Centre, Keighley, West Yorkshire BD21 1AG, UK.

A.R. Michell, Dept of Large Animal Medicine and Surgery, The Royal Veterinary College, University of London, UK.

M.A.E. Rex, (deceased) University of Queensland, Dept of Companion Animal Medicine & Surgery, Brisbane, Qld 4072, Australia.

E.P. Steffey, University of California, Dept of Surgery and Radiological Sciences, School of Veterinary Medicine, Davis, CA 95616, USA.

P.M. Taylor, University of Cambridge, Dept of Clinical Veterinary Medicine, Madingley Road, Cambridge CB3 0ES, UK.

C.M. Trim, University of Georgia, College of Veterinary Medicine, Athens, Georgia 30602, USA.

Preface

For many years the cat has appeared as an also-ran in veterinary textbooks. There are many reasons that the cat should be considered in its own right but the main one is that it is not simply, as it has so often in the past been considered to be, a 'small dog'. Its temperament is unique among the domestic animals and so is its metabolism of many drugs. This book puts the focus on the cat itself — at least as far as anaesthesia is concerned.

Of particular note is the wealth of information relating to feline anaesthesia in physiological and other non-clinical literature not readily available to veterinarians. The invited authors have dug deeply into these various sources and the relevant material has now been brought together in the appropriate chapters in this book. We believe that as a result everything relevant to feline anaesthesia is covered for the first time in one volume.

Our thanks are due to Katharine Hinton of Baillière Tindall for encouraging us to complete this work when we could so easily have given up. We are also extremely grateful to our colleagues at the Cambridge University Department of Clinical Veterinary Medicine, and the Animal Health Trust, Newmarket, for their forbearance and help. We are especially grateful to the patient models, both two and four-legged, who appear in many of the photographs and to all the contributors of the chapters who so willingly completed the tasks we asked of them.

L.W. Hall
P.M. Taylor

M.A.E. Rex

1
Anatomy

Introduction

This chapter provides descriptions of the anatomy of those regions of the domestic cat which are of particular importance to the anaesthetist.

The Respiratory Tract

In any consideration of general anaesthesia, the respiratory tract is of paramount importance as the well-being of the cat is dependent on the maintenance of a clear airway throughout anaesthesia.

Nares and Pharynx

The nasal cavity of the cat is bounded laterally by the facial bones and has a longitudinal partition dividing it into two halves. These cavities are almost completely filled on each side by the ethmoturbinate caudally, the nasoturbinate which extends ventrally from the ventral surface of the nasal bone and the maxilloturbinate which extends medially from the medial surface of the maxilla. The turbinates are covered with mucosa and are well endowed with sensory nerve endings from the olfactory nerve and from the branches of the trigeminal nerve emanating from the Gasserian ganglion.

The nasal cavities perform an important function in the humidification and warming of the inspired air and it is important to realize that these mechanisms are bypassed when an endotracheal tube is inserted (Fig. 1.1). Sensory nerves in the nasal cavities and nasopharynx have receptors which are sensitive to irritants and to volatile anaesthetics. Their stimulation may provoke respiratory reflex effects of importance during general anaesthesia.

Mouth and Pharynx

The anatomy of the oral cavity is important, as endotracheal intubation in the cat is normally performed by the oral route.

The roof of the mouth is formed by the hard and soft palates, the teeth, gums and cheeks form the walls and the floor is formed mainly by the tongue which extends caudally to the isthmus faucium. The free end of the tongue is joined to the floor of the mouth by the frenulum. At its caudal end the glossoepiglottic frenulum passes from the dorsal surface of the tongue to the cranial aspect of the epiglottis.

This is an important anatomical relationship for intubation, as pulling the tongue rostrally tends to move the tip of the epiglottis ventrally, exposing the aditus laryngis and vocal cords (Fig. 1.2).

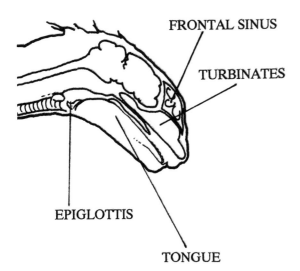

FRONTAL SINUS

TURBINATES

EPIGLOTTIS

TONGUE

Fig. 1.1 Longitudinal section of cat's head to show nares and pharynx.

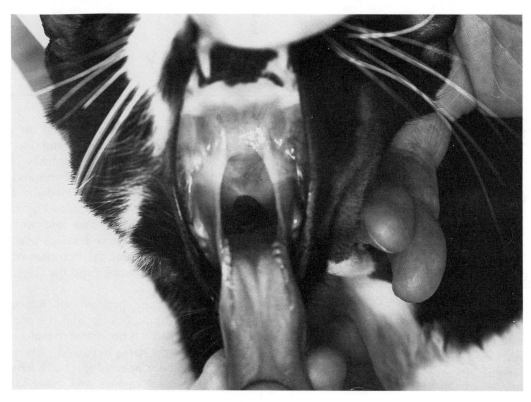

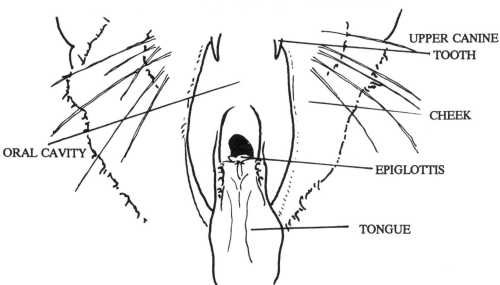

Fig. 1.2 Relationship of tongue to epiglottis.

The Pharynx

The pharynx is an important region, as it is here that the food passage and respiratory passage cross over. At the cranial end, the mouth is ventral and the nasal cavity dorsal, but further back the entrance to the oesophagus is dorsal whereas the laryngeal opening is ventral. This is therefore a potential site for obstruction of the airway due to food material, vomitus or other foreign bodies. During swallowing in the conscious cat, the free edge of the soft palate is pushed against the wall of the pharynx dorsally and the caudal part of the pharynx moves forward to form a continuous passage with the mouth. Food being swallowed does not pass into the nasopharynx, which communicates cranially with the nasal cavity, because it has been effectively sealed off by the soft palate. As this mechanism does not occur during general anaesthesia there is a potential for vomited or regurgitated food material to enter the nasopharynx dorsal to the soft palate.

The pharynx is well provided with sensory receptors whose afferent pathways are in the maxillary branch of the trigeminal nerve, the hypoglossal nerve and the vagus nerve.

The Larynx

The larynx is the major structure protecting the airway. It is made up of three unpaired cartilages, the thyroid, cricoid and epiglottic and the paired arytenoid cartilages. They articulate with each other and their movement is controlled by the intrinsic laryngeal muscles. The lumen of the larynx is lined with mucosa. There are three structures which are of particular importance in the protection of the airway:

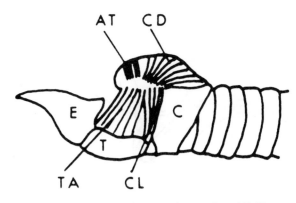

Fig. 1.3 The intrinsic laryngeal muscles. AT, Transverse arytenoid muscle; CD, dorsal arytenoid muscle; TA, thyroarytenoid muscle; CL, lateral cricoarytenoid muscle; E, epiglottis; T, thyroid cartilage; C, cricoid cartilage.

the cricoepiglottic folds which join the dorsal aspect of the rostral border of the cricoid cartilage to the sides of the epiglottis; the arytenoid cartilages; and the vocal cords which stretch from the apices of the arytenoid cartilages to the thyroid cartilage near the base of the epiglottis. The width of the glottis can be varied by the action of the intrinsic laryngeal muscles (Fig. 1.3).

The intrinsic laryngeal muscles are striated in character, are bilaterally disposed and can be grouped as adductors or abductors of the glottis and tensors of the vocal cords. The lateral cricoarytenoid muscle, thyroarytenoid muscle and transverse arytenoid muscle produce adduction of the vocal cords and arytenoids when they contract. Contraction of the cricothyroid muscle increases the tension of the vocal cords, and contraction of the dorsal cricoarytenoid muscle produces abduction of the cords.

In normal quiet respiration the abductor (dorsal cricoarytenoid) is active during inspiration, so that the cords move laterally, widening the glottis. The abductor group is active during expiration, so that the cords move towards the midline during expiration, narrowing the glottis.

Motor Innervation of the Intrinsic Laryngeal Muscles

The intrinsic laryngeal muscles receive a motor nerve supply from the external branch of the cranial laryngeal nerve and recurrent laryngeal nerves on each side. The cranial laryngeal nerves innervate the cricothyroid muscle, while the recurrent laryngeal nerve provides the motor supply to the other intrinsic muscles.

Because the intrinsic laryngeal muscles are striated muscles, injection of neuromuscular blocking agents such as suxamethonium or vecuronium will paralyse them. This is clinically useful in providing relaxation of the laryngeal musculature and preventing laryngeal spasm during endotracheal intubation.

Afferent Nerve Pathways Involved in Intrinsic Laryngeal Muscle Activity

Stimulation of a wide variety of receptors in the body may result in reflex contraction of the

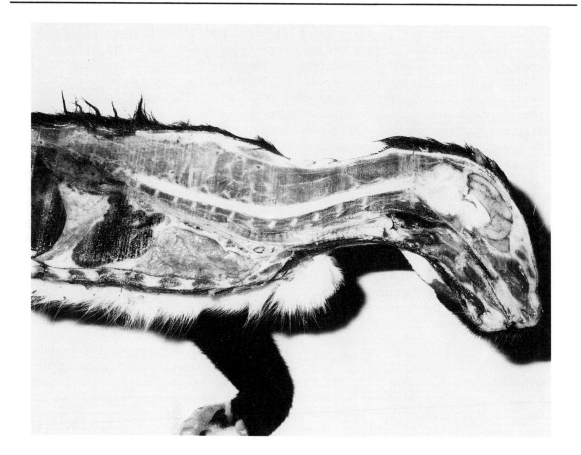

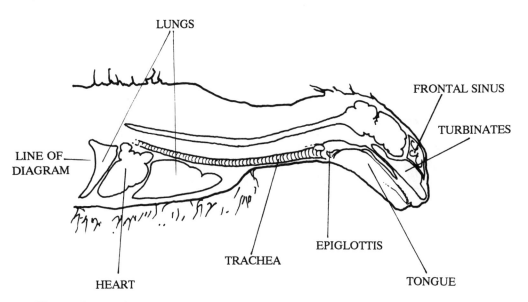

Fig. 1.4 Longitudinal section of head, neck and thorax of cat to show respiratory tract.

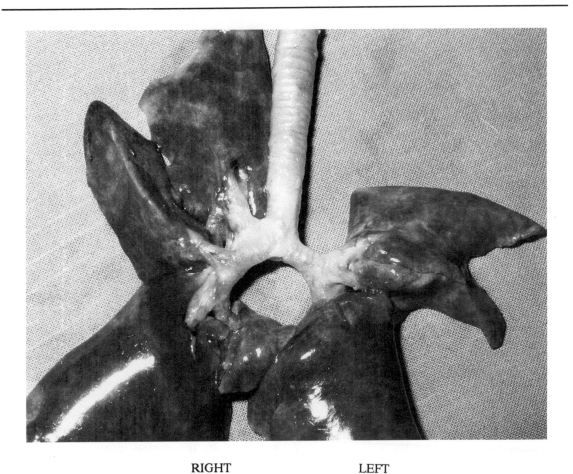

RIGHT   LEFT

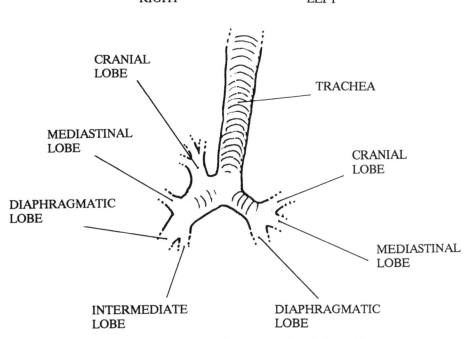

Fig. 1.5 Ventral view of trachea and main bronchi.

intrinsic laryngeal adductor muscles. Changes in respiratory rhythm and laryngeal muscle activity may result from afferent impulses travelling not only in the vagus nerves, but also in the cranial laryngeal, trigeminal, auditory, phrenic, splanchnic and other sensory nerves (Rex, 1970). A knowledge of the anatomy of the larynx and of the nerves innervating its intrinsic muscles provides a sound basis for the prevention or alleviation of laryngeal spasm and other respiratory reflex problems during anaesthesia.

The Trachea

The trachea of the cat extends from the larynx to the bronchi and has an internal diameter of about 5 mm. It lies ventral to the oesophagus for the first 3–4 cm at its cranial end, but more caudally it is related dorsally to the longus coli muscles. On its ventral aspect, the trachea is related to the sternohyoid muscles in its cranial half and more caudally it is related to the sternothyrohyoid and sternocephalic muscles. Laterally, the trachea is related to other long muscles of the neck and has the common carotid artery, the vagosympathetic trunk, the recurrent laryngeal nerves and the internal jugular vein lying dorsally on each side. Within the thorax, the trachea lies in the cranial and middle mediastinum with the oesophagus and major vessels and nerves. The trachea has a lining of ciliated mucosa and is covered by connective tissue which encloses the tracheal cartilages. The tracheal cartilages are ring-shaped structures which are incomplete dorsally. The gap on the dorsal aspect is filled by connective tissue and the trachealis muscle. The presence of the gap and the trachealis muscle means that the trachea does not have a fixed diameter, because this can be increased or diminished by the activity of the trachealis muscle. Rhythmic contractions of the trachealis muscle during anaesthesia have been reported. The blanket of mucus on the lining of the trachea is constantly being changed as the beating of the cilia moves it towards the pharynx. This forms a protective mechanism, eliminating small particles which may have entered the airway. When an endotracheal tube

is inserted into the trachea a large area of this protective mucosa is bypassed. At its distal end the trachea bifurcates to form the two main bronchi at about the level of the sixth rib (Fig. 1.5).

The blood supply to the trachea is from branches of the common carotid arteries and the broncho-oesophageal artery. Venous drainage is mainly via branches of the external and internal jugular vein. The trachea is innervated by parasympathetic nerve fibres from the recurrent laryngeal nerves and sympathetic nerve fibres from the sympathetic trunk and middle cervical ganglia. Sensory receptors are more abundant in the area of trachea close to its bifurcation to form the main bronchi and less in number in the mid-tracheal region. This provides a rational basis for the recommendation that the tip of the endotracheal tube should lie in the mid-tracheal region.

The Lungs

The main lobes of the lungs are separate from each other and lie on each side of the thorax, separated by the mediastinum. There are four lobes in the right lung and three lobes in the left (Fig. 1.5). There is a cranial lobe, mediastinal lobe and diaphragmatic lobe on each side, and in addition an intermediate lobe on the right. The cranial bronchus on the right side lies cranial to the pulmonary artery, whereas all the other bronchi to the lung lobes lie caudal to

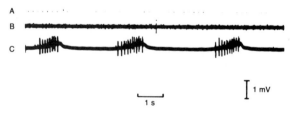

Fig. 1.6 A record of intrathoracic pressure in the cat superimposed on the electromyogram signal from the diaphragm. A, Time marker 0.2 s.; B, electromyogram from cricothyroid muscle; C, electromyogram from the diaphragm with intrathoracic pressure record superimposed.

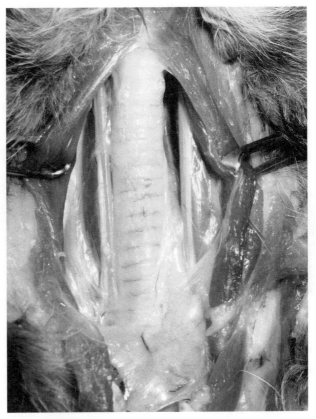

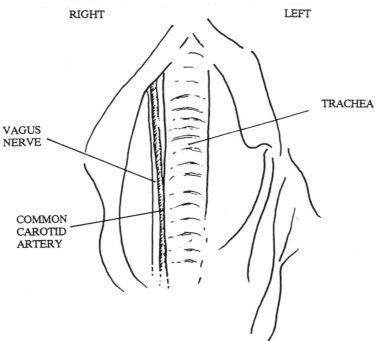

RIGHT   LEFT

TRACHEA

VAGUS NERVE

COMMON CAROTID ARTERY

Fig. 1.7 Ventral view of the trachea, showing its relationship with the right common carotid artery and right vagus nerve.

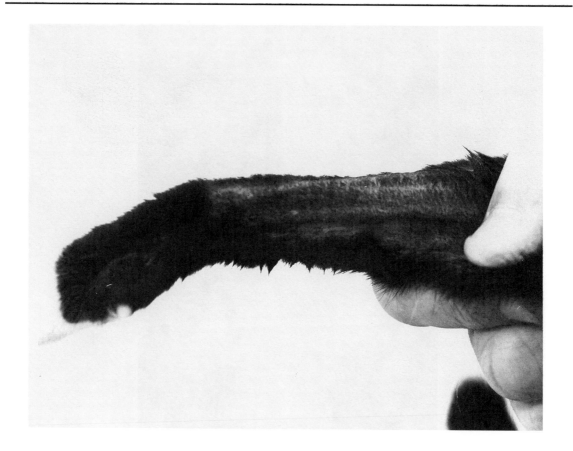

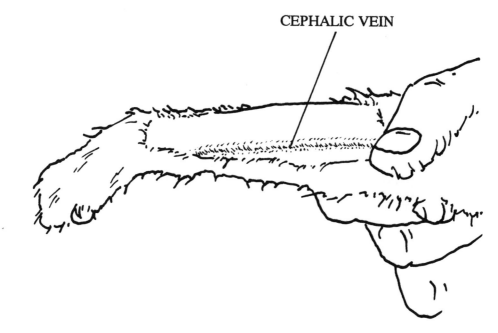

CEPHALIC VEIN

Fig. 1.8 Cat's foreleg, showing distended cephalic vein.

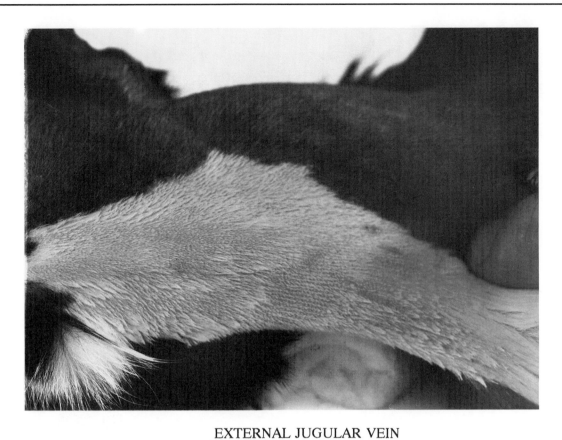

EXTERNAL JUGULAR VEIN

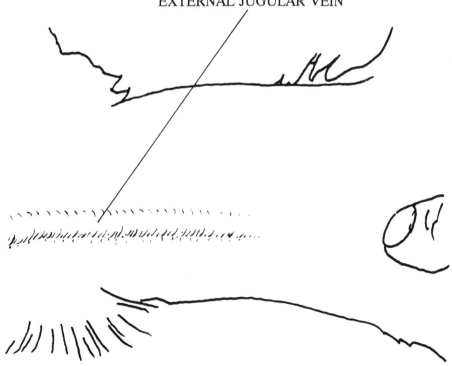

Fig. 1.9 Cat's neck showing distended external jugular vein.

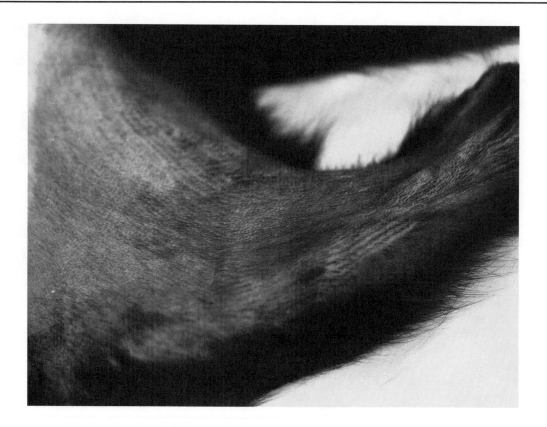

SAPHENOUS VEIN

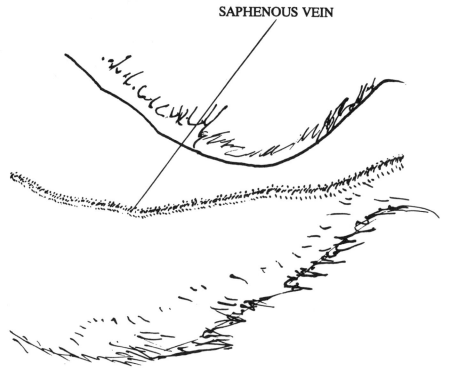

Fig. 1.10 Medial aspect of cat's hind leg showing distended saphenous vein.

the pulmonary artery (Fig. 1.5 shows branching of the main bronchi).

The Diaphragm

The diaphragm is a musculotendinous structure which separates the pleural cavity from the peritoneal cavity. It is dome-shaped, with its convex surface facing the pleural cavity. It is covered by the pleura on its thoracic aspect and by the peritoneum on the abdominal side. The diaphragm has both muscular and tendinous parts. Dorsally, the crura arise from a combined tendon on the ventral aspect of the lumbar vertebrae and the muscle fibres join the muscular costal diaphragm on each side. The central part of the diaphragm is tendinous and is surrounded by the muscular costal diaphragm. There are a number of hiatuses in the diaphragm. The aortic hiatus allows the passage of aorta, azygos vein and thoracic duct; the oesophageal hiatus contains the oesophagus, vagus nerve and small oesophageal vessels; and the ventral hiatus allows the passage of the caudal vena cava and some branches of the right phrenic nerve.

Motor innervation of the diaphragm is by the phrenic nerves, which arise from the fourth, fifth and sixth cervical nerves. Rhythmic activity of the diaphragm, together with activity of the intercostal muscles is responsible for the inspiratory phase of respiration (Fig. 1.6)

This activity is controlled by the respiratory centre in the medulla. Sensory receptors in many parts of the body may cause reflex effects in the activity of the diaphragm. Nerve pathways involved are similar to those involved in laryngeal reflexes.

The Cardiovascular System

The Arteries

Arteries of interest to the anaesthetist are the common carotids (see Fig. 1.7), which is easily palpable in the cervical region just dorsal to the trachea on each side and the femoral artery, which lies on the medial aspect of the hind leg in a depression between the bellies of the sartorius and gracilis muscles. Both these arteries may be used for monitoring the pulse during anaesthesia and for direct measurement of arterial blood pressure. The radial artery may be palpated over the dorsomedial aspect of the distal radius and the carpus, while in the hind leg, the dorsal pedal artery, which is the continuation of the cranial tibial artery may be palpated over the dorsal aspect of the hind paw, dorsomedially just distal to the hock. These are useful arteries for monitoring the peripheral circulation.

The Veins

The two most important veins for the administration of intravenous fluids in the cat are the cephalic vein (Fig. 1.8) and the external jugular vein (Fig. 1.9).

If access to the hind leg vein is required, the saphenous vein is easily identified on the medial aspect between the bellies of the sartorius muscle anteriorly and the gracilis muscle posteriorly (Fig. 1.10). Proximally it drains into the femoral vein which is also accessible in the cat on the medial aspect of the femoral region. The recurrent tarsal vein is also used for intravenous access; it has a short section on the medial aspect of the hock and then runs obliquely across the lateral aspect of the leg above the hock. This vein is easily accessible, particularly on the lateral aspect, although it it very mobile at this site.

Acknowledgements

Paul Fabbri was responsible for the photography.

References

Rex, M.A.E. (1970) A review of the structural and functional basis of laryngospasm and a discussion of the nerve pathways involved in the reflex and its clinical significance in man and animals. *Brit. J. Anaesth.* **42**, 891–899.

A.R. Michell

2
Physiology

Introduction

During anaesthesia, the main physiological concerns are adequate circulatory and respiratory function, in particular the maintenance of adequate arterial pressure, peripheral perfusion, blood gases and circulating volume. Haemostasis is also important while adequate respiratory, renal and hepatic function are essential for excretion of drugs used for or during anaesthesia. Analgesia and muscle relaxation are key attributes of the effects of anaesthesia, as is the tendency of anaesthetic agents to reach the foetal circulation. Anaesthesia and surgery have important effects on endocrine function, some of which affect the appropriate use of supportive fluids. In addition, anaesthesia, shock and the use of unwarmed parenteral fluids can all affect temperature regulation. Even digestive function is potentially affected both by pre-anaesthetic food deprivation and the effects of hypovolaemia on enteric circulation. The anaesthetist, directly or indirectly, may therefore be concerned with the physiology of almost any organ system except, perhaps, the special senses.

A single chapter on physiology, in the context of anaesthesia, must necessarily be highly selective. Selection rests not so much on which systems as which aspects of their function to include. This, in turn, must reflect their contribution to the anaesthetist's ability to maintain the stability of the patient and to detect or avoid complications. Within each section of this chapter the correct title should be 'selected aspects of physiological function' and the latter certainly includes both adaptive and maladaptive pathophysiological responses.

The prime physiological concerns for the anaesthetist, other than maintenance of effective analgesia and muscle relaxation, are to ensure adequate circulatory and respiratory function. These are reflected in adequate circulating volume, normal cardiac function, effective tissue perfusion and normal blood gases. These are expressions of cardiovascular, pulmonary and renal physiology together with their neural and endocrine controls.

Body Fluids

Water represents 70% of lean mass, 60% of adult weight and the majority (40% body weight) is intracellular fluid (ICF). Extracellular fluid (ECF) (20%) differs mainly in its low concentration of potassium (4–5 mmol/l) and its high concentration of sodium (140–150 mmol/l), compared with ICF. This contrast is maintained by the energy expended by the sodium pump (Na–K ATPase) which supplies cells with potassium and restricts sodium predominantly to ECF. Sodium thus acts as the osmotic skeleton of ECF, maintaining its volume (against the osmotic pull of the cells). Changes in body sodium primarily cause parallel changes in ECF volume. The sodium concentration in ECF is stabilized by thirst and arginine vasopressin (AVP or ADH, antidiuretic hormone); that is, via water balance. Sodium depletion only indirectly depresses plasma sodium concentration when it causes sufficient hypovolaemia to divert thirst and AVP towards the defence of circulating volume, at the expense of plasma Na^+ concentration. Adequate ECF volume, plasma volume in particular, is the key to normal circulatory function (Michell et al., 1989; Michell, 1991a). Circulating volume in cats (slightly less than 70 ml/kg; Table 13.5) is somewhat less than in dogs (90 ml/kg) and this is an important factor underlying some differences in the distribution and effect of drugs (Boothe, 1990). Others result from differences in hepatic metabolism (see below). ECF volume in cats may be up to 30% bodyweight, 300 ml/kg (Di Bartola, 1992).

Table 2.1 Representative haematological data (based on Wills & Wolf, 1993 and Jain, 1986)

Total red cells	$5–10 \times 10^6$ /µl
PCV	25–45%
Haemoglobin	80–150 g/l
Total white cells	$6–20 \times 10^3$ /µl
Neutrophils	$5–15 \times 10^3$ /µl
Lymphocytes	$1–5 \times 10^3$ /µl
Eosinophils	0–750 /µl
Basophils	0–200 /µl
Monocytes	0- 800 /µl

Circulation

Arterial pressure, important though it is, merely subserves the essential function of the circulatory system; that is, maintenance of adequate tissue perfusion. As the word implies, perfusion depends on adequate flow through capillaries which, in turn, depends on:

1. The pressure head (arterial pressure).
2. Arteriolar resistance (hence the residual pressure in the capillaries).
3. Pre- and postcapillary tone (hence the pattern of vasomotion, the rate and duration of capillary flow, and the capillary pressure).
4. Blood viscosity – mainly determined by packed cell volume (PCV) and red cell (RBC) elasticity – though white cells (WBC) may contribute because, though fewer in number, they are much less pliable (Table 2.1).
5. Any abnormal obstruction to venous outflow (e.g. tight bandages, casts or raised venous pressure due to inadequate cardiac function).

Capillary Perfusion: Exchange with Interstitial Fluid (ISF)

Adequate capillary perfusion allows the replenishment of interstitial fluid and this renews the environment of the cells. While the actual volume of ISF is much greater than plasma (3:1), there is normally little free fluid, much being adsorbed on to structural components of the tissue spaces. Accumulation of free fluid

underlies the common form of oedema and its adverse effects include an increase in diffusion distances between cells and capillaries. On the other hand, cell swelling is particularly important in brain oedema since the effect of small volume changes is exacerbated by the rigid cranium; the interstitial compartment in brain is small compared with most tissues.

The normal balance between plasma and interstitial fluid depends on the flux supplying ISF (as a result of the higher pressure within capillaries) and the flux draining it in response to the higher oncotic (protein osmotic) pressure within plasma. Interstitial fluid functions both as a reservoir and an overflow for plasma, thus expansion of ECF volume is compensated by a fall in peripheral resistance (mainly arteriolar) which:

1. Limits any rise in arterial pressure.
2. Transmits a greater pressure to the capillaries and favours outflow of excess fluid into ISF. This is also helped by dilution of plasma protein (particularly albumin which contributes most of the oncotic pressure).

Conversely, contraction of ECF volume (e.g. caused by haemorrhage, diarrhoea or alimentary obstruction) leads to increased peripheral resistance (protecting arterial pressure) and reduced pressure transmission to the capillaries, thus favouring uptake of fluid from ISF, provided colloid osmotic pressure is adequate. As long as it is not too extreme, this natural haemodilution response to hypovolaemia improves rather than impedes tissue oxygenation because the fall in PCV reduces viscosity (Biro, 1980). This is particularly important at low flow rates because blood is thixotropic (its viscosity is reduced by accelerated flow, like 'non-drip' paint). Thus, haemodilution has been shown to improve retinal and brain blood flow for feline surgery (Roth, 1992; Muizelear *et al.*, 1992) and this may be especially important after head injury when autoregulation of cerebral circulation is impaired (De Witt *et al.*, 1992; Sutin *et al.*, 1992).

Apart from a rise in capillary pressure (increased transmission of arterial pressure or obstruction to venous outflow), the main cause of tissue oedema is disruption of the oncotic pressure gradient. In theory, this can result from hypoalbuminaemia whether iatrogenic (excess fluid therapy with crystalloids) or caused by impaired synthesis (hepatic disease) or enhanced loss of albumin (glomerulonephritis, protein-losing enteropathy, burns). Certainly, hypoalbuminaemic animals are at greater risk of hypovolaemia but the fall in albumin has to be substantial to cause gross oedema. This is because of the 'safety factor' provided by the normally negative (subatmospheric) interstitial pressure. Until sufficient oedema fluid accumulates to eliminate it, the immediate effect of excess flux into ISF is to accelerate lymphatic drainage (Guyton, 1991). The key oncotic factors contributing to peripheral oedema are thus lymphatic obstruction or capillary damage and it is worth emphasizing that the impact of the latter is mainly increased leakage of albumin to ISF, since water moves freely through normal capillaries.

These concepts, though almost traditional in circulatory physiology, are incomplete. First, it is not just capillary pressure which matters for adequate perfusion but the balance of time between increased and decreased precapillary resistance. Capillaries are thus subject to periods of generous or less generous flow and this pattern (vasomotion) depends partly on local metabolic demand (autoregulation of blood flow). Secondly, capillary permeability varies greatly between tissues and although ISF contains a lower albumin concentration than plasma, it is also a larger compartment. As a result, acceleration of lymphatic drainage can restore substantial amounts of albumin to the circulation and this may be beneficial in post-traumatic hyperglycaemia and perhaps in the use of hypertonic saline in the treatment of shock; the rise of interstitial osmolality will favour water outflow from cells, expansion of ISF and thus promote lymphatic drainage (Michell, 1985, 1989).

It is particularly important to recognize that the balance of forces across pulmonary capillaries, and therefore the factors predisposing to oedema, are quite different from those in peripheral capillaries. The double circulation of mammals allows high flows at lower pressures in pulmonary capillaries. It would also mean, however, that the balance of fluxes was heavily in favour of fluid uptake into pulmonary capillaries. In fact this is offset by a reduced oncotic uptake gradient; since the albumin concentration of pulmonary capillaries cannot greatly differ from other capillaries, this reduced gradient can only result from greater leakage of albumin and a higher concentration in ISF (Michell, 1985). Thus, while we can readily observe tissue oedema in response to excess saline, it is too facile to assume that this represents the parallel onset of pulmonary oedema, a much more serious condition since it impedes both pulmonary ventilation (by stiffening the lungs) and gas exchange. The lungs gain some degree of protection from the higher albumin concentration in their ISF; onset of oedema dilutes it and steepens the oncotic gradient favouring absorption of fluid into capillaries. Pulmonary oedema results not so much from oncotic dilution as from raised venous pressure with excessive infusion rates. Rate for rate, therefore, excessive infusion of colloids would be *more* hazardous than electrolyte solutions despite their lesser impact on oncotic pressure (Michell, 1985). Trauma, inhalation, for example of blood, and other factors likely to increase capillary permeability greatly potentiate any tendency towards pulmonary oedema.

Regulation of Blood Flow

The regulation of blood flow is vitally dependent on the maintenance of an adequate and stable arterial pressure. The patency and resistance of the peripheral circulation, however, is under both central and local control, responsive to the needs of adequate circulating volume and arterial pressure and those of local tissue activity. It is also under the control of nerves (particularly sympathetic), hormones (particularly catecholamines) and metabolites. In recent years, the importance of local regulators, for example prostaglandins, has been increasingly appreciated and, in the latest wave of progress, it has become clear that the blood vessels modulate their own tone via constrictors such as the endothelins and dilators such as EDRF (endothelium-derived relaxing factor, most of which is probably nitric oxide derived from arginine; Vanhoutte & Eber, 1991). These insights are important not only because of their physiological and pathophysiological implications but the opportunities which they offer for deliberate or unintended modulation by drugs. The whole picture is far more dynamic than the former view of a pump and a system of conduits largely under the external control of nerves and hormones. Instead, the vascular system is responsive not only to changes in local tissue demand but changes in its own function (Harrison *et al.*, 1992). Thus, for example, EDRF may modulate arterial pressure in response to the stress in the vessel walls (Persson *et al.*, 1992).

The main factors determining tissue blood flow are metabolic activity in the area supplied and the defence of arterial pressure. The volume of blood is much smaller than the total capacity of the circulatory system, thus generous perfusion of more active tissues usually implies less generous perfusion of less active regions. This effect is intensified by hypovolaemia when, under the influence of sympathetic tone, catecholamines and other vasoconstrictors such as AVP and angiotensin, blood flow to less 'important' areas (such as subcutaneous tissue and muscle) is restricted while coronary and cerebral circulation is maintained. However, if the restriction is severe, it ceases to be innocuous as muscles, even when inactive, leak potassium; intestinal capillaries become leaky and exacerbate the hypovolaemia and hypoxic tissues leak potassium and generate acid, particularly lactic acid. The latter is usually briskly metabolized by the liver, provided it is healthy, but not when the liver is poorly perfused. Such changes are part of the progression from vasoconstriction as a homeostatic defence of arterial pressure to a major contributory factor in circulatory shock.

The local factors mediating increased blood flow during enhanced metabolic activity are not fully defined and may differ between tissues but probably include vasodilators (EDRF, CO_2, lactic acid, adenosine compounds, histamine, K^+, H^+) and perhaps factors reflecting demand for nutrients (e.g. glucose) and oxygen. Moreover, all tissues have the ability to maintain some stability of blood flow in the face of modest changes in arterial pressure. This 'autoregulation' is especially effective in the kidneys and also the brain (where CO_2 is a key determinant of blood flow, hence the reduced perfusion associated with hypocapnia). Barbiturates, however, undermine autoregulation of brain blood flow and increase cerebral vascular resistance (Sato *et al.*, 1992). Moreover, shock may impair EDRF-dependent vasodilation in feline renal arteries (Szabo *et al.*, 1992). Even if anaesthetics reduce renal perfusion, this may be well tolerated provided that autoregulation remains active (Gelman *et al.*, 1984). Beyond autoregulation, there is scope for the effects of vascular occlusion to be offset by enhanced circulation through collateral vessels; this varies substantially between tissues.

Neural and Humoral Effects on Blood Vessels: Autonomic System

Balancing of the 'rival' demands of different tissues depends on the overriding influence of neural and humoral regulation of blood flow. In particular, the dominant control is sympathetic constrictor tone maintained by the reticular vasomotor centres of the medulla and pons. These also accelerate heart rate and increase contractility via cardiac sympathetic nerves. Normally the heart rate is restrained by vagal parasympathetic tone, still under the influence of the vasomotor centres, which are themselves stimulated or inhibited by various other brain areas, notably the hypothalamus. The vasomotor centres differentially affect perfusion of different tissues (Dean *et al.*, 1992).

Vascular tone is maintained by the sympathetic neurotransmitter, noradrenaline, acting mainly on α-receptors, whereas the adrenal medulla produces adrenaline which has additional dilator effects on β-receptors in blood vessels and bronchioles (β_2) as well as increasing heart rate and contractility (β_1). Neurally mediated vasodilation is especially important in skeletal muscle. Vasodilation thus depends on reduced activation of α-receptors or stimulation of β_2-receptors. A few sympathetic dilator nerves utilize cholinergic transmission but acetyl choline serves mainly as the transmitter for parasympathetic nerves: in both cases the muscarinic cholinergic receptors are involved. Autonomic ganglia (both sympathetic and parasympathetic) and the neuromuscular junctions also utilize cholinergic transmission (nicotinic receptors). Dopaminergic receptors (D_1) are also important, particularly in increasing splanchnic and renal perfusion; there are also D_2- and α_2-receptors which cause presynaptic inhibition of the release of noradrenaline (Foex, 1989). At higher dosage, dopamine also stimulates β_1-receptors, with α-receptors only affected at even higher doses (Hosgood, 1990).

The effects of the autonomic nervous system are widespread, for example parasympathetic stimulation of secretions (including saliva and tears) and also dual control of pupillary aperture (sympathetic dilation, parasympathetic constriction). Both sympathetic stimulation and adrenaline also have important effects on metabolism, notably mobilization of glucose and raised metabolic rate.

Cardiac Output

All flow within a hydraulic system results from pressure gradients: the pressure in the circulatory system, like the voltage in an electrical system, is a store of energy. In both cases this store is dissipated across resistances which thus reduce the voltage or pressure beyond them. Ohm's law applies well to both electrical and vascular circuits:

$$V/I = R$$

where V is voltage/pressure; R is resistance; and I is current/flow. In this electrical analogy, the veins are well represented as capacitors – stores of the charge/fluid volume which normally provide the flow.

Just as the flow of current into an electric appliance does not create energy, but transmits the energy resulting from the work done at the generator, the main work of the circulatory system is done by the heart. There is an additional important but small contribution from vascular tone.

The atria merely serve to augment ventricular filling and the key determinants of cardiac output are venous return, filling pressure (atrial pressure) and ventricular systole. Cardiac output can increase via stroke volume (hence reduction of end diastolic volume) or acceleration of heart rate. Cardiac work is exerted in accelerating the volume of blood received and raising its pressure ('preload') and in ejecting it against the resistance of the arterial 'tree' ('afterload').

Within limits, increased stretch of the myocardium increases its force of contraction (Frank–Starling law) but in heart failure, overstretching reduces the force of contraction. In particular, La Place's law reminds us that within an elastic container, pressure is inversely related to radius and directly to tension. Thus, as the heart enlarges, it takes greater tension (work) to sustain the same pressure. Work is also increased by pumping against a greater resistance, hence it rises in parallel with arterial pressure and the vascular factors sustaining it.

Catecholamines not only accelerate the heart, they increase its force of contraction (positive chronotropic and inotropic effects). However, any agents which increase cardiac work also raise oxygen consumption and, unless myocardial perfusion is also enhanced to match, the result may be cardiac damage. This is a particular risk with hypoxia or severe anaemia.

Conduction disturbances and arrhythmias reduce the efficiency of cardiac work by disrupting the co-ordination between filling and emptying of the ventricles and also the pattern of ventricular contraction. Valvular stenosis increases the resistance against which the preceding chamber must contract. Valvular incompetence increases the work of the preceding chamber by partially recycling blood into it.

The hallmarks of cardiac failure are inadequate tissue perfusion ('forward failure') and raised venous pressure ('backward failure'). This is manifest as venous congestion (right heart failure) or pulmonary congestion and oedema (left heart failure). Commonly, heart failure becomes bilateral because

1. Pulmonary congestion (left failure) overloads the right ventricle.
2. Right-sided failure impairs left ventricular filling, hence impeding cardiac output and coronary perfusion.

Pulmonary disease can exacerbate right-sided failure because alveolar hypoxia causes local vasoconstriction and raises pulmonary vascular resistance, thus increasing afterload.

The defining feature of heart failure is not simply that cardiac output is inadequate; in the early stages it may be sustained but only *at the price of a raised filling pressure*. The failing heart, therefore, cannot sustain an adequate cardiac output at a normal filling pressure.

Increased work load, as in any muscle, may cause cardiac hypertrophy as opposed to dilation or overstretching. The workload may be physiological (e.g. athletic) or pathological (e.g. caused by valvular incompetence). Hypertrophy is not purely benign as it may also encroach on the volume available for filling and reduce ventricular compliance, as seen in hypertrophic cardiomyopathy. It may also produce areas of less adequately perfused muscle (Henderson, 1983).

Apart from its role as a pump, the heart is also an endocrine gland, producing atrial natriuretic peptide (ANP) in response to atrial stretch. This reduces arterial pressure and, by enhancing renal sodium excretion, it also reduces ECF volume; it thus defends the heart against volume overload. Clearly, in congestive heart failure, this defence is insufficient to prevent oedema or ascites (Michell, 1991a).

Circulatory Pressures

Capillary pressure has already been discussed. For cardiovascular monitoring, the central venous pressure and the various arterial pressures are the most important.

The veins are the storage side of the circulation and are normally very compliant; that is, they expand with a small rise in intraluminal pressure. Measurement of central venous pressure (CVP) represents the filling pressure of the right atrium. It is reduced by inadequate venous return (e.g. caused by peripheral pooling of blood in shock or underfilling of the circulation in hypovolaemia). Conversely, hypervolaemia will tend to raise CVP. Equally, CVP is affected by cardiac performance and a failing heart, or one which is overloaded, will only sustain cardiac output at the price of a raised filling pressure (CVP). Thus excessive CVP warns of fluid therapy which is too fast or inappropriate to the level of cardiac function. Nevertheless, the veins themselves respond to constrictor stimuli including increased sympathetic tone and, in particular, metabolic acidosis heightens the tendency for CVP to rise despite persistent hypovolaemia; this is because it dilates arterioles but constricts veins (Carroll & Oh, 1978). CVP is also affected by changes in intrathoracic pressure, for example during positive pressure ventilation of the lungs (Hillman, 1989).

Arterial pressure is complex, depending not only on cardiac output and peripheral resistance, but on the reinforcing or cancelling effects of pressure waves reflected from branch points in the arterial tree (Michell, 1993a). Thus, even direct measurements with intra-arterial catheters reveal different pressures in different arteries. All pressure measurements must allow for the difference in height between the point at which the measurement is made and the reference or zero point – conventionally the level of the tricuspid (right AV) valve.

Indirect measurements depend on occlusion of an artery (usually limb or tail) and the detection of changes in the behaviour of the vessel wall or in blood flow as the pressure of the occluding cuff falls from suprasystolic to subdiastolic.

The peak pressure during left ventricular ejection is the 'systolic pressure'. The minimum level during ventricular relaxation, sustained substantially by the elasticity of the great vessels, is the 'diastolic pressure'. They do not always change in parallel; for example, a loss of vascular elasticity may raise systolic but lower diastolic pressure (Michell, 1993a). The difference between systolic and diastolic pressure is the 'pulse pressure'. Mean arterial pressure is a good representation of the predominant filling pressure for the peripheral circulation during the cardiac cycle. It is not, however, the average of systolic and diastolic because systole is faster than diastole. Moreover, since acceleration of heart rate encroaches on diastole rather than systole, mean pressure rises with heart rate.

The encroachment on diastole at high rates also underlies the loss of cardiac efficiency when they are extreme; diastole is the time of optimum myocardial perfusion (free of the external resistance imposed on the coronary circulation by the contracting myocardium), hence shortening of diastole restricts the time available for both myocardial perfusion and ventricular filling.

The approximation of right atrial pressure by CVP is relatively simple but determination of left atrial pressure is anatomically more elusive; it can be approximated by measuring the pulmonary wedge pressure. This involves the passage of a venous catheter to the pulmonary artery via the right heart; it is then allowed to wedge in a small branch of the artery. The supposition is that wedging stops the arterial flow in that branch and converts it into a tube measuring the pressure transmitted from beyond; that is, the pressure in the pulmonary veins (hence the left atrium).

Cardiac Sounds

The physical origin of the sounds associated with cardiac function is a matter of continuing debate; it is certainly not the slamming of valves but changes in the blood flow, notably turbulence, which accompany or fractionally precede valve closure. Physiologically or clinically, however, it is essential to be clear that the first and second sounds demarcate, approximately, the beginning and end of ventricular systole. They are, therefore, associated with closure of the entry valves (AV valves; 1st sound) or exit valves (aortic or pulmonic; 2nd sound) respectively.

Atrial fibrillation may make the pattern of 1st and 2nd sounds very irregular in rhythm and intensity (by disrupting the regular depolarization of the AV node which ought to signal ventricular contraction) but it does *not* eliminate first sounds.

Regulation of Arterial Pressure

The long-term regulator of arterial pressure is the kidney because supranormal pressures readily enhance sodium excretion and thus reduce ECF volume. However, the immediate response to changes in circulating volume depends on neural and humoral control of peripheral resistance, cardiac output and tissue perfusion. In particular, vasoconstriction in response to hypovolaemia which:

1. Maintains the upstream (arterial) pressure.
2. Drops the downstream pressure and facilitates transcapillary uptake of fluid from ISF into circulation.
3. Helps to redistribute blood flow away from the least vital tissues.
4. Reduces the amount of blood in the venous (storage) side of the circulation by venoconstriction.
5. In the aftermath of haemorrhage, assists haemostasis by vasoconstriction.

The rapid vasoconstrictor response to hypovolaemia depends on feedback from the baroreceptors of the aorta, main arteries and carotid sinus (ideally placed to protect cerebral blood flow from the risk of hypotension). It also depends on the chemoreceptors of the aortic and carotid bodies (which respond to hypoxia) and the central nervous system ischaemic response. The chemoreceptors respond to hypotension because a reduction in their perfusion reduces their oxygenation even if blood PO_2 remains normal. The baroreceptor response to hypotension is depressed by anaesthesia; in cats a comparison of three anaesthetics (Sellgren *et al.*, 1992) showed isoflurane the most and propofol the least potent depressant with methohexitone only depressant at high dose. The antihypotensive effect of vasoconstriction is reinforced by increased heart rate and contractile strength. In cats, however, hypoxia stimulates the parasympathetic as well as the sympathetic system and can, therefore, increase or reduce heart rate (O'Donnell & Bower, 1992). Heart rate is also increased by atrial stretch, thus helping the heart to balance increased venous return by increased output.

The ischaemic response of the CNS, which mainly reflects the accumulation of CO_2 and H^+, is especially effective in raising arterial pressure (through vasoconstriction) when hypotension is severe. Ultimately, however, ischaemia depresses the activity of the vasomotor centre and arterial pressure falls steeply. The role of chemoreceptors in breathing is discussed below.

The main role of AVP is in the regulation of

water balance and plasma sodium concentration, and that of angiotensin is directly and indirectly (via aldosterone) in the regulation of renal sodium excretion (also in thirst responses to hypovolaemia); however, during severe hypovolaemia both hormones reach concentrations which are effective in reinforcing vasoconstriction.

Haemostasis

An important defence against hypovolaemia lies in the ability of blood to seal both minor and major damage to the vessels and the ability of arteries, by retraction, to limit haemorrhage. Sequentially, the defence against haemorrhage comprises:

1. Vascular spasm.
2. Platelet plugging – the extensive petechial haemorrhages associated with thrombocytopaenia reveal the importance of this mechanism not only in major injury but everyday 'wear and tear', for example in the intestine.
3. Clotting.
4. Clot stabilization.

Clotting depends on intrinsic (changes within blood) and extrinsic (changes in vessels or surrounding tissues) mechanisms and consists of a complex, self-accelerating (positive feedback) cascade of reactions. Rapid acceleration of clotting is especially powerful via the extrinsic pathway. Intrinsic clotting *in vitro* or in catheters depends on damage to blood at contact surfaces and is reduced when these are physiologically inert.

Everyone remembers the existence, if not the detail, of these cascades without necessarily being so aware of the importance of fibrinolytic mechanisms responsible for the dissolution of 'unwanted' or excessive clots, especially microemboli, free in circulation. There are also numerous natural anticoagulants, most notably heparin which acts by complexing antithrombin. The extreme example of thromboembolism in small animals is possibly the feline condition affecting the aorta, the iliac arteries and other vessels, probably as a result of cardiac damage (see Chapter 4). In septicaemic shock and other conditions there can be excessive activation of clotting mechanisms and suppression of fibrinolysis; initially this causes 'disseminated intravascular coagulation' (widespread distribution of microthrombi) (DIC) and may eventually impair clotting by consumption of precursors ('consumptive coagulopathy').

The process of clot formation depends on the formation of prothrombin activator, which leads to thrombin generation. This converts fibrinogen to fibrin and the resulting mesh traps platelets and cells. The clot stabilizes and retracts under the influence of platelets exuding serum; this retraction reduces the surface area of the wound, further limiting haemorrhage and facilitating repair.

Clotting can occur in tissue spaces because damaged capillaries leak the necessary precursors. Clotting within vessels is generally limited to the damaged area by the diluting effect of continued blood flow within the vessels but excessive clotting readily occurs in regions of very low blood flow. Circulating precursors are also removed by the macrophage system and, as new thrombin forms, it tends to adhere to fibrin, thus increasing the clot rather than forming emboli.

Both the intrinsic and extrinsic pathways are highly calcium-dependent (hence the effectiveness of calcium chelators such as EDTA or citrate as anticoagulants) and both are dependent on vitamin K for the hepatic formation of prothrombin and other factors, hence the haemorrhagic effects of warfarin and similar compounds.

Severe anaemia or haemorrhage, especially with clotting disorders, may require not only restoration of circulating volume but also supplementation of RBC by transfusion. Cats have fewer known blood groups than dogs but apart from the difficulty of obtaining adequate volumes of donor blood, it is harder to find universal donors; that is, those whose blood type confers least risk of adverse reactions to mismatched transfusions (Autheneil, 1992; Cotter, 1992). These are most likely with a second transfusion when there has been time for antibody formation to be stimulated but prior history is not always completely known and there is always the risk of natural antibodies to alien erythrocytes without prior exposure

(Giger, 1992). Full details of blood transfusion in cats are described in Chapter 13.

Shock

The greatest catastrophe of circulatory function, other than acute heart failure, is shock. The main problem is a failure of capillary perfusion usually caused by hypovolaemia or endotoxaemia, sometimes by neurogenic, vasogenic or cardiac failure. Cardiac output is usually reduced, though in endotoxic shock it may increase due to futile overperfusion of affected capillary beds – hence not all shocked patients are pale and vasoconstricted. Nevertheless, overperfusion implies vasoconstriction and underperfusion in other capillary beds, hence most forms of shock converge on a final common path characterized particularly by widespread and excessive vasoconstriction, with its adverse effects causing damage to capillaries and the tissues supplied. In addition, endotoxic shock often causes hypovolaemia through capillary leakage while hypovolaemic shock may cause endotoxaemia via gut capillaries damaged by splanchnic constriction (Michell, 1985, 1989). Leakage from plasma raises PCV and viscosity of blood, an effect intensified during low flow rates, and the aggregation of RBC which also become more rigid as plasma acidity increases.

Since the normal response to hypovolaemia or reduced cardiac output is vasoconstriction, the outcome is further damage and this is only one of the characteristic vicious cycles (positive feedback loops) which build up and intensify, the longer shock persists. Early treatment, or preferably prevention, is thus essential because therapy which may succeed if given early will often fail if delayed and some drugs, for example corticosteroids, are much more effective at preventing shock than reversing it once it is established.

While the peripheral vascular effects are emphasized and remain the most responsive to treatment, cardiac output is also reduced in most cases of shock, partly because of myocardial depressant agents generated by pancreatic damage associated with splanchnic vasoconstriction (and reinforcing the tendency towards

shock in acute pancreatitis). Shock also interferes with clotting (DIC), though not in every case, and in addition has widespread effects on cell metabolism which remain the least understood though perhaps the most intractable in irreversible shock. Among these, the simplest are lactic acidosis and hyperkalaemia (caused both by acidosis and K^+ leakage from damaged or underperfused cells). In severe injury there is also an acceleration and distortion of metabolic activity (metabolic response to injury; Michell, 1985; Gann & Kenney, 1990) which can raise body temperature in the absence of infection. Normally, however, shock depresses body temperature (see below). In recent years, some of the greatest progress in understanding the basis of shock, and increasing the scope for therapeutic intervention, has been the detailed analysis of the local and systemic mediators, both normal (e.g. EDRF) and abnormal (e.g. leukotrienes and thromboxanes) contributing to successive stages in its development (Michell, 1993b, c).

Respiratory Function

Respiration is centred on the cellular events which generate high energy phosphates, notably ATP, and thus on the supply and utilization of substrates for the mitochondrial electron transport chain, the stage at which oxygen is utilized. The Krebs cycle is the key source of substrates for aerobic metabolism. Anaerobic metabolism generates less ATP and involves the accumulation of lactic acid (which titrates plasma bicarbonate). The lactic acid can be readily remetabolized, particularly by the liver, once oxygen supply improves, so regenerating the equivalent amount of bicarbonate (and underlying the therapeutic use of lactate as a bicarbonate precursor).

Since the CNS is peculiarly dependent on both oxygen and glucose, it is essential that neither surgery nor anaesthesia impede the maintenance of adequate cerebral blood flow and blood gases. In this sense, the focus of respiratory function is pulmonary gas exchange and capillary delivery and uptake of oxygen and carbon dioxide. The adverse effects of anaesthesia may be on pulmonary blood flow, on the respiratory muscles, the nerves supplying them or the centres controlling their activity (Kazemi & Hitzig, 1987).

Oxygen Delivery

The shape of the haemoglobin–oxygen dissociation curve in cats is similar to that in all mammals: as oxygen tension increases along the abscissa, haemoglobin saturation rises on the ordinate in a sigmoid curve characterized particularly by a sharp rise to a sustained virtual plateau. This means that supranormal oxygen tensions cannot bind more oxygen to haemoglobin though they may dissolve more in plasma (a minor effect at normal pressure but sometimes important, and at hyperbaric tensions it can reach dangerous concentrations). The sharp rise reflects the 'positive co-operativity' of oxygen binding (oxygen affinity increased by the oxygen already bound). Functionally it means that haemoglobin loads or unloads oxygen over a relatively narrow range of oxygen tensions. Moreover, the further to the right (i.e. towards high oxygen) the curve and particularly this steep portion lie, the more readily oxygen is unloaded, that is, low saturation is compatible with high oxygen tension. A shift to the left assures that high saturation is achieved even at low tension; that is, it facilitates loading. Liberation of oxygen at the capillaries is favoured by:

1. The low oxygen tension created by metabolic activity, which also creates a favourable diffusion gradient towards areas of need.
2. Right-shifting of the curve by CO_2, H^+ (and temperature).
3. The metabolite 2,3,DPG binds competitively with oxygen and also right-shifts the curve and facilitates oxygen delivery in the capillaries. Except during anaemia cats have low levels of 2,3,DPG (Jain, 1986).

Conversely, oxygen uptake in the lungs is favoured by left-shifting of the curve which results from removal of CO_2 (diffusion towards the lower CO_2 tension in the alveoli). Alkalosis impedes unloading of oxygen in the tissue

capillaries. Hypoxia impedes tissue perfusion by increasing RBC rigidity, especially in cats (Hakin & Maceli, 1988). Feline haemoglobin is susceptible to oxidative damage by drugs resulting in conversion to methaemoglobin (Boothe, 1990).

Cyanosis

Normally venous blood is only about 25% desaturated, thus if tissue oxygen tension falls very low, or blood flow is very sluggish, substantially more oxygen can be extracted from haemoglobin. Extreme desaturation imparts a blue colour to haemoglobin, hence cyanosis is caused by an unusually low oxygen tension either from sluggish peripheral circulation or admixture of venous blood into the arterial supply (right-to-left shunts, which are less usual because the pressure gradients for left-to-right shunts are more favourable). Severe disruption of either pulmonary ventilation or gas exchange, or inadequate oxygen supply can also cause cyanosis. Anaemia does not; it restricts maximum oxygen delivery because there is less haemoglobin but it does not increase desaturation.

Carbon Dioxide

More than 90% of carbon dioxide transport results from rapid conversion to carbonic acid by the carbonic anhydrase of the RBC. The acid dissociates weakly with the resulting H^+ buffered by haemoglobin while the HCO_3^- diffuses into plasma in exchange for Cl^- ('chloride shift'). The remaining carbon dioxide transport is predominantly in simple solution with a smaller fraction bound to haemoglobin and other proteins.

The carbon dioxide tension of plasma is a key component of successful homeostasis because of its decisive role in the regulation of pulmonary ventilation, cerebral blood flow and acid–base balance. 'Tension' or partial pressure (PCO_2) measures the pressure contributed by an individual gas in a gas mixture and thus reflects the pressure of the mixture and the percentage of the gas in it. The partial pressure of CO_2 or O_2 in arterial blood is that of the gas mixture which would be in exact equilibrium; that is, alveolar air in a normal individual (in fact there is normally a minute gradient across the alveolar membrane but this can increase in pulmonary disease).

Pulmonary Gas Exchange and Blood Gases

Abnormal blood gases (i.e. PCO_2 or PO_2) indicate abnormal composition of alveolar air, interference with alveolar gas exchange or circulatory abnormalities, notably 'shunts'. The analysis requires anaerobically drawn arterial blood since venous blood is affected by local tissue activity; however, venous blood is suitable for assessment of metabolic acid–base disturbances (see below) and will give some indication of respiratory disturbances. Normal values in feline arterial and [venous] blood respectively are PO_2: 13.7 [5.2] kPa (103 [39] mmHg) and PCO_2 4.5 [5.6] kPa (34 [42] mmHg); the corresponding values for pH and total CO_2 (TCO_2, see below) are 7.34 [7.30] and 18 [20] mmol/l (Middleton et al., 1981) (see also Table 13.5).

Alveolar air is not identical to atmospheric air since it is humidified and is not completely replaced at every breath and thus has less O_2 and more CO_2. As a result, alveolar air has some stability against changes in the composition of inspired air or changes in breathing pattern. The effect of increased pulmonary ventilation during increased tissue activity is to offset the increased removal of alveolar oxygen into blood and maintain a stable alveolar PO_2. Normally, blood is fully equilibrated before it leaves the alveolar capillaries, however large the cardiac output. In anaemia (insufficient haemoglobin), hyperventilation does not normally occur and would not help as the residual haemoglobin reaches normal saturation. The compensatory response is an increased resting heart rate and an enhanced cardiac output. This emphasizes the primacy of *circulatory* function in oxygen *delivery*, but *respiratory* function in oxygen *supply*.

Carbon dioxide diffuses much more readily across the alveolar membrane than does oxygen. Thus if the cause of a blood gas abnormality is alveolar thickening, PCO_2 can remain deceptively normal when PO_2 is dangerously low. Conversely, if there is severe obstruction to gas exchange and this is counteracted by oxygen therapy, PO_2 may be maintained while PCO_2 is abnormally high. Blood PCO_2 must always rise if its rate of metabolic production exceeds its rate of alveolar removal.

Not all the air moved by pulmonary ventilation reaches the exchange surfaces of the alveoli. Anatomically, there is a fixed 'dead space' to be filled, comprising the airways (upper respiratory tract, trachea, bronchi and bronchioles), through which gases move but do not exchange with blood; this is increased by the external tubing of anaesthetic circuits which therefore should be as short as convenient (though the intratracheal tube bypasses the dead space of the upper respiratory tract).

While the same volume of air can be moved by rapid-shallow or slow-deep breathing, the effects are quite different:

1. In shallow breathing, the same volume is required to fill the dead space; that is, dead space becomes a greater proportion of the total air exchanged and less is available for alveolar exchange. At supranormal ventilation this would minimize the disturbance of blood gases (lowering of PCO_2, respiratory alkalosis). At subnormal ventilation, it would impede the replenishment of oxygen and removal of CO_2 from circulation.
2. When air movement is slow but deep, most of the work is done in expanding the lungs and chest, whereas with rapid air movement (especially if breathing is shallow), most of the work is against the resistance of the airways. Resistance is greatly increased by constriction or the rippling effect of abnormally accumulating secretions. This may be enhanced by the reduced pressures generated as air flows beyond a resistance. Such effects are particularly disrupting when the lungs lose their elasticity and expiration becomes dependent on muscular effort. Upper airway obstruction increases inspiratory effort and if the larynx is unable to relax normally, the additional resistance may generate a further drop in airway pressure and thus a vicious

cycle with a further rise in resistance (Robinson, 1992).

It is easily and widely imagined that most disturbances of respiratory function result from direct interference with gas exchange (diffusion) or breathing. Pulmonary oedema, for example, restricts gas exchange. Diffusion problems are actually much less usual than disturbances of the normally excellent match between changes in alveolar ventilation and consequent changes in perfusion; they result from vasoconstriction in hypoxic areas of the lung. When this fails (e.g. as it may when vasodilators, including some anaesthetics are used; Nunn, 1989), the resulting disturbance of 'ventilation perfusion ratio' ('V/Q') has the effect either on 'physiological shunting' or physiological dead space. The latter results from generous ventilation of alveoli unable to contribute to effective gas exchange (analogous to the generous ventilation of the trachea). The former results from generous perfusion of poorly ventilated alveoli so that some blood reaches the left heart and arterial circulation still with its venous blood gas characteristics ('venous admixture'). The plateau of the haemoglobin dissociation curve means that no compensatory activity of normal alveoli can offset the delivery of desaturated haemoglobin into arterial blood caused by shunting. Oxygen-rich gas mixtures can collapse poorly ventilated alveoli if the delivery of O_2 is outpaced by its absorption (Benumof, 1990).

The uppermost areas of the lung tend to have less ventilation and perfusion, with perfusion particularly affected (greater physiological dead space) whereas dependent areas are less well ventilated in relation to their greater blood flow (increased shunting). Lateral recumbency also encourages transudation into the dependent lung (especially if the patient receives excess fluids) and reduces its ability to oxygenate the blood; turning every 30 min may prevent this, whereas intervals of an hour fail to do so in humans (Benumof, 1990). The supine position causes impedance of diaphragmatic movement by abdominal viscera. Posture thus affects pulmonary efficiency. These effects are probably small in normal cats compared with humans, horses or large dogs, but they do occur (Henik *et al.* 1987).

The main alveolar impediments to exchange result from membrane thickening, accumulation of local secretions, flooding with exudates from the airways (or aspirated vomit or blood), or collapse. During the respiratory pause between inspiration and expiration, there may normally be some redistribution of air between different alveoli, along small pressure gradients caused by differences in alveolar radius. If this were extreme, some alveoli might collapse once they contracted below a certain size; this would be because the contained pressure (P) would no longer be sufficient to resist their own wall tension (T) at low radius; again, La Place's law $P = T/R$; that is, if radius falls, P needs to be bigger to offset T. Once alveoli collapse, very large expansion forces may be needed to reopen them. Fortunately, these La Place effects are greatly reduced by the low and variable surface tension of the surfactant which normally coats the alveoli.

Normal alveolar function also depends on the protection against large particles afforded by the upper respiratory tract and against smaller (<10 μm) particles by the cough reflex and tracheobronchial ciliary movement of mucus. Excess secretions disrupt the normal viscosity of the mucus and, by increasing airway resistance, may cause coughing to propel material towards some alveoli. Tracheostomy or intratracheal tubes remove the protective and humidifying effects of the upper respiratory tract, as do dehydration and dry anaesthetic gas mixtures (Benumof, 1990).

Artificial ventilation of the lungs can replace or reinforce spontaneous breathing. Commercial ventilators maintain either set pressures or set volumes of air exchange. The latter becomes important when damage to the chest or lungs prevents adequate air exchange at normal pressures. A variety of pressure patterns is used, for example IPPV (intermittent positive pressure ventilation) which uses intermittent inflation pressures, while PEEP (positive end expiratory pressure) raises the pressure at the end of expiration; CPPV (continuous positive pressure ventilation) combines both. PEEP, by preventing complete contraction of the lungs to

Table 2.2

Total lung capacity	Volume of gas at the end of maximal inspiration
Functional residual capacity	Volume of gas at the end of *normal* expiration (FRC)
Residual volume	Volume of gas after *maximal* expiration (RV)
Vital capacity	Maximal volume *exhaled* after maximal inspiration
Expiratory reserve volume	Difference between FRC and RV
Inspiratory capacity	Maximum feasible inspiration following tidal expiration
Inspiratory reserve volume	Maximum feasible inspiration beyond tidal inspiration

their normal expiratory volume, may help to prevent alveolar collapse, maintain alveolar surfactant and may assist some ventilation perfusion abnormalities. It does, however, reduce cardiac output (Murray, 1981).

It is far from routine to measure the functional volumes of the lung in non-research animals, moreover some measurements require patient co-operation to a degree only likely in humans, hence their definitions are merely summarized in Table 2.2. The forced vital capacity of cats is 90–100 ml/kg (Fujita *et al.*, 1990). Recently, relationships between expiratory or inspiratory flow rates and lung volumes (flow–volume loops and maximal expiratory flow volumes) have started to be evaluated in the diagnosis of causes of respiratory dysfunction in small animals (Robinson, 1992).

Regulation of Breathing

The main functional features of normal breathing are its rate, depth and rhythm; the total volume of air exchanged is important but its effect depends on the rate and depth by which it is achieved (see above). The rhythmic pattern of inspiration and expiration is established by respiratory centres in the brain (medulla and pons), detailed views on which continue to develop (Schneerson, 1990). There are also important reflexes protecting against excessive pulmonary inflation and reflexes triggered from specific sites which potently stimulate breathing, especially after a period of cessation (apnoea), for example the nasal philtrum in cats (Ruckebusch *et al.*, 1991).

Stability of blood gases normally depends on parallel changes in pulmonary ventilation whenever arterial PCO_2 rises or falls. Thus hypercapnia generally stimulates an increased rate and depth of breathing, through its effects on PCO_2 and pH in the cerebrospinal fluid (CSF). This rapid equilibration between CO_2 in plasma and CSF is important because most ions, notably H^+ and bicarbonate, only change slowly, if at all, in CSF when their plasma concentration alters. Thus, in an established metabolic acidosis (see below), over-fast infusion of bicarbonate rapidly corrects the subnormal plasma bicarbonate, whereas CSF bicarbonate recovers more slowly. The correction of the acidosis should also terminate the compensatory hyperventilation (see below) but as PCO_2 rises towards normal in plasma it also rises in CSF. This leaves CSF with a normal PCO_2 but still with subnormal bicarbonate; as a result, it remains acidic and sustains an unwanted hyperventilation.

A rise in PCO_2 and H^+ concentration stimulates both the peripheral chemoreceptors and the CNS respiratory centres. In contrast, hypoxia stimulates ventilation via the chemoreceptors but has little effect on ventilation via the respiratory centres. Although the normal control of ventilation is based on CO_2 rather than O_2, artificial ventilation may keep CO_2 so low that hypoxia is the only drive to spontaneous breathing. When hypoxia results from poor diffusion, PCO_2 may be less affected because CO_2 diffuses more freely; any increase in ventilation may thus rest on hypoxia rather than hypercapnia. Nevertheless, in chronic hypoxia, when there is sustained hyperventilation, the respiratory centres become less sensitive to hypocapnia which would otherwise undermine the continued increase in pulmonary ventilation. Equally, however, chronic hypercapnia is a less effective drive to increased ventilation than acute rises in PCO_2. The reason may be a parallel rise in plasma and CSF bicarbonate, moderating the fall in CSF pH (Hanning, 1989).

Activation of the vasomotor centre (e.g. in response to hypotension) generally activates the respiratory centres as well. The activity of the respiratory centres is readily depressed by deep anaesthesia. It is also depressed by excessively high PCO_2. Volatile anaesthetics and opiates reduce the CO_2-responsiveness of ventilatory drive (Paulin & Hornbein, 1986; Hanning, 1989). Anaesthesia also depresses the peripheral chemoreceptors and thus weakens this essential defence against hypoxia; patients already dependent on hypoxic drive (e.g. the chronic bronchitic) are then at particular risk (Nunn, 1989). The response to acidosis is also depressed, undermining the compensation of metabolic acidosis (see below). In addition, anaesthesia impairs the normal response whereby increased respiratory workload stimulates increased respiratory effort.

Anaesthesia affects the mechanics of breathing as well as its regulation. It increases the active muscular component of expiration, and depresses the intercostal component of inspiration rather than diaphragmatic function; unfortunately intercostal activity is particularly important in the response to increased PCO_2 (Nunn, 1989). In addition, the diaphragm of anaesthetized animals has less tone at the end of expiration (i.e. FRC is reduced); this is important because pulmonary vascular resistance is minimal at normal FRC and increases above or below (Hanning, 1989). A lower FRC also increases the risk of airway collapse. Pain, particularly chest pain, can also impede breathing. Both pain and the effect of anaesthesia may continue to interfere with breathing during recovery from surgery; as well as respiratory depression, pain and anxiety can cause hyperventilation and respiratory alkalosis. Among the important effects of the latter may be redistribution of K^+ and cardiac arrhythmias (Gann & Kenney, 1990).

Renal Function

Most aspects of renal function are not of specific interest to anaesthetists but a few concern them

very deeply. In particular, these are the effects of prerenal failure, whether caused by hypovolaemia, hypotension or cardiac failure, the risks associated with acute renal failure (ARF) and the insidious nature of chronic renal failure (CRF). Assessment of renal function merits discussion because it is a matter of tradition rather than logic that so many cats, especially older animals, are subjected to anaesthesia without the most rudimentary attempt to check their kidneys. Therefore, the following section focuses, in turn, on the renal regulation of water, electrolytes and acid–base balance, on renal dysfunction and on the detection of renal failure.

Anaesthesia suppresses both consciousness and pain perception but does not abolish neural or humoral responses, for example to visceral traction or neural and humoral influences on renal function, indeed it may considerably affect endocrine function. The potential influences of surgery on renal function or fluid and electrolyte balance are therefore through:

1. Pre-anaesthetic food and water restriction.
2. Losses (wounds, respiratory, pooling in damaged tissues, haemorrhage, enteric secretions, excised tissues or organs).
3. Effects on cardiovascular function, renal perfusion and interference with autoregulation of renal blood flow.
4. Effects of surgery on renal function.
5. Effects of anaesthesia and associated medication on renal function (Michell, 1983; Altman & Suki, 1987; Gann & Kenney, 1990).
6. Nephrotoxicity of anaesthetics or other drugs including older contrast agents (Michell, 1981; Altman & Suki, 1987).
7. Effects of anaesthesia on renal nerves (Stoetling & Dierdorf, 1988).

Normal renal function has excretory, endocrine and regulatory components but the latter are the most important and those most likely to be distorted by surgical procedures and their aftermath.

Renal Perfusion and Glomerular Filtration: Acute Renal Failure

The kidneys receive approximately a quarter of cardiac output and convert about 20% of their plasma flow (filtration fraction, FF) to primitive urine by glomerular filtration. Maintenance of stable glomerular filtration rate (GFR) is an essential feature of renal function and depends substantially on autoregulation of renal blood flow (RBF) and tubuloglomerular feedback. As a result:

1. RBF is reasonably stable despite hypotension until it becomes severe. Lowering of GFR by hypotension or reduced cardiac output is 'prerenal failure' and the renal defence against it depends crucially on constriction of the efferent arterioles. This raises the pressure in the preceding capillaries (i.e. the glomeruli) and raises the FF. The constriction is induced by secretion of renin by the afferent arterioles and the resulting generation of angiotensin (renin and angiotensin thus act predominantly as a single hormone system with a variety of effects). The renal defence against hypovolaemia or hypotension is thus undermined by ACE-inhibitors because they block the angiotensin converting enzyme which generates angiotensin in response to renin.
2. Changes in GFR are balanced by parallel changes in tubular reabsorption unless they are fast or extreme (glomerulotubular balance).

Although GFR is stable in the face of moderate hypotension, it is increased by amino acids following protein digestion and this effect is particularly important in carnivores, of which the cat is a prime example.

The main work of the kidney is reabsorption of the vast majority (>95%) of glomerular filtrate; a day's primitive urine, without reabsorption, would be equivalent to several months' output of final urine. This matching of GFR to reabsorption is, therefore, vital because even a minor mismatch could rapidly cause dangerous fluid retention or hypovolaemia. Thus, potent diuretics will cause hypovolaemia and hypotension at excessive dosage; that is when they mobilize urine faster than oedema fluid (Michell, 1988a).

Acute renal failure (ARF) always reduces GFR and usually reduces urine output but the latter can sometimes rise if reabsorption is not as severely depressed. The renal cortex includes the glomeruli and the proximal and distal convoluted tubules. Their function is dependent on the highest tissue perfusion rate in the body (Michell, 1988b). In contrast, the medulla has the lowest soft tissue perfusion rate and this is equally important for its function in producing concentrated urine. In ARF there is a catastrophic diversion of RBF from the cortex to the medulla, crippling the function of both and causing the production of minimal volumes of urine which nevertheless remains dilute and rich in sodium. Normally, reduction of urine output is a response to dehydration and hypovolaemia, hence both water and sodium are conserved (concentrated urine, virtually Na^+-free).

As well as producing the potent vasoconstrictor angiotensin (via output of renin), the kidneys produce vasodilators, including prostaglandins, mainly from the medulla. These protect against the effects of excessive vasoconstriction; cats on non-steroidal anti-inflammatory drugs (NSAID) are therefore susceptible to renal damage caused by hypotension (see Chapters 7 and 12).

Provided the glomeruli are intact, proteins larger than albumin are retained in plasma and they, and substances bound to them, are absent from urine; glomerular restraint of proteins also depends on their negative charge. Smaller proteins, including hormones and enzymes, enter primitive urine but are catabolized in the proximal tubule, following reabsorption. Proteinuria thus indicates:

1. Non-renal urinary tract haemorrhage or inflammation.
2. Glomerular damage.
3. Leakage of tubular proteins (enzymes) or failure of tubular reabsorption of small proteins. Unlike (1) and (2), this is likely to cause very slight proteinuria requiring specific detection techniques.

Glomerular leakage of proteins, for example haemoglobin following haemolysis or myoglobin following muscle damage, can lead to proximal tubular damage. The proximal tubules are also susceptible to the nephrotoxic effects of drugs and poisons because they are important in the secretion of many substances which are less readily excreted by glomerular filtration.

Regulation of ECF Volume and Composition

The main expenditure of renal energy is on reabsorption of sodium. This underlies the reabsorption of water and various solutes which are either cotransported (glucose, amino acids) or whose reabsorption is facilitated by the concentration gradients created by the associated reduction in urine volume. Other ions (K^+, H^+) may be more readily secreted as a result of the electrical gradients caused by sodium reabsorption.

In the proximal tubule, sodium and water are reabsorbed at plasma concentration and reabsorption increases or decreases according to the need to expand or reduce plasma volume. Since primitive urine resembles the electrolyte composition of plasma, reabsorption of proximal tubular fluid is ideally suited to the defence of plasma volume. In severe hypovolaemia, however, excessive proximal reabsorption can sufficiently restrict delivery of sodium to the loop and distal nephron to interfere with their crucial role in the regulation of plasma composition. Specifically, by interfering with secretion of K^+ and H^+ and with the production of either fully concentrated or fully dilute urine (hence with maintenance of water balance) it impedes the regulation of the plasma concentration of K^+, H^+ and Na^+. Thus parenteral fluids similar in composition to normal plasma can nevertheless correct disturbances of plasma composition. Correction of ECF volume is the key to correction of plasma composition because it restores normal renal perfusion and the normal segmental balance of sodium reabsorption.

Sodium reabsorption in the ascending thick limb of the loop of Henlé creates dilute urine suitable for the excretion of excess water; additional dilution occurs in the distal nephron, facilitated by aldosterone from the adrenal cortex. Aldosterone also promotes the excretion of K^+ and H^+ and the stimuli for its secretion are:

1. Sodium depletion – the resulting fall in ECF volume and renal perfusion stimulates the production of angiotensin which is the actual stimulus for aldosterone secretion.

2. Hyperkalaemia – which directly stimulates aldosterone secretion.

Aldosterone also promotes colonic sodium conservation and potassium excretion.

The sodium reabsorbed in the loop generates high concentrations of sodium in medullary interstitial fluid (as a result of countercurrent multiplication; Chou *et al.*, 1993). These promote water conservation from urine in the collecting duct when its permeability is increased by AVP (an effect opposed by glucocorticoids, hypokalaemia or hypercalcaemia; Schrier, 1976) and thus allow production of concentrated urine. Cats are better concentrators than dogs (maximal urinary osmolality close to 3000 mOsm/kg vs. 2800 mOsm/kg). Maximum concentration depends on fully concentrated medullary ISF which is impeded by excessive medullary blood flow ('medullary washout') which can occur as a result of ARF or polydipsia.

Urea is also partially reabsorbed and concentrated in the medulla; its reabsorption increases in response to AVP during dehydration and its presence in the medullary ISF assists the formation of fully concentrated urine. At the simplest, this is because the necessary high concentration of urea in final urine does not create osmotic opposition to water conservation since urea is also at high concentration in the ISF surrounding the collecting ducts. The real involvement of urea transport in urine concentration is more complex and more fundamental (Gillin & Sands, 1993) and inadequate hepatic urea synthesis undermines water conservation. The other major nitrogenous waste product (creatinine) is normally excreted almost solely by glomerular filtration without significant reabsorption or secretion (though this varies slightly between species and non-renal excretion may become detectable in CRF). Thus, in ARF or CRF, the fall in GFR raises the plasma concentration of both, whereas in prerenal failure the reduced GFR affects both but plasma urea, unlike creatinine, is further increased by absorption under the influence of AVP (Michell, 1988b).

The main renal defence against sodium depletion and reduced ECF volume is thus enhanced proximal reabsorption reinforced by production of almost Na^+-free urine in the distal nephron under the influence of aldosterone. The renal defence of plasma sodium concentration is via changes in water reabsorption under the influence of AVP (reinforced by thirst). The main defence against excess ECF volume is the fall in proximal sodium absorption and the effects of natriuretic hormones including ANP. This increases GFR, reduces arterial pressure (via reduced peripheral resistance), promotes transfer of fluid towards ISF and reduces renal reabsorption of sodium substantially by opposing the effects of the renin–angiotensin system (Atlas & Maack, 1992; Gunning & Brenner, 1992; Awazu & Ichikawa, 1993). Whereas ANP originates from the heart, similar peptides originate from the brain and the kidneys themselves. These peptides do not block the sodium pump, but circulating transport inhibitors (ASTI) originate from the brain; other natriuretic factors may originate in the feline gut (Lundgren & Hansson, 1991; Michell, 1991). Healthy kidneys in unanaesthetized animals with normal circulation are well able to excrete excess sodium in response to volume expansion and this is the main protection against excessive parenteral fluid therapy; it is undermined by ARF.

Whether or not surgery and the preceding events cause hypovolaemia, surgery and anaesthesia tend to stimulate production of AVP, angiotensin and aldosterone and thus promote irrelevant retention of water and sodium. The water retention tends to predominate; that is, the patient is predisposed to hyponatraemia (Hall, 1980; Michell et al., 1989; Gann & Kenney, 1990). Parenteral fluids during surgery should therefore be those which restore ECF volume (sodium concentration similar to plasma sodium concentration) rather than those which exacerbate hyponatraemia. Where possible, hypovolaemia should be corrected prior to surgery because it enhances the depression of RBF and GFR associated with anaesthesia (Michell et al., 1989).

Potassium and Magnesium

Hypovolaemia, if mild (e.g. chronic vomiting), promotes urinary loss of potassium and predisposes to hypokalaemia. In severe hypovolaemia, reduced distal delivery of sodium impedes this aldosterone-induced kaliuresis and hyperkalaemia is likely, especially where acidosis drives potassium out of cells. Because the concentration of K^+ in ICF is so high compared with ECF, transcellular distribution is as important an influence on plasma K^+ as renal excretion. Catecholamines and insulin encourage uptake into ICF, as does aldosterone, and insulin secretion rises with plasma K^+; that is, both hormones participate in the regulation of plasma K^+ concentration (Michell, 1991b). Diabetes mellitus may predispose to hyperkalaemia as a result of catabolism, acidosis and reduced secretion or effectiveness of insulin. β-Blockers may predispose to hyperkalaemia, as may ACE-inhibitors (by reducing aldosterone secretion) and depolarizing muscle relaxants (release of cell K^+).

Diuretics tend to cause K^+ depletion (enhancement of aldosterone secretion in response to Na^+ loss), hence they are often used alongside potassium-boosted diets or drugs which restrict K^+ secretion in the distal nephron (K^+-sparing diuretics, e.g. amiloride or spironolactone). It is easy for a combination of factors among the above, for example high-K diet, β-blocker, ACE-inhibitor to produce hyperkalaemia where each alone would not.

ARF is generally associated with hyperkalaemia (substantially due to acidosis) whereas CRF generally does not cause hyperkalaemia until it is far advanced (or decompensated) because there is time for an adaptive increase in potassium secretion in the surviving nephrons. Indeed, some cats with CRF may be predisposed to hypokalaemia, especially where dietary intake is poor, and this presents as muscle weakness but also impairs renal function (Dow et al., 1987; Jones, 1990).

The use of diuretics in the treatment of cardiac failure does not only predispose to hypokalaemia; there may also be hypomagnesaemia, especially with diuretics primarily affecting the loop because this is the main site of magnesium reabsorption (De Rouffignac, 1992). Both are potentially causes of acute and serious ventricular arrhythmias (Cobb & Michell, 1992).

Potassium and magnesium are both predominantly intracellular ions, thus plasma concentration is an imperfect predictor of deficits. This is especially true in the absence of pH data, thus, for example, diarrhoea (and inappetance) create potassium deficits in ICF but acidosis may still cause hyperkalaemia. Potassium and sodium ions are freely dissolved in plasma whereas much calcium or magnesium is bound (to albumin) or complexed (e.g. with citrate) and does not contribute to physiological responses. It thus functions as a reserve (which also escapes renal excretion). Ion-specific electrodes measure purely the active fraction which governs the effects of hypomagnesaemia or hypocalcaemia whereas other techniques include the inactive fractions. Unless albumin is also measured, such measurements can be deceptive.

Acid–Base Balance

Normal plasma pH is maintained by the combined effects of the kidneys, the respiratory system and the liver, plus the effects of chemical buffering in plasma and cells. The main intracellular buffers are proteins (including haemoglobin) and phosphate; the main ECF buffer is bicarbonate. Like most buffer systems, this comprises a weak acid and its sodium salt (carbonic acid and bicarbonate). Since weak acids are only partially dissociated, removal of H^+ increases dissociation and (within limits) replaces the lost H^+. Conversely, added H^+ can combine with excess anion (bicarbonate) to form undissociated acid and avoid a change in the concentration of free H^+:

$$H_2O + CO_2 \rightarrow H_2CO_3 \dashrightarrow H^+ + HCO_3^-$$

The concentration of free H^+ thus depends on the ratio of $CO_2 : HCO_3^-$ and provided this ratio is normal, so is plasma pH. The importance of these facts is as follows:

1. Unlike an *in vitro* buffer system, the major components (CO_2 and HCO_3^-) can be regulated by the lungs and kidneys respectively and H^+ can also be renally excreted; this confers power on bicarbonate buffering beyond that expected from its chemical concentration.
2. Since all other buffers will parallel the changes in bicarbonate buffering, assessment

of this system allows general statements concerning acid–base disturbances.

3. Primary disturbances of CO_2 are defined as 'respiratory acidosis' (rise) or 'respiratory alkalosis' (fall) respectively. Primary disturbances of bicarbonate are defined as 'metabolic acidosis' (fall) or 'metabolic alkalosis' (rise) respectively.
4. Either a metabolic or respiratory disturbance is more tolerable if the ratio (and thus plasma pH) remains close to normal. The compensatory response to a change in bicarbonate is thus a parallel change in CO_2, for example hyperventilation to reduce CO_2 during metabolic acidosis (reduced bicarbonate). This is impeded by anaesthesia or respiratory dysfunction. The compensatory response to a change in CO_2 is correspondingly a parallel change in renal bicarbonate reabsorption (more slowly than respiratory compensation). This could be impeded by renal disease or loss of bicarbonate (e.g. due to diarrhoea); these conditions could therefore intensify any respiratory acidosis caused by pulmonary dysfunction or anaesthesia. There is a widespread assumption that respiratory disease always causes respiratory acidosis but it often causes reflex hyperventilation and respiratory alkalosis.

Acid–base disturbances thus present as simple, compensated or mixed conditions (e.g. metabolic acidosis due to diarrhoea plus respiratory alkalosis due to hyperventilation during fever), predictable to a limited degree from history and hardly at all from clinical signs.

The renal role in pH regulation mainly comprises reabsorption of filtered bicarbonate and secretion of hydrogen ions (both dependent on carbonic anhydrase). The secreted H^+ lowers urine pH but, more important, it loads the urinary buffers (filtered phosphate and secreted ammonia) and since urine pH cannot fall much below 4.5, most of the excreted hydrogen ions are carried by urinary buffers. Renal excretion of excess bicarbonate is a powerful protection against metabolic alkalosis except in two important circumstances:

1. Hypovolaemia – when sodium conservation may necessitate parallel absorption of bicar-

bonate, especially when the main alternative, chloride, has been depleted by vomiting.
2. Cell potassium depletion – this favours the loss of H^+ rather than K^+ during sodium conservation; this increases the alkalosis.

Metabolic alkalosis can therefore be corrected by bicarbonate-free solutions which restore ECF volume (e.g. NaCl) and helped by the inclusion of K^+; it does not require the provision of acid. This emphasizes the difference between a physiologically regulated *in vivo* system and a chemical buffer solution *in vitro* – much neglected by the exponents of 'strong ion difference' (see below). Metabolic alkalosis increases the protein binding of calcium, here only bicarbonate can lower the plasma concentration of free (active) calcium (Chew *et al*. 1989).

Since the main anions available for reabsorption with sodium are predominantly chloride and bicarbonate, loss of bicarbonate (as in diarrhoea) tends to raise plasma chloride (hyperchloraemic acidosis: 'hyperchloraemia' is descriptive, not causal). Metabolic acidosis can also occur because bicarbonate is reduced by accumulation of acid. The bicarbonate is titrated by the accumulated H^+ but chloride is unaffected because the anions of the acids increase instead. Since the sum of $Na^+ + K^+$ normally exceeds $Cl^- + HCO_3^-$, this difference ('anion gap') which mainly reflects the routinely unmeasured anions of organic acids, is diagnostically useful; for example in lactic acidosis, it increases whereas in diarrhoea it does not.

Quantitation of Acid–Base Disturbances

Conventionally this is done by measuring pH and PCO_2 in an anaerobically drawn blood sample using ion-specific electrodes in a blood gas machine, which also calculates plasma bicarbonate. These are too expensive for routine veterinary clinical use and a much more affordable approach is via the use of total CO_2 (TCO_2). This can be done with the Harleco *Micro* CO_2 apparatus (Groutides & Michell, 1990) which is not t the same as the glass Harleco syringe cited by Gentry and Black (1975) and Chew (1989) or other analysers

based on the same principle (Naylor, 1987; Michell, 1990a).

The measurement of TCO_2 depends on the fact that there is much more bicarbonate than CO_2 in normal blood; addition of strong acid converts both to free CO_2. Measurement of this liberated CO_2 and comparison with standard bicarbonate solutions thus quantitates bicarbonate in blood rather than the CO_2. Since fluid therapy is directed towards metabolic disturbances, this serves as an adequate clinical guide and can use whole venous blood. However, it does not allow any reliable insight into respiratory disturbances for which estimates of PCO_2 and preferably PO_2 are necessary preferably in arterial blood.

Recently there has been considerable American enthusiasm for 'strong ion difference' (SID) as the basis of acid–base interpretation (Stewart, 1983; Eicker, 1990; Jones, 1990; de Morais, 1992). It is hard to see why. The concept has made little impact on human medicine, despite some impact in respiratory physiology. It is simplistic in equating *in vitro* and *in vivo* responses, can be clinically misleading and is highly impractical, requiring three measurements (plasma concentration of Na^+, K^-, Cl^-) with the cumulative errors of each. Because it is a hybrid of anion gap and bicarbonate it precludes the useful insights from each. It is also undermined by the fact that Na^+ and K^+ can be separately regulated or disturbed (without acid–base disturbances) and that the former is a reflection of water balance rather than sodium balance. Since both lactate and chloride are strong ions, neither, supposedly, affects SID – yet lactate improves metabolic acidosis whereas chloride improves metabolic alkalosis. Hydrogen ion concentration is supposedly unimportant – whereas many physicochemical and physiological processes relate precisely to pH, as does the change in the buffering capacity of haemoglobin with temperature (Rahn *et al.*, 1975). Proton pumps supposedly would not work – yet Peter Mitchell was awarded his Nobel Prize substantially for his research on proton pumps. Closer to earth, as acidosis worsens in animals with diarrhoea, their SID may 'improve', not least because of hyperkalaemia. On practical, clinical and theoretical grounds, including the sheer complexity of the concept, SID is best ignored for clinical purposes.

Quantitation of Renal Function

The basis of renal function is glomerular filtration and the hallmark of renal failure is the decline in GFR. Renal failure can occur without sufficient glomerular damage to cause proteinuria; the cause of the fall in GFR with CRF is the loss of whole nephrons (Michell, 1988b, 1990b). In ARF, it is diversion of blood flow away from the glomeruli (see above). Therefore, the ideal measure of renal function is GFR, but it is not easily done.

There are other indices of renal function, for example concentrating capacity or tubular reabsorptive capacity, but they are not suitable as single diagnostic indicators for CRF or ARF. Some enzymes (e.g. amylase, lipase) are renally excreted and their plasma concentration can rise in renal failure but with insufficient specificity for diagnostic use. Plasma urea and creatinine rise but the normal range is wide because of individual variation and these are insensitive indicators of CRF. This is especially true of urea which also depends on dietary protein, hepatic function and dehydration. Moreover, with progressive loss of nephrons, as in CRF, the rise is initially insidious and essentially logarithmic; that is, accelerates progressively. Thus loss of 50% of GFR may scarcely elevate plasma creatinine beyond the upper limits of normal and by the time clinical signs are obvious, two-thirds to three-quarters of renal function has probably been lost. The key point is that an asymptomatic cat may have less than half its renal function and hypotension or excessively deep anaesthesia may readily decompensate what is left, causing 'acute-on-chronic' failure. The additional hazard posed by NSAIDs has been noted and while ACE-inhibitors may benefit patients with CRF, those that have both heart failure and compensated CRF are at risk since they depend on angiotensin for the maintenance of their GFR (see above).

Determination of GFR requires measurement of the clearance of a solute such as inulin which is excreted solely by filtration, without reabsorp-

tion. Clearance is the excretion rate per plasma concentration (and is thus an expression of excretory efficiency). But it also represents the volume of plasma which would carry that amount of marker per minute, thus if (like inulin) the transfer to urine occurs solely by filtration, this volume is also the GFR.

$$U/P \times F = C$$

where U is concentration in urine; P is concentration in plasma; F is urine flow rate (ml/min); and C is clearance (ml/min). The problem is the need for a timed urine collection during a period of stable plasma concentration following inulin infusion. Creatinine clearance avoids some of the problem since it is endogenously present in plasma but the timed urine collection is still needed (and the precision of the calculated clearance is undermined by the errors of analysing low creatinine concentrations). In cats, exogenous creatinine clearance is feasible but has the same problems described for inulin (though the analysis is simpler); however, it is hard to obtain a sterile supply of creatinine.

To avoid the need for urine collection various 'one-shot' techniques have been tried, measuring the disappearance of markers such as phenol red within a set period following i/v injection. Exogenous creatinine has also been used in this way (Labato & Ross, 1991). Usually these markers are substantially excreted by secretion rather than filtration, nevertheless, since CRF involves progressive loss of whole nephrons, the results should reflect the fall in GFR without actually measuring it.

Techniques based on the relatively safe isotope, technetium ($T_{1/2} = 6$ h), bound to a filtration 'marker' such as DTPA, allow assessment of renal function by:

1. True clearance (with the advantage of simple quantitation at low concentration (Rogers *et al.*, 1991).
2. Renal imaging (which can allow estimates of GFR and gives additional information regarding shape and perfusion (Uribe *et al.*, 1992).

The problem with these techniques is their dependence on expensive equipment (scintillation counter or gamma-camera respectively).

Currently the clinical usefulness of measuring Tc-DTPA disappearance from circulation using an external radiation monitor is being evaluated (Gleadhill & Michell, 1992). Except for a small injection, the technique is totally non-invasive and requires neither blood nor urine samples – a great potential benefit in cats. While the current evaluation is mainly centred on CRF in dogs, there is no reason why the technique should not work in cats and some have already been studied. The final expression of GFR from external counting is per ECF volume but this seems at least as valid as the conventional use of scaling factors such as weight or calculated surface area. It would probably take a very large and undetected source of oedema or ascites to cause serious misinterpretation.

Renal Dysfunction and Anaesthesia

Pre-existing renal disease poses pathophysiological problems for the anaesthetist. Heavy proteinuria may sufficiently reduce plasma albumin to predispose to hypovolaemia and decreased protein binding of anaesthetic agents. ARF is predisposed by hypovolaemia but undermines the normal defence against excess parenteral fluids and causes metabolic acidosis and hyperkalaemia, as well as uraemia (the clinical signs of a rise in plasma urea, creatinine and other nitrogenous end-products of protein breakdown: the rise is azotaemia).

Advanced CRF causes anaemia (through lack of erythropoietin, a renally synthesized hormone ensuring normal maturation of RBC) and secondary hyperparathyroidism, which may also have toxic effects beyond those on mineral metabolism (Michell, 1983). Uraemia can cause coagulation disturbances and these, together with shorter RBC survival, reinforce the anaemia. The excretion of many drugs is affected by renal failure but the response to non-renally excreted drugs may also be affected as a result of changes in their volume of distribution or the responsiveness of target tissues affected by uraemia, electrolyte disturbances or pH abnormalities (Michell, 1981). The uraemic environment and associated disturbances also depress cardiovascular function. Above all,

hypotension, hypovolaemia or drugs may decompensate what remains of renal function.

Hepatic Function

The main impact of anaesthesia and surgery on liver function in cats is via the effects of hypovolaemia or hypotension on hepatic perfusion, together with the hepatotoxicity of some drugs in susceptible individuals. Reduced hepatic perfusion slows the excretion of many drugs; hepatic blood flow is adversely affected by splanchnic vasoconstriction and positive pressure ventilation (Walton, 1987). The effects of pre-existing liver disease are potentially numerous including susceptibility to hypoglycaemia, reduced urea synthesis and increased blood ammonia, endocrine disturbances caused by reduced hormone breakdown, malabsorption of lipids and fat-soluble vitamins, impaired coagulation, reduced albumin synthesis predisposing to hypovolaemia. In addition, hepatic dysfunction affects other organs, notably the brain (hepatic encephalopathy) and kidney, which may be predisposed to ARF as in human hepatorenal syndrome (Michell, 1983). Accumulation of ascitic fluid may interfere with breathing. Hypoalbuminaemia not only predisposes to ascites or oedema but affects the distribution of drugs which normally bind to albumin. Excessive use of diuretics predisposes to metabolic alkalosis as a result of contraction of ECF volume and this is particularly dangerous with liver disease because it favours the existence of ammonia in the uncharged form (rather than NH_4^+) which crosses more readily into the CNS.

The liver is also involved in acid–base regulation and the fact that this goes far beyond its role in metabolizing excess lactate is a fairly recent perception. Thus, while ammonia functions as a urinary buffer, the synthesis of the glutamine from which ammonia is produced also affects acid–base balance (Halperin et al., 1990). In fact, both flux through the urea cycle and glutamine synthesis give the liver a central role, alongside the kidney, in acid–base homeostasis. The clinical implications, including changes in hepatic function during anaesthesia, are only beginning to be considered (Haussinger *et al.*, 1988).

Hepatic metabolism in cats is characterized by low levels of glucuronyl transferases which normally make morphine, salicylates and aceto-minophen into more water-soluble compounds, facilitating both urinary and biliary excretion (Baggot, 1988). On the other hand, cats are better acetylators than dogs. Not all drugs dependent on glucuronide conjugation are toxic to cats because not all transferases are deficient and alternative pathways, for example sulphate conjugation, may compensate (Boothe, 1990). However, such alternatives may make other drugs more toxic. Cats are unable to synthesize arginine and this predisposes them to acute ammonia intoxication on inadequate intakes; it may also predispose them to hepatic lipidosis which impedes drug metabolism (O'Donnell & Hayes, 1987; Zawie & Shaker, 1989; Boothe, 1990). The inability of the feline liver to synthesize taurine is well known and predis-poses cats to blindness and cardiomyopathy on inadequate diets. Cats are totally dependent on taurine for bile salt conjugation (Armstrong & Havel, 1989) and it may also be important in protecting brain cells from the effects of hypertonic dehydration, providing 'idiogenic osmoles' to prevent the shrinkage which would otherwise occur (Trachtman *et al.*, 1988).

While the liver plays an essential role in detoxification of many foreign compounds including drugs, some metabolic intermediates are more toxic than the parent compound. Since a wide range of compounds may be metabolized by the same pathway (e.g. cytochrome P-450), drugs affecting that pathway may reduce the toxicity of some compounds, enhance the toxicity of others (Zimmerman & Maddrey, 1987). Adverse effects of anaesthesia on hepatic function are seldom those of true hepatotoxicity (as with older agents such as chloroform or ether), nor of cholestasis; they are most often idiosyncratic hepatic injury (due to individual susceptibility resulting from hypersensitivity to metabolites, unusual metabolites, or immune responses) or the result of inadequate perfusion.

Temperature Regulation

Cats are small compared with most veterinary patients and thus face the problem of a relatively large surface area for heat loss and a small tissue mass (especially liver and muscle) for thermogenesis; this is simply a matter of geometry. Changes in blood flow and the neuromuscular and metabolic effects of drugs may impede thermogenesis during anaesthesia and recovery, and the thermoregulatory centres in the brain may also be depressed; thus shock causes both impaired thermoregulation and a regulated fall in the 'set point' (Michell, 1982).

This is the opposite of fever which involves a regulated rise in set point so that the cat's current 'normal' temperature is above its usual normal temperature and it responds as if in a cold environment. When set point returns to normal spontaneously, or under the influence of NSAIDs, the cat responds as if in a warm environment, until its temperature falls to normal. The early phase therefore comprises superficial vasoconstriction, erection of the fur, shivering, etc., whereas recovery involves cuta-neous vasodilation (and increased respiratory heat loss). There may be several such cycles during the course of an infection, corresponding to proliferation or death of microorganisms. Heat stroke, unlike fever, implies that set point is normal but the cooling mechanisms cannot cope with the existing heat load; NSAIDs will not help whereas gradual cooling will (during fever it would simply increase shivering, etc.).

Non-primates, including cats, depend greatly on panting as opposed to sweating for their evaporative cooling, even where it is not the obvious and specialized open-mouth, resonant-frequency panting typified by the dog. The efficiency of all evaporative cooling depends on sufficiently dry air, hence the greater stress when high temperature is accompanied by high humidity. Exposed wounds provide an abnormal source of evaporative cooling.

The main insulation comes from fat and the air trapped in fur; replacement by water in wet fur (e.g. due to secretions, spilled fluids, urine, etc.) greatly undermines its efficiency and predisposes to hypothermia. During recovery from anaesthesia the aim should be to limit heat losses, since the patient is susceptible to hypothermia, but not to overwarm, which might cause excessive vasodilation and exacerbate any tendency towards hypotension. Limitation of heat loss can involve both insulation (to reduce losses caused by conduction and radiation) and use of reflective materials to limit radiation to cooler surroundings. Warming of parenteral fluids is important, especially in shock when large volumes are used (see Chapter 12).

While anaesthesia generally predisposes to hypothermia, a peculiar form of hyperthermia (malignant hyperpyrexia) is seen in susceptible individuals exposed particularly to halothane or stress (Ording, 1989; O'Brien *et al.*, 1990). It has mainly been seen in humans and pigs; despite its interest (and lethal potential) it is unusual even in these species and only one or two cases have been recorded in cats (Bellah *et al.*, 1993). The more usual elevation of body temperature, in fever, is mediated by the effect of prostaglandin E_2 within the hypothalamus (hence its correction by NSAID) and depends mainly on the effects of endogenous pyrogens. These are induced by exogenous pyrogens (which do not reach the brain), including bacterial toxins and agents associated with viral and neoplastic cell damage, as well as some chemicals (Coceani *et al.*, 1986). The production of endogenous pyrogens by leucocytes, in response to these various factors, stimulates the change in hypothalamic set point underlying the rise in body temperature. This is generally but not invariably an adaptive rather than a maladaptive response to infection (Michell, 1982; Barnet, 1986; Kluger, 1986). It could reasonably be regarded as an endocrine response and endogenous pyrogen (interleukin-1) as a hormone.

Endocrine Disturbances

Most non-sexual endocrine disturbances potentially affect the response to surgery and anaesthesia and both major surgery and extensive trauma can trigger changes in the secretion or breakdown of a variety of hormones, especially those associated with metabolism (e.g. catecholamines, insulin, ACTH, cortisol, GH, etc.). Cellular responsiveness may also be affected. However, some important disturbances are not particularly common in cats. Thus hypothyroidism and adrenal insufficiency (except perhaps as a result of excess steroids) are unusual. Cushing's syndrome occurs but cats are resistant to iatrogenic steroid excess (Peterson & Randolph, 1989). The most important endocrine disturbances in the present context are probably diabetes mellitus and hyperthyroidism (see Chapter 11).

Hyperthyroidism

Hyperthyroid cats have an accelerated metabolic rate and a hyperdynamic circulation with increased cardiac output, high heart rate, increased GFR and, in many cases, hypertrophic cardiomyopathy (Peterson & Randolph, 1989; Salisbury, 1991). They are also prone to cardiac arrhythmias and the arrhythmogenic effects of catecholamines (Muir & Swanson, 1989). Overperfusion of the renal medulla with consequent 'washout' of interstitial solute may cause polyuria (Malkovic-Basic & Kleeman, 1991). Polydipsia, polyuria (often without renal disease), vomiting and diarrhoea are all liable to cause dehydration. The hyperdynamic circulation raises GFR (Malkovic-Basic & Kleeman, 1991) thus, if anything, it is the aftermath of surgery that is likely to precipitate or decompensate renal failure (Peterson & Randolph, 1989). Anaesthesia of cats with hyperthyroidism is described in Chapter 11.

Diabetes Mellitus

Type I diabetes mellitus primarily involves inadequate secretion of insulin (equivalent to human 'juvenile onset'). Type II (equivalent to human 'maturity onset') involves both impaired insulin secretion in response to hyperglycaemia and tissue resistance to insulin which, in humans, is usually associated with obesity (Felig *et al.*, 1981; Lewis *et al.*, 1987; Bjorntorp, 1992; MacEwen, 1992; De Fronzo *et al.*, 1992). Insulin resistance may also result from antibodies to injected insulin and increased secretion of other hormones, notably glucagon. Clear differentiation between these types of diabetes is difficult in cats (Peterson & Randolph, 1989).

The severest consequence of diabetes is ketoacidosis (with increased anion gap), while other metabolic disturbances include decreased glucose tolerance (due to hepatic and peripheral failure of glucose uptake), elevation of plasma lipids and impairment of amino acid uptake and protein synthesis; this impedes wound healing (Altman & Suki, 1987). Diabetics are also prone to hyperkalaemia, not only because of ketoacidosis, should it occur, but because of impaired cell uptake of potassium (Michell, 1991b). On the other hand, insulin therapy may cause hypokalaemia. Cerebral glucose uptake is not impaired by lack of insulin. Sustained hyperglycaemia leads to glycosylation of haemoglobin which thus serves as an index of therapeutic control. The stress associated with surgery exacerbates hyperglycaemia by raising secretion of catecholamines, ACTH and glucocorticoids.

Polyuria (and secondary polydipsia) result from osmotic diuresis because the high concentration of glucose in plasma and glomerular filtrate exceeds the maximum rate of tubular reabsorption. While osmotic diuresis usually promotes sufficient water loss to raise plasma sodium concentration, it may also fall as a result of water held in circulation by the additional glucose (Michell *et al.*, 1989). In fact, measured plasma sodium concentration should be corrected to allow for depression by hyperglycaemia (Ellis, 1990). The combination of hyperglycaemia and dehydration may cause hyperosmolar coma in the absence of ketoacidosis; although this is unusual, it is serious (Peterson & Randolph, 1989).

As well as hyponatraemia, diabetes can cause increased urinary loss of sodium and contraction of ECF volume; like hyperkalaemia, this probably results substantially from loss of the stimulatory effect of insulin on Na–K ATPase. ECF volume may be further depressed as blood glucose falls and fluid shifts towards ICF. Treatment of hypovolaemia is thus an essential priority (May & Watlington, 1990).

Anaesthesia, Analgesia and Stress

Despite a rapid growth of knowledge concerning the interactions of anaesthetics and analgesics with neurotransmitter systems such as glutamate/NMDA, neurokinins and endogenous opioids, the basis of anaesthesia still awaits explanation (Headley & Lodge, 1993). The concept that it lay in non-specific effects on membrane lipids has been substantially superseded by the demonstration of rather specific effects on target proteins. As a result, excitatory synaptic transmission is depressed (e.g. NMDA by dissociative anaesthetics) or inhibitory transmission potentiated (e.g. GABA by barbiturates). Most anaesthetics seem to affect several transmitters.

There is perhaps better understanding of the effects of analgesics, especially those affecting opioid receptors (Sackman, 1991), and a growing realization that the physiology of pain is different once it becomes chronic. There is also growing appreciation of the various chemicals released by injured cells which raise the sensitivity of nociceptors, for example prostaglandins (hence the analgesic effects of NSAIDs) and also leukotrienes and mediators such as serotonin, bradykinin and substance P which originates from nerves (Sackman, 1991). The phenomenon of referred pain is also better, though incompletely, understood and attributed to superficial and deep structures sharing the same dorsal root innervation or convergence of nociceptive pathways within the spinal cord.

The physiology of pain overlaps with that of stress, which has major effects on behavioural, endocrine, cardiovascular and immune responses (Michell, 1987). Among these, the best known are the increases in the secretion of catecholamines, ACTH and corticosteroids and the rises in sympathetic activity, heart rate and arterial pressure. No single response is a reliable indicator of stress, though corticosteroid secretion is often interpreted as though it were. Nor can stress be predicted simply from the characteristics of the stressor, since it depends on the perception of the individual involved, especially the extent to which the situation seems uncontrollable or unpredictable. The social context is also important; isolation is generally stressful but grouping with unfamiliar animals or people is also potentially stressful, as are unfamiliar surroundings for some individuals, or surroundings in which pain or fear have previously been experienced. There are thus physiological reasons, as well as concern for patient welfare, to understand the factors which underlie stress and to minimize them both prior to induction of anaesthesia and during recovery.

References

Altman, M. & Suki, W.N. (1987) Preoperative fluid management of the surgical patient. In: *Clinical Disorders of Fluid and Electrolyte Metabolism* (ed. M.H. Maxwell & C.R. Kleeman), pp. 897–916. McGraw Hill, New York.

Armstrong, P.J. & Havel, M.A. (1989) Nutritional disorders. In: *The Cat: Diseases and Clinical Management* (ed. R.G. Sherding), pp. 141–161. Churchill Livingstone, New York.

Atlas, S.A. & Maack, T. (1992) Atrial natriuretic factor. In: *Handbook of Physiology: Renal Physiology* (ed. E.E. Windhager), pp. 1577–1673. Oxford, New York.

Autheneil, J.L. (1992) Blood transfusion therapy. In: *Fluid Therapy in Small Animal Practice* (ed. S.P. Di Bartola), pp. 371–383. W.B. Saunders, Philadelphia.

Awazu, M. & Ichikawa, I. (1993) Biological significance of atrial natriuretic peptide in the kidney. *Nephron* **63**, 1–14.

Baggot, J.D. (1988) Disposition and fate of drugs in the body. In: *Veterinary Pharmacology* (ed. N.H. Booth & L.E. McDonald), pp. 38–72. Iowa State University Press, Iowa.

Barnet, M. (1986) Fever in mammals: is it beneficial? *Yale J. Biol. Med.* **59**, 117–124.

Bellah, J.R., Robertson, S.A., Buergect, C.D. & McGavin, A.D. (1993) Suspected malignant hyperthermia after halothane anaesthesia in a cat. *Vet. Surg.* **18**, 483–488.

Benumof, J.L. (1990) Respiratory physiology and respiratory function during anaesthesia. In: *Anaesthesia* (ed. R.D. Miller), pp. 505–556. Churchill Livingstone, New York.

Biro, G.P. (1980) Anaesthesia and haemodilution. In: *The Circulation in Anaesthesia* (ed. C. Prys-Roberts), pp. 327–350. Blackwell, Oxford.

Bjorntorp, P. (1992) Biochemistry of obesity in relation to diabetes mellitus. In: *International Textbook of Diabetes Mellitus* (ed. K.G.G.M. Alberti, R.A. DeFronzo, H. Keen & P. Zimmet), pp. 551–568. John Wiley, Chichester.

Boothe, D.M. (1990) Drug therapy in cats: mechanisms and avoidance of adverse drug reactions. *J. Am. Vet. Med. Assoc.* **196**, 1297–1307.

Carroll, H.J. & Oh, M.S. (1978) *Water, Electrolyte and Acid–Base Metabolism* J.B. Lippincott, Philadelphia.

Chew, D.J. (1989) Parenteral fluid therapy. In: *The Cat: Diseases and Clinical Management* (ed. R.G. Sherding), pp. 35–80. Churchill Livingstone, New York.

Chew, D.J., Leonard, M. & Muir, W. (1989) The effect of sodium bicarbonate infusion on carried calcium and total calcium concentration in serum of clinically normal cats. *Am. J. Vet. Res.* **50**, 145–150.

Chou, C.L., Knepper, M.A. & Layton, H.E. (1993) Urinary concentrating mechanism. *Sem. in Nephr.* **13**, 168–181.

Cobb, M. & Michell, A.R. (1992) Electrolyte changes in dogs during diuretic therapy for cardiac failure. *J. Small Anim. Prac.* **33**, 526–529.

Coceani, F., Bishai, I., Lees, J. & Sirko, S. (1986) Prostaglandin E$_2$ and fever: a continuing debate. *Yale J. Biol. Med.* **59**, 169–174.

Cotter, S.M. (1992) Clinical transfusion medicine. *Adv. Vet. Sci. Comp. Med.* **36**, 187–223.

Dean, C., Seagard, J.L., Hopp, F.A. & Kampwe, J.P. (1992) Differential control of sympathetic activity to kidney and skeletal muscle by ventral medullary neurons. *J. Autonomic Nerv. System* **37**, 1–10.

De Fronzo, R.A., Bonadonna, R.C. & Ferranini, E. (1992) Pathogenesis of NIDDM; a precarious balance between insulin action and insulin secretion. In: *International Textbook of Diabetes Mellitus* (ed. K.G.G.M. Alberti, R.A. De Fronzo, H. Keen & P. Zimmet), pp. 569–634. John Wiley, Chichester.

De Morais, H.S.A. (1992) A non-traditional approach to acid–base disorders. In: *Fluid Therapy in Small Animal Practice* (ed. S.P. Di Brtola), pp. 297–320. W.B. Saunders, London.

De Rouffignac, C. (1992) Regulation of magnesium excretion. In: *Disorders of Bone and Mineral Metabolism* (ed. F.L. Coe & M.J. Favus), pp. 42–55. Raven Press, New York.

De Witt, D.S., Prough, D.S., Taylor, C.L. & Whitley, J.M. (1992) Reduced cerebral blood flow, oxygen delivery and electroencephalographic activity after traumatic brain injury and mild haemorrhage in cats. *J. Neurosurg.* **76**, 812–821.

Di Bartola, S.P. (1992) *Fluid Therapy in Small Animal Practice* W.B. Saunders, Philadelphia, P. 5.

Dow, S.W., Le Couteur, R.A., Fettman, M.J. & Spurgeon, T.L. (1987) Potassium depletion in cats: hypokalemic polymyopathy. *J. Am. Vet. Med. Assoc.* **191**, 1563–1573.

Eicker, S.W. (1990) An introduction to Strong Ion Difference. *Veterinary Clinics of North America (Food Animal Practice)* **6**(1), 45–50.

Ellis, E.N. (1990) Concepts of fluid therapy in diabetic ketoacidosis and hyperosmolar hyperglycemic non-ketotic coma. *Pediat. Clin. North America* **37**(2), 313–321.

Felig, P., Havel, R.J. & Smith, L.H. (1981) Metabolism and nutrition. In: *Pathophysiology* (ed. L.H. Smith & S.O. Thier), pp. 479–652. W.B. Saunders, Philadelphia.

Foex, P. (1989) Heart and autonomic nervous system. In: *Anaesthesia* (ed. W.S. Nimmo & G. Smith), pp. 115–161. Blackwell, Oxford.

Fujita, M., Orima, H., Shimizu, M., Motoyoshi, S., Katayama, M. & Miyasaka, K. (1990) Forced vital capacity in cats. *Jap. J. Vet. Sci.* **52**, 1097–1098.

Gann, D.S. & Kenney, P.R. (1990) Special problems of fluid and electrolyte management in surgery. In: *Kidney Electrolyte Disorders* (ed. J.C.M. Chan & J.R. Gill), pp. 343–361. Churchill Livingstone, New York.

Gelman, S., Fowler, K.C. & Smith, L.R. (1984) Regional blood flow during isoflurane and halothane anaesthesia. *Anesth. Analg.* **63**, 557–565.

Gentry, P.A. & Black, W.D. (1975) Evaluation of Harleco CO_2 apparatus: comparison with the Van Slyke method. *J. Am. Vet. Med. Assoc.* **167**, 156–157.

Giger, V. (1992) The feline AB blood group system and incompatibility reactions. In: *Current Veterinary Therapy XI* (ed. R.W. Kirk), pp. 470–474. W.B. Saunders, Philadelphia.

Gillin, A.G. & Sands, J.M. (1993) Urea transport in the kidney. *Sem. Nephr.* **13**, 146–154.

Gleadhill, A. & Michell, A.R. (1992) Towards earlier diagnosis of canine renal disease. *Proceedings, XVIIth WSAVA World Congress (Rome)*, pp. 999–1004.

Groutides, C.P. & Michell, A.R. (1990) Evlauation of acid–base disturbances in calf diarrhoea. *Vet. Rec.* **126**, 29–31.

Gunning, M.E. & Brenner, B.M. (1992) Natriuretic peptides and the kidney: current concepts. *Kidney Int.* **42** (Suppl. 8), S127–S133.

Guyton, A.C. (1991) *Textbook of Medical Physiology*, 8th edn. W.B. Saunders, Philadelphia.

Hakin, T.S. & Maceli, A.S. (1988) Effect of hypoxia on erythrocyte deformation in different species. *Biorheology* **25**, 857–868.

Hall, L.W. (1980) Preliminary investigations of the effects of injury on the body fluids of cats and dogs. *J. Small Anim. Pract.* **21**, 679–689.

Halperin, M.L., Ethier, J.H. & Kamel, S.K. (1990) The excretion of ammonium ions and acid–base balance. *Clinic. Biochem.* **23**, 185–188.

Hanning, C.D. (1989) Respiratory physiology. In: *Anaesthesia* (eds. W.S. Nimmo & G. Smith), pp. 162–190. Blackwell, Oxford.

Harrison, D.G., Kurz, M.A., Quillen, J.E., Sellke, F.W. & Mugge, A. (1992) Normal and pathophysiological considerations of endothelial regulation of vascular tone and their relevance to nitrate therapy. *Am. J. Cardiol.* **70**, 11B–17B.

Haussinger, D., Meijer, A.J., Gerok, W. & Sies, H. (1988) Hepatic nitrogen metabolism and acid–base homeostasis. In: *pH Homeostasis; Mechanisms and Control* (ed. D. Haussinger), pp. 337–378. Academic Press, London.

Headley, P.M. & Lodge, D. (1993) Neurotransmitters and neurotransmission; relevance to anaesthetic actions and analgesic therapy. In: *The Advancement of Veterinary Science, Vol. 4 (Veterinary Science – Growth Points and Comparative Medicine* (ed. A.R. Michell), pp. 211–225. C.A.B. International, Wallingford.

Henderson, A.H. (1983) Basic mechanisms of myocardial contraction in health and disease. In: *Scientific Foundation of Cardiology* (ed. P. Sleight & J. Vann Jones), pp. 1–10. W. Heinemann, London.

Henrik, R.A., Wingfield, W.E., Angleton, G.M. & Porter, R.E. (1987) Effects of body position and ventilation: compression ratios during cardiopulmonary resuscitation in cats. *Am. J. Vet. Res.* **48**, 1603–1606.

Hillman, K. (1989) Fluid therapy. In: *Recent Advances in Anaesthesia and Analgesia* 16 (ed. R.S. Atkinson & A.P. Adams), pp. 105–123. Churchill Livingstone, Edinburgh.

Hosgood, G. (1990) Pharmacologic features and physiologic effects of dopamine. *J. Am. Vet. Med. Assoc.* **197**, 1209–1211.

Jain, N.C. (1986) *Veterinary Hematology*. Lea & Febiger, Philadelphia.

Jones, B.R. (1990) Hypokalaemia in the cat. *Cornell Vet.* **80**, 13–15.

Jones, N.L. (1990) A quantitative physicochemical approach to acid–base physiology. *Clin. Biochem.* **23**, 189–195.

Kazemi, H. & Hitzig, B. (1987) Control of ventilation: central chemical drive. In: *Clinical Disorders of Fluid and Electrolyte Metabolism* (ed. M.H. Maxwell &

C.R. Kleeman), pp. 147–157. McGraw Hill, New York.

Kluger, M.J. (1986) Is fever beneficial? *Yale J. Biol. Med.* **59**, 89–95.

Labato, M.A. & Ross, L.A. (1991) Plasma disappearance of creatinine as a renal function test in the dog. *Res. Vet. Sci.* **50**, 253–258.

Lewis, L.D., Morris, M.L. & Hand, M.S. (1987) *Small Animal Clinical Nutrition III* 6.

Lundgren, O. & Hansson, G.C. (1991) Is there an intestinal natriuretic factor? *Acta Physiol. Scand.* **141**, 19–25.

MacEwen, E.G. (1992) Obesity. In: *Current Veterinary Therapy XI* (ed. R.W. Kirk), pp. 313–318. W.B. Saunders, Philadelphia.

Malkovic-Basic, M. & Kleeman, C.R. (1991) The kidneys and electrolyte metabolism in thyrotoxicosis and hypothyroidism. In: *The Thyroid* (ed. L.E. Braverman & O.R.D. Utiger), pp. 771–779; 1009–1016. J.B. Lippincott, Philadelphia.

May, J.M. & Watlington, C.O. (1990) Special problems of fluid and electrolyte metabolism in diabetic patients. In: *Kidney Electrolyte Disorders* (ed. J.C.M. Chan & J.R. Gill), pp. 363–420. Churchill Livingstone, New York.

Michell, A.R. (1981) Anaesthesia and the kidney. *Proc. Assoc. Vet. Anaesth. Great Britain and Ireland* **9**, 111–124.

Michell, A.R. (1982) Current concepts of fever. *J. Small Anim. Prac.* **23**, 185–193.

Michell, A.R. (1983) Abnormalities of renal function. In: *Veterinary Nephrology* (ed. L.W. Hall), pp. 189–210. Heinemann Veterinary Books, London.

Michell, A.R. (1985) What is shock? *J. Small Anim. Prac.* **26**, 719–738.

Michell, A.R. (1987) The pathophysiology of malaise and malingering. In: *Animal Disease – A Welfare Problem* (ed. T.E. Gibson), pp. 8–21. B.V.A. Animal Welfare Foundation, London.

Michell, A.R. (1988a) Diuretics and cardiovascular disease. *J. Vet. Pharmacol. Therap.* **11**, 246–253.

Michell, A.R. (1988b) In: *Renal Disease in Dogs and Cats: Comparative and Clinical Aspects*, pp. 5–29. Blackwell, Oxford.

Michell, A.R. (1989) Shock in companion animals. *Veterinary Annual*, 29th edn, pp. 45–58. Bailliere, London.

Michell, A.R. (1990a) Evaluation of acid–base disturbance. *Vet. Rec.* **126**, 173.

Michell, A.R. (1990b) From renal physiology to renal failure: a subtle progression. *Proceedings, 5th Annual Symposium, European Society for Veterinary Nephrology and Urology, Milan*, pp. 1–8.

Michell, A.R. (1991a) Regulation of sodium and water balance in dogs and cats. *J. Small Anim. Pract.* **32**, 135–145.

Michell, A.R. (1991b) Intracellular cations: out of sight, out of mind? *J. Nutrit.* **121**, S97–98.

Michell, A.R. (1993a) Hypertension in companion animals. In: *Veterinary Annual* (ed. M-E Raw & T.J. Parkinson), Baillière Tindall, London pp. 11–23.

Michell, A.R. (1993b) Circulatory shock: pathophysiology and management. In: *Proc. Assoc. Vet. Pharmacol. Therap.* (in press).

Michell, A.R. (1993c) Circulatory shock: new developments in therapy. In: *Proc. Assoc. Vet. Pharmacol. Therap.* (in press).

Michell, A.R., Bywater, R.J., Clarke, K.W., Hall, L.W. & Waterman, A.E. (1989) *Veterinary Fluid Therapy.* Blackwell, Oxford.

Middleton, D.J., Ilkiw, J.E. & Watson, A.D.J. (1981) Arterial and venous blood gas tensions in clinically healthy cats. *Am. J. Vet. Res.* **42**, 1609–1611.

Muir, W.R. & Swanson, C.R. (1989) Techniques and complications of feline anaesthesia and chemical restraint. In: *The Cat: Diseases and Clinical Management* (ed. R.G. Sherding), pp. 81–116. Churchill Livingstone, New York.

Muizelear, J.P., Bouma, G.J., Levasseur, J.E. & Kontos, H.A. (1992) Effect of haematocrit variations on cerebral blood flow and basilar artery diameter *in vivo. Am. J. Physiol.* **262**, H949–954.

Murray, J.F. (1981) Respiration. In: *Pathophysiology* (ed. L.H. Smith & S.O. Thier), pp. 921–1071. W.B. Saunders, Philadelphia.

Naylor, J.M. (1987) Evaluation of the total carbon dioxide apparatus and pH meter for the determination of acid–base status. *Canad. Vet. J.* **28**, 45–48.

Nunn, J.F. (1989) Effect of anaesthesia on respiration. In: *General Anaesthesia* (ed. J.F. Nunn, J.E. Utting & B.R. Brown), pp. 185–199. Butterworth, London.

O'Brien, P.J., Klip, A., Britt, B. & Kalow, B.I. (1991) Malignant hyperthermia susceptibility: biochemical basis for pathogenesis and diagnosis. *Canad. Vet. J.* **54**, 83–92.

O'Donnell, C.P. & Bower, E.A. (1992) Heart rate changes evoked by hypoxia in the anaesthetized, artificially ventilated cat. *Exp. Physiol.* **77**, 271–284.

O'Donnell, J.A. & Hayes, K.C. (1987) Nutritional disorders. In: *Diseases of the Cat* (ed. J. Holzworth), pp. 15–42. W.B. Saunders, Philadelphia.

Ording, H. (1989) Pathophysiology of malignant hyperthermia. *Ann. Franc. Anesth. Reanim.* **8**, 411–416.

Paulin, E.G. & Hornbein, T.F. (1986) Anaesthesia and the control of ventilation. In: *Handbook of Physiology: Respiratory System* (Section 3). Vol. 2. *Control of*

Breathing, Part 2 pp. 793–813. American Physiological Society, Bethesda.

Persson, P.B., Baumann, J.E., Ehmke, H., Nafz, B., Wittman, V. & Kirchheim, H.R. (1992) Phasic and 24-hour blood pressure control by endothelium-derived relaxing factors in conscious dogs. *Am. J. Physiol.* **262**, H1395–H1400.

Peterson, M.E. & Randolph, J.F. (1989) Endocrine diseases. In: *The Cat: Diseases and Clinical Management* (ed. R.G. Sherding), pp. 1095–1161. Churchill Livingstone, New York.

Rahn, H., Reeves, R.B. & Howell, B.J. (1975) Hydrogen ion regulation, temperature and evolution. *Am. Rev. Resp. Dis.* **112**, 165–172.

Robinson, N.E. (1992) Airway physiology. *Veterinary Clinics of North America: Small Animal Practice* **22**(5), 1043–1064.

Rogers, K.S., Komkov, A., Brown, S.A., Lees, G.E., Hightower, D. & Russo, E.A. (1991) Comparison of four methods of estimating glomerular filtration rate in cats. *Am. J. Vet. Res.* **52**, 961–964.

Roth, S. (1992) The effects of isovolaemic hemodilution on ocular blood flow. *Exp. Eye Res.* **55**, 59–63.

Ruckebusch, Y., Phaneuf, L.P. & Dunlop, R. (1991) *Physiology of Small and Large Animals.* B.C. Decker, Philadelphia.

Sackman, J.E. (1991) Pain: its perception and alleviation in dogs and cats. *Compendium on Continuing Education for the Practising Veterinarian (European Edition)* **13**, 35–40; 81–92.

Salisbury, S.K. (1991) Hyperthyroidism in cats. *Compendium on Continuing Education for the Practising Veterinarian (European Edition)* **13**, 606–613.

Sato, M., Niiyama, K., Kuroda, R., Ioku, M., Kanai, N. & Hayakawa, T. (1992) Experimental study on the indications for barbiturate therapy; change in haemodynamics and the influence of dopamine. *Acta Neurochirurg. Wein* **117**, 200–205.

Schneerson, J. (1989) Ventilatory control. In: *Disorders of Ventilation* pp. 3–13. Blackwell, Oxford.

Schrier, R.W. (1976) *Renal and Electrolyte Disorders.* Little Brown & Co., Boston.

Sellgren, J., Biber, B., Henriksson, B.A., Martner, J. &

Ponten, J. (1992) The effects of propofol, methohexitone and isoflurane on the baroreceptor reflex in the cat. *Acta Anaesth. Scand.* **36**, 784–790.

Stewart, P.A. (1983) Modern quantitative acid–base chemistry. *Canadian J. Physiol. Pharmacol.* **61**, 1444–1461.

Stoetling, R.K. & Dierdorf, S.F. (1988) Renal disease. In: *Anaesthesia and Coexisting Disease* 2nd edn (ed. R.K. Stoelting, S.F. Dierdorf & R.L. McCammon), pp. 415–443. Churchill Livingstone, London.

Sutin, K.H., Ruskin, K.J. & Kaufman, B.S. (1992) Intravenous fluid therapy in neurologic surgery. *Critical Care Clinics* **8**, 367–408.

Szabo, C., Farago, M., Horvath, I., Lohinai, Z. & Kovach, A.G. (1992) Haemorrhagic hypotension impairs endothelium-dependent relaxation in the artery of the cat. *Circulatory Shock* **36**, 238–241.

Trachtman, H., Barbour, R., Sturman, J. & Finberg, L. (1988) Taurine and osmoregulation: taurine is a cerebral osmoprotective molecule in chronic hypernatraemic dehydration. *Pediatric Res.* **23**, 35–39.

Uribe, D., Krawiec, D.R., Twardock, A.R. & Gelberg, H.B. (1992) Quantitative renal scintigraphic determination of the glomerular filtration rate in cats with normal and abnormal kidney function using ^{99}Tc-diethylenetriamine pentacetic acid. *Am. J. Vet. Res.* **53**, 1101–1107.

Vanhoutte, P.M. & Eber, B. (1991) Endothelium-derived relaxing and contracting factors. *Wiene Klinische Wochenschrift* **14**, 405–411.

Walton, B. (1987) The liver. In: *Hazards and Complications of Anaesthesia* (ed. T.H. Taylor & E. Major), pp. 85–100. Churchill Livingstone, Edinburgh.

Wills, J. & Wolf, A. (1993) *A Handbook of Feline Medicine.* Pergamon, Oxford.

Zawie, D.A. & Shaker, F. (1989) Nutrition. In: *The Cat: Diseases and Clinical Management* (ed. R.G. Sherding), pp. 1015–1036. Churchill Livingstone, New York.

Zimmerman, H.J. & Maddrey, W.C. (1987) Toxic and drug induced hepatitis. In: *Diseases of the Liver* (ed. L. Schiff & E.R. Schiff), pp. 591–629. J.B. Lippincott, London.

R.J. Evans

3
Pharmacology

Introduction

This chapter discusses the principles which underlie drug usage in the cat in the specific context of anaesthetic practices. Pharmacokinetic processes are dealt with in the first section of this chapter and pharmacodynamics in the second. Emphasis is placed on the general aspects of drug metabolism rather than on the pharmacokinetics of specific agents and on the developing understanding of neuropharmacology and the effects of drugs used in anaesthetic practice on neurotransmission rather than on the clinical pharmacology of the individual compounds, which is described in Chapters 7–9. It is hoped that such an approach will equip the reader to assimilate subsequent developments as they appear.

Pharmacokinetics

The fate of any chemical agent administered to an animal is complex. Its absorption will be influenced by the route of administration, by the physiological state of the recipient and by the chemical and physical nature of the material itself as well as its pharmaceutical formulation.

For the agents used in anaesthetic practice, the route of administration is of major concern and is determined by the nature of the agent. Administration by inhalation results in a particular form of pharmacokinetic behaviour where factors determining bulk flow of the agent in the airways, across the lung epithelium and in the blood stream dominate rather than the first order (exponential) processes which are generally of prime importance following administration by the oral route or by non-respiratory parenteral routes (see Hladky, 1990 and Pratt & Taylor, 1990 for useful expositions).

Once absorbed, any compound will be distributed in one or more body compartments. It may be confined to the circulation, may permeate the extracellular compartment, may enter the intracellular compartment and approach distribution through the total body water, or it may be concentrated selectively in particular organs. The pattern of distribution may change with time as drug movements between compartments, metabolism and elimination occur.

Wherever it has access to a specific site of action or receptor, the agent will exert its pharmacological and/or toxicological actions in a dose-dependent fashion provided that its concentration exceeds any necessary threshold level and is in an appropriate range for receptor occupancy to vary with ligand concentration. This is determined by the affinity of the agent for the binding site. Side-effects may arise from subsidiary actions at other receptors or sites than those resulting in the desired action, or from undesirable consequences of the primary action. A detailed account of the mathematics of drug–receptor interactions will not be given here (see Dean, 1987 and Pratt & Taylor, 1990 for useful expositions). In the case of inhalational agents, which do not interact with specific receptors, drug action theoretically shows continuously grade effect with increasing concentration, although there will be a defined concentration window within which anaesthetically useful actions are obtained.

Drug Metabolism and its Influence on Pharmacokinetics in the Cat

Drug circulating in the vascular compartment is continually exposed to the processes of metabolism and elimination, which generally inactivate the compound and clear it from the blood and then from the body (see Gibson & Skett, 1986 and Hladky, 1990 for surveys of these areas). Most drugs are lipophilic organic compounds and the levels attained in the tissues are markedly influenced by their rate of metabolism. In some cases metabolism may result in the formation of an active principle from an inactive precursor (prodrug) or to the conversion of one active compound to another and, again, rates of enzymic conversion critically determine tissue levels of active metabolites. The major site of drug metabolism is the liver. Drug excretion occurs mainly via the urine and bile. Many drugs partition into milk and it is wise to recognize this if dealing with nursing queens. Many of the therapeutic difficulties encountered in the cat are the consequence of an unusual pattern of hepatic drug metabolism in this species. This may represent an adaptation to extreme carnivorism: in free-living animals the major source of unusual foreign compounds will be their food and particularly ingested plant material because of the wide range of metabolic end-products synthesized and stored by plants.

In all cases, it has to be recognized that, while blood concentrations are an index of whole-body handling of drug and may be a useful guide to tissue concentration, sequestration of drug in particular compartments, slow transfer processes or slow receptor kinetics may lead to marked divergence of the duration and intensity of drug action from those predicted from plasma concentration.

Where drug metabolism is limited by the activity of hepatic enzymes, this may account for significant differences in pharmacological or toxicological responses between species. In this circumstance alterations in enzyme activity due to induction or inhibition may have dramatic effects on the duration and or intensity of drug effects. In the cat, unusual features of hepatic drug metabolism, which in turn influence pharmacokinetic parameters, are a major determinant of drug usage.

Inhalational anaesthetic agents, of course, are a special case, much of their pharmacokinetics being determined by processes of mass transport and diffusional processes in the airways and across the alveolar wall as well as the pulmonary blood flow. For inhalational agents, metabolism usually makes little or no contribution to elimination and does not need detailed consideration in predicting duration of action but active metabolites may be responsible for adverse or toxic reactions.

Hepatic Drug Metabolism

Hepatic drug metabolism has two phases. Phase I, functionalization, is a catabolic reaction. The reactions in this phase involve oxidation, reduction or hydrolysis and are most commonly catalysed by the P-450-mixed function microsomal mono-oxygenase system of the liver, but other oxygenase enzymes also contribute, notably flavine mono-oxygenases. Hepatic microsomal mono-oxygenase (HMO) activity is due to many isoenzymes and isoforms of cytochrome P-450 (Nebert & Gonzalez, 1987). HMOs can oxidize the majority of lipophilic drugs. In consequence of phase I, the drug may be changed in activity, may be inactivated or, in some cases, an inactive precursor may be changed to an active metabolite. The parent compound is generally metabolized to a more reactive compound as a substrate for phase II reactions. Species variation is encountered in phase I reactions (Walker, 1978, 1980). In general, there is a good correlation across species between HMO activity and the rate of phase I drug metabolism and activity is inversely related to body size (Walker, 1978). The cat, however, has low HMO activity relative to other mammals of similar metabolic mass (Walker, 1992).

Phase II is the anabolic component of drug metabolism and generally involves the coupling of the drug, or a product of phase I, to an endogenous compound such that the product is water soluble. The conjugate is then excreted by way of the biliary or renal routes. The endogenous substrates commonly employed as conjugating agents in mammals are carbohydrates, amino acids, acetic acid or inorganic sulphate. Conjugation through the glucuronide pathway is the most important phase II reaction in most mammalian species, for example, in man around 95% of a therapeutic dose of aspirin is excreted as the glucuronide (Caldwell, 1982).

Compared to herbivores or omnivores, there is deficiency in the glucuronide pathway in carnivores, presumably because of their reduced exposure to plant-derived compounds, and this deficit is manifested to its most extreme degree in cats. For example, the formation of glucuronide from phenol, proceeds 65 – 100 times as fast in many species (e.g. pig and goat) as it does in the cat (Smith, 1978; Gibson & Skett, 1986). Glucuronide formation is also limited, although less severely so, in other carnivores including the dog and ferret. Interestingly, the cat's conjugation deficit is not absolute: while only 1–3% of doses of phenol, 1-naphthol or paracetamol undergo glucuronide conjugation, 60% of a similar dose of phenolphthalein is glucuronidated. Progesterone and testosterone also undergo substantial glucuronic acid conjugation. The major part of the poorly glucuronidated compounds is converted to the sulphate conjugate which is a much slower reaction. Possibly as a further compensation for its glucuronidation deficiency, the cat also makes some unusual conjugates, notably phosphate and glycyltaurine derivatives.

These drug metabolism pathways and particularly the phase II conjugation reactions have been discussed in some detail because the cat's limited capacity to metabolize xenobiotics and particularly the glucuronidation defect is a significant determinant of the pharmacokinetic behaviour of many drugs.

Pharmacodynamics

Action potential propagation along axons in the mammalian CNS is essentially the same as was originally described by Hodgkin and Huxley (1952) for the squid giant axon. Depolarization is due to the opening of time- and voltage-dependent sodium channels with repolarization being due to voltage-operated potassium channels. We now know much of the molecular structure of such voltage-operated channels and the mechanisms by which local anaesthetic agents block axon potential propagation by

interaction with voltage-operated sodium channels (Courtney, 1975; Ritchie & Green, 1992; Wann, 1993). Although there is evidence for interaction of general anaesthetic agents with voltage-operated sodium and potassium channels, in general voltage-gated channels are relatively insensitive to anaesthetics, particularly the volatile agents, and it is too early in the investigations to draw firm conclusions and at present it seems doubtful whether these are relevant to the clinical actions of general anaesthetics (Franks & Lieb, 1993; Frenkel *et al.*, 1993; Urban, 1993).

It would seem that effects on chemical transmission at central synapses are of much greater relevance to the mechanisms of general anaesthesia than any modification of axon potential propagation. Synaptic transmitters in the CNS may presently be classified as biogenic amines, amino acids, purines and peptides. Some 50 such molecules which are confirmed or candidate CNS transmitters are now recognized and, since there is growing evidence of heterogeneity of receptors for many and possibly all transmitters, receptors and other putative ligand-binding sites run into hundreds.

One general theme which will be apparent is the large degree of heterogeneity amongst receptors for virtually any known mediator which has been revealed by recent pharmacological and cloning studies. The full functional and pharmacological consequences of this heterogeneity are likely to take some time to clarify; however, it is already obvious that it may allow a previously unexpected subtlety in signalling and modulation mechanisms within the CNS and elsewhere. It also offers the opportunity for the development of receptor subtype-specific drugs which may much improve the precision with which desired clinical effects can be achieved whilst also minimizing side-effects which are often due to drugs interacting with multiple receptors.

A further area of neurotransmitter handling, in which cloning is unmasking a large superfamily of related proteins, is that of transporter molecules for transmitters. Centrally acting drugs which are presently used in anaesthetic practice have known interactions with a limited range of these channels, transport systems, transmitters, receptors and intracellular signalling mechanisms (Hille, 1992; Griffith & Norman, 1993; Kress & Tass, 1993; Terrar, 1993). Since the available evidence suggests that interaction with neurotransmission is of particular significance, this section concentrates on such effects (Pocock & Richards, 1993). It concerns itself only with those transmitters and receptors with which neuroleptic, sedative, analgesic and anaesthetic drugs are known to have interactions and thus examines an eclectic grouping based on current, and probably therefore flawed, perceptions of importance and of drug mechanisms. The systems chosen for discussion are glutamate and the NMDA receptor, γ-aminobutyrate (GABA) and the $GABA_A$ and $GABA_B$ receptors, the α_2- and D_2 catecholamine receptors, and the opioid peptides and their receptors. Emphasis has been placed on receptors rather than other aspects of signal transmission since current developments are particularly focused in that area and are revealing more concerning mechanisms of relevant drugs than are other aspects of neuropharmacology. Evidence for interactions with other elements of the signal transmission process are very briefly reviewed, but for further information the reader may wish to consult the *British Journal of Anaesthesia*, Volume 71, part 1, which includes comprehensive review and discussion of these other aspects.

Synaptic Transmission

The following criteria must be satisfied for any mediator in order to establish its validity as a central synaptic neurotransmitter or neuromodulator:

1. A pathway for synthesis of the material must be present in appropriate nerve terminals.
2. Storage of the material in appropriate nerve terminals must be demonstrable or, in the case of those mediators that are synthesized on demand, storage of a precursor.
3. Calcium-dependent release must occur on appropriate stimulation.

4. The postjunctional membrane must bear receptors for the proposed mediator.
5. Antagonists of transmission should produce identical modification of the response whether it is induced by presynaptic stimulation or by application of the putative transmitter.
6. A mechanism which terminates the action of released mediator should be demonstrable.

Although these criteria still have to be satisfied for many of the putative neurotransmitters, they have been established for all of the mediators discussed in this section and these aspects are therefore discussed here only when this is essential. The reader is referred to Cooper *et al.* (1992) for an overview of transmitter identification and biochemistry.

Classification of Membrane Receptors

Membrane-associated receptors activated by endogenous mediators and drugs receptors are currently classified into four main types on the basis of the intracellular signalling mechanisms which they utilize:

1. Those that directly operate ligand-gated ion channels, for example, N_1 and N_2 nicotinic acetylcholine receptors, and are characteristically responsible for fast neurotransmitter-mediated effects.
2. Those that are linked to metabolic mechanisms or to ion channels by guanine nucleotide-binding regulatory proteins (G-proteins), for example, the cholinergic $M_1 - M_5$ muscarinic receptors and the β-adrenoceptors and which mediate slower effects.
3. Those with endogenous tyrosine kinase activity, which phosphorylate other cellular proteins and also autophosphorylate on tyrosine residues, and mainly comprise growth factor and metabolic hormone receptors.
4. Those with endogenous guanylyl cyclase activity, which directly synthesize cyclic GMP, for example $ANP_{A \& B}$ atrial natriuretic peptide receptors.

The receptors discussed in this chapter all fall into the first two categories. The former are sometimes referred to as ionotropic receptors, the latter as metabotropic or collision-coupled receptors. Much is now known, albeit in general terms, of their molecular biology and physiology. In each case it seems that all receptors in each class may be coded by an evolutionarily-related gene superfamily, so that much homology of amino acid sequence and of secondary, tertiary and quaternary protein structure is to be found between the various superfamily members. The nicotinic receptor has a hetero-oligomeric structure composed of subunits each of which has four transmembrane sequences of alpha helix-forming hydrophobic amino acids (Stroud & Finer-Moore, 1985; Brisson & Unwin, 1985; Galzi *et al.*, 1991). On the basis of the presently known structural homologies, it seems likely that all other mammalian ligand-gated ion channels have a similar hetero-oligomeric composition and function in like fashion to the nicotinic receptor (Langosch *et al.*, 1988). The β_2-adrenoceptor is the archetype of the G-protein-linked receptor and has seven transmembrane domains which form the ligand-binding site (Lefkowitz & Caron, 1988; Schwinn, 1993). Amino acid residues in the second and third intracellular loops and the intracellular carboxy terminal portion contribute to interaction with members of another superfamily of gene products, the heterotrimeric G-proteins. A diversity amongst heterotrimeric G-proteins allows great flexibility in coupling patterns and therefore the responses which can be generated by different receptors or by the same receptor in different cells or tissues (Kaziro *et al.*, 1991). In most cases G-protein-linked receptors of importance for CNS function act by one or more of four main mechanisms:

1. Activation of adenylyl cyclase thus increasing cellular cyclic AMP (cAMP) levels.
2. Inhibition of adenylyl cyclase thus reducing cellular cyclic AMP levels.
3. Activation of one of a family of phospholipases – in the context of CNS transmitter action perhaps the most important of these are the phospholipases C which liberate

inositol trisphosphate (IP$_3$) and diacylglycerol (DAG) from membrane phospholipids.
4. Modulation of the conductance of ion channels.

More detailed discussion of G-proteins or any consideration of the subsequent steps in intracellular signalling mechanisms and the cellular effector mechanisms which these regulate in order to transduce ligand binding to receptor into a co-ordinated cellular response are beyond the scope of this chapter and the reader is referred to Taylor (1990), Kaziro *et al.* (1991) and Lambert (1993) for an overview and entry points to the literature. Direct biochemical evidence for the disposition of transmembrane segments and intra- and extracellular loops and terminal sequences is presently available for only a handful of receptors. However, in view of the high degree of sequence homology between proteins within superfamilies and their functional similarities, it is generally thought appropriate to make predictions of the expected configuration on the basis of hydrophobicity (hydropathy) analysis of the known or predicted amino acid sequence. The majority of such descriptions which follow are therefore predictions awaiting experimental confirmation. For the current status of any receptor type the reader would do well to refer to the compilation of Watson and Girdlestone (1993) and its annual successors. Receptor desensitization and mechanisms and consequences of control of receptors by phosphorylation, understanding of which is in its infancy, is not discussed.

Glutamate as a Central Transmitter

Glutamate and aspartate are dicarboxylic amino acids which are found in high concentration in the CNS. They have potent stimulatory activity when applied to neurons (Curtis & Watkins, 1960, 1963) and are believed to be the major neurotransmitters mediating fast excitatory processes in the CNS of mammals (see Cooper *et al.*, 1992 for discussion). The unequivocal identification of these excitatory amino acids

(EAAs) as neurotransmitters has been hindered by their importance in general metabolic reactions, but the detailed characterization and classification of EAA receptors and the study of excitotoxicity have done much to legitimize their case in recent years.

Much more is known about the role of glutamate than that of aspartate. Glutamate metabolism is linked that of GABA (see below) and to the tricarboxylic acid cycle. The major source of glutamate in CNS is transamination of α-ketoglutarate by GABA-transaminase but it can also be derived from glutamine and from ammonia and α-ketoglutarate. Glutamate is stored in synaptic vesicles and released by a calcium-dependent mechanism. Glutamate is involved in developmental plasticity, learning and memory, sensory transmission, and control of respiratory and cardiovascular function (Kemp & Sillito, 1982; Rauschecker & Hahn, 1987; Lodge, 1988; Wong & Kemp, 1991).

The EAAs have two discrete types of action producing on the one hand fast depolarization responses lasting 1–2 ms and on the other longer depolarizing events with a duration of 10–15 ms accompanied by other effects. There appear at the present count to be five receptor types for EAAs in the CNS. These are the NMDA, AMPA, kainate, LAP-4 and metabotropic receptors and many neurons bear more than one type of receptor (Monaghan *et al.*, 1989). The receptors are identified by the use of selective agonists and antagonists and by their actions, signalling pathways and locations.

Receptor Types for Excitatory Amino Acids (Glutamate, Aspartate and Congeners)

NMDA receptors are excitatory receptors producing the slower (~10 ms) depolarizations physiologically induced by glutamate, and at which *N*-methyl-D-aspartate (NMDA) is the eponymous selective agonist. *Trans*-2,3 PDA is also a selective agonist whilst aspartate, quinolate and ibotenic acid have agonist activity at this site. Selective antagonists include D-2-amino-5-phosphonovalerate (D-AP5), CPP, CGS19755 and D-CPPene. Other antagonists include ketamine, dizocilpine, phencyclidine (PCP) and SKF 10047 which block by binding to a discrete site (the PCP site) within the ion channel. Opiates can also interact with this site which may correspond to the σ-opiate receptor at least as initially conceived, if not as presently defined (Johnson & Jones, 1990). In addition to the glutamate binding site, this receptor also carries a regulatory glycine recognition site at which D-serine may also bind. Glycine binding is necessary in addition to glutamate binding for channel opening to occur. Glycine thus potentiates EAA responses as well as being an inhibitory transmitter in its own right.

The NMDA receptor complex has at least three distinct binding sites other than the two already mentioned and has an integral non-selective ligand-gated cation channel with high conductance which provides the mechanism of depolarization. The channel has a particularly high conductance for calcium which is responsible for the major ion flux through it. Channel opening is modulated in a voltage-dependent manner by a Mg^{2+} binding site on the inner face of the receptor which leads to channel block when Mg^{2+} is bound. Thus under physiological conditions, Mg^{2+} ions are bound and small membrane depolarizations are without effect. Agonist-induced currents are greatest at mildly depolarized membrane potentials of -20 to -30 mV (Flatman *et al.*, 1983).

Once the channel is open this voltage dependence produces a feedback effect which tends to maintain the channel in the open state and resulting in the prolonged response characteristic of NMDA receptors. One implication of this is that activation of other depolarizing receptors may be necessary for opening of the NMDA receptor ion channel and this, in turn, may require tetanic presynaptic stimulation to release sufficient glutamate for kainate and AMPA receptors to become active. An external Zn^{2+} binding site also regulates channel function. Zinc is concentrated in presynaptic terminals and is released on stimulation: it may therefore play a modulatory role in central neurotransmission at NMDA and a number of other receptor types. Five genes, nmdar1 and nmdar2A–2D, have been identified but the precise protein structure of naturally formed channels is not known.

NMDA receptors are found throughout the brain, with a high density in the cerebral cortex and the hippocampus. They may play an important part in synaptic plasticity, short-term memory and the underlying phenomenon of long-term potentiation (LTP) for which their Mg^{2+}-modulated voltage-dependence and calcium conductance ideally fit them (Lodge, 1988). Calcium ion entry activates a wide range of other intracellular messenger pathways including: protein kinase C; calmodulin-dependent kinase II; protein phosphatases; phospholipase C with consequent generation of IP_3 and DAG; and nitric oxide synthesis. NMDA receptors are also implicated in seizure generation, degenerative processes, motor function and cardiovascular regulation (Lodge, 1988). They have a role in nociception: activation of NMDA receptors results in wind up of responses by spinal projection neurons in the pain pathway resulting in recurrent discharges. C fibre input to the CNS leads to increased excitability associated with increased EAA, tachykinin and opioid peptide levels. The sensitized state and consequent hypersensitivity/hyperalgesia outlasts the painful lesion and the alterations in transmitter levels.

NMDA can increase CNS hypersensitivity to pain. Cyclohexylamines, including ketamine and tiletamine, interact with the PCP site and can prevent this, particularly if administered prior to the onset of the painful stimulus, for example, surgical intervention. Similarly, reduction in the nocisensory input to higher centres by prior use of local anaesthetics or opiates can prevent the development of hyperalgesia. NMDA receptors are also involved in the pathogenesis of excitotoxicity and in ischaemic neuronal death, an essentially excitotoxic event, with the large calcium influx through NMDA receptor channels being a important contributory process (Olney, 1990). NMDA antagonists such as dizocilpine are protective in animal models. Many antagonists binding at the PCP site have dissociative anaesthetic actions (e.g. ketamine, tiletamine, and phencyclidine) but may also produce perceptual alterations and

behavioural stimulation (ketamine, phencyclidine, dizocilpine) which, in man, result in undesirable psychotomimetic manifestations.

The physiological role of the site to which these reagents bind is as yet obscure. The detailed physiological and pathological significance of the glycine-binding site and the mechanisms of its modulatory role similarly remain to be identified (Kemp & Leeson, 1993) but are of great interest since it is now apparent that glycine is an obligatory coagonist for activation of NMDA receptors (Wong & Kemp, 1991). It seems likely that there is sufficient free glycine in the CNS extracellular space to saturate the site under normal conditions and thus NMDA responses occur readily and raised glycine concentrations produce little potentiation.

AMPA (formerly quisqualate) and kainate receptors have been difficult to differentiate (McLennan, 1988; Watkins & Olverman, 1988) and have often been referred to simply as non-NMDA receptors. They have associated integral cation channels which are more selective than that of the NMDA receptor and have lower calcium conductance or allow only Na^+ and K^+ currents to flow and are responsible for fast depolarizations. Development of newer selective agonists and antagonists have, however, allowed discrimination between AMPA and kainate receptors (Davies & Watkins, 1981). AMPA receptors were originally named quisqualate receptors after that agonist but AMPA and fluorowillardine are also selective agonists. NBQX, a quinoxalinedione, and GYK152466 are selective antagonists. The cloned receptor has 860–890 amino acids and is predicted to have four transmembrane domains. At kainate receptors there is no good selective agonist or antagonist. In addition to glutamate, kainate, domoate and 5-bromowillardine are agonists. AMNH has weak selective antagonist activity and CNQX, DNQX and kynurenate are amongst other antagonists at the site. Nine genes coding for AMPA and kainate receptor subunits (*glur1–7* and *ka* 1 & 2) have been cloned. Two different forms (flip and flop) of *glur1–4* exist due to differing splicing and the flip variants show larger sustained currents on L-glutamate-induced activation. Differential editing of RNA also gives rise to variants of *glur2, 5 & 6* differing in channel calcium conductance. *Glur1–4* encode receptors at which AMPA has higher binding affinity than does kainate while the converse is the case for the glur5–7 and ka1 & 2 gene products. Both AMPA and kainate receptor activation results in fast (1–3 ms) excitatory transmission which shows rapid desensitization. AMPA receptors are widespread in the CNS with a distribution which tends to parallel that of NMDA receptors. They are responsible for rapid EPSPs in many excitatory pathways in the CNS. AMPA antagonists reduce neuronal loss in ischaemic damage to the cerebral cortex. Kainate receptors have a distribution which is almost the inverse of that of NMDA and AMPA receptors and they are therefore localized in particular regions of the CNS. The dorsal horn is one area where they may have an important role being the only ionotropic EAA receptor on C fibre terminals. Kainate and domoate are neurotoxic and potent convulsant agents.

L-AP$_4$ receptors are probably responsible for presynaptic inhibition mediated by glutamate and have the eponymous selective agonist l-2-amino-4-phosphonobutyrate (L-AP$_4$, also known as LAPB) and are probably presynaptic autoinhibitory receptors acting to reduce transmitter release at glutamatergic terminals (Davies & Watkins, 1982). Glutamate and L-*O*-phosphoserine are also agonists but there are no selective antagonists.

Five metabotropic glutamate receptors (mGluR) of size 870–1200 amino acids belonging to the seven-transmembrane domain superfamily have been identified in the rat and a sixth cloned (Schoepp & Conn, 1993). mGluRs$_1$ and $_5$ act via activation of phospholipase C with mobilization of inositoltrisphosphate and diacylglycerol as second messengers. mGluRs$_{2-4}$ reduce adenylyl cyclase activity and decrease cyclic AMP levels. Activation increases the opening of NMDA- and AMPA-gated channels. A number of other effects have also been reported including: activation of phospholipases D and A$_2$; decreased opening of voltage gated potassium channels and of N-type calcium channels; increased opening of calcium-activated potassium and chloride chan-

nels. At mGluR$_1$ and $_5$, quisqualate is the most potent agonist, 1s,3R-ACPD is so at mGluR$_2$ and $_3$ and L-AP$_4$ at mGluR$_4$. No selective antagonists have yet been identified. Metabotropic receptors are able to enhance NMDA receptor–response coupling and are involved in long term (~100 ms) processes including synaptic modulation, long-term potentiation and depression. Their physiological roles include regulation of nociceptive pathways within the CNS, cardiovascular and extrapyramidal motor control. They are also implicated in seizure generation and excitotoxic neuronal degeneration.

γ-Aminobutyrate (GABA) as a Neurotransmitter

γ-Aminobutyrate (GABA) is now well validated as one of two major inhibitory amino acid transmitters encountered in the CNS, the other being glycine (Cooper *et al.* 1991). Glycine performs this function in the spinal cord, brain stem and retina whereas GABA is found in the cerebrum and cerebellum. In these brain regions, GABA accounts for transmission at some 25–40% of synapses. GABA is formed from glutamate by α-decarboxylation catalysed by glutamate decarboxylase (GAD) and is stored in synaptic vesicles in the prejunctional terminal. GAD is a pyridoxal phosphate-containing enzyme and is inhibited by a variety of structural analogues of glutamate, carbonyl trapping reagents (notably hydrazides) which react with the pyridoxal phosphate, sulphydryl reagents and thiols. GAD inhibition lowers brain GABA levels and can precipitate seizures as can lack of the pyridoxal phosphate coenzyme due to dietary deficiency of vitamin B$_6$. However there is no simple relation between GABA levels and seizure activity.

There is evidence that the degree of association of pyridoxal phosphate with the apoenzyme may be regulated by glutamate, GABA and adenine nucleotides and that variation in saturation of the enzyme by the cofactor may be of physiological significance for the control of GABA levels. GABA release is induced in a calcium-dependent fashion by action potentials in inhibitory pathways *in vivo* and by depolarization of brain slices *in vitro*. Termination of action is due to re-uptake by a sodium-dependent GABA transporter located on pre- and postsynaptic neurones and astroglia. GABA is degraded by transamination with α-ketoglutarate, catalysed by γ-aminobutyrate: α-ketoglutarate transaminase (GABA-transaminase: GABA-T). GABA-T is also pyridoxal phosphate-dependent and has a mitochondrial localization in neurons and astrocytes. GABA-T is inhibited by gabaculine, hydroxylamine, aminooxyacetic acid and hydrazinopropionic acid. The product of GABA-T is succinic semialdehyde which is extremely rapidly converted to succinate by succinic semialdehyde dehydrogenase (SSA-DH), an NAD-dependent enzyme. The resultant succinate re-enters Krebs cycle and thus GABA metabolism forms a shunt across the tricarboxylic acid cycle which is unique to CNS tissue.

GABA Receptors

The two major receptors described for γ-aminobutyrate are the $GABA_A$ and $GABA_B$ receptors (Hill & Bowery, 1981) . Both $GABA_A$ and $GABA_B$ receptors are found at pre- and postsynaptic sites. They differ in their signalling mechanisms. $GABA_A$ receptors have an integral ligand-gated chloride channel leading to rapid membrane hyperpolarization (Stevenson, 1988). The $GABA_B$ receptor is variously coupled to Ca^{2+} or K^+ channels by a G-protein (G_i) dependent mechanism, the receptor is thus likely to belong to the seven-transmembrane domain superfamily (Hill, 1985; Bowery, 1993). There is evidence of heterogeneity of coupling, some $GABA_B$ receptors acting via adenylate cyclase and cAMP levels, others through alterations in phosphatidyl inositol turnover. Inhibition results from opening of the potassium channels or closing of calcium channels (Robertson & Taylor, 1986). Currently most evidence supports the possibility that the calcium channels are of the N type, that is voltage-dependent

and dihydropyridine-insensitive. Pharmacological discrimination between $GABA_A$ and $GABA_B$ receptors relies on the actions of selective agonists and antagonists and also of modulatory agents. At the $GABA_A$ receptor muscimol and isoguvacine are selective agonists, picrotoxin, bicuculline and SR95531 are selective antagonists and benzodiazepines and barbiturates, amongst other agents exert a modulatory effect. While at the $GABA_B$ receptor, phaclofen and 2-hydroxysaclofen are selective agonists and baclofen, saclofen, 3-aminopropylphosphinic acid, 3-aminopropylmethylphosphinic acid, CGP35348 and CGP36742 are selective antagonists. γ-Hydroxybutyrate also has agonist activity at $GABA_B$ receptors. A $GABA_C$ receptor has also been described in the retina.

Presently there is much more detail concerning the $GABA_A$ receptor: a number of agents of importance in anaesthetic practice, including barbiturates and benzodiazepines, interact with this receptor.

The $GABA_A$ Receptor

$GABA_A$ receptor Cl^- channels can be discriminated from those of the glycine receptor by the ability of strychnine to block the latter and not the former. The $GABA_A$ receptor has been the subject of much study using electrophysiological, ligand-binding and behavioural methods. These have revealed remarkable complexity with at least eight interacting binding sites being present (Sieghart, 1992). The $GABA_A$ binding site is also the locus of interaction for muscimol, isoguvacine and a number of competitive antagonists including bicuculline and SR95531. This site exists in two affinity states, that with the lower affinity being antagonist-preferring. Otherwise the drug selectivity of the two forms is similar. Pentobarbitone increases the proportion of states in the high affinity form. The significance of the two states is not yet established, but it may be that the high affinity form is a desensitized state since the range of GABA concentrations that are physiologically active is compatible with binding to the low affinity variant. Picrotoxin is also an antagonist at $GABA_A$ receptors (Hill *et al.*, 1972).

Benzodiazepines

A large number of electrophysiological studies have demonstrated that benzodiazepines, for example diazepam and flunitrazepam, potentiate the actions of GABA at the $GABA_A$ receptor and that they do so by increasing the frequency of chloride channel opening. Ligand-binding studies have revealed high affinity binding sites for benzodiazepines associated with $GABA_A$ receptors. There is a reciprocal interaction by which GABA and the benzodiazepines each increase the binding of the other agent. There is a very good correlation between the binding affinities of benzodiazepines to this site and their clinical potencies and it is therefore assumed that this is the site at which they produce their important effects.

There are a number of complexities relating to interactions at this site. Firstly some compounds appear to discriminate two classes of such site, BZ_1 and BZ_2, and as many as six variants may exist (Doble & Martin, 1992). The ligand interactions with BZ sites are also unusual in that three categories of action can be identified. Agents such as diazepam which increase GABA binding and also GABA-induced Cl^- current are regarded as agonists. A number of agents exist, notably the β-carbolines, βCCE and DMCM, which interact with the site but reduce GABA binding and GABA-induced chloride flux. These are known as inverse agonists. A third group of compounds (e.g. flumazenil) have no efficacy at the site but bind and are thus genuine antagonists of both agonists and inverse agonists (Gardner, 1988; Goodchild, 1993). There is considerable speculation that endogenous ligands for this site may be involved in the regulation of anxiety levels but no convincing candidate has yet been identified (Goodchild, 1993). Recent evidence suggests that some anxiolytic cyclopyrrolones which were previously thought to bind here may interact with an overlapping or discrete binding site.

Barbiturates

Generally, barbiturates are sedative and hypnotic and most are anticonvulsant. However, some (e.g. phenobarbitone) suppress seizures at doses well below those required for hypnosis and thus have selective anticonvulsant activity, suggesting that different mechanisms are involved in the hypnotic and antiepileptic effects.

Like benzodiazepines, barbiturates enhance the inhibitory actions of GABA and have been shown to interact with $GABA_A$ receptors. However, patch-clamping has shown that the action of barbiturates is to increase the mean opening time of the chloride channel, rather than affecting channel opening frequency, and thus differs from that of the benzodiazepines (Twyman *et al.*, 1989). The binding affinity appears to be low and thus ligand-binding studies have not proved possible. In the presence of barbiturates, the binding affinities of both GABA and benzodiazepines are increased and the potency of barbiturates in this respect is well correlated with anaesthetic and hypnotic potency.

At high concentrations barbiturates open the channel in their own right, having a GABA-mimetic effect to increase chloride conductance, and also reduce the excitatory action of glutamate, decrease calcium action potentials and calcium-dependent transmitter release. Pentobarbitone is much more effective than phenobarbitone at producing these latter effects. They may be due to binding at one or more other sites and may make an important contribution to hypnotic actions. Selectively anticonvulsant barbiturates may interact with a different site on the GABA receptor complex than hypnotic barbiturates, since phenobarbitone is less potent than pentobarbitone at enhancing the binding of GABA and benzodiazepines and is very weak in displacing dihydropicrotoxinin binding. Barbiturates have also been described which are excitatory and convulsant (e.g. 5,5 dibenzylbarbiturate) and their action appears to be mediated via yet another site (Rall, 1991). Barbiturates are known to modulate a number of other neurotransmitter–receptor interactions in the mammalian CNS. These include antagonism of nicotinic actions of acetylcholine and antagonism of glutamate and aspartate. The significance of these for their clinical effects is presently obscure.

Other Interactions

A further discrete site which modulates GABA-binding and chloride conductance is that to which the macrocyclic lactone antiparasitic avermectins (e.g. ivermectin) bind with high affinity. The 4′-chloro-derivative of diazepam (Ro54864) has been regarded as the archetypical ligand for so-called peripheral benzodiazepine receptors. However, recent investigations have revealed the existence of a class of low affinity modulatory site on the central GABA$_A$ receptor complex with which this compound interacts. Ro54864 is a potent convulsant. Subsequently two phenylquinolines (PK8165 & PK9084) and an isoquinoline carboxamide derivative (PK1195) have been shown to interact with the same site. PK1195 antagonizes the actions of Ro54864. The physiological and pharmacological significance of these sites is presently obscure.

In addition to the binding of GABA antagonists at the GABA site, there is a further site which is associated predominantly with antagonist action and with convulsant activity. Ligands at this site include picrotoxinin and a number of bicyclic cage compounds including TBPS. Binding of these compounds at the picrotoxinin/TBPS-binding site impairs the chloride conductance of the channel, probably by a direct action. Since a number of agonists at the benzodiazepine binding site decrease the binding affinity of TBPS for its site, while inverse agonists increase it, it seems likely that the TBPS-binding site may be associated with the closed configuration of the Cl$^-$ channel.

There is evidence for the interaction of at least three other classes of pharmacologically important agents with the GABA$_A$ receptor complex although none of the interactions or sites involved is yet well characterized. Propofol (2,6-diisopropylphenol) can both potentiate GABA-induced chloride currents in a dose-dependent manner and directly open the channel at high dose. Chlormethiazole, a sedative–hypnotic, anticonvulsant and anxiolytic, does likewise and it is possible that it interacts with the same site. Ethanol can also

enhance GABA-induced chloride conductance. As with the NMDA receptor, there is a zinc-binding site which may play an important modulatory role. Evidence has also accumulated that Cl$^-$ and other halide ions and some other anions (notably NO_3^-, SCN^-, ClO_4^-) can modulate the properties of many of the other ligand-binding sites on the receptor complex. The physiological significance of this is currently uncertain.

Molecular Biology

A great deal is also now known about the molecular biology of the GABA$_A$ receptor as a result of receptor isolation and subsequently cloning and expression of the genes coding for this (Martin, 1992; Doble & Martin, 1992; Sieghart, 1992). The receptor belongs to the superfamily of ligand-gated ion channels which are multi-subunit receptors each subunit having at least four membrane-spanning hydrophobic domains of around 21 amino acids and a long (200–250 amino acid) *N*-terminal domain which is believed to be on the exterior face of the cell membrane.

The 16 subunit variants which have been cloned thus far can be divided into five classes, α, β, γ, δ and ρ. Any one class of subunit can form an ion channnel but the naturally occuring forms of the receptor involve more than one subunit class and the properties of the receptor depend on the combination of subunits, there being at least two subclasses due to regional variations in the subunit structure in different parts of the brain. The ρ subunits have been found only in retina. The α subunit appears to determine the structural recognition of benzodiazepines but γ-subunits are a requirement to obtain benzodiazepine-induced responses. Expression of α1β1γ2 yields a receptor with binding characteristics compatible with the BZ$_1$ receptor subtype whereas the α3β1γ2 combination resembles the BZ$_2$ subtype in its properties. However much further information is required about the phenotypically expressed variants of the receptor, their pharmacology and their brain distribution in order to relate the molecular biological findings to actions in intact animals with security.

The GABA$_B$ Receptor

GABA$_B$ receptors are defined by demonstrating concentration-dependent responses to GABA which are insensitive to anatgonism by bicuculline (Bowery *et al.*, 1980, 1981). Selective agonists and antagonists for GABA$_B$ receptors are discussed above. There is presently no molecular biological information about this receptor subclass. GABA$_B$ receptors are found in the periphery on sympathetic nerve terminals in a wide variety of sites and pre- and postjunctionally, as well as on glial cells, in the CNS (Bowery, 1993). Within the CNS, GABA$_A$ and GABA$_B$ receptors coexist in many sites. However, areas are known where GABA$_B$ receptors predominate, for example the interpeduncular nucleus. GABA$_B$ sites are absent from the cerebellar granule cell layer. High densities of GABA$_B$ receptors are found in the cerebral cortex and in the medial and dorsolateral geniculate nuclei. The density is low in the pyramidal cell layer of the hippocampus. Otherwise in the hippocampus moderate densities are found, as they are in the globus pallidus, habenular nucleus, amygdala and superior colliculi.

In many brain regions, GABA$_B$ receptors are found primarily presynaptically. This is the case in the interpeduncular nucleus, the molecular layer of the cerebellum and the pyramidal cell layer of the hippocampus. In the rat spinal cord, there is a high density in the dorsal horn and evidence for both pre- and postjunctional localization. This may be important for both synaptic plasticity and nociceptive imformation processing (see below). The physiological roles of the GABA$_B$ receptor are still poorly defined. Activation of GABA$_B$ receptors produces hyperpolarization at postjunctional sites and reduced transmitter release at prejunctional sites. In higher centres activation has been shown to inhibit release of catecholamines, GABA, glutamate and somatastatin, in the spinal cord release of glutamate, substance P (SP), somatostatin and calcitonin gene-related peptide (CGRP) is reduced whilst in the periphery acetylcholine (ACh), catecholamines, SP, CGRP and eicosanoids are affected. In the thalamus and hippocampus the late K$^+$ current is potentiated (Soltesz *et al.*, 1988).

In the spinal cord much attention has been paid to the localization of GABA$_B$ receptors on C-fibre terminals in relation to the possible antinociceptive effects of GABA$_B$ agonists such as baclofen. While analgesia has been demonstrated in rats and may involve supraspinal as well as spinal sites of action, there is little evidence for such an action in man except in the case of trigeminal neuralgia. Other effects identified in mamalian tissues or intact animals (generally rat, rabbit or guinea pig) include decreased release or circulating levels of a number of pituitary hormones, decreased gastric acid secretion, increased food intake, decreased gut and bladder contractility and skeletal muscle relaxation. The latter action underlies the major therapeutic use of baclofen in man which is as a muscle relaxant in multiple sclerosis, spinal trauma, and focal dystonic conditions.

The Glycine Receptor

Much less is known of the glycine receptor and its interactions than of the GABA receptors. There is, however, evidence that interactions with glycine receptor-operated channels may be of some significance for general anaesthesia. It has been known for two decades that increased atmospheric pressure was capable of reversing anaesthesia due to volatile anaesthetics and this has been interpreted as evidence for the importance of non-specific membrane expansion as a mechanism of general anaesthesia due to these agents. It has been assumed that hyperbaric conditions compress the membrane to its original volume and/or eject the anaesthetic agent into the aqueous environment. It would now seem that raised pressure has more specific effects. The glycine-operated channel is highly pressure sensitive in its responses and there is speculation that this may be related to the pressure-reversal of anaesthesia but a tangible link is presently lacking (Daniels & Smith, 1993).

α_1-Adrenoceptors

α_1-Receptors may be distinguished by sensitivity to both adrenaline and noradrenaline, to selective agonists (phenylephrine, methoxamine and cirazoline) and antagonism by prazosin and corynanthine. They are members of the seven transmembrane domain superfamily (Harrison et al., 1991) and G-protein linked to formation of inositol trisphosphate and the mobilization of intracellular calcium. Four subtypes have been identified by a combination of selective ligands and gene-cloning studies. The main importance of α_1-receptors for anaesthetic practice is in the genesis of cardiovascular side-effects of agents such as acepromazine. The major central actions of such neuroleptic agents are mediated via other monoamine receptors notably D_2 receptors. α_1-Receptors are found, amongst many other sites, on the smooth muscle of blood vessels and airways, agonists producing constriction of these. The neuroleptic drugs show great variability in their potency as blockers of α_1-receptors but the marked hypotensive effect of acepromazine, clozapine and thioridazine is mediated via such antagonism.

α_2-Adrenoceptors

α_2-Adrenoceptors may be defined by sensitivity to both adrenaline and noradrenaline, to selective agonists (e.g. xylazine, metomidine, medetomidine, clonidine, UK-14,304 or B-HT 933) and antagonism by yohimbine, idazoxan, rauwolscine and atipamezole. They are members of the superfamily of G-protein-linked receptors with seven hydrophobic transmembrane domains, three intracellular and three extracellular hydrophilic loops, an extracellular N-terminal segment and intracellar C-terminal segment (Harrison, 1991). It seems likely that the agonist binding site is formed by the transmembrane domains. α_2-Receptors inhibit adenylate cyclase via coupling through G_i. Subsequent effector mechanisms are: (1) decreased adenylyl cyclase activity, with reduced

cyclic AMP accumulation, protein kinase A activity and attenuated phosphorylation of substrate proteins; (2) potassium channel opening with cell hyperpolarization resulting in inhibition of neuronal firing; and (3) suppression of calcium channel opening, particularly in nerve terminals where the effect is to reduce neurotransmitter release.

Three non-congruent subdivisions of α_2-adrenoceptors are proposed on the basis of: (1) potency ratios for agonists and differential sensitivities to antagonists as determined from functional studies; (2) binding affinities as determined by radioligand binding studies; and (3) the results of cloning and expression of genes encoding the receptors (Bylund, 1988; Ruffolo et al., 1993).

Functional studies on NG108 and HT29 cells discriminate between α_2A and α_2B subtypes of receptor on the basis of greater potency of the antagonist prazosin at the latter sites. This would be consistent with radioligand-binding studies. However it seems that most physiologically identified responses are mediated by α_2A receptors, which is not surprising since many of these were identified as α_2 responses on the basis of sensitivity to yohimbine and insensitivity to prazosin. In rat cortex, submandibular salivary gland and atrium there is, however, evidence for prejunctional α_2B receptors. However, the identification of antagonists, such as SKF 104078, SKF 104856, Abbott-65265 and naftopidil, which discriminate between pre- and postjunctional α_2-adrenoceptors has raised the possibility of an alternative functional classification which shows no correlation with ligand-binding studies available to date. This is further complicated by the possibility of heterogeneity of prejunctional α_2-receptors in rat vas deferens.

Radioligand-binding studies provide evidence for the existence of two well-defined types of α_2 site (α_2A and α_2B) and a further two putative examples (α_2C and α_2D). The latter two presently appear to have no functional correlates. When binding sites for tritiated rauwolscine are examined, it is clear that they can be divided into sites which are insensitive to prazosin (α_2A) and others for which prazosin exhibits high affinity (α_2B). A number of other selective agents can be used to discriminate these sites. Imiloxan; ARC-239; SKF104856 and chlorpromazine are α_2B-selective and, with the exception of imiloxan, also bind avidly to α_1-receptors. Benoxathian, BRL4408 and oxymetazoline are α_2A selective. Binding displacement curves reveal the presence of both subtypes in rodent and human CNS. It is possible that two subtypes of α_2B exist on the basis of binding studies with the radioligand [^{3}H] RX 821002 but only one compound has so far been identified which appears to discriminate between them. α_2C sites are characterized by very high, and α_2D sites by very low affinity for rauwolscine by comparison with α_2A and α_2B sites but have, as yet, only been identified on a few cell types.

Cloning and expression of the genes for α_2-adrenoceptors has provided evidence for three or possibly four subtypes each of which is separately encoded (Harrison *et al.*, 1991; Ruffolo *et al.*, 1993). Studies were performed using oligonucleotide probes prepared using the sequences of peptides from the purified human platelet α_2-adrenoceptor. Application of the probes has identified three distinct genes which are located on chromosomes 2, 4 and 10. That on chromosome 10 encodes the platelet receptor and is probably an α_2A receptor. The gene on chromosome 4 codes for a receptor expressed in kidney and CNS which is probably of the α_2B type and that on chromosome 2 a peripheral α_2B or an α_2C receptor. Three genes have also been identified in rats two of which are clearly homologues of the human chromosome 2 and chromosome 4 clones. The third rat gene shows considerable homology in protein sequence when compared with the chromosome 10 clone from man. However, when expressed, the gene product has pharmacological properties which are appropriate for the functionally described α_2D receptor type. It may well be that additional genes for α_2-adrenoceptor subtypes have yet to be identified.

Functions of α_2-Adrenoceptors

α_2-Adrenoceptors mediate a variety of functions. Peripheral effector cell α_2-adrenoceptors contribute to the control of vascular tone, renal excretory function, platelet aggregation , intest-

inal motility and secretion, insulin release, control of the release of endothelium-derived relaxing factor (EDRF; nitric oxide: NO) and metabolism of lipoproteins (Hayashi & Maze, 1993; Ruffolo *et al.*, 1993). Prejunctional peripheral α_2-adrenoceptors have a key role in local modulation of neurotransmitter release in all tissues with sympathetic innervation and similar prejunctional receptors occur in the CNS (Hayashi & Maze, 1993; Ruffolo *et al.*, 1993). CNS postjunctional α_2-adrenoceptors are implicated in many roles including control of arousal and pain/nociception, sleep–waking cycle, cardiovascular regulation and modulation of pituitary hormone release. In the dorsal horn of the spinal cord both pre- and postjunctional α_2-receptors inhibit transmission from C-fibres to projection neurones. The effects on arousal and pain sensation and those on cardiovascular regulation will be discussed further in view of their relevance to anaesthetic practice.

Arousal and Pain

The central catecholaminergic and α-receptor-bearing neurones of which we presently know most are those of the locus coeruleus. This is the most prominent nucleus containing noradrenergic neurones in the brain stem. Its projections, which run in five main tracts, are widespread including the cerebral cortex, olfactory bulb, thalamic and hypothalamic nuclei, the cerebellum and hippocampus together with the spinal cord. These projections appear mainly to be inhibitory on their targets via activation of β-receptors and increased adenylate cyclase activity. Noradrenaline and adrenaline inhibit firing of locus coeruleus cells via α_2 autoreceptors and this feedback loop is an important mechanism of synaptic homeostatsis. The locus coeruleus is the principal site at which the marked sedative effect of α_2-agonists is exerted (de Saro *et al.* 1981). Selective α_2-agonists depress locus coeruleus cell firing rate and this effect is overcome by α_2-antagonists. Thus clonidine or xylazine decrease activity, whereas yohimbine and idazoxan markedly increase it. In rodents, the rate of firing of locus coeruleus cells is well correlated with brain levels of 3-methoxy-4-hydroxy-phenylethyleneglycol (MOPEG) and noradrenaline turnover. In rats, stress increases MOPEG levels and noradrenaline turnover by a mechanism which is dependent on the locus coeruleus. As would be expected, α_2-agonists decrease and α_2-antagonists increase MOPEG levels and, by inference, noradrenaline turnover. The main function of the locus coeruleus in conscious animals appears to be to regulate the brain's level of activation in response to sensory stimuli and, as yet, more defined functions have not been specifically attributed to the locus coeruleus (Ruffolo *et al.*, 1993).

Activation of central α_2-adrenoceptors produces a powerful analgesic effect which can be more potent than that of morphine (Hayashi & Maze, 1993). This appears to involve both supraspinal and spinal sites. There is evidence for the involvement of brain and spinal α_2-receptors in the analgesic action of clonidine in the cat (Murata *et al.*, 1989). Morphine and opioid peptides also inhibit locus coeruleus cell firing rate. The analgesic action of α_2-agonists is synergistic with that of the opiates (Wilcox *et al.*, 1987) and there is evidence to suggest that the two transmitter systems are closely interrelated and may regulate the same potassium channel (Koob & Bloom, 1988).

Cardiovascular Function and Blood Pressure Regulation

The contribution of α_2-receptors in the regulation of cardiovascular function and blood pressure involves at least four sites (Ruffolo *et al.*, 1993). These are at central catecholaminergic synapses particularly in the ventrolateral medulla, in the periphery where prejunctional α_2-receptors regulate noradrenaline release, postjunctional receptors on vascular smooth muscle directly regulate tone and endothelial receptors may do so indirectly by stimulating release of endothelium-derived relaxing factor (EDRF: nitric oxide).

Central actions
Activation of central α_2-adrenoceptors in the region of the vasomotor centres decreases sympathetic outflow to the periphery, increases parasympathetic discharge and thus induces bradycardia and hypotension (Dashwood *et al.*,

1985). Clonidine and other centrally acting α_2-agonists are able to bring about such a reduction in blood pressure and heart rate and this is long-lasting and well-correlated with their α_2 potency appropriately corrected for ability to penetrate the blood–brain barrier. The α_2-receptors responsible appear to be postjunctional and not on catecholaminergic neurones since chemical destruction of catecholaminergic neurones using 6-hydroxydopamine or catecholamine depletion using reserpine do not abolish the hypotensive response to α_2-agonists.

Peripheral actions
Prejunctional peripheral α_2-receptors provide a local feedback loop modulating noradrenaline release and thus may be expected to reduce the effect on vascular tone of increasing sympathetic outflow. It is now clear that postjunctional α_2-adrenoceptors exist on vascular smooth muscle, and are vasoconstrictors. These α_2-receptors are remote from the neuroeffector junctions whereas postjunctional α_1-receptors are in close proximity to the innervation sites. These receptors have an important role in the regulation of venous capacitance (Bentley & Widdop, 1987) and do appear to be responsive to sympathetic tone. It has been suggested that postjunctional arteriolar α_2-receptors may respond to circulating catecholamines during stress and pathological conditions where high catecholamines are encountered and thus increase peripheral resistance. In dog and pig, it has been shown that endothelial α_2-adrenoceptors can induce release of EDRF, an effect which antagonizes the vasoconstrictor actions The characteristic blood pressure response to intravenous administration of an α_2-adrenoceptor agonist is an immediate pressor response due to the peripheral actions. This is followed by centrally induced hypotension and bradycardia.

Xylazine and medetomidine are α_2-agonists used in feline practice. The analgesic and cardiovascular effects have been discussed above. The α_2-agonists can markedly reduce the requirements for inhalational anaesthetics. The sedative effect of α_2-adrenoceptor agonists is potentiated by benzodiazepines. α_2-Agonists are emetics: the exact mode of this action has not been described. Yohimbine is an antagonist at

α_2-receptors and yohimbine sensitivity has, in some cases, been used as a definition of the involvement of α_2 sites in physiological mechanisms of drug actions. As such, yohimbine can be used to reverse the actions of α_2-agonists in clinical practice. Recently, however, the more selective antagonist, atipamezole, has been developed and marketed specifically for this purpose.

Opioids as Neurotransmitters or Neuromodulators

Amongst the neurotransmitter/neuromodulator compounds responsible for slow regulatory signalling in the CNS are three classes of opioid peptide, the enkephalins, endorphins and dynorphins. These three families are derived from polyfunctional precursor proteins which are coded for by separate, but none the less evolutionarily related genes, and which can be differentially cleaved to yield a number of bioactive peptides including pituitary and neurohormones. Three precursor proteins exist: (1) proopiomelancortin (POMC), which gives rise to β-endorphin as well as ACTH, α- and γ-MSH and β-lipotropin; (2) proenkephalin (proenkephalin A: PE) which gives rise to the enkephalin pentapeptides met^5-enkephalin and leu^5-enkephalin; and (3) prodynorphin (pro-enkephalin B: PD) which gives rise to four main active peptides, dynorphins A & B and neodynorphins α & β, all of which are variants of leu^5-enkephalin with C-terminal extensions (see Akil *et al.*, 1984 or Cooper *et al.*, 1992 for more detailed overviews).

There is differential expression and, in some cases, alternate proteolytic cleavage patterns of these precursors to yield distinct spectra of active peptide products in various tissues as shown by the following examples. POMC is expressed in the anterior and intermediate lobes of the pituitary and in the hypothalamic arcuate nucleus. In the anterior pituitary it is mainly cleaved to ACTH, whilst in the other two sites it is processed to yield β-endorphin and α-MSH. The β-endorphin-containing neurons form long

projection pathways with predominantly neuroendocrine functions. POMC-derived peptides are also found in the pancreatic islets. PE is expressed in a widely distributed array of neurons which fall into a number of categories including dorsal horn interneurones (particularly in lamina I and the substantia gelatinosa, lamina II), in cells of the trigeminal nucleus and the periaqueductal grey matter. Most of these are short-axon or interneurones but enkephalins are also found in long descending pathways from the brain stem to the cord, running in the dorsolateral funiculus (Jaffe & Martin, 1992). In addition to these areas associated with nociception and control of traffic in pain pathways, PE is found in brain areas associated with behavioural responsiveness, and neuroendocrine and autonomic regulation. It is also expressed in the enteric plexuses and in the adrenal medulla. PD is expressed in other spinal interneurones and in intrahippocampal neurones projecting from the dentate gyrus to synapse on CA_3 pyramidal cells. From the perspective of this chapter, the most important opioid peptidergic neurones are those involved in regulation of pain transmission and perception.

Spinal interneurones release, amongst other mediators, GABA, glycine, enkephalin and dynorphin which inhibit transmitter release from C-fibre terminals and firing of postsynaptic projection neurones. For example, morphine inhibits Substance P release from cat spinal cord. Both projection and interneurones in the dorsal horn are influenced by Aδ and C-fibre inputs and by descending serotoninergic and noradrenergic pathways which originate in the pons and midbrain. Other descending pathways release enkephalins, thyrotropin-releasing hormone, SP and GABA. C-fibre terminals are subject to modulation of transmitter release by the descending pathways and via the interneurones. These descending pathways are themselves subject to control involving excitatory actions of opioid peptides.

Opioid Receptors

Three main classes of opioid receptor have been characterized, μ, δ and κ, and in some cases subtypes are now beginning to be recognized (Lord *et al.*, 1977; Loew *et al.*, 1986; Iyengar *et al.*, 1986; Jaffe & Martin, 1992; Traynor & Elliott, 1993). Morphine is active at all three types of site and naloxone and naltrexone have antagonist activity. The classes are distinguished on the basis of the potency order for endogenous ligands, the specificity of selective agonists and by selective antagonists. At μ-receptors the potency order for endogenous ligands is β-endorphin>dynorphin A>met^5-enkephalin>leu^5-enkephalin. Selective agonists at this site are DAMGO, sufentanil and PL017, CTAP is a selective antagonist. For δ-receptors the potency order of endogenous ligands is β-endorphin > met^5 - enkephalin > leu^5-enkephalin >dynorphin A. DPDPE, DSBULET and [DAla^2] deltorphin I and II are selective agonists whilst ICI174864 and naltrindole are selective antagonists. The potency order for endogenous ligands at κ-receptors is dynorphin A >> β-endorphin > met^5-enkephalin~leu^5-enkephalin. Bremazocine, U69593, C1977 and ICI197067 are selective agonists whilst norbinaltorphimine is a selective antagonist. σ-Receptors have also been described but are no longer considered to be opioid-selective binding sites (Johnson & Jones, 1990). Their definition has been a vexed question for a number of years. The σ site was originally named after the ligand SKF10,047, but this was subsequently found to bind to two discrete sites:

1. The PCP (previously designated the σ or PCP/σ site) site. This is now known to be the site borne by the NMDA receptor at which PCP, ketamine and dizocilpine modulate the NMDA receptor ion channel and which has already been described above. The site has a much higher affinity for PCP than for benzomorphans.
2. A site, now known as the σ site, which displays lower affinity for PCP than for the benzomorphans. This site is much less securely delineated since there are no actions which fully correlate with binding affinity to the receptor. A number of opioid agents, for example nalorphine but notably the benzomorphans including pentazocine and cyclazocine, produce marked dysphoria in man

and behavioural effects in animals which are not antagonized by naloxone. These agents have at least two distinct binding sites in the CNS, one of which is the PCP site and the other is the σ site. It is because naloxone is inactive at this site that it is now questionable whether it should be regarded as an opioid receptor and many authors exclude it. Evidence is emerging for subclasses of σ-receptor.

Generally opioids exert inhibitory modulation of synaptic transmission often by a prejunctional action to decrease release of neurotransmitters, but they also have postjunctional effects to cause hyperpolarization of the majority of responsive neurones. Excitatory responses are also documented but it is not clear to what extent these may represent disinhibition rather than a direct depolarizing action. The μ-, δ- and κ-receptors all appear to act via G-protein-linked mechanisms. In the case of μ- and δ-receptors there is inhibition of adenylate cyclase activity and a decrease in basal cAMP levels as well as in monoamine- and eicosanoid-induced cAMP formation. There is also activation of an inward rectifier potassium channel which is responsible for the hyperpolarization. The κ-receptors appear to differ in their mechanism, being G-protein coupled to inhibition of N type Ca^{2+} channels. These known mechanisms would lead to the prediction that the receptors should belong to the seven-transmembrane domain superfamily of receptors.

Progress in purifying and cloning opioid receptors has been slower than that for other mediators because of a number of technical difficulties and little is yet known about their molecular propertes (Loh & Smith, 1990). A number of proteins have been identified with which opioids interact, but the majority of these have structural features or biochemical and pharmacological properties which make it improbable that they are genuine opioid receptors. However, one gene, with a 372 amino acid seven-transmembrane domain product, which may be the δ-receptor, has been cloned from the mouse. Further cloning and expression of putative receptors together with the development of better selective ligands and antibodies will be critical for a better understanding of the diversity, distribution and function of opioid receptors.

Presently, control of pain pathways, and consequently the analgesic actions of morphine and the opioids, is thought to be mediated primarily by μ- and κ-receptors. Supraspinal μ-receptors are thought to be relatively more important but there is certainly a contribution at spinal level. The important κ-receptors are principally located within the spinal cord. It seems likely that δ-receptors are also involved but there is dispute as to the relative importance of spinal and supraspinal sites. There is some difficulty in any case in discriminating μ and δ contributions and this may be partly attributable to synergism between μ and δ actions (Traynor & Elliott, 1993). The μ-receptors are also responsible for some of the adverse effects of morphine including respiratory depression.

In cats, morphine causes pupillary dilatation and excitation, effects which have generally been attributed to σ actions and which in any case represent overdosage. As will be seen from the discussion of σ sites above, this is presently difficult to interpret. Morphine and other opiates also induce vomiting by an action on the chemoreceptor trigger zone to activate the vomiting centre, most probably due to an action on μ-receptors. This is discrete from the emetic effect of apomorphine which is due to its action as a D_2 agonist. In the myenteric plexus of the gut μ-, κ- and δ-receptors are present. The effects of opiates on gut activity are complex and partly due to central as well as peripheral actions. Overall there is inhibition within the myenteric plexus with a consequent reduction in motility and a marked increase in smooth muscle tone leading to constipation.

Dopamine as a Central Neurotransmitter

The CNS functions of dopamine are better understood than those of the other catecholamines. Three major neurone systems have around three quarters of the total brain content of dopamine. These are:

1. The A9 neurones in the substantia nigra and their projection to the corpus striatum.
2. The A8 and A10 neurones in the ventral tegmentum which project to the nucleus accumbens and the limbic system.
3. The tuberoinfundibular neurone system arising from the arcuate nucleus of the hypothalamus and projecting to the median emminence and the anterior pituitary.

Other dopaminergic neurone systems are found in the chemoreceptor trigger zone, the retina and the olfactory cortex.

Dopamine Receptors

Dopamine receptors are probably of prime importance in the action of neuroleptic drugs including the phenothiazines (e.g. acepromazine, trifluphenazine, thioridazine), thioxanthines (e.g. flupenthixol), butyrophenones (e.g. haloperidol, fluanisone), benzamides (e.g. sulpiride), diphenylbutylpiperazines (e.g. pimozide) and dibenzodiazepines (e.g. clozapine).

Until recently two main types of dopamine receptor have been distinguished, namely D_1 and D_2 receptors. Recent cloning and expression studies have given rise to three more gene products which were initially numbered, in order of discovery D_3 to D_5 (Sibley, 1991; Civelli *et al.*, 1993) but there is considerable confusion over nomenclature. Subsequently it has become apparent that D_3 and D_4 are similar in properties to the original D_2 receptor and thus, D_2, D_3 and D_4 have subsequently been classified as D_{2A}, D_{2B} and D_{2C} respectively and this terminology will be used in this section in those cases where discrimination is possible. Similarly, D_5 has proved to be D_1-like and thus D_1 and D_5 have been alternatively designated D_{1A} and D_{1B} and these designations will be used here in those cases where the distinction is possible since they emphasize the relatedness of the two proteins.

All of the cloned products are consistent with these receptors being members of the seven-transmembrane domain receptor superfamily, with 387–477 amino acid residues, and this is compatible with the findings from electro-physiological and neurochemical studies of endogenous dopamine receptors. D_{1A} receptors are G-protein coupled to activation of adenylyl cyclase and thus increase the synthesis of cyclic AMP. Selective agonists are fenoldopam and SKF38393, while SCH23390, SKF83566 and SCH39166 are selective antagonists, D_{1B} has been reported to have a similar pharmacological profile but some reports suggest that differences may emerge. D_{2A} receptors are also G-protein coupled but to inhibition of adenylyl cyclase, to activation of potassium channels, inactivation of calcium channels and possibly inhibition of phosphatidyl inositol turnover. Selective agonists are bromocriptine and N-0437 and domperidone, (-)sulpiride and YM091512 are selective antagonists. Long and short isoforms of the human, rat, mouse and bovine D_{2A} receptors, due to differential splicing, have been reported and may show some functional and pharmacological differences. Both isoforms appear to be naturally expressed. D_{2B} has AJ76 and UH232 as selective antagonist, no other functional correlates are yet established. It may, however, be significant that these antagonists are selective for presynaptic autoreceptors. D_{2C} has clozapine as a weak selective agonist and also couples to inhibition of adenylyl cyclase. In common with many other seven-transmembrane domain receptors, the C-terminal segment of D_{2A} has a conserved cysteine residue which probably serves as a site for post-translational palmitoylation and thereby anchors this residue to the cell membrane. D_{2A} also has a large third cytoplasmic loop which is a frequent feature of receptors which inhibit adenylyl cyclase.

All D_2 clones have possible glycosylation sites, consistent with biochemical evidence for D_2 receptors being glycoproteins. The regional distribution of D_{2A} mRNA and protein reveals high concentrations in most regions where dopaminergic cell bodies and terminals are found and is compatible with both presynaptic autoreceptor and postjunctional roles for these receptors. D_{2B} expression appears to be much more restricted in distribution being mainly in the limbic sytem and possibly consistent with a predominantly presynaptic autoreceptor role. Present evidence suggests that D_{2C} is expressed predominantly in the cortex, amygdala, midbrain and medulla, a finding which is consistent with the lack of motor effects characteristic of clozapine.

The molecular biology of the D_1 receptors is less secure than that of the D_2 receptors because of some ambiguities about the initiation point for translation. However D_{1A} has a short third cytoplasmic loop and long C-terminus which are features characteristic of receptors which activate adenylyl cyclase. There are two possible glycosylation sites, compatible with evidence for the natural receptor being a glycoprotein, and a potential palmitoylation site. Studies of mRNA and protein levels indicate a high degree of physiological gene expression in the caudate-putamen, the olfactory tubercle and the nucleus accumbens. Lower levels are observed in the cerebral cortex, hypothalamus and thalamus and in the limbic system. Cloned D_{1B} receptor shows considerable homology with D_{1A} and has similar pharmacological properties except that dopamine is about an order of magnitude more potent at the former. Studies of expression indicate high levels in the hippocampus, hypothalamus, mammillary bodies and the pretectal area, although there is disparity between rat and human data which may be due to technical considerations.

Although the currently used neuroleptic agents interact with a wide range of monoamine receptors and uptake systems, all are blockers of D_2 dopamine receptors and neuroleptic potency parallels activity at and affinity for D_2 sites as measured both *in vitro* by displacement of D_2-selective radioligands such as spiroperidol and *in vivo*. Unfortunately, detailed information is not yet available about the functional correlates of the D_2 receptor subtypes. The neuroleptics all acutely increase the turnover of dopamine in the corpus striatum and limbic system and increase spike activity in presynaptic dopaminergic neurons, features consistent with blocking of negative feedback by effective presynaptic D_2 blockade. However in view of complex interactions which are known to occur between D_1 and D_2 receptors and regional variations in these, much more detailed information about receptor expression at the cellular level and also receptor mechanisms and their interrelationships is needed for secure interpretation of these findings. The motor effects of these drugs are believed to relate to the striatal dopaminergic projections whereas behavioural effects are associated with limbic system actions. However, all these agents also block a wide variety of other monoamine receptors albeit with lesser potency than for D_2 antagonism.

Many of the neuroleptic agents, for example chlorpromazine, also have antiemetic activity because of both the presence of D_2 receptors in the chemoreceptor trigger zone of the area postrema of the medulla and also, in some cases, due to actions to relax the pyloric sphincter and to co-ordinate peristalsis which are thought to be related to dopaminergic control of acetylcholine release in the enteric nerve plexuses. The antihistaminergic activity shown by many of these agents may also contribute to their antiemetic actions. Some atypical newer agents such as the dibenzodiazepines, for example clozapine, act mainly on dopaminergic sites but show some selectivity for D_1 over D_2 receptors.

Conclusion

Despite the eclectic nature of this account it will be apparent that the considerable recent advances in understanding of the CNS have begun to shed meaningful light on the mechanism of action of centrally acting drugs. It is to be expected that the further development of molecular and cellular neurobiology will reveal further sites and mechanisms of action which will rapidly make the propositions of this chapter appear naive and dated. None the less, the general principles underlying the identification, delineation and differentiation of sites and mechanisms of action should be applicable to any specific ligand–receptor interaction and thus to any future proposed mechanism which displays molecular structural selectivity.

References

Akil, H., Watson, S.J., Young, E,. Lewis, M.E., Khachaturian, H & Walker, J.M. (1984) Endogenous opioids: biology and function. *Annu. Rev. Neurosci.* **7**, 223–255.

Bentley, G.A. & Widdop, R.E. (1987) Postjunctional α_2-receptors mediate venoconstriction in the hindquarters of anaesthetised cats. *Brit. J. Pharmacol.* **92**, 121–128.

Bowery, N.G. (1993) GABA$_B$ receptor pharmacology. *Annu. Rev. Pharmacol. Toxicol.* **33**, 109–148.

Bowery, N.G., Hill, D., Hudson, A.L., Doble, A. & Middlemiss, D.N. (1980) Baclofen reduces transmitter release in the mammalian CNS by an action at a novel GABA receptor. *Nature* **283**, 92–94.

Bowery, N.G., Doble, A., Hill, D., Hudson, A.L. & Shaw, J.S. (1981) Bicuculline-insensitive GABA receptors on peripheral autonomic nerve terminals. *Eur. J. Pharmacol.* **71**, 53–70.

Brisson, A. & Unwin, P.N.T. (1985) Quaternary structure of the acetylcholine receptor. *Nature* **315**, 474–477.

Bylund, D.B. (1988) Subtypes of α_2-adrenoceptors: pharmacological and molecular biological evidence converge. *Trends Pharmacol. Sci.* **9**, 356–361.

Caldwell, J. (1982) Conjugation reactions in foreign compound metabolism: definition, consequences and species variations. *Drug Metab. Rev.* **13**, 745–778.

Civelli, O., Bunzow, J.R. & Grandy, D.K. (1993) Molecular diversity of the dopamine receptors. *Annu. Rev. Pharmacol., Toxicol.* **33**, 281–308.

Cooper, J.R., Bloom F.E. & Roth R.H. (1991) *The Biochemical Basis of Neuropharmacology*, 6th edn. Oxford University Press, New York.

Courtney, K.R. (1975) Mechanism of frequency dependent inhibition of sodium currents in frog myelinated nerve by the lidocaine derivative GEA968. *J. Pharmacol. Exp. Therap.* **195**, 225–236.

Curtis, D.R. & Watkins, J.C. (1960). The excitation and depression of spinal neurons by structurally-related amino acids. *J. Neurochem* **6**, 117–141.

Curtis, D.R. & Watkins, J.C. (1963). Acidic amino acids with strong excitatory actions on mammalian neurons. *J. Physiol.* **166**, 1–14.

Daniels, S. & Smith, E.B. (1993) Effects of general anaesthetics on ligand-gated ion channels. *Brit. J. Anaesth.* **71**, 59–64.

Dashwood, M.R., Gilbey, M.P. & Spyer, K.M. (1985) The localization of adrenoceptors and opiate receptors in regions of the cat nervous system involved in cardiovascular control. *Neuroscience* **15**, 537–551.

Davies, J. & Watkins, J.C. (1981) Differentiation of kainate and quisqualate receptors in cat spinal cord by selective antagonism with with D- (and L-) glutamylglycine. *Brain Res.* **206**, 172–177.

Davies, J. & Watkins, J.C. (1982) Actions of D- and L- forms of 2-amino-5-phosphonovalerate and 2-amino-4-phosphonobutyric acid in the cat spinal cord. *Brain Res.* **235**, 378–386.

Dean, P.M. (1987) *Molecular Foundations of Drug Receptor Interaction*. Cambridge University Press, Cambridge.

de Saro, G.B., Ascioti, C, Froio, F., Libri, V. & Nistico, G. (1987) Evidence that the locus coeruleus is the site where clonidine and drugs acting at alpha$_1$ and alpha$_2$ receptors affect sleep and arousal mechanisms. *Brit. J. Pharmacol.* **90**, 675–685.

Doble, A. & Martin, I.L. (1992) Multiple benzodiazepine receptors: no reason for anxiety. *Trends Pharmacol. Sci.* **13**, 76–81.

Flatman, J.A., Schwindt, P.C., Crill, W.E. & Strafstrom, C.E. (1983) Multiple actions of N-methyl-D-aspartate on cat neocortical neurons *in vitro*. *Brain Res.* **266**, 169–173.

Franks, N.P. & Lieb, W.R. (1993) Selective actions of volatile general anaesthetics at molecular and cellular levels. *Brit. J. Anaesth.* **71**, 65–76.

Frenkel, C., Duch, D.S. & Urban, B.W. (1993). Effects of i.v. anaesthetics on human brain sodium channels. *Brit. J. Anaesth.* **71**, 15–24.

Gardner, C.R. (1988) Functional *in vivo* correlates of the benzodiazepine agonist–inverse agonist continuum. *Prog. Neurobiol.* **31**, 425–476.

Galzi, J-L, Revah, F., Bessis, A. & Changeux, J-P. (1991) Functional architecture of the nicotinic acetylcholine receptor: from the electric organ to the brain. *Annu. Rev. Pharmacol. Toxicol.* **31**, 37–72.

Gibson, G.G & Skett, P (1986) *Introduction to Drug Metabolism*. Chapman & Hall, London.

Goodchild, C.S. (1993) GABA receptors and benzodiazepines. *Brit. J. Anaesth.* **71**, 127–133.

Griffiths, R. & Norman, R.I. (1993) Effects of anaesthetics on uptake, synthesis and release of transmitters. *Brit. J. Anaesth.* **71**, 96–107.

Harrison, J.K., Pearson, W.R. & Lynch, K.R. (1991) Molecular characterization of α_1- and α_2-adrenoceptors. *Trends Pharmacol. Sci.* **12**, 62–67.

Hayashi, Y. & Maze, M. (1993) Alpha$_2$ adrenoceptor agonists and anaesthesia. *Brit. J. Anaesth.* **71**, 108–118.

Hill, D.R. (1985) GABA$_B$ receptor modulation of adenylate cyclase activity in rat brain slices. *Brit. J. Pharmacol.* **84**, 249–257.

Hill, D.R. & Bowery, N.G. (1981) ^{3}H-baclofen and ^{3}H-GABA bind to bicuculline-insensitive GABA$_B$ sites in the brain. *Nature* **290**, 149–152.

Hill, R.G., Simmonds, M.A. & Straughan, D.W. (1972) Antagonism of GABA by picrotoxin in feline cerebral cortex. *Br. J. Pharmacol.* **44**, 807–809.

Hille, B. (1992) *Ionic Channels of Excitable Membranes*, 2nd edn. Sinauer, Sunderland, Mass.

Hladky, S.B. (1990) Pharmacokinetics. Manchester University Press, Manchester, UK.

Hodgkin, A.L. & Huxley, A.F. (1952) Currents carried by sodium and potassium ions through the membrane of the giant axon of Loligo. *J. Physiol.* **116**, 449–472.

Iyengar, S., Kim, H.S., & Wood, P.L. (1986) Effects of kappa opiate antagonists on neurochemical and neuroendocrine indices: evidence for kappa receptor subtypes. *J. Pharmacol. Exp. Therap.* **238**, 429–436.

Jaffe, J.H. & Martin, W.R. (1992) Opioid analgesics and antagonists. In: *The Pharmacological Basis of Therapeutics*, 8th edn. (ed. A.G. Gilman, T.W. Rall, A.S. Nies & P. Taylor), pp. 485–521. McGraw Hill, New York.

Johnson, M. K. & Jones, S.M. (1990) Neuropharmacology of phencyclidine: basic mechanisms and therapeutic potential. *Annu. Rev. Pharmacol. Toxicol.* **30**, 707–750.

Kaziro, Y., Itoh, H., Kozasa, T., Nakafuku, M. & Satoh, T. (1991) Structure and function of signal-transducing GTP-binding proteins. *Annu. Rev. Biochem.* **60**, 349–400.

Kemp, J.A. & Leeson, P.D. (1993) The glycine site of the NMDA receptor – five years on. *Trends Pharmacol. Sci.* **14**, 20–25.

Kemp, J.A. & Sillito, A.M. (1982) The nature of the excitatory transmitter mediating X and Y cell inputs to the cat dorsal lateral geniculate nucleus. *J. Physiol.* **323**, 377–391.

Koob, G.F. & Bloom, F.E. (1988) Cellular and molecular mechanisms of drug dependence. *Science* **242**, 715–723.

Kress, H.G. & Tass, P.W.L. (1993) Effects of volatile anaesthetics on second messenger Ca^{2+} in neurones and non-muscular cells. *Brit. J. Anaesth.* **71**, 47–58.

Lambert, D.G. (1993) Signal transduction: G proteins and second messengers. *Brit. J. Anaesth.* **71**, 86–89.

Langosch, D., Thomas,L. & Betz, H. (1988) Conserved quaternary structure of ligand-gated ion channels: the postsynaptic glycine receptor is a pentamer. *Proc. Natl. Acad. Sci. USA* **85**, 7394–7398.

Lefkowitz, R.J. & Caron, M.G. (1988) Adrenergic receptors: models for the study of receptors coupled to guanine nucleotide regulatory proteins. *J. Biol. Chem.* **263**, 4993–4996.

Lodge, D. (1988) (ed.) *Excitatory Amino Acids in Health and Disease.* Wiley, Chichester.

Loew, G., Keys, C., Luke, B., Polgar, W. & Toll, L. (1986) Structure–activity relationships of morphiceptin analogs: receptor binding and molecular determinants of mu-affinity and selectivity. *Mol. Pharmacol.* **29**, 546–553.

Loh, H.H. & Smith, A.P. (1990) Molecular characterisation of opioid receptors. *Annu. Rev. Pharmacol. Toxicol.* **30**, 123–147.

Lord, J.A.H., Waterfield, A.A., Hughes, J. & Kosterlitz, H.W. (1977) Endogenous opioid peptides: multiple agonists and receptors. *Nature* (Lond.) **267**, 495–499.

Martin, I.L. (1992) Isolation and molecular studies of drug receptors. *Proc. Assoc. Vet. Pharmacol. Therap.* **14**, 79–89.

McLennan, H. (1988) The pharmacological characterization of excitatory amino acid receptors. In: *Excitatory Amino Acids in Health and Disease.* (ed. D. Lodge), pp. 1–11. Wiley, Chichester.

Monaghan, D.T., Bridges, R.J. & Cotman, C.W. (1989) The excitatory amino acid receptors: Their classes, pharmacology and distinct properties in the function of the central nervous system. *Annu. Rev. Pharmacol. Toxicol.* **29**, 365–402.

Murata, K., Nakagawa, I., Kumenta, Y., Kitahata, L. & Collins, J.G. (1989) Intrathecal clonidine suppresses noxiously evoked activity of spinal wide dynamic range neurons in cats. *Anesth. Analg.* **69**, 185–191.

Nebert, D.W. & Gonzalez, F. (1987) The cytochrome P450 gene superfamily. *Annu. Rev. Biochem.* **56**, 945–993.

Olney, J.W. (1990) Excitotoxic amino acids and neuropsychiatric disorders. *Annu. Rev. Pharmacol. Toxicol.* **30**, 47–71.

Pocock, G. & Richards, C.D. (1993) Excitatory and inhibitory mechanisms in anaesthesia. *Brit. J. Anaesth.* **71**, 134–145.

Pratt, W.B. & Taylor, P. (1990) *Principles of Drug Action: the Basis of Pharmacology,* 3rd edn. Churchill-Livingstone, Edinburgh.

Rall, T.W. (1992) Hypnotics and sedatives; ethanol. In: *The Pharmacological Basis of Therapeutics,* 8th edn (ed. A.G. Gilman, T.W. Rall, A.S. Nies & P. Taylor), pp. 345–382. McGraw Hill, New York.

Rauschecker, J.P. & Hahn, S. (1987) Ketamine-xylazine anaesthesia blocks consolidation of ocular dominance changes in kitten visual cortex. *Nature* **326**, 183–185.

Ritchie, J.M & Greene, N.M. (1992) Local anaesthetics.

In: *The Pharmacological Basis of Therapeutics,* 8th edn. (ed. A.G. Gilman, T.W. Rall, A.S. Nies & P. Taylor), pp. 311–331. McGraw Hill, New York.

Robertson, B. & Taylor, W.R. (1986) Effects of γ-aminobutyric acid and (-) baclofen on calcium and potassium currents in cat dorsal root ganglion neurones *in vitro. Br. J. Pharmacol.* **89**, 661–672.

Ruffolo, R.R. Jr, Nichols, A.J., Stadel, J.M. & Hieble, J.P. (1993) Pharmacological and therapeutic application of α_2-receptor subtypes. *Annu. Rev. Pharmacol. Toxicol.* **33**, 243–280.

Schoepp, D.D. & Conn, P.J. (1993) Metabotropic glutamate receptors in brain function and pathology. *Trends Pharmacol. Sci.* **14**, 13–20.

Schwinn, D.A. (1993) Adrenoceptors as models for G protein-coupled receptors: structure, function and regulation. *Brit. J. Anaesth.* **71**, 77–85.

Sibley, D.R. (1991) Cloning of a 'D₃' receptor subtype expands dopamine receptor family. *Trends Pharmacol. Sci.* **12**, 7–9.

Sieghart, W. (1992) $GABA_A$ receptors: ligand-gated Cl^- ion channels modulated by multiple drug binding sites. *Trends Pharmacol. Sci.* **13**, 446–450.

Smith, R.L. (1978) Extrapolation of animal results to man. In: *Drug Metabolism in Man* (eds J.W. Gorrod & A.W. Beckett), pp. 97–118 Taylor & Francis, London.

Soltesz, I., Halby, M., Leresche, N. & Crunelli, V. (1988) The GABAb antagonist phaclofen inhibits the late K^+-dependent IPSP in cat and rat thalamic and hippocampal neurons. *Brain Res.* **448**, 351–354.

Stevenson, F.A. (1988) Understanding the $GABA_A$ receptor: a chemically gated ion channel. *Biochem. J.,* 249, 21-32.

Stroud, R.M. & Finer-Moore, J. (1985) Acetylcholine receptor structure, function and evolution. *Annu. Rev. Cell. Biol.* **1**, 317–351.

Taylor, C.W. (1990) The role of G-proteins in transmembrane signalling. *Biochem. J.* **272**, 1–13.

Terrar, D.A. (1993) Structure and function of calcium channels and the action of anaesthetics. *Brit. J. Anaesth.* **71**, 39–46.

Traynor, J.R. & Elliott, J. (1993) δ-Opioid receptor subtypes and cross-talk with μ-receptors. *Trends Pharmacol. Sci.* **14**, 84–85.

Twyman, R.E., Rogers, C.E. & Macdonald, R.L. (1989) Differential regulation of γ-aminobutyric acid receptor channels by diazepam and phenobarbital. *Ann. Neurol.* **25**, 213–220.

Urban, B.W. (1993) Differential effects of gaseous and volatile anaesthetics on sodium and potassium channels. *Brit. J. Anaesth.* **71**, 25–38.

Walker, C.H. (1978) Species differences in microsomal

mono-oxygenase activity and their relationship to biological half-lives. *Drug Metab. Rev.* **7**, 295–323.

Walker, C.H. (1980) Species differences in some hepatic microsomal enzymes that metabolise xenobiotics. *Prog. Drug Metab.* **5**, 118–164.

Walker, C.H. (1992) Comparative drug metabolism in domestic animals. *Proc. Assoc. Vet. Pharmacol. Therap.* **14**, 144–152.

Wann, K.T. (1993) Neuronal sodium and potassium channels: structure and function. *Brit. J. Anaesth.* **71**, 2–14.

Watkins, J.C. & Olverman, H.J. (1988) Structural requirements for activation and blockade of EAA receptors. In: *Excitatory Amino Acids in Health and Disease* (ed. D. Lodge), pp. 13–45. J. Wiley, Chichester.

Watson, S.P. & Girdlestone, D. (1993) *Trends in Pharmacological Sciences Receptor Nomenclature Supplement 1993*. Elsevier Trends Journals, Cambridge.

Wilcox, G.L., Carlsson, K.H., Jochim, A. & Jurna, I. (1987) Mutual potentiation of antinociceptive effects of morphine and clonidine on motor and sensory responses in rat spinal cord. *Brain Res.* **405**, 84–93.

Wong, E.H.F. & Kemp, J.A. (1991) Sites for antagonism on the *N*-methyl-D-aspartate receptor channel complex. *Annu. Rev. Pharmacol. Toxicol.* **31**, 401–425.

4
Pathology

A.R. Jefferies

Introduction

The purpose of a chapter on pathology in a text on feline anaesthesia is three-fold. First, to increase the anaesthetist's awareness of the significant pathology underlying the clinical signs which may be detected in the pre-anaesthetic examination of the cat. Secondly, to remind the anaesthetist of the common pathological conditions of the cat which may be relevant to anaesthesia. Thirdly, to provide some guidance on the pathology likely to be encountered in the event of an anaesthetic or post-anaesthetic death being investigated by an anaesthetist rather than a pathologist. Only those anaesthetists in veterinary school practice are likely to have ready access to expert necropsy examination. Nevertheless, all anaesthetic deaths should be followed by post-mortem examination and on occasions the anaesthetist may gain some comfort from this examination. If this chapter both helps and encourages these aims then it will have achieved its purpose.

It is probably true to say that all pathological lesions and most disease processes occur in all species at one time or another. In comparative pathology it is the differences in incidence or presentation of disease that are of most interest and importance. This chapter is, therefore, most concerned with those conditions particularly prevalent in the cat or those which are of particular significance in that species and especially those of interest to the anaesthetist. Consideration of feline pathology in this text is thus restricted to the cardiovascular system, the respiratory system, the urinary system, the endocrine system, the haemopoietic system and the liver.

Of most immediate concern in the provision of safe and stable anaesthesia are disorders of the cardiovascular and respiratory systems. A predictable, complete and rapid recovery may be influenced by hepatic, renal and endocrine function. More generalized disorders such as those of the haemopoietic system are also of fundamental importance by influencing the oxygen carrying capacity of the blood. This chapter therefore considers the pathology of these body systems, drawing attention to those conditions of particular importance in the cat. Of particular concern to the anaesthetist is the unexpected death during or following anaesthesia. A consideration of the necropsy examination in these cases would seem useful here.

In the pathological investigation of any disease process, and anaesthetic accidents in particular, it is of as much importance to recognize those incidental pathological findings which are of little clinical significance, as to recognize those lesions producing disease and possibly contributing to the animal's death.

It is important to say at this stage that in those anaesthetic deaths due to idiosyncratic reactions and excessive or inappropriate use of anaesthetic agents there may be few if any gross pathological changes visible at necropsy. At the histological level the changes seen are often only those associated with cardiopulmonary failure and tissue hypoxia. These agonal changes are common to the process of death from any cause.

The importance of the necropsy following death associated with anaesthesia is to establish the presence or absence of any conditions likely to have contributed to death. To assess whether any variation in the anaesthetic technique could have improved the chances of survival, and to monitor the occurrence of conditions overlooked at the time of the pre-anaesthetic examination. Last but not least, the results of the examination may be of considerable comfort to the animal's owner in coming to terms with the loss of a valued pet if it can be shown that some undetected underlying condition contributed to that death or that the animal was in fact suffering from some incurable illness. It should also be borne in mind that litigation may sometimes follow occurrences of this type and it is essential that the necropsy is conducted in a competent manner and accurate records kept even if a definitive diagnosis cannot be reached.

Post-mortem Examination

The post-mortem examination should be thorough but need not take an inordinate length of time. Descriptions of standard techniques are available (Kelly *et al.*, 1982) and attention is therefore drawn only to points particularly relevant to the necropsy following anaesthetic death.

It is, of course, important that the person undertaking the autopsy is familiar with the appearance of agonal changes; that is, those changes that occur in the short time immediately preceding death, at the time of irreversible circulatory failure. The commonest change is vascular congestion and this is seen especially in the lungs which may be darker and heavier than normal, particularly the dependant lung. Limited pulmonary oedema is common, probably as a result of agonal impairment of venous return from the lungs to the left atrium.

It should be remembered that barbiturate solutions are mildly irritant, producing hyperaemia and sometimes haemolysis around the site of injection. Barbiturates injected into solid tissues produce a characteristic brown–red discoloration around the injection site. Associated with this there may be deposition of white crystalline material resembling snowflakes. Animals killed by an overdose of intravenous barbiturate may have this type of barbiturate deposit in the right atrium and ventricle. Barbiturate anaesthesia may also produce striking splenomegaly but this is not an invariable finding and its absence does not preclude death from barbiturate overdose.

Initial necropsy examination should pay particular attention to airway obstruction. This may be complete, or more frequently partial, and is particularly associated with tracheostomy tubes where mucus and inflammatory exudate can build up sufficiently to cause significant hypoxia. The obstructing mass can form either on the end of the tube itself or on the damaged endothelium distal to the end of the tube. Pieces of this exudate may break free, be inhaled and impact further down the bronchial tree leading to collapse of lung lobes. External pressure from tumours or enlarged lymph nodes may lead to partial airway obstruction and hypoxia which may be of critical importance under anaesthesia.

The presence of gastric contents within the trachea is a common post-mortem finding due to manipulations of the body after death. If gastrointestinal contents are present in the trachea before death respiratory efforts will pull the foreign material deeper into the lung, particularly under anaesthesia and this will rapidly lead to an acute inflammatory reaction and pulmonary oedema. Occasionally this will lead to reflex cardiac arrest. The appearance of pulmonary oedema is described in the section on lung disease. The presence of inhaled foreign material can completely obstruct the airway

In addition to the examination for airway obstruction the presence or absence of pneumothorax should be ascertained. This can be carried out by radiographic examination of the chest. Alternatively the thorax can be opened under water when bubbles of gas can be detected in the thoracic cavity. This has the added advantage that small punctures or lacerations of the lung can be detected by the presence of gas bubbles appearing on the visceral pleura over the puncture site. If this procedure is not feasible then the trachea can be tightly tied so as to make it airtight and the chest cavity opened. The lungs should then appear in the state of inflation they were in before death and any discrepancies between the degree of lung inflation and thoracic expansion can be noted.

A careful examination should be made of the heart and great vessels *in situ*, beginning with an incision into the pulmonary artery. The purpose of this examination is the detection of pulmonary thrombosis or embolism. The pulmonary trunk may need to be opened to its bifurcation. A careful examination of the jugular veins at the site of any cannulation should also be made for the presence of thrombi. The heart can be examined in detail following removal of the thoracic viscera from the chest. It should be opened completely and in a logical manner, preferably following the direction of blood flow. The chambers should be examined carefully for the presence of thrombi. Ante-mortem thrombi must be differentiated from post-mortem clot. The former are rougher, drier, irregular and may have a layered appearance on close examination. Post-mortem clots are smooth, shiny and form a cast of the chamber or vessel in which they form. They may also be divided into a red and white portion due to cellular sedimentation. The significance of cardiac thrombi is not so much that they may be a cause of death but that they may indicate failing cardiac function or the development of cardiac arrythmias, such as atrial fibrillation, that may in themselves have been fatal.

The cardiac muscle should be inspected for evidence of infarction, haemorrhage or fibrosis and transverse incisions of the ventricles used to assess evidence of ventricular hypertrophy. This is of necessity a subjective examination and precise weighing and measuring of cardiac parameters and comparison with normal matched controls is necessary for accurate evidence of cardiac hypertrophy. A method such as that described for the dog could be used (Turk & Root, 1983)

Gross examination of abdominal viscera may indicate severe underlying organic disease but histological examination is usually necessary to detect diffuse degenerative changes in liver or kidney likely to be significant in altering the course of an anaesthetic.

Examination of the brain both grossly and histologically is desirable, but unless this is done with care artefactual changes are likely to render the examination valueless. The brain should be removed and fixed whole. The external surface is examined for presence of haemorrhage and the fixed brain is sliced and examined for gross abnormalities. In the case of anaesthetic deaths changes are likely to be restricted to anoxic lesions.

All but the most intrepid anaesthetist is likely to rely on a pathologist for histological interpretation and the provision of adequate specimens is paramount if time and the client's money are not to be wasted. The following would be the minimum material submitted for a useful histological examination following an anaesthetic death in the absence of a definitive gross diagnosis:

1. Lung—portions from ventral and dorsal parts of right and left sides.
2. Myocardium—complete transverse slice through the centre of both ventricles and septum. Portions of both atria. (Examination of the conduction system is sometimes rewarding but requires submission of the whole heart, is time consuming and expensive.)
3. Portion of liver.
4. Slice of both kidneys to include cortex and pelvis.
5. Both adrenal glands—whole.
6. Both thyroid glands—whole.
7. Slice of spleen.
8. Whole brain.
9. Samples from other organs only if they appear abnormal or the clinical history indicates their involvement.

It is sometimes possible to understand the reason for an anaesthetic death following the gross necropsy examination. Airway obstruction and gross cardiac anomalies would fall into this category but often there is no gross evidence of disease. Histological examination may reveal lesions in heart, lung, liver, kidney or endocrine glands that would have contributed to death. In a substantial number of cases, despite extensive and expert investigation no morphological lesions can be found.

A re-examination of the circumstances surrounding the case can sometimes be of help but one can still be left with the possibility of anaesthetic drug overdose or idiosyncratic response to anaesthetic agents. Examination of tissue residues for anaesthetic agents or drugs is rarely practical or very rewarding. A significant proportion of deaths remain a mystery despite all efforts.

Incidental Findings

It may be useful at this stage to review a number of incidental post-mortem findings some of which are normal for the cat and some which might be considered pathological. These are generally of no clinical significance but serve as a trap for the inexperienced or unwary.

Alimentary system

In the cat the oesophagus contains in its lower third distinct transverse striations; these are normal structures. In the stomach can often be found small stress ulcers. These consist of multiple small punctate erosions or ulcers, sometimes haemorrhagic which extend no more than a millimetre below the epithelial surface. Small amounts of blood can sometimes be seen on the epithelial surface. These lesions occur in association with a variety of primary illnesses and stressful conditions and have no particular significance. In the small bowel there is normally darkening of the top of the intestinal mucosal folds.

Pancreas

In older cats a nodular hyperplasia of the pancreas is frequently found. The hyperplastic nodules can be up to 1 cm in diameter and compress adjacent normal pancreatic tissue. They are of no clinical significance. The pancreas in older cats may also have a finely granular appearance with a pale, firm cut surface. Histologically there is chronic interstitial inflammation and fibrosis. Rarely does this produce clinical signs.

Punctate chalky white foci may occur in the mesenteric, omental and perirenal fat of clinically normal cats. These lesions histologically are granulomatous inflammatory foci indistinguishable from the lesions of pansteatitis, suggesting that subclinical forms of this condition are not infrequent.

Kidney

The capsule of the kidney is readily detachable from the cortex in the cat, even in a severely scarred kidney. The radial stellate cortical veins are very prominent in this species. The cortex of the cat kidney is usually pale due to the deposition of intracytoplasmic lipid droplets in the epithelial cells of the tubules. The medulla adjacent to the pelvis often has a streaked appearance accentuated by medullary calcification which is common in the cat (Lucke & Hunt,

1967). All of these changes can be seen in cats with normal renal function (Jeraj et al., 1982).

Upper airway

Focal grittiness within the cartilage of the larynx, trachea and bronchi is another common occurrence, due to focal calcification in these organs. Within the lung gritty calcified foci are found in the absence of metastatic calcification elsewhere and are of no clinical consequence. Black carbon pigmentation in the lung and drainage lymph nodes is common in urban cats. The anterior lung lobes may be the site of subpleural emphysema and there is no clinical or pathological evidence to suggest that this limited area of damage has any deleterious effect on lung function.

Circulatory system

Focal intimal arterial lesions sometimes with calcification or ectopic bone formation are common in older animals but are not associated with thrombotic disease.

Endocrine system

Calcification of the adrenal cortex is extremely common in the cat producing gritty white foci easily detected grossly. It is associated with focal cortical necrosis but is without clinical effect.

The thyroid glands in older animals are the site of small non-functional nodules and cysts as well as the more prominent nodular hyperplasia that is considered later.

The following sections consider the pathology of the cat on a systems basis with emphasis on those conditions relevant to anaesthesia. Although no claim is made that these are comprehensive, they include those conditions of most significance.

Cardiovascular System

Congenital Anomalies

These disorders are most often seen in the young animal but clinical signs of cardiac dysfunction in the cat are often manifest only as poor growth and general dullness. Cardiac disease may not be the first diagnosis that comes to mind. Although most types of congenital defect can be seen in the cat (Van Mierop, 1970), some are more commonly encountered than others. The most common abnormalities are patent ductus arteriosus (Cohen *et al.*, 1975), ventricular septal defects, the Tetralogy of Fallot and atrioventricular valve defects (Liu, 1976; Bolton & Linu, 1977).

Patent ductus arteriosus
The ductus arteriosus develops from the sixth left branchial arch and serves in foetal life to divert blood from the pulmonary artery to the aorta. This channel normally closes rapidly after birth due to changes in oxygen tension in the blood. Failure of closure may, depending on the size of the defect, result in sequelae that are of clinical importance particularly at the time of anaesthesia. Initially after birth blood will flow from the aorta to the pulmonary artery due to the pressure differential between these vessels. In response to the increased pulmonary perfusion pressure there is reflex vasoconsriction in the pulmonary bed, leading to increased resistance in the vasculature of the lung. If this pressure exceeds that in the aorta there may eventually be reversal of flow so that blood now flows from pulmonary artery to aorta. This results in the development of hypoxia and cyanosis. These changes in blood flow produce a pressure overload on the right side of the heart and a volume overload on the left. The compensatory response of the heart is to develop ventricular hypertrophy. There may also be dilatation of the left atrium due to increased blood flow. Depending on the size of the patent ductus these changes may be sufficiently severe to produce congestive heart failure.

Another unfortunate sequel to patency of the ductus is turbulence in the blood flow through this abnormal opening. This may result in fibrous intimal scarring in the aorta or pulmonary artery, the so called 'jet' lesions. More seriously this intimal damage may lead to the development of thrombosis either in the ductus, pulmonary artery or aorta.

Septal defects
These most commonly involve the ventricular septum, in either the membranous or muscular portions. Small defects may produce few clinical signs but large defects may result in considerable left to right shunting of blood (because of the pressure differential) and development of right ventricular hypertrophy. Heart failure may occur, particularly if the animal is put under cardiorespiratory stress of some kind. It should be noted that some defects in the membranous septum can be high up underneath the septal valve leaflets and are easily missed. Careful post-mortem examination is indicated in all cases of suspected cardiac anomaly but is particularly important when this defect is suspected.

Tetralogy of Fallot
The four pathological changes seen in this condition represent three congenital abnormalities and one secondary change. They are:

1. Ventricular septal defect.
2. Pulmonic stenosis.
3. Overriding aorta.
4. Secondary hypertrophy of the right ventricle because of the pulmonary outflow stenosis.

The changes represent a malformation in the development of the conotruncal septum. The critical clinical factor is the degree of pulmonic stenosis but the condition almost invariably results in cardiac failure. Animals are often poorly grown, cyanotic and polycythemic due to chronic hypoxia.

A–V valve defects
Malformations of the mitral valve complex are probably the commonest congenital anomaly in the cat. The annulus is enlarged with short thick leaflets, short thickened chordae tendinae, upward malpositioning of atrophic or hypertrophic papillary muscles and enlargement of left atrium and ventricle. There may be accompanying diffuse endocardial fibrosis. Clinically this defect will produce a mixed frequency holosystolic murmur, with maximum intensity on the left caudal sternal border.

Dysplasia of the tricuspid valve is also seen in the cat with greater frequency than in other species (Lin & Tilley, 1976). The appearance of the valve is variable with diffuse or focal thickening of the leaflets. Portions of the leaflets may be absent. There may be shortening and thickening of the chordae tendinae and parts of the valve may be fused to the ventricular wall.

Pericardial Disease

Pericardiodiaphragmatic hernia, a relatively common defect, consists of a communication of varying size between the pericardial sac and the abdominal cavity (Evans & Biery, 1980). Abdominal viscera may pass through the diaphragm to lie within the pericardial sac. In addition to effects on cardiorespiratory function this may result in strangulation of loops of bowel or liver lobes.

Pericardial effusion

Hydropericardium may occur as part of a general anasarca in congestive heart failure or with cachectic illness. It can also occur with local disease such as lymphosarcoma of the myocardium or in association with feline infectious peritonitis. Percarditis or inflammatory pericardial disease is uncommon in the cat but suppurative pericarditis is occasionally seen as part of a general empyaema.

Myocardial Disease

Cardiomyopathy

This term is strictly used to denote a primary disease of the myocardium of unknown cause. It is used in veterinary medicine in a rather looser manner to denote both primary and secondary disorders resulting in damage to or failure of the myocardium (Liu, 1970, 1977; Fox, 1988). In the cat cardiomyopathy is the commonest of the cardiac disorders and the idiopathic cardiomyopathies can be divided into five categories:

1. Endomyocardial.
2. Congestive.
3. Symmetric hypertrophic.
4. Asymmetric hypertrophic.
5. Restrictive.

The endomyocardial form appears predominantly inflammatory in nature but with no evidence of an aetiological agent. There are subendocardial and myocardial inflammatory cell infiltrates predominantly of neutrophils with deposits of fibrin on the endocardium. There may be myocardial cell necrosis. Atrial thrombi are common. Sometimes the condition is more chronic with fibrosis dominant.

The congestive form shows a grossly enlarged heart which is thin walled due to dilation of atria and ventricles. Papillary muscles are atrophied (Van Vleet *et al.*, 1980; Kimman & Van der Molen, 1984; Liu & Maron, 1990). Histologically there may be mild interstitial oedema and fibrosis. The incidence of atrial thrombosis is low with this form.

In symmetrical hypertrophy (70% of cases in the cat) the left ventricle and septum are affected equally with a resultant reduction in left ventricular volume. The right ventricle is unaffected. Myofibres are hypertrophied with large nuclei and there is sometimes fibre disarray. There is diffuse myocardial fibrosis.

Asymmetric hypertrophy consists of septal thickening with apparent encroachment on the left-sided aortic outflow tract, although this may not result in actual functional obstruction to flow. Muscle fibres are disorientated. Left atrial thrombosis may occur and lead to aortic thromboembolism.

The main mechanical problem in both forms of hypertrophic cardiomyopathy is reduced compliance of the ventricular wall and diastolic filling problems. Added to this is poor myocardial perfusion due to compression of the intramural coronary vessels which are attempting to perfuse an increased thickness of myocardium (Liu *et al.*, 1975).

Finally, restrictive cardiomyopathy presents with severe endocardial thickening due to fibrosis and the deposition of hyalinized material beneath the endocardium. Left atrial enlargement is marked and there may be atrial thrombosis (Paasch & Zook, 1980).

Excess left ventricular moderator bands

Another type of restrictive endocardial lesion is the presence of excessive left ventricular moderator bands (Liu *et al.*, 1982). This has been described in all ages of cat and results in impaired diastolic function.

Although the pathogenesis of cardiomyopathies as a group remains unknown, one form of dilated cardiomyopathy in the cat has been shown to be associated with a taurine deficiency in the diet (Pion *et al.*, 1987). Some drug toxicities are also associated with dilated cardiomyopathy, notably doxorubicin. Dilated cardiomyopathies not associated with taurine or drug toxicities do, however, still occur. Hypertrophic cardiomyopathy in man has a genetic component (Liu & Maron, 1990).

Cardiomyopathies have a wide range in the age of onset from 7 months to 24 years. Presenting clinical signs include lethargy, anorexia, dyspnoea, tachypnoea and occasional abdominal distension. Murmurs and arrythmia are common. About one-third of cats present with thromboembolic disease, most usually uni- or bilateral hind limb ischaemia. Emboli (Fig. 4.1) usually originate in the left atrium and impact at the bifurcation of the aorta as 'saddle' emboli (Fig. 4.2) or sometimes in the femoral arteries themselves (Butler, 1971; Olmstead & Butler; 1977). Other major vessels which can become obstructed include the renal artery and vessels supplying forelimb, gut and brain. Physical occlusion of the vessels is only partly responsible for the clinical signs observed. Release of vasoactive mediators such as serotonin from the thrombus leads to profound vasoconstriction in the distal vascular bed which curtails collateral supply. This ischaemia will often result in infarction. In fatal cases of thromboembolic disease there may be infarcts of differing ages found in many organs at postmortem, indicating silent episodes of infarction preceding the final fatal occurrence.

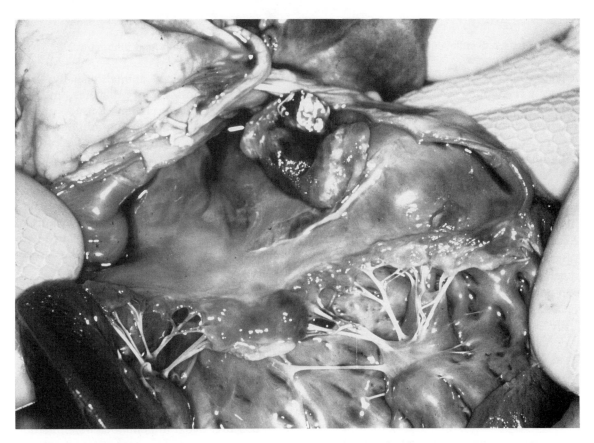

Fig. 4.1 Thrombus on right atrial wall of cat with dilated cardiomyopathy and atrial fibrillation.

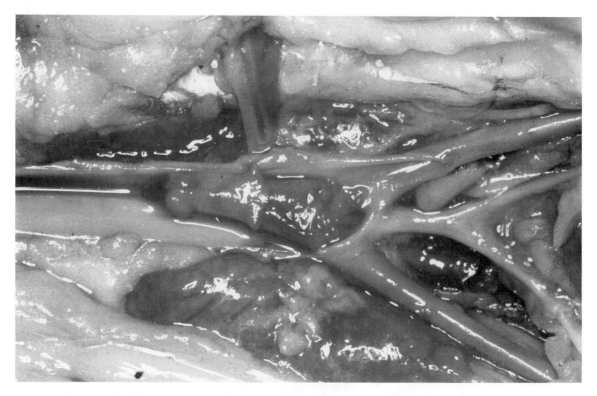

Fig. 4.2 'Saddle' embolus at bifurcation of abdominal aorta in cat with hind limb paresis.

Secondary cardiomyopathies

These are of common occurrence in the cat. Most usually the primary disorder is hyperthyroidism (Liu *et al.*, 1984). The cardiac changes are those of symmetric hypertrophic cardiomyopathy due to the increased basal metabolic rate and heart rate associated with hyperthyroidism. The cardiac changes may regress following treatment of the thyroid disorder and cardiac function usually returns to normal. The thyroid lesions are discussed with the endocrine system.

Systemic hypertension may also result in hypertrophic cardiomyopathy. This hypertension may be due to hyperthyroidism or chronic renal failure. Systemic arterial pressure is not easily measured in the cat and hypertension may only be suspected because of the presence of its secondary effects, hypertrophic cardiomyopathy and retinal detachment sometimes with hyphaema.

Hypertrophic cardiomyopathy has also been reported associated with acromegaly in the cat. Acromegaly occurs in older cats with pituitary adenomas and affected animals usually show signs of insulin-resistant diabetes mellitus (Lichensteiger *et al.*, 1986). Raised growth hormone concentrations in the adult result in soft tissue overgrowth once the epiphyseal plates have closed. Enlargement of liver, kidneys and tongue may occur in addition to cardiomegaly. There may also be appositional growth of new bone involving the flat bones, particularly of the skull. In the cat, deformity of the bones of the skull can also be associated with the mucopolysaccharidoses, one of the lysosomal storage diseases.

Ventricular hypertrophy may also develop if the outflow tract is restricted (Fig. 4.3).

Inflammatory cardiac disease

This condition is uncommon in the cat but bacterial endocarditis does occur and spread to the myocardium can follow. Primary myocarditis occurs uncommonly and the aetiology is often obscure. Pyogranulomatous inflammation and vasculitis can be seen as part of the pathology of feline infectious peritonitis, usually affecting the pericardium but with frequent spread to the myocardium. The gross and microscopic appearances of this condition are considered later.

Thromboembolic disease is relatively common in the cat due to its propensity to develop cardiac diseases, particularly the cardiomyopathies which result in atrial dilatation. Alterations in blood pressure and flow in the heart follow with the creation of foci of turbulence. This leads to damage to the cardiac endothelium and the development of intracardiac thrombosis. The dilated atria, most usually the left, are common sites for thrombi to develop. Thrombi are pale and compact and firmly attached to the endocardium. It may be possible to distinguish

laminations in them grossly as an aid to differentiation from ante-mortem thrombi but this may only be apparent histologically. The presence of intracardiac thrombi is often associated with infarcts in other viscera. In the kidney these take the form of wedge-shaped lesions with their base under the capsule and their apex at the corticomedullary junction. Initially they may be haemorrhagic but with time become pale with a peripheral red rim of hyperaemia. They then progress to a pale contracted wedge-shaped scar. Cerebral infarcts may occur and recent infarcts in this site are visible as pale yellow areas usually within the grey matter of the cerebral cortex. With time these lesions become necrotic with liquefaction of nervous tissue and the formation

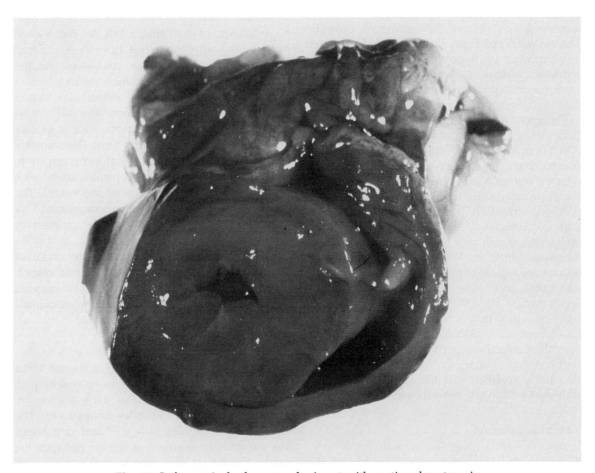

Fig. 4.3 Left ventricular hypertrophy in cat with aortic valve stenosis.

of cystic cavities. Clinical presentation is variable depending on the site of the lesion.

Obstruction of the terminal aorta or femoral arteries has already been mentioned in the context of thromboembolic disease. Loss of hindleg function is a common clinical presentation in cats with this condition (Butler, 1971).

Disseminated Intravascular Coagulation

This thrombotic disorder is not a disease in itself but is a frequent accompaniment of many severe systemic disorders and is potentially life threatening (see Chapter 2). The problem is one of inappropriate activation of the intravascular clotting mechanism which can be local or generalized. There is consumption of clotting factors, particularly platelets. The pathological picture is a composite of thrombotic and haemorrhagic phenomena. The haemorrhagic component is usually only seen in those animals which survive the thrombotic episode. The clinical picture is dominated by the development of hypovolaemic shock due to reduced venous return to the heart plus systemic and pulmonary arterial hypertension due to thrombosis.

The gross appearance of an animal suffering from disseminated intravascular coagulation (DIC) is of widespread petechial and echymotic haemorrhages in the serosa, mucosa, skin and internal organs. Gross thrombi are not seen but there are microthrombi in many organs with a patchy distribution. It is important to remember that microthrombi can be rapidly lysed even after death which may make confirmation of the diagnosis difficult. Widespread haemorrhagic lesions are typical of many systemic septicaemic infections and toxaemias. Not all will be accompanied by DIC but many will and the latter condition may account for a fatal outcome. Conditions often associated with DIC in the cat are feline infectious peritonitis, Gram-negative septicaemias, leukaemia, disseminated neoplasia, shock, acidosis, vascular stasis, postsurgical state and prolonged anaesthesia.

Vascular Lesions

Although vascular lesions, particularly of the arteries, are quite common in cats they appear with one or two exceptions to be of little clinical significance. Arteriosclerosis means hardening and luminal narrowing of arteries. The cause is proliferative and degenerative changes of the intima and media. These are common in the cat but rarely lead on to lipid deposition and atheroma or to thrombosis.

There is a specific medial arterial hypertrophy of the pulmonary arteries in the cat which is of dramatic and characteristic appearance but appears to be of no clinical significance even when severe and generalized (Hamilton, 1966; Rogers et al., 1971). The change is seen with equal frequency in germ-free and conventional cats of all ages and sexes. The presence of nematode parasites in the lung including *Aleurostrongylus abstrusus* and *Ascaris* species was thought to be the cause of this change. The mechanism suggested is increased levels of histamine in lung tissue producing chronic vasoconstriction. The condition can occur with no evidence of parasitism but as the lesions persist long after parasites have been cleared from the lung, parasitism may well be the primary cause. There is no increase in pulmonary blood pressure and no ventricular hypertrophy associated with the condition. The most severely affected vessels may be visible grossly on the cut surface of the lung. Histological changes vary from mild medial hypertrophy to severe medial and intimal proliferation with encroachment on the lumen of the vessel. The arterial changes may be accompanied by fibromuscular hyperplasia of the pulmonary parenchyma and alveolar ducts.

Vasculitis can occur from a wide range of causes, viral, bacterial, fungal, parasitic, chemical and immunological. The commonest cause in the cat is the immunological reaction associated with feline infectious peritonitis.

Feline infectious peritonitis
This disease is associated with a corona virus infection and has a chronic course resulting in death after 1–3 months. The early stages are often insidious and clinically unapparent. The disease can be divided into 'wet' and 'dry' forms but the only distinguishing feature between the two is the extent of fibrinous peritonitis which may be only apparent grossly in about 60–70%

of cases. The pathological lesions in this disease are due to immune reactions occurring in the walls of blood vessels and the associated inflammatory results. All serous surfaces throughout the body may be involved in this inflammatory process and fluid accumulates in the peritoneal and pleural cavity. The fluid is usually clear and deep yellow although it may contain flocules and strands of fibrin. There are white foci of necrosis or raised granulomatous cellular infiltrates on the serosal surfaces and extending from the serosa into the substance of parenchymatous organs. The foci of inflammation vary in size from a few millimetres to 1 cm in diameter. These lesions can be found separately within the substance of parenchymatous organs as well as in extensions from the serosal surface. Lesions in the central nervous system and the eye are not uncommon.

Histologically the central lesion is a generalized vasculitis (Fig. 4.4), perivasculitis and focal pyogranulomatous inflammation that occurs in the serous membranes, nervous system and in the connective tissue of the parenchymatous organs. These vascular lesions result in fibrinonecrotic and pyogranulomatous reaction around blood vessels. The vessel changes are of proliferation and desquamation of the endothelium followed by medial necrosis, narrowed lumina and thrombophlebitis. There are accumulations of neutrophils, lymphocytes, plasma cells and macrophages in and around the affected vessels. Changes may be seen in the omentum and mesentery as well as the serosa and can be mild or severe. The mild changes may appear as mesothelial proliferation with small amounts of fibrin exudation, a scattering of inflammatory cells and fibroblast proliferation. Severe changes may result in a thick layer of fibrin with necrosis and cuboidal metaplasia with syncytial formation in the serosa. Lesions in specific parenchymatous organs are due to the vascular damage in the capsule and interstitial stroma. They may be found throughout

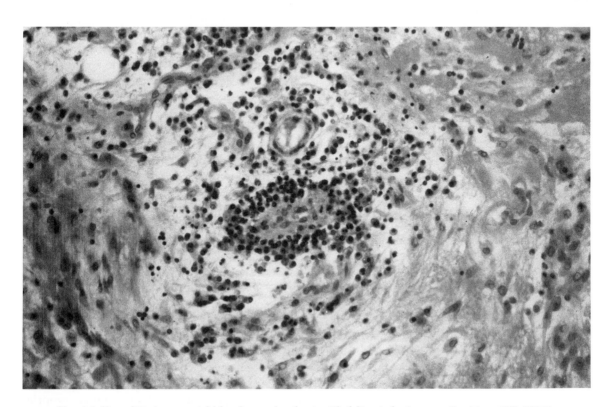

Fig. 4.4 Vasculitis in omental blood vessels of cat with feline infectious peritonitis. ×200. H&E.

the body. In the lung, in addition to focal lung lesions there may a diffuse interstitial pneumonia. Similarly a focal or diffuse interstitial nephritis may develop.

Cellular infiltration in the cerebral or spinal meninges and perivascular spaces tend to be mononuclear and diffuse rather than pyogranulomatous. Degenerative and necrotic lesions in the parenchyma of the central nervous system appear to be related to the vasculitis.

The pathogenesis of the disease appears to be that the virus is phagocytosed and taken to the local lymph nodes where viral multiplication takes place. There is then a generalized infection of monocytes and a second cell associated viraemia. The development of neutralizing antibody results in deposition of antigen–antibody complexes in vessel walls (type III hypersensitivity) that fix complement and trigger the inflammatory vascular lesions.

Arteritis may occur with conditions other than feline infectious peritonitis but is uncommon.

Veins and Lymphatics

Congenital anomalies of veins occur uncommonly but may be of clinical significance. Portosystemic anastamoses have been recorded in the cat (Blaxter *et al.* 1988). These lead to shunting of blood away from the liver and into the posterior vena cava. The most prominent clinical signs are poor growth and central nervous system disturbances due to the failure of the liver to deal adequately with ammonia and other substances that are normally metabolized by the liver. This diversion of blood away from the liver may be of importance to the anaesthetist when recovery from anaesthesia depends on metabolism of drug by the liver.

Portosystemic shunts can also occur as an acquired disease as will be discussed in the section on hepatic disease.

Thrombophlebitis and lymphadenitis occur in association with sepsis from bite wounds which are common in the cat, but otherwise, apart from feline infectious peritonitis, are seldom encountered.

Respiratory System

Upper Respiratory Tract

Feline respiratory disease is a common clinical problem with a complex and variable aetiology. The disease has two major components, infection by Feline Herpes virus I and Feline Calicivirus. Feline Reovirus and the feline-adapted strain of *Chlamydia psittaci* (Hoover *et al.*, 1978) are minor components.

Feline Herpes I, the cause of feline rhinotracheitis, is primarily an upper respiratory tract pathogen. An initial serous inflammation of nasal passages, conjunctiva, pharynx, tonsils and sometimes trachea rapidly becomes mucopurulent or fibrinous within a few days. This may in severe cases extend to a viral pneumonia. This manifests as a focal necrotizing bronchitis , bronchiolitis and interstitial pneumonia with serofibrinous flooding of air spaces. Viral multiplication with cell necrosis is at its height from 2 to 7 days postinfection. During this period large acidophilic inclusion bodies are present in the nuclei of affected cells. Calicivirus infections have an affinity for the epithelium of mouth and lung. Oral ulceration is a common feature of this infection (Wardley & Povey, 1977).

Bronchitis of viral or bacterial aetiology is usually self-limiting and even severe ulcerative lesions may heal with little residual scarring. The development of chronic bronchitis and bronchiectasis is rare in the cat (Moses & Spaulding, 1985). There is one form of chronic bronchitis which is not uncommon and is frequently referred to as allergic bronchitis or asthma. Clinical diagnosis depends on the presence of coughing, wheezing, respiratory distress, eosinophils in blood or tracheobronchial exudates and alleviation of signs by sympathomimetic drugs and corticosteroids. The significant pathological feature is a narrowing of the bronchiolar lumen by prominent hyperplasia of mucosal glands and goblet cells in the epithelium. Eosinophils infiltrate the epithelium and oedematous lamina propria. The lumen of the bronchus is filled with mucous and sloughed cells. Hypertrophy of bronchial smooth muscle is common but not always present. The pathogenesis is unclear but environmental allergens may be involved in some cases.

Rhinitis

A chronic non-specific rhinitis occurs in the cat, presenting as a mucopurulent unilateral or bilateral nasal discharge. The epithelium of the nasal cavity is ulcerated, hyperplastic or metaplastic with oedema of the underlying fibrous stroma. There is a heavy infiltration of this tissue by lymphocytes and plasma cells and the glandular tissue is hyperplastic. The pathogenesis is unclear but initial viral infection is probably rapidly followed by secondary proliferation of normally non-pathogenic resident flora. This begins a self-perpetuating inflammation associated with release of mediators from the many inflammatory cells in the area. Sinusitis is the most common sequel to this process, but inflammatory exudate may be inhaled to produce a bronchopneumonia, particularly under anaesthesia.

Granulomatous rhinitis in the cat can be due to infection with *Cryptococcus neoformans*. The lesions are rather gelatinous due to the massed organisms having an abundant mucopolysaccharide capsule. They take the form of polypoid nodules or more diffuse slowly destructive space occupying masses (Palmer, 1980).

Polyps are protruberant masses with a chronically inflamed oedematous core and an ulcerated or metaplastic covering epithelium. They are usually a sequel to chronic inflammation and are quite common in the nasopharyngeal area of the cat either in the eustachian tube or in the middle ear.

Pleural Cavity

Pneumothorax

Diagnosis of this condition at necropsy has been dealt with earlier. Causes are usually traumatic although infective processes can result in perforation of the lung and the establishment of a permanent sinus allowing air to leak out into the pleural cavity.

Pleuritis and Pyothorax

Non-suppurative pleuritis is uncommon in the cat. Inflammation in the pleural cavity usually arises as a result of bite wounds from fighting and the organisms involved are often *Pasteurella* or *Nocardia*, producing a thick foul-smelling purulent exudate. Lung collapse is almost inevitable although the cat often shows little clinical evidence of respiratory embarrassment and the condition can be missed prior to anaesthesia. If the infection is overcome healing is by fibrous organization with development of extensive adhesions between visceral and parietal pleura (Creighton & Wilkins, 1975; Sherding, 1979).

Lungs

Atelectasis

This term was originally used to describe defective aeration of the foetal lung at birth, but it is now applied to collapse of previously air-filled lung. Lung collapse is commonly seen due to occlusion of bronchi by inflammatory exudates in bronchitis and bronchopneumonia. Space-occupying lesions of the pleural cavity such as haemothorax, hydrothorax, chylothorax (Lindsey, 1974; Fossum *et al.*, 1991), exudative pleuritis and mediastinal tumours are common causes of atelectasis in the cat. Hypoproteinaemia and cardiac causes of oedema in the cat frequently lead to hydrothorax rather than to accumulations of fluid in other sites. Pneumothorax will also lead to massive atelectasis.

In the context of anaesthesia almost total atelectasis can be seen in animals breathing 80–100% oxygen as part of intensive care. By the time the thorax is examined post-mortem the lungs are usually completely degassed and are uniformly shrunken, dark red, flabby and ooze blood. Concentrations of oxygen as high as this are also directly toxic to the lung causing damage to type I alveolar epithelial cells and vascular endothelium (Tams, 1985).

Emphysema

Although frequently seen at post-mortem in the apices and sharp ventral border of the lung, this emphysema is very rarely of clinical significance.

Pneumonia

This is uncommon in cats as a primary disease and when it occurs is usually a sequel to the respiratory disease syndrome described under diseases of the upper respiratory tract. The pulmonary inflammatory response varies according to the nature of the inciting agent, the way in which they reach the lung and their persistence. They can most usefully be categorized according to their initial site of involvement and their pattern of spread. Most disease then falls into one of three categories:

1. Bronchopneumonia.
2. Lobar pneumonia.
3. Interstitial pneumonia.

Bronchopneumonia

This begins with inflammation of the bronchiolar–alveolar junction. This correlates with an aerogenous portal of entry. There is involvement of the cranioventral regions of the lung and a patchy or variegated gross appearance. In the cat *Pasteurella multocida* and a variety of Gram-negative organisms are found but are almost certainly secondary to a viral infection, severe stress or some other precipitating factor. Occasionally *Pasteurella multocida* will result in a lobar pneumonia in the cat. In this situation entire pulmonary lobes or major portions of the lobes are consolidated.

In both these types of pneumonia consolidated lung varies in appearance from dark red, through grey–pink to predominant grey. Palpable firmness is the single most important criteria of pneumonias. In bronchopneumonia the cut surface of the lung reveals areas of exudation centred on bronchi and surrounded by areas of hyperaemia. The centre of these areas can contain frank abscessation. Histologically in bronchopneumonia the predominant response is a filling of the alveoli around the bronchi and bronchioles with exudate consisting of neutrophils, cell debris, mucus and fibrin. Depending on the aetiological agent involved there may be changes to the bronchiolar epithelium, varying from necrosis to hyperplasia. The inflammation may spread out from

these areas to involve large areas of lung parenchyma and sometimes whole lung lobes to become a lobar pneumonia. The time sequence of these inflammmatory events can vary greatly but as a guide the red stage of consolidation will only last 2–3 days while the grey stage is reached in 5–7 days. Proliferation of type II pneumocytes can occur at this stage producing an appearance that can be confused with interstitial pneumonia which will be considered later. Resolution of pneumonia takes a variable course but mild bacterial pneumonias can resolve in 7–10 days and the lung returns to normal in 3–4 weeks. Death in pneumonias is due to a combination of hypoxia and toxaemia and death can occur when only a relatively small part of the lung is diseased (Pechman, 1985).

Interstitial pneumonia

This is characterized by diffuse or patchy damage to the alveolar septa. There is usually a short exudative intra-alveolar phase followed by a proliferative and fibrotic response. A wide variety of agents can cause the acute pulmonary injury, including acute viral infections, chemical lung injury (Breeze & Carlson, 1982), acute pancreatitis, shock and septicaemia. Commonly there may be secondary toxic damage caused by high concentrations of oxygen used therapeutically. This is often superimposed on the lung pathology that necessitated the oxygen administration leading to a rather complex and sometimes confusing appearance. Concentrations of oxygen greater than 50% can produce damage in already compromised lung. The mechanism of damage is thought to be by the generation of reactive oxygen radicles (superoxide, hydroxyl and singlet oxygen). These cause lipid peroxidation of cell membranes, inactivation of sulphydryl enzymes and damage to various macromolecules such as DNA. The enhanced sensitivity of damaged lung to the effects of high oxygen concentrations obviously has important implications for anaesthetists.

Interstitial pneumonia can be differentiated from bronchopneumonia by the absence of a distribution around airways. Grossly the lesions are widely distributed throughout the lung often in the dorsocaudal regions. This is in sharp contrast to the anterioventral distribution of the infective pneumonias. In most cases the respiratory insult is blood borne although inhaled toxic gases can be diffusely distributed in the lung with little concentration gradient between the alveoli and the small airways. The damage to the alveolar wall affects predominantly the type I cells and capillary endothelium causing necrosis and an acute inflammatory response. This is rapidly followed by regeneration on intact basement membranes by proliferation of type II pneumocytes. This produces a cuboidal epithelial lining to the alveolus which is characteristic of interstitial pneumonia. Resolution is by differentiation of type II cells to type I pneumocytes. The critical factor in the progression of interstitial pneumonia is the development of fibrosis. It can occur early in the inflammatory process and is potentially irreversible. The degree of fibrosis depends on the intensity of the inflammation and the subsequent balance between formation and degradation of collagen.

In the cat interstitial pneumonia is seen most commonly following infection with feline calicivirus. The main features of this disease are ulceration of the oral cavity, particularly the tongue, and serous rhinitis and conjunctivitis. Pneumonia commonly occurs but is usually mild and resolves in 7–10 days unless bacterial complications ensue. The virus has a strong tropism for alveolar type I epithelial cells. Grossly the pneumonia involves the cranioventral parts of the lung with irregular patches elsewhere. This is a pattern more reminiscent of bronchopneumonia rather than interstitial pneumonia but histologically the changes are typical of an interstitial pneumonia. Resolution usually occurs without residual fibrosis.

Parasitic lung disease
Aleurostrongylus abstrusus is the commonest and most widespread parasitic lung disease of the cat. Clinical signs are not marked but there may be coughing and some weight loss. The lesions are characteristic and consist of yellowish firm nodules 1–10 mm in diameter that represent nests of eggs and larvae. They are distributed throughout the lung but particularly in the peripheral portions. The nodules contain a thick creamy exudate. The marked medial proliferation of pulmonary blood vessels and bronchiolar smooth muscle has been mentioned previously. This change is very persistent and will far outlast the presence of the adult parasite which may remain for up to 9 weeks.

Neoplasia
As in other sites in the cat neoplastic disease of the thoracic cavity is dominated by lymphoid tumours. Mediastinal lymphosarcoma occurs particularly in young cats and may be of significance to the anaesthetist, presenting as a space-occupying lesion of the pleural cavity. It may also displace the heart and compress the large vessels of the thorax leading to pleural effusion. The fluid, which is often white and creamy in consistency, contains large numbers of neoplastic lymphocytes. This condition is often referred to as thymic lymphosarcoma but the most usual sites for neoplastic transformation are the mediastinal and bronchial lymph nodes. Involvement of the thymus with the production of a thymoma is much less common. The tumour masses are soft white or grey, lobulated and usually lie within the anterior mediastinum. Lymphosarcoma can also occur as a pulmonary tumour with widespread infiltration in the lung around airways and in association with blood vessels. The radiographic appearance can give the appearance of an interstitial inflammatory lesion. Lung lavage or aspiration can provide cytological material, which is dominated by neoplastic lymphoid cells.

Urinary System

Developmental Disease

Renal hypoplasia results in small kidneys but even in the young animal most abnormally small kidneys are not hypoplastic. Strictly speaking hypoplastic kidneys result from a reduced mass of metanephric blastema or incomplete induction of nephron formation. If the amount of blastema is normal but there is malfunction of the ureteral bud, then renal dysplasia results and this is probably the commoner congenital defect resulting in abnormally small kidneys. It should be remembered that the commonest cause of small irregular kidneys even in the young is postinflammatory scarring.

Renal dysplasia can be congenital but has been associated with disease in the early postnatal period, particularly panleucopaenia in the cat. Renal dysplasia is usually only detected when a young animal goes into renal failure. Both kidneys are usually shrunken and fibrosed with cystic cavities in the parenchyma and tortuous ureters. Microscopically, the characteristic of renal dysplasia is the presence of structures inappropriate to the stage of development of the animal or the development of clearly anomalous structures. These include areas of undifferentiated mesenchyme in cortex or medulla, groups of undifferentiated glomeruli in adult animals and primitive ducts lined by cuboidal or columnar epithelium lying in undifferentiated mesenchyme. There are often superimposed inflammatory and fibrotic changes as these kidneys are particularly susceptible to pyelonephritis.

Polycystic Disease

This is thought to be a congenital condition in the cat (Crowell *et al.*, 1979). Functional renal tissue is reduced by multiple cystic cavities varying in size from microscopic to several centimetres in diameter (Fig. 4.5). If both kidneys are involved there is progressive irreversible destruction of renal tissue and renal failure will ensue. Surprisingly large amounts of renal tissue can be lost before renal failure occurs. The pathogenesis of the condition is unclear.

Glomerular Disease

Pathological changes in the glomerulus are very common in cats and are probably a common ageing change in all species. Diffuse and wide-

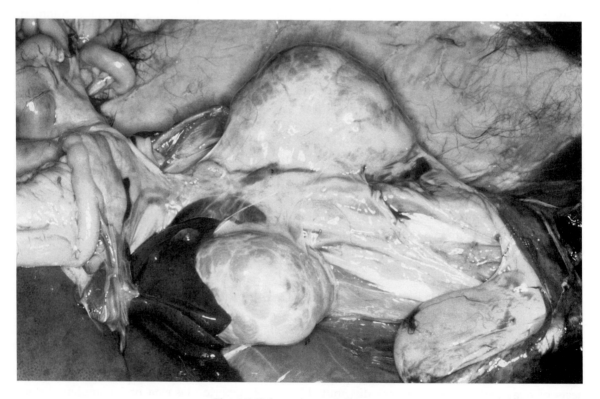

Fig. 4.5 Polycystic renal disease.

spread glomerular lesions which result in renal failure are much less common. Glomerular disease can be divided into the following groups (Lucke, 1968; Glick *et al.*, 1978; Jergans, 1987):

1. Membranous.
2. Proliferative.
3. Membrano-proliferative.
4. Glomerulosclerosis.

Glomeruli frequently exhibit a spectrum of lesions and terminology depends on the dominant type of pathological change present. In the cat, although all types of lesion do occur, membranous glomerulonephritis dominates the picture, particularly in clinically apparent disease.

Membranous glomerulonephritis
The predominant lesion is thickening of the glomerular basement membrane (Wright *et al.*, 1981). This can vary from mild change, with little clinical effect, to severe disease with marked thickening, distortion and significant fibrous scarring of the glomerulus. There is generally good correlation in the cat between the severity of the pathological lesions and the clinical signs of renal disease. However, caution should be exercised in interpretation of kidney biopsies as sometimes mild morphological renal changes can result in marked glomerular dysfunction, the so-called minimal change disease.

Proliferative glomerulonephritis
There is an increased cellularity of the glomerulus due to accumulation of inflammatory cells in the tuft. There is also multiplication and swelling of epithelial, endothelial and mesangial cells of the glomerulus. The stimulus for this increase in cell numbers is often the presence of immune complexes within the glomerulus (Bishop *et al.*, 1991).
Membrano-proliferative is a complex of the above forms.

Glomerulosclerosis
In this condition the glomerular structure is partly or completely lost due to the accumulation of hyaline deposits in the glomerular tuft. The chemical nature of these deposits is variable but they are usually proteinaceous in character and distinguished from glomerular fibrosis.

Grossly, kidneys affected by glomerulonephritis may appear normal, be slightly swollen or appear scarred and shrunken. Light microscopy with the aid of stains such as periodic acid Schiff or methenamine silver can demonstrate thickened glomerular basement membranes. Definitive diagnosis requires electron microscopy to demonstrate the deposition of electron-dense material in subendothelial, intramembranous or subepithelial locations. These electron-dense deposits are usually immune complexes. This marked thickening of the basement membrane is paradoxically associated with increased permeability of the glomerular capillaries and marked proteinuria, probably due to changes in electrical charge and slit pore size in the glomerular filtration barrier (Bishop *et al.*, 1991). The loss of protein into the urine results in the nephrotic syndrome which is a common clinical entity in cats suffering from glomerular disease.

The immune complexes found in the glomerular basement membrane are commonly of non-glomerular origin. In the cat, formation and deposition of these complexes has been associated with feline leukaemia, feline infectious peritonitis, feline progressive polyarthritis and other virus infections. In many cases it is not possible to substantiate the cause of the immune complex formation.

The nephrotic syndrome
In the cat, this is associated with severe proteinuria leading to weight loss, oedema, hypoalbuminaemia and hypercholesterolaemia (Nash *et al.*, 1979). A hypercoagulable state is associated with the nephrotic syndrome in man and cases of pulmonary artery thrombosis have also been seen in the cat with nephrotic syndrome. Hypertension is also associated with human glomerular disease and evidence of left ventricular hypertrophy suggestive of renal hypertension has been found at autopsy in cats with glomerulonephritis.

Tubular Disease

This is reflected morphologically in changes to the lining epithelial cells of the tubule. The tubule and interstitium are intimately related and damage to one results in damage or dysfunction of the other. Some disorders are thus termed tubulo-interstitial disease (Lucke & Hunt, 1965).

Normally the renal tubular epithelial cells of cats contain considerable amounts of lipid, giving a pale appearance to the kidney cortex. Tubular damage can be produced in a number of ways and the tubular epithelium is particularly sensitive to ischaemia which may result in acute tubular necrosis. Damage may thus follow a period of hypertension or haemorrhage with reduced renal vascular perfusion and hypoxia. Reflex renal vasoconstriction may follow severe hypertension and this may result in complete cortical necrosis. Histologically, there is focal necrosis of epithelial cells along the nephron. The basement membrane may be disrupted and the tubular lumen may be filled with proteinaceous cast material and cell debris. If the cause of the tubular damage is relieved then epithelial regeneration occurs and the tubules become lined with flattened epithelial cells.

A variety of chemicals and drugs can cause tubular necrosis in the cat. Notably, ethylene glycol (Grauer et al., 1982), which is present in antifreeze, is palatable to cats. Certain antibiotics, including neomycin, amphoterecin B, kanamycin and gentamycin are also toxic to renal tubular cells. Grossly, acute tubular damage may produce a slightly swollen kidney in which the cut surface bulges. The animal will either go into acute renal failure resulting in death or if the damage is less severe will recover completely in 2–3 weeks as the tubular epithelium is regenerated. If the interstitium is affected and the abuse is prolonged but insufficient to result in acute renal failure, secondary ischaemia may occur due to compression of blood vessels by inflammatory exudate or resultant fibrosis. This will result in glomerular lesions and further scarring of the cortex because of impairment of blood supply. In this way the condition can become chronic and progressive leading eventually to chronic renal failure.

Pyelonephritis

Acute pyelonephritis has been produced experimentally in cats with temporary obstruction of the ureter, by using intravenous infusions of *Escherichia coli* (Kelly et al., 1979). In naturally occurring cases both ascending and haematogenous infections probably occur but, as in all species, interruption of free urine flow is of critical importance in the development of this condition. Pyelonephritis is by definition inflammation of the renal pelvis and renal parenchyma. There is inflammation, necrosis and deformity of the calices in association with areas of tubulointerstitial nephritis. The condition is typically asymmetric and has a tendency to become chronic and intermittent. This results typically in irregular contraction of the kidneys with pelvic deformities which serves to differentiate it from other forms of nephritis. Although the true incidence of pyelonephritis in the cat is not known, chronic renal scarring in the older cat is common and may progress to end-stage renal disease and renal failure. It is believed that a significant proportion of renal scarring in the cat is due to chronic pyelonephritis. Large irregular scars are often interspersed with normal renal tissue.

The commonest type of renal disease by far in the cat is that presenting as chronic renal failure (DiBartola et al., 1987). The causes of this are many and varied but the resultant pathology is often very similar with the appearance of the 'end-stage' kidney. These kidneys are shrunken, sometimes misshapen and fibrosed. It is often difficult to identify the underlying pathological process. It has been suggested that the majority of these cases are of infective aetiology, some showing evidence of pyelonephritis and some interstitial nephritis. A few appear to have vascular origins. In distinction to the situation in the dog, leptospirosis does not appear to be a major cause of renal disease in the cat.

Renal amyloidosis

The exact pathogenesis of amyloidosis is often unknown, but it occurs with chronic inflammatory conditions and multiple myeloma as well as in an idiopathic form. Grossly, deposits of amyloid give a firm and rather opaque character to tissues. Microscopically, the material is amorphous, structureless and eosinophilic with a hyalinized appearance. The filamentous character of the material can be seen with the electron microscope. The unusual feature of renal amyloidosis in the cat is that it occurs mainly in the renal papillae and outer medulla rather than the cortex. Glomerular deposits do occur in the cat but are more common in other species. Because of this difference marked proteinuria is much less common in cats with amyloidosis than it is in dogs. The kidneys in this condition are very firm, shrunken and coarsely nodular due to fibrosis extending from medulla to capsular surface. In this respect they resemble kidneys with chronic pyelonephritis. Microscopically, the basement membranes of tubules and capillaries are thick and hyaline with deposition of amyloid fibrils. The ischaemia and tubular obstruction this produces leads to fibrosis in the medullary rays. The prevalence of amyloidosis is much increased in cats on diets providing excess vitamin A.

Hydronephrosis
This is dilatation of the renal pelvis due to chronic partial obstruction to urine outflow with subsequent pressure atrophy of the kidney parenchyma. The condition is relatively uncommon in the cat which is at first sight surprising in view of the propensity for the male cat to suffer from urethral obstruction due to urolithiasis. Obstruction in this condition is usually complete and acute so there is little opportunity for hydronephrosis to develop as the animal will either die or the obstruction will be relieved.

Sometimes a type of hydronephrosis occurs in which there is a large accumulation of fluid between the capsule and the cortex. The pathogenesis is unclear but may involve obstruction of lymphatics.

Neoplasia
Primary tumours of renal tissue are uncommon in the cat but it is a common site for the development of lymphoma. These tumours occur as one or more circumscribed solid grey or white masses displacing normal renal tissue and often bulging from the cortical surface. Histologically they consist of sheets of neoplastic lymphoid cells disrupting the normal renal architecture. Tumour cells may be present in the renal lymph node and other organs but disease is often restricted grossly to the kidneys.

Resection of isolated tumour masses or nephrectomy is not likely to be therapeutically successful as other masses subsequently develop. Despite the apparent localization of lymphoma in the cat it should probably always be considered a multisystem disease.

The Lower Urinary Tract

The pathology of the lower urinary tract in the cat is dominated by the so-called 'feline urological syndrome'. This clinical description probably embraces a number of pathological conditions resulting in the signs of dysuria, haematuria, cystitis–urethritis, urolithiasis and urethral obstruction. The condition occurs most commonly in cats between 2 and 5 years of age.

Urolithiasis is the most important manifestation of disease particularly in the male where it leads to urethral obstruction, which is life threatening with a mortality of up to 25%. In the female, urolithiasis occurs as bladder calculi which may attain a considerable size. In the male, microcalculi some 2 mm in diameter sometimes occur but usually the urolith in the male is a sabulous plug composed of proteinaceous material and crystals. The commonest crystalline material is struvite or magnesium ammonium phosphate hexahydrate. Microcalculi and plugs become impacted where the musculomembranous urethra narrows to become the penile urethra. Sometimes the sabulous plugs extend the whole length of the urethras. The pathogenesis of these uroliths in the cat is obscure. Among the possible predisposing factors are viral infections, exclusive use of dried food, inhibition of urethral growth following castration, infrequent urination in cold weather and imbalance in dietary levels of magnesium and phosphate. None of these adequately explains the aggregation of struvite crystals to form calculi. Crystals alone can be found in normal animals. Cystitis is a common antecedent to urolithiasis in other animals and cystitis associated with bacterial infections does occur in the cat but other cases of cystitis in this species are bacteriologically sterile.

A haemorrhagic cystitis may occur in animals treated for neoplastic or immunological diseases with cyclophosphamide, metabolites of the drug causing oedema, haemorrhage and ulceration in the bladder.

The Liver

Pathological conditions affecting the liver can predominantly involve the vasculature, the hepatic parenchyma or the biliary excretory system. These component parts of the organ are intimately connected and disease in any one component will also tend to produce changes in other parts.

The liver parenchyma, although rather sensitive to injury, has an enormous capacity for regeneration provided the basic reticulin framework of the liver remains intact and the cause of the abuse is removed. If the framework is destroyed then healing involves fibrosis with distortion of liver architecture and the efforts of the parenchyma to regenerate without rigid guidance leads to hyperplastic nodularity. This distortion of architecture disturbs blood flow leading to hepatic hypertension and possible ascites (Greenaway & Oshiro, 1972).

Parenchymal Disease

Hepatic lipidosis
The accumulation of fat in hepatocytes can occur under a variety of circumstances both physiological and pathological. These may concern abnormalities of synthesis, utilization or mobilization of lipid. There may be an excess of lipid in the form of free fatty acids, in the blood being brought to the liver. This tends to overwhelm the liver's metabolic capabilities. There may be a defect in the protein synthesizing capabilities of the hepatocyte so that lipid cannot be exported from the hepatocyte as lipoprotein. While the circumstances leading to hepatic lipidosis may not be injurious in themselves, other functions of the liver may be impaired leading to signs of disease.

Fatty liver syndrome
This occurs in obese, nutritionally stressed animals (Thornburg et al., 1982). There is hypertriglyceridaemia and a high mortality rate. Clinically, jaundice is frequently observed. Grossly, the liver is pale, swollen and the cut surface has a greasy appearance with a friable texture. There is severe fatty accumulation in all hepatocytes and there may be severe periacinar hepatocellular necrosis. The pathogenesis is unclear. Excess lipid in the liver and blood is in the form of triglyceride which implies that the liver is capable of esterification of fatty acids but that eventually the plasma transport mechanisms are overwhelmed and lipid begins to accumulate in the hepatocyte.

Hepatocyte necrosis
Necrosis of individual hepatocytes or of large groups of cells within the liver occurs for a variety of reasons. Individual cell necrosis or apoptosis is common in the liver and probably is part of the normal turnover of hepatic tissue. Large areas of tissue can become necrotic due to ischaemia, toxins and a variety of infectious agents.

Grossly, hepatic necrosis can appear as pale areas of coagulation or perhaps more often as areas of haemorrhage. The spaces left when hepatocytes necrose become filled with blood. This gives a mottled red appearance to the liver. Microscopically, these necrotic areas consist of pools of blood surrounded by hepatocytes with degenerative changes and infiltrating inflammatory cells. Coagulative necrosis results in hepatocytes showing loss of definition with dissolution of nuclei and disappearance of cell boundaries.

The pattern of distribution of necrosis within the liver can be diagnostically helpful. Hypoxia associated with anaemia or congestive heart failure leads to centrilobular or periacinar degeneration of hepatocytes as these cells are the last to receive oxygenated blood from the hepatic artery. Toxic agents frequently produce centrilobular or periacinar necrosis as these cells contain the highest concentration of mixed function oxidase enzymes which are capable of transforming certain exogenous compounds into reactive metabolites which may be hepatotoxic. It is often difficult to prove which hepatotoxin has been involved in naturally occurring cases of hepatic necrosis in the cat.

Treatment of sick cats with acetaminophen (paracetamol) by owners may produce areas of hepatic necrosis. There is also anaemia, haemoglobinuria and intravascular haemolysis in these cases. Cyanosis may also occur due to anoxia associated with conversion of haemoglobin to methaemoglobin. Acetylsalicylic acid may also result in hepatotoxicosis together with bone marrow hypoplasia.

Mycotoxins have been associated with liver damage and aflatoxin from the fungus *Aspergillus flavus* will cause hepatic necrosis in high doses. In lower doses given over a prolonged period, proliferation of biliary epithelium is seen. These toxins may occur in poorly stored dry food.

Infective disease can result in hepatic necrosis. Feline Herpes virus which causes rhinotracheitis in adult animals can produce a generalized viraemia in the neonate. This is associated with a patchy hepatic necrosis. Infected hepatocytes may show herpetic intranuclear inclusion bodies. It should be remembered that the coronavirus causing feline infectious peritonitis can produce pyogranulomatous foci in the liver with central areas of heptocyte necrosis.

Toxoplasmosis can also result in focal areas of hepatic necrosis in the cat. The organism has its natural cycle in the gut epithelium of the cat but occasionally tachyzoites can be carried to the liver in lymph or blood and produce focal necrosis. *Bacillus pisiformis*, the cause of Tyzzers disease, has been reported to cause focal necrotic hepatitis in the cat. The organism cannot be grown in culture so diagnosis depends on the demonstration of large long rod shaped bacilli in the cytoplasm of hepatocytes at the periphery of the necrotic lesion. It seems likely that this infection is associated with some form of immunological insufficiency.

Jaundice

Jaundice occurs for two basic reasons, either overproduction of bile due to excessive breakdowns of red cells or impaired excretion of the pigment by the liver. Impaired excretion can occur either due to failure of hepatocytes to conjugate bilirubin and then excrete it, or due to obstruction to the free flow of bile in ductules or extrahepatic ducts.

Any of the diseases causing hepatocyte necrosis can result in hepatocellular jaundice in the cat if the disease is of sufficient severity. Haemolytic jaundice in the cat may occur in babesiosis with intravascular haemolysis and the presence of haemoglobin in the urine. It can also occur with extravascular haemolysis where there is no haemoglobinuria. This type of haemolytic jaundice may occur with feline infectious anaemia and autoimmune haemolytic anaemia. In both cases anaemia may be a more prominent sign than jaundice. There is often increased urobilinogen in the urine and dark-staining faecal material.

The Biliary Tree

Obstructive jaundice can be either intra- or extrahepatic in origin. Conjugated bilirubin does not enter the gut and so urobilinogen is not formed and is absent from the urine. Faeces also tend to be pale and greasy. The obstruction to bile flow can occur within the hepatic parenchyma when it is due to hepatocyte swelling with occlusion of cholangioles. This type of obstruction occurs in hepatic lipidosis. Obstruction can also be associated with disease affecting the larger bile ducts in the portal areas of the liver or occlusion of the extrahepatic ducts.

Cholecystitis, cholangitis and cholangiohepatitis appear to be quite common in the cat and are predominantly subclinical conditions. They are often accompanied by a low-grade inflammation of the pancreas and pancreatic duct (Kelly *et al.*, 1975). In view of the common opening of the pancreatic and bile duct in the cat it is assumed that the cause of the inflammation in both pancreatic and biliary system is ascending infection from the bowel.

The clinical course and pathological changes in cholangiohepatitis vary greatly from an acute fulminating suppurative infection (Hirsch & Doige, 1983) to a chronic mild infection which over a period of months or years leads to progressive portal fibrosis (Fig. 4.6). In the cat cholangiohepatitis more often takes the latter form, is chronic and of ill-defined pathogenesis

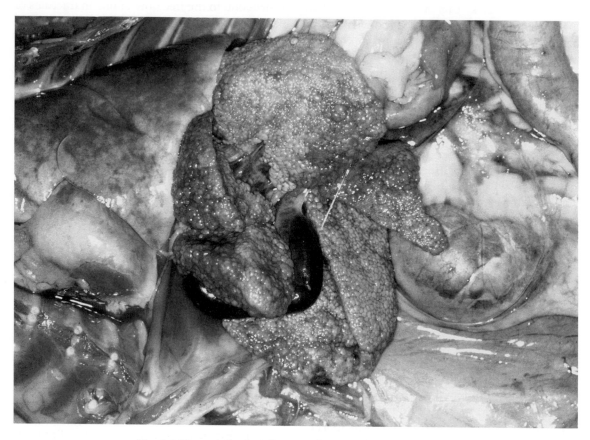

Fig. 4.6 Liver cirrhosis following chronic cholangiohepatitis.

(Prasse *et al.*, 1982). In severe cases jaundice may develop. The liver may be enlarged but is usually of normal shape although in advanced cases a granularity may appear on the capsular surface. Eventually there may be distortion of the liver architecture by fibrosis and regenerative hyperplasia. Histologically there is fibrosis in the portal areas accompanied by infiltration of lymphocytes and a few neutrophils. There is usually proliferation of biliary epithelium which can become quite marked. The lesions may regress following prednisolone therapy.

Endocrine System

In general terms dysfunction of the endocrine system can be manifest either by symptoms resulting from overproduction of hormones or those resulting from insufficient hormone production. Alternatively, in the presence of normal hormone secretion, there may be altered sensitivity of the target organs or altered breakdown of secreted hormone. Owing to the fact that the pituitary gland has a central regulating function in hormonal homeostasis, the primary pathological lesion may reside in this organ even though the clinical signs may be produced by failure of a peripheral endocrine gland (for example the thyroid).

Pituitary Gland

Pituitary disease appears to be relatively rare in cats. Neoplasia is the commonest disorder encountered but tumours rarely appear to be functionally secretory and therefore exert their effects by compression of adjacent structures as they enlarge. This compression may affect the optic chiasma resulting in visual impairment. It may also affect the hypothalamus resulting in abnormal appetite and weight gain. Abnormalities of sexual and other behaviour may also occur. Tumours of the anterior pituitary may also compress the pars nervosa, infundibular stalk or supraoptic nucleus of the hypothalamus. This may disrupt synthesis, secretion or transport of antidiuretic hormone. This leads to failure to resorb water in the distal convoluted tubules and collecting ducts of the kidney. The excretion of large volumes of hypotonic urine obliges the animal to take in large amounts of water, a condition known as diabetes insipidus. Clinically the condition may be confused with chronic renal disease in the cat. Water deprivation testing will result in an increased urine specific gravity above 1.011 in diabetes insipidus. Cats with chronic renal disease, on the other hand, will be unable to concentrate urine on water deprivation. Injection of pitressin in oil will produce a substantial increase in urine specific gravity in diabetes insipidus, indicating that the condition is of neurogenic origin. Occasional cases of diabetes insipidus occur due to failure of the renal tubular cells to respond to antidiuretic hormone. The cause is believed to be a lack of the adenylate cyclase enzyme in the plasma membrane of the tubular cells.

Thyroid Gland

Gross abnormalities of the thyroid gland are a common finding in cats particularly with increasing age (Lucke, 1964). The thyroid is often enlarged and nodular, sometimes with cystic areas. In some cases the condition is bilateral. The nodules are tan or white and of variable size. The nodules consist of hyperplastic follicular cells which are arranged into variable-sized follicles sometimes with papillary ingrowths. The colloid content of the follicles is very variable. The distinction between hyperplasia and adenoma is very difficult and probably artificial. A single, encapsulated lesion with compression of surrounding thyroid tissue can be termed an adenoma, but the situation is seldom so simple. Multiple hyperplastic nodules compres-

sing surrounding thyroid tissue are sometimes referred to as adenomatous hyperplasia. In practice it is more important to distinguish benign and malignant neoplasia. Fortunately this is more easily achieved.

If the new tissue is endocrinologically active the adjacent thyroid follicles, which are often compressed, show colloid involution. This is due to inhibition of thyrotrophin release from the pituitary, via the negative feedback exerted by a raised level of thyroid hormone in the blood. This change may also be seen in the contralateral thyroid when one gland is involved in a hyperplastic or neoplastic process. Nodular hyperplasia can be seen in cats of any age, while adenomas and occasional carcinomas are seen in older cats, usually more than 10 years of age (Clark & Merier, 1958).

A syndrome of hyperthyroidism occurs in cats associated with multinodular hyperplasia, adenoma or adenocarcinoma (Holzworth *et al.,* 1980; Liu *et al.,* 1984). It is most common in aged cats but can occur at any age. Clinically there is weight loss, polydipsia, polyuria, increased frequency of defecation and increased activity. There may be tachycardia with premature beats and/or a systolic murmur. These signs are associated with an increased metabolic rate in these animals. The increased work load for the heart leads to cardiac hypertrophy and cardiomegaly due to left ventricular hypertrophy and this may be evident on radiographs. This type of hypertrophic cardiomyopathy may be complicated by intracardiac thrombosis and secondary iliac thrombosis as mentioned earlier.

Hypothyroidism appears to be very uncommon in the cat and has only been recorded in association with an iodine deficiency when cats were fed an all meat diet.

Adrenal Cortex

Hyperadrenocorticism (Cushing's syndrome) has seldom been reported in the cat but does appear to occur both with adrenocortical adenoma and with pituitary-dependent hyperadrenocorticism (Nelson *et al.,* 1988). The clinical signs appeared to be as for the dog, with alopecia over the trunk, dull lustreless hyperpigmented skin, pendulous abdomen and emaciation. Poly-phagia, polydipsia, polyuria and depression also occurred. In the pituitary-dependent case the adrenals showed nodular hyperplasia of the cortex with cortical tissue extending through the capsule in places. Laboratory examination revealed leucopenia with eosinophilia, hyper-glycaemia, glycosuria and ketonuria. Plasma cortisol levels were elevated.

Adrenocortical insufficiency appears to be relatively uncommon in the cat and when it does occur the pathogenesis is unclear (Petersen *et al.*, 1989). Areas of calcification in the adrenal cortex are common incidental findings (Howell & Pickering, 1964) as mentioned previously and do not appear to have any functional signifi-cance. Grossly the foci are yellow–white and gritty. They may impinge on the adrenal medulla. Histologically there are large areas of necrosis with mineral deposition adjacent to areas of nodular regeneration.

Hyperplastic nodules are relatively common in older cats but appear to have no functional significance.

Endocrine Pancreas

Diabetes mellitus due either to failure of insulin secretion or to unresponsiveness of the periph-eral target cells is uncommon in the cat (Fig. 4.7). It has been associated with lesions in the pancreatic islets consisting of disruption of their structure and the accumulation of amy-loid-like material (Yano *et al.*, 1981; Kranek *et al.*, 1984; Westermark *et al.*, 1987).

Haemopoietic System

Disease of the haemopoietic system is of fundamental importance to the anaesthetist, particularly disease affecting the erythroid compartment. Anaemia will affect the oxygen

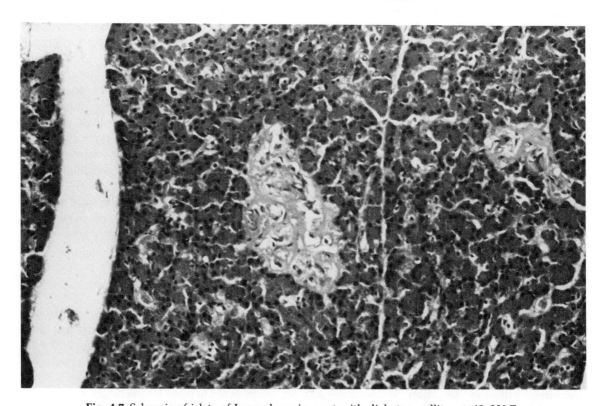

Fig. 4.7 Sclerosis of islets of Langerhans in a cat with diabetes mellitus. ×40. H&E.

carrying capacity of the blood and will also produce clinical signs such as hyperpnoea, tachycardia and heart murmurs which may suggest cardiorespiratory disease. Polycythemia and myeloid disease may lead to thrombotic episodes. Thus, no discussion of the pathology of the cat in relation to anaesthesia would be complete without a brief mention of diseases of the blood.

Anaemia may occur because of defective red cell production or because of increased red cell loss. Excessive blood loss can result from external trauma which is usually self evident or from internal bleeding. The loss in the latter case may be insidious and chronic particularly if loss is into the gastrointestinal tract with conditions such as coccidiosis, hookworm or ulcerated alimentary tract neoplasms.

Changes indicating blood loss can be detected in the peripheral blood. In acute blood loss there is within a few hours a reticulocytosis and neutrophilia with a 'left shift', as immature haemopoietic cells are released from the marrow. In 3–4 days immature red blood cells appear in the peripheral blood as a regenerative response begins in the bone marrow. Blood films at this time may show anisocytosis, polychromatophilic macrocytes, normoblasts and red cells containing Howell Jolly bodies.

If the blood loss is chronic in nature, the peripheral blood picture may become microcytic and hypochromic, with small nucleated red cells and poikilocytosis. This occurs because the marrow is unable to keep up with the demand for red cells, and iron particularly becomes in short supply.

In haemolytic anaemia there is again a fall in red cell numbers in the blood and the presence of immature red cells in the peripheral circulation. Haemoglobin may be released into the blood and this may subsequently appear in the urine.

The causes of haemolytic anaemia are varied. Feline leukaemia virus infection is often associated in its early stages with haemolytic anaemia. This may then lead to bone marrow depression. Toxins such as phenol can cause haemolysis and some drugs such as methylene blue and acetaminophen have been associated with this type of anaemia.

Autoimmune haemolytic anaemia is less common in the cat than in the dog. There is often splenomegaly, hepatomegaly, icterus and epistaxis, the latter being due to the accompanying thrombocytopaenia.

Haemolytic anaemias also occur with protozoan blood parasites such as *Haemobartonella felis* and *Babesia felis*. Parasites can be identified in Giemsa-stained smears of peripheral blood.

Defective red cell production accounts for the majority of cases of anaemia in the cat. A number of factors are known to cause bone marrow depression in this species. The drugs chloramphenicol and acetylsalicylic acid are known marrow depressants and may cause aplastic anaemia. Feline leukaemia virus infection may cause a refractory normocytic normochromic anaemia. This may progress to myelofibrosis in which the marrow is replaced by fibrous tissue. In some cases of hypoplastic anaemia the marrow may be hypercellular due to large numbers of erythroid precursors, indicating a defect in maturation or release of red cells.

Anaemia is also a common finding in chronic renal disease thought to be due to reduced erythropoietin production by the kidney together with reduced red cell survival time and red cell loss into the urinary tract. A common reason for anaemia is the occupation of the marrow compartment by neoplastic haemopoietic cells. There may be an accompanying frank leukaemia but sometimes neoplastic cells are confined to the marrow and the presenting syndrome is of anaemia.

Haemopoietic neoplasia in the cat is dominated by lymphoid tumours (Hardy, 1981). In decreasing order of frequency these can be classified as mediastinal, alimentary, multicentric, leukaemic and miscellaneous. The degree of differentiation of the neoplastic cells may differ but, as yet, no reliable correlation between histological appearance and behaviour exists in the cat. The commonest type, (under the Rappaport classification) appears to be the poorly differentiated lymphocytic form. About 10% of haemopoietic neoplasms in the cat are of myeloid derivation. Acute and chronic forms of myeloid leukaemia are seen and some tumours differentiate along monocytic lines.

Bone marrow examination is required for accurate diagnosis. Erythremic myelosis and polycythemia vera affecting the red cell lineage have been recorded but are very rare.

Mast cell neoplasia is distinctive in the cat. It is seen in the cutaneous form as in other species but also as an alimentary condition and as a systemic disease (Liska *et al.*, 1979). In the systemic form the clinical presentation is of vomiting, diarrhoea and anorexia. Splenomegaly is a consistent finding and deposits of neoplastic mast cells are found in many organs. Alimentary mastocytosis most commonly affects the small intestine with metastasis to liver and local lymph nodes. With both systemic and visceral forms of the disease there is often ulceration of stomach and duodenum associated with the release of histamine from the neoplastic mast cells.

References

Bishop, S.A., Lucke, V.M., Stokes, C.R. & Grwffydd Jones, T.J. (1991) Plasma and urine biochemical changes in cats with experimental immune complex glomerulonephritis. *J. Comp. Path.* **104** (1), 65–76.

Blaxter, M.C., Holt, P.E., Pearson, G.R., Gibbs, C. & Gryffydd-Jones, J.J. (1988) Congenital portosystemic shunts in the cat. Report of 9 cases. *J. Small Anim. Pract.* **29** (10), 631-645.

Bolton, G.R. & Linu, S.K. (1977) Congenital heart disease in the cat. *Vet. Clin. N. Am. Small. Anim. Pract.* **7**, 341.

Breeze, R.G. & Carlson, J.R. (1982) Chemical-induced lung injury in domestic animals. *Adv. Vet. Sci. Comp. Med.* **26**, 201–232.

Butler, H.C. (1971) An investigation into the relationship of aortic embolus to posterior paralysis in the cat. *J. Small. Anim. Pract.* **12**, 141.

Clark, S.T. & Merier, H. (1958) A clinicopathological study of thyroid disease in the dog and cat. Part I. Thyroid pathology. *Zentralbl Vet. Med. [A]* **5**, 17.

Cohen, J.S., Tilley, L.P., Liu, S.K. & De Hoff, W.D. (1975) Patent ductus arteriosus in five cats. *J. Am. Anim. Hosp. Ass.* **11**, 95.

Creighton, S.R. & Wilkins, R.J. (1975) Thoracic effusions in the cat. Aetiology and diagnostic features. *J. Am. Anim. Hosp. Ass.* **11**, 66.

Crowell, W.A.S., Hubbard, J.J. & Riley, J.C. (1979) Polycystic renal disease in related cats. *J. Am. Vet. Med. Assoc.* **175**, 286-288.

DiBartola, S.P., Rutgers, H.C., Zak, P.M. & Tarr, M.J. (1987) Clinico-pathologic findings associated with chronic renal disease in cats. 74 cases (1973–1984). *J. Am. Vet. Med. Assoc.* **190**, 1196-1202.

Evans, S.M. & Biery, D.N. (1980) Congenital peritaneopericardial diaphragmatic hernia in the dog and cat. A literature review and 17 additional case histories. *Vet. Radiol.* **21**, 108.

Fossum, T.W., Forrester, S.D., Swenson, C.L., Miller, M.W., Cohen, N.D., Boothe, H.W. & Birchard, S.J. (1991) Chylothorax in cats. 37 cases 1969–1989. *J. Am. Vet. Med. Assoc.* **198** (4), 672–678.

Fox, P.R. (ed.) (1988) *Feline Myocardial Disease in Canine and Feline Cardiomyopathy*. Churchill Livingston, New York.

Glick, A.D., Horn, R.G., Holscher, M., Holzworth, J., Theran, P., Carpenter, J.L., Harpster, N.K. & Todoroff, R.J. (1978). Characterization of feline glomerulonephritis associated with viral induced haemopoietic neoplasms. *Am. J. Pathol.* **92**, 321–332.

Grauer, G.F. & Thrall M.A. (1982) Ethylene Glycol poisoning in the dog and cat. *J. Am. Anim. Hosp. Ass.* **18**, 492–497.

Greenaway, C.V. & Oshiro, G. (1972) Intrahepatic distribution of portal hepatic arterial blood flow in anaesthetised cats and dogs and the effect of portal occlusion, raised venous pressure and histamine. *J. Physiol (Lond.)* **227**, 473–485.

Hamilton, J.M. (1966) Pulmonary arterial disease of the cat. *J. Comp. Path.* **76**, 133–145.

Hardy, W.D. (1981) Haemopoietic tumours of the cat. *J. Am. Anim. Hosp. Ass.* **17**, 921.

Hirsch, V.M. & Doige C.E. (1983) Suppurative cholangitis in cats. *J. Am. Vet. Med. Ass.* **138**, 1223.

Holzworth, J. *et al.* (1980) Hyperthyroidism in the cat: ten cases. *J. Am. Vet. Med. Assoc.* **176**, 345–353.

Hoover, E.A., Kahn, D.E. & Langloss, J.M. (1978) Experimentally induced feline chlamydial infection (feline pneumonitis). *Am. J. Vet. Res.* **39**, 451–548.

Howell, J.M. & Pickering, C.M. (1964) Calcium deposits in the adrenal glands of dogs and cats. *J. Comp. Path.* **74**, 280.

Jeraj, K., Osborne, C.A. & Stevens, J.B. (1982) Evaluation of renal biopsy in 197 dogs and cats. *J. Am. Vet. Med. Assoc.* **181**, 367–369.

Jergens, A.E. (1987) Glomerulonephritis in dogs and cats. *Compend. Cont. Ed. Pract. Vet.* **9** (9), 903–911.

Kelly, D.F., Baggot, D.G. & Gaskell, C.J. (1975) Jaundice in the cat associated with inflammation of the biliary tract and pancreas. *J. Small. Anim. Pract.* **16**, 163.

Kelly, D.F., Lucke, V.M. & McCullagh, K.G. (1979) Experimental pyelonephritis in the cat. *J. Comp. Path.* **89**, 125–139, 563–579.

Kelly, D.F., Lucke, V.M. & Gaskell, C.J. (1982) *Notes on Pathology for Small Animal Clinicians.* Wright P.S.G.

Kimman, T.G. & Van der Molen, E.J. (1984) Pathological findings in nineteen cats with idiopathic cardiomyopathy. *Tijdschr Diergeneeskd* **109**, 132.

Kranek, B.A., Moise, N.S. & Cooper, B. *et al.* (1984) Neuropathy associated with diabetes mellitus in the cat. *J. Am. Vet. Med. Assoc.* **184**, 42.

Lichensteiger, C.A., Wortman, J.A. & Eigermann, J.E. (1986) Functional pituitary acidophil adenoma in a cat with diabetes mellitus and acromegalic features. *Vet. Path.* **23**, 513.

Lindsey, F.E.F. (1974) Chylothorax in the domestic cat. A Review. *J. Small Anim. Pract.* **15**, 241.

Liska, W.D., MacEwen, E.G. & Zak, F.A. *et al.* (1979) Feline Systemic Mastocytosis: A review and results of splenectomy in 7 cases. *J. Am. Anim. Hosp. Ass.* **15**, 589.

Liu, S.K. (1970) Acquired cardiac lesions leading to congestive heart failure in the cat. *Am. J. Vet. Res.* **31**, 2071.

Liu, S.K. (1977) Pathology of feline heart disease 1977. *Veterinary Clinics of North America: Small Animal Practice* **7**, 323.

Liu, S.K. & Maron, B.J. (1990) Comparison of hypertrophic cardiomyopathy in humans, cat and dog. *Lab. Investigation* **62** (1), 58A.

Liu, S.K. & Tilley, L.P. (1976) Dysplasia of the Tricuspid valve in the dog and cat. *J. Am. Vet. Med. Assoc.* **169**, 623.

Liu, S.K., Tilley, L.P. & Tashjian, R.J. (1975) Lesions of the conduction system in the cat with cardiomyopathy. *Recent Adv. Stud. Card. Struct. Metab.* **10**, 681.

Liu, S.K., Fox, P.R. & Tilley, L.P. (1982) Excessive moderator bands in the left ventricle of 21 cats. *J. Am. Vet. Med. Assoc.* **178**, 1215.

Liu, S.K., Petersen, M.E. & Fox, P.R. (1984) Hypertrophic cardiomyopathy and hyperthyroidism in the cat. *J. Am. Anim. Hosp. Ass.* **185**, 52.

Lucke, V.M. (1964) An histological study of thyroid abnormalities in the domestic cat. *J. Small Anim. Pract.* **5**, 351.

Lucke, V.M. (1968) Renal disease in the domestic cat. *J. Path. Bact.* **95**, 67–91.

Lucke, V.M. & Hunt, A.C. (1965) Interstitial nephropathy and papillary necrosis in the domestic cat. *J. Pathol. Bact.* **89**, 723–728.

Lucke, V.M. & Hunt, A.G. (1967) Renal calcification in the domestic cat. A morphological and x-ray diffraction study. *Pathol. Vet.* **4**, 120–136.

Moses, B.L. & Spaulding, G.L. (1985) Chronic bronchial disease of the cat. *Veterinary Clinics of North America.* **15**, 929.

Nash, A.S., Wright, N.G., Spencer, A.J., Thompson, H. & Fisher, E.W. (1979) Nephrotic syndrome in the cat. *Vet. Record.* **105**, 71.

Nelson, R.W. & Fellman, E.C. (1988) Spontaneous hyperadrenocorticism in cats. 6 cases (1978–1986) *J. Am. Vet. Med. Assoc.* **193**, 245–250.

Olmstead, M.L. & Butler, H.C. (1977) Five-hydroxytryptamine antagonists and feline aortic embolism *J. Small. Anim. Pract.* **18**, 247.

Paasch, L.H. & Zook, B.C. (1980) The pathogenesis of endocardial fibroelastosis in Burmese cats. *Lab Investigation.* **42**, 187.

Palmer, G.H. (1980) Feline upper respiratory disease. A review. *Vet. Med. Small Anim. Clin.* **75**, 1156–1158.

Pechman, R.D. (1985) Newer knowledge of feline bronchopulmonary disease. *Veterinary Clinics of North America. (S.A. Pract.)* **14** (5), 1007–1019.

Petersen, M.E., Greco, D.S. & Orth, D.N. (1989) Primary hypoadrenocorticism in ten cats. *J. Vet. Int. Med.* **3** (2), 55–58.

Pion, P.D., Kittleson, M.D., Rogers, Q.R. & Morris J.G. (1987) Myocardial failure in cats associated with low plasma taurine: a reversible cardiomyopathy. *Science* **237** (4816), 764–768.

Prasse, K.W., Mahaffey, E.A. & Denovo R. (1982) Chronic lymphocytic cholangitis in three cats. *Vet. Path.* **19**, 99.

Rogers, W.A., Bishop, S.P. & Rohovsky M.W. (1971) Pulmonary artery medial hypertrophy and hyperplasia in conventional and specific pathogen free cats. *Am. J. Vet. Res.* **32**, 767.

Sherding, R. (1979) Pyothorax in the cat. *Compend. Cont. Ed. Pract. Vet.* **1**, 247–253.

Tams, T.R. (1985) Aspiration pneumonia and complications of inhalation of smoke and toxic gases. *Vet. Clin. N. Am.* **15**, 971.

Thornburg, L.P., Simpson, S. & Diglio, K. (1982) Fatty liver syndrome in cats. *J. Am. Anim. Hosp. Ass.* **18**, 397–400.

Turk, J.R. & Root, C.R. (1983) Necropsy of the canine heart: A simple technique for quantifying ventricular hypertrophy and valvular alterations. *Compend. Contin. Education* **11**, 905–910.

Van Mierop, L.S.H. (1970) Pathology and pathogenesis of the common cardiac malformations. *Cardiovascular Clin.* **2**, 28.

Van Vleet, J.F., Ferrnas, V.J. & Weirich, W.E. (1980) Pathologic alterations in hypertrophic and congestive cardiomyopathy of cats. *Am. J. Vet. Res.* **41**, 2037.

Wardley, R.C. & Povey, R.C. (1977) The pathology and

sites of persistence associated with three different strains of feline calicivirus. *Res. Vet. Sci.* **23**, 15–19.

Westermark, P., Wernstedt, C., O'Brien, T.D., Hayden, D.W. & Johnson, K.H. (1987) Islet amyloid in type II human diabetes mellitus and adult diabetic cats contain a novel putative polypeptide hormone. *Am. J. Pathol.* **127**, 414.

Wright, N.G., Nash, A.S., Thompson, H. & Fisher E.W. (1981) Membranous nephropathy and follow up of 16 cases. *Lab. Investigation* **45**, 269–277.

Yano, B.L., Hayden, D.W. & Johnson, K.A. (1981) Feline insular amyloid: Association with diabetes mellitus. *Vet. Pathol* **18**, 621.

L.W. Hall

5
Handling and Restraint

Introduction

It is to be regretted that all too often cats are regarded as opponents to be forcibly subdued so that the most undignified and painful procedures can be performed on them without retaliatory damage being inflicted on the veterinarian. There can be no doubt that when provoked by rough, unsympathetic handling, cats may be formidable adversaries. Their teeth are razor sharp and their mouths often harbour organisms (e.g. *Pasteurella* species) that are pathogenic for man and cause very unpleasant sepsis in anyone unfortunate enough to be bitten. A cat's claws are admirably suited to removing slivers of human skin and subcutaneous tissue from anyone attempting to restrain the cat against its will. These claws are on four paws that can move incredibly fast and an apparently placid cat can turn in the space of almost milliseconds into a biting scratching creature struggling vigorously to evade all restraint.

The cat also has a quite amazing ability to sense insecurity in its handlers; this ability may result in it becoming apprehensive and very uncooperative. It may also have had a previous unpleasant experience when being handled by a veterinarian. Fortunately for the clinician, most pet cats respond extremely well to gentle persuasion and minimal physical restraint imposed by a relaxed person who is not anticipating trouble he or she is not capable of handling in a quiet, competent way. Petting the animal, speaking to it in a relaxed, quiet manner, calling it by its name and avoiding sudden movements of the hands will usually ensure its tolerance if not active co-operation. Thus, the expert feline anaesthetist seldom uses force and avoids violent conflict with the animal, thereby ensuring that the cat will not develop fearful or hostile reactions to all veterinary procedures and will at least tolerate, even if not actually co-operate, in its treatment.

Cat scratch disease is a well known hazard of feline practice although its aetiology seems still to be rather uncertain. Rather more than 58 papers, clinical reports and articles have been published on 'cat scratch fever' or 'cat scratch disease' in the past 20 years and a good review of the literature has been published by Shinall (1990). More recently, Zangwill *et al.* (1993) claim to have identified the causal organism as *Rochalimaea henselae* or a closely related organism. This organism is genetically similar to the Bartonellaceae family (Welch *et al.*, 1992; Regenery *et al.*, 1992a,b) and because *Bartonella bacillformis* is transmitted by the sandfly and another *Rochalimaea* species known to cause human disease, *R. quintana* (trench fever), is transmitted by lice, Zangwill *et al.* propose that arthropods may play a part in cat scratch disease. They also claim, from their data on the seroprevalence of *R. henselae*, that cats may frequently be infected with *Rochalimaea* or a related organism and that, at least in Connecticut, USA, ownership of a kitten is the risk factor most strongly associated with the development of cat scratch disease. In man, the spectrum of illness ranges from mild self-limited adenopathy to severe systemic disease – hepatosplenomegaly, encephalopathy, osteolytic lesions, splenic abscesses, mediastinal masses and neuroretinitis (Ulrich *et al.*, 1992). Gentamycin treatment is said to be effective in most cases (Lewis & Wallace, 1991).

Cat scratch disease is a much more serious condition in HIV (human immunodeficiency virus) positive subjects (Arlet & Perol, 1990) and, since there is no way of knowing whether an owner or animal attendants may be HIV positive, it is clear that today extreme care needs to be taken to avoid situations where cats may scratch or bite those handling them for examination or treatment.

In countries where rabies is endemic and both the history and the immunological status of an obviously excited or resentful cat may be unknown, there is a often a desire on the part of the veterinarian to don thick leather gauntlets before attempting to grasp the animal. It must be recognized, however, that wearing thick leather gloves makes grasping a struggling cat much less easy, the cat can often wriggle free, and a partially restrained cat may successfully attack an unprotected part of the handler's body. In such potentially dangerous situations the use of a crush cage or chemical restraint administered without actually having to handle the cat is much to be preferred to the use of thick handling gloves.

Removal of Cats From Transport Cages and Baskets

The majority of cats are presented for treatment after transportation in a travel cage, basket or box. This travel container may be made of wire mesh, hard impervious plastic or, in the case of disposable types, stiff cardboard. The design of the cage or basket is important and often not enough thought is given to their design. It is usually much easier to remove a cat from a basket that incorporates a hinged lid or at least one that can be opened up. It can be very difficult to remove a recalcitrant cat from a container that has only an end door or opening.

Cats vary in their reaction to being confined in a cage. Some are eager to escape from confinement and try to emerge as soon as the cage is opened, others are reluctant to leave, crouch down and resist removal. Thus, the first problem facing the anaesthetist is usually the removal of the patient from the container without allowing it to escape or causing excitement or fear. This can be very simple or very difficult, depending on the temperament of the cat and the design of the basket or cage.

After ensuring that there are no escape routes from the room by shutting all doors, windows, etc., the best procedure for removing a cat from a cage with a lid or top opening is to raise the lid or open it just enough to allow the confident, but cautious, insertion of a hand to stroke the cat's head. The animal's reaction to this initial approach is easily ascertained and this determines the subsequent actions of the owner, nurse or anaesthetist.

Most pet cats respond to this initial approach in a friendly manner and the cage lid or opening can be fully opened while the hand is kept on the cat's head or neck. The hand can then be slid

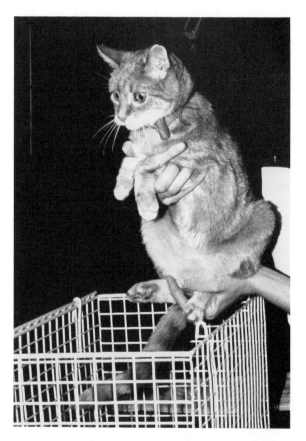

Fig. 5.1 Lifting a placid cat from a top-opening cage or basket. The fingers of one hand are entwined between the cat's fore legs while the other hand supports the weight of the cat and at the same time restrains the hind limbs and the tail. Speaking to the cat quietly and calmly does much to maintain the cat's confidence in the handler.

around to under the cat's thorax while the fingers are entwined between the fore legs. The other hand may next be introduced into the cage so that its palm is on the tail with its fingers between the hind limbs; the cat may then be gently lifted from the cage (Fig. 5.1) and placed on a table. Sometimes the cat's claws will retain their hold on bedding or paper lining the floor of the cage and if the cat does not release its hold spontaneously the claws will need to be gently disengaged. The importance of a gentle, reassuring approach to the whole procedure as an aid to the smooth induction of general anaesthesia or the administration of premedication cannot be over-emphasized.

If the cat's response to the initial approach is not obviously friendly, the hand introduced into the cage should gently grasp the scruff of the cat's neck but, except in obviously aggressive animals, no attempt should be made to lift the cat from the container by the scruff. The other hand should be introduced as with friendly cats and used to support the weight of the cat as it is taken from the container (Fig. 5.2), the fingers again being used to prevent movement of the cat's front paws. When carrying even an apparently friendly, calm cat it is advisable to maintain a gentle grip on the skin on the scruff of the neck so that instant firm restraint can be applied if some stimulus causes the cat to panic or struggle. It is always important to ensure that the weight of the animal is supported from beneath as shown in Fig. 5.3.

An aggressive response to the initial approach as shown by hissing or spitting should encourage a firm grasp to be taken on the scruff of the

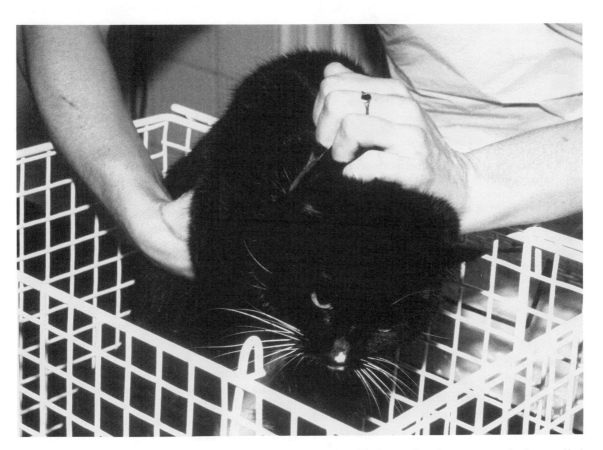

Fig. 5.2 When the handler is not sure of the cat's nature it is advisable for one hand to grasp gently the scruff of the neck as the cat is removed from the cage or basket. The other hand should be used to support the weight of the cat and to restrain the fore limbs.

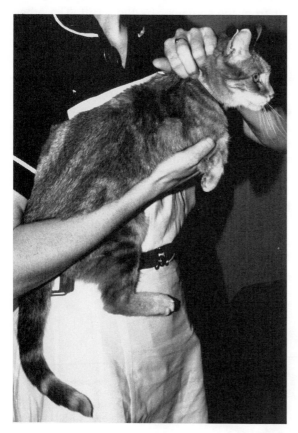

Fig. 5.3 Cats are always best transported in a wire mesh carrying cage but if one is not available, or to transfer the cat from the carrying cage to a table or a kennel, the weight of the animal should be taken on the fore arm, pressing the cat gently into the body. The cat's fore limbs should be restrained by the fingers of this hand while the other hand exerts gentle control from a light grip on the scruff of the neck.

neck – and only one attempt at this may be possible without the risk of injury to the nurse or anaesthetist. The cat should be lifted from the container by this hand and the hind legs secured as soon as possible with the other hand approaching from behind the legs and out of reach of the cat's claws. It is wise to remember that a firm grip on the scruff of the neck does not preclude the infliction of considerable damage

on that gripping hand and arm by unrestrained hind-limb claws.

Should the cat show violent resentment when a hand is introduced into the cage it is generally safer to abandon attempts to remove it from the cage before it is anaesthetized but, if one is available, it may be possible to manipulate the carrying cage in such a manner that the cat moves into a crush cage where it can be pressed against the front of this cage for the administration of parenteral drugs (Fig. 5.4) with no danger to the administrator. Escape of the cat into the room during the transfer manoeuvre is always a risk and for this reason many prefer to enclose the carrying cage in a transparent bag and introduce volatile anaesthetic agents volatilized in a stream of oxygen until the cat loses consciousness. This method of administering volatile anaesthetics is probably the method of choice for anaesthesia of totally unhandleable or feral cats but the scavenging of waste gases is difficult so the procedure is best performed out-of-doors.

Removing a cat from a front-opening cage or basket can present problems, for even placid cats may retreat to the furthest end and use their claws to prevent being dragged out by whatever part may be grasped by a hand introduced through the cage opening. Raising the far end of the basket and shaking it gently may encourage the cat to emerge voluntarily but sometimes even violent shaking will fail to produce the desired effect and recourse will have to be taken to grasping the cat by the scruff of the neck and forcibly withdrawing it (often accompanied by its bedding) from the basket or cage – a procedure which can almost be guaranteed to upset even a friendly, placid cat. With unfriendly or vicious cats the hand introduced into the cage is very vulnerable to injury by both claws and teeth of the cat. Again, enclosing the cage or basket in a transparent plastic bag and anaesthetizing the cat prior to removal by introducing a volatile anaesthetic agent into the bag may be the only safe, atraumatic method of extracting the cat from what it obviously regards as its lair.

Restraint for Pre-anaesthetic Examination

The assistance of a trained nurse for restraint of the cat during the pre-anaesthetic examination can be most helpful but this is not always possible and, indeed, many veterinarians prefer to work without assistance.

It is most important to avoid exciting or frightening the cat to avoid spurious observations of pulse and respiratory rates. In general, this is best accomplished by allowing the cat moderate freedom of movement thus giving it the impression that it is not being subjected to any restraint. When carrying out the examina-tion, the examiner should allow the cat to move around a very restricted area of the table top but ensure that his or her hands are always in contact with the cat's body, stroking it and gently deflecting the animal from any attempt to escape or explore other regions of the table. Any sudden violent movements can usually be anticipated and countered appropriately if this hand contact is continuously maintained. A skilled examiner usually has no difficulty in measuring the body temperature by the inser-tion of a well lubricated rectal thermometer when a cat is handled in this manner.

Obviously, vicious cats need firmer handling and the assistance of a trained nurse can be essential if a thorough pre-anaesthetic examina-

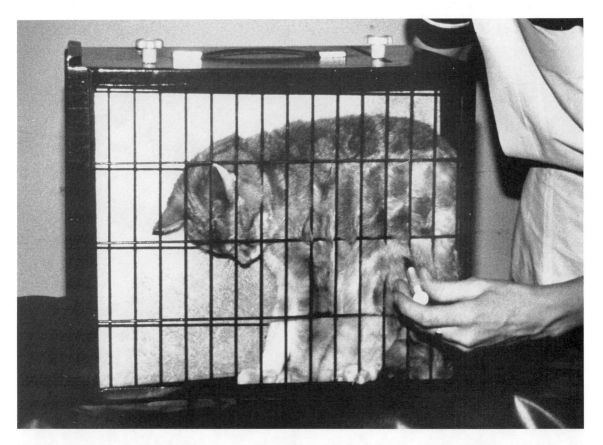

Fig. 5.4 Wild, vicious, unhandleable cats can be restrained in a crush cage to enable injections to be made without danger to the handler. Once the cat is transferred to this cage, the back of it is pushed in and locked in a position to press the cat tightly against the wire mesh front of the cage. The procedure usually enrages the cat and it is best to release the pressure and leave the cat in the crush cage until any sedative drug administered has taken effect.

tion is to be carried out. Feral cats can usually only be examined visually by inspection whilst in a cage if violent confrontations are to be avoided.

Clipping over the site of future venepuncture may be carried out at the conclusion of the examination. Clippers should be started and the cat allowed to become accustomed to their noise before attempting to clip the hair.

Restraint for the Administration of Drugs

Once transfer to the table has been affected the cat should be pressed gently but firmly down on to the surface by the hand on the scruff of the neck and pressure on the hind end by the other hand (Fig. 5.5) so that parenteral drugs can be administered. Even with reasonably placid cats restraint on the table top in this way may be necessary for drug injections, although subcutaneous injections between the shoulder blades can often be made with minimal restraint (Fig. 5.6). An alternative method for intramuscular injection into the vastus muscles that may be useful for the more difficult cat is shown in Fig. 5.7.

When the restrained cat has been given premedication, or a parenterally administered anaesthetic, outside of a cage or basket it should be returned whilst the drug takes effect. This should be done as gently as possible and the animal left undisturbed by bright lights or loud noises in its immediate vicinity, but it is most

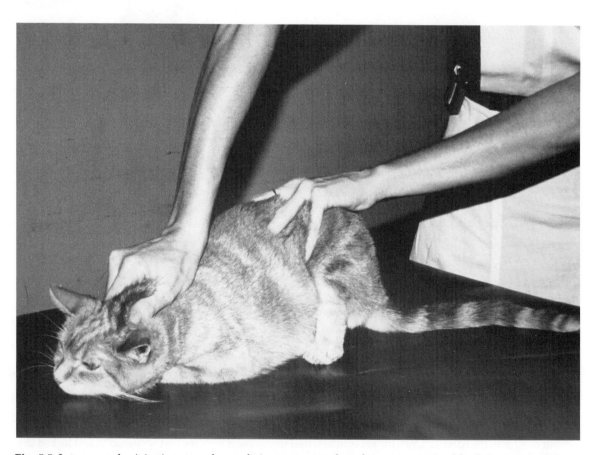

Fig. 5.5 Intramuscular injections may be made in most cats when they are restrained by being pressed down on the table. Handling needs to be firm for if the hind limbs are allowed any movement their claws can inflict scratches on the hand holding the scruff of the neck.

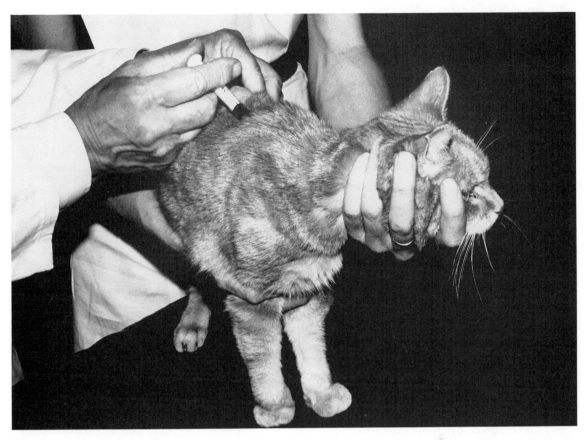

Fig. 5.6 In most pet cats subcutaneous injections can be made in the region between the shoulder blades with only minimal restraint of the animal.

important to keep the cat under observation for it may collapse unconscious against the cage or basket wall in such a way as to flex its head on its neck and obstruct its airway.

Restraint for the Induction of Anaesthesia

The most controllable way of inducing anaesthesia is undoubtedly by the intravenous administration of an anaesthetic drug such as thiopentone, thiamylal, propofol or 'Saffan' (see Chapter 8). This usually causes no problems for the anaesthetist, especially if sedative premedication has been given. Most intravenous injections are made into the cephalic vein but some anaesthetists prefer the femoral vein. As a result of the thin skin over these veins they are easily visible if the overlying hair is clipped. If clipping causes the cat to become upset it should be allowed time to regain its composure before being restrained for the intravenous injection.

The minimum of restraint usually suffices for injections into the cephalic vein (Fig. 5.8). The animal is placed in a sitting position on a table of convenient height and for injection into the right cephalic vein the nurse stands on the left side of the cat raising and supporting its head between the thumb and fingers of the left hand. In this position the nurse can usually keep the animal's attention away from the venepuncture site by gently tickling below its ears. The nurse's right hand is placed so that the middle, third and fourth fingers are behind the olecranon and the thumb is around the front of the right fore

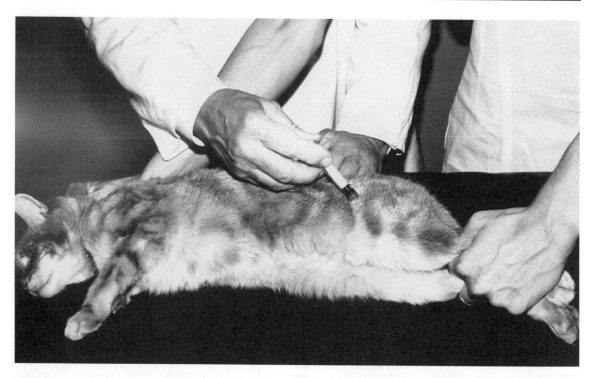

Fig. 5.7 An alternative way of restraining a cat for an intramuscular injection into the vastus muscles is to stretch it on its side by holding the nape of the neck while drawing the hind limbs as far backwards as possible. Depending on the nature of the cat and its reaction to the injection, it may be advisable not to release the grip on the cat until it has been replaced in a cage or kennel.

limb. The limb is extended by gently pushing on the olecranon and the vein is raised by gentle pressure with the thumb. The limb must not be held in a vice-like grip because this can cut off the arterial supply and, in any case, distresses the cat.

It is most important that the needle should be sharp (and modern, disposable needles are) and of minimum bore. A 25 G needle about 1.5 cm long is probably ideal for intravenous injections in cats and it should be introduced through the skin and into the vein in one smooth continuous movement without any stabbing motion. Intravenous catheterization is described in Chapter 8.

Should it become obvious that more restraint is needed to enable venepuncture to be carried out, the nurse can provide this rapidly by squeezing the cat between the right arm and body while preventing use of its hind-limb claws by pressing the cat firmly on to the surface of the table. The cat's head needs no

more restraint than to be held firmly in the nurse's left hand. Cats with active front and hind limbs may be restrained by being confined in a blanket (Fig. 5.9) which is less confining than a cat bag, but which allows greater freedom for exposure of one limb. Should even this amount of restraint be insufficient for successful venepuncture, it is probably best to abandon attempts at intravenous injection until an appropriate intramuscular premedication has had time to take effect, or to induce anaesthesia by other means.

Restraint for injection into the femoral, saphenous or medial section of the recurrent tarsal vein (see Chapter 1) is shown in Fig. 5.10 and it will be obvious that this site of venepuncture can only be used in fully conscious animals without provoking resentment in quiet, easily handled cats. The cat is held in a similar manner without raising the upper hind leg for injection into the recurrent karsel vein on the lateral

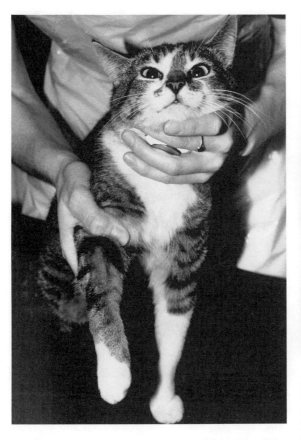

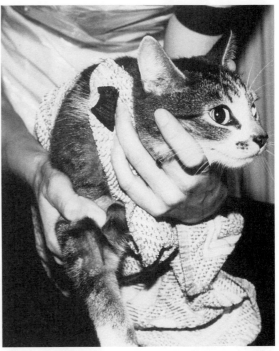

Fig. 5.9 Restless, but generally good-natured cats can be confined in a blanket wrapped around the head end of the body. This will protect the nurse from injury due to sudden, unexpected, escape-directed, movement of the cat.

Fig. 5.8 Restraint for venepuncture using the right cephalic vein. For most cats, provided a sharp, fine bore needle is used and the operator is skilled, only the minimum of restraint is necessary. For injection into the right cephalic vein the nurse usually stands on the left side of the cat, supporting its head between the thumb and fingers of the left hand. The nurse's right hand is placed so that the middle, third and fourth fingers are behind the cat's olecranon and the thumb is around the front of the limb to exert gentle pressure to raise the vein. The nurse's right fore arm can then be used to press the cat's body gently into his or her body. It is most important for the nurse not to grip the cat's limb in a vice-like manner and the more secure the cat can be made to feel by body contact, the less likely is it to become distressed by venepuncture.

aspect of the limb. It is helpful if a second assistant holds the limb in extension and raises the vein by pressure in the popliteal region. The jugular vein is particularly useful for the administration of intravenous fluid therapy and when comparatively large blood samples

are needed for diagnostic or other purposes. Injection into the jugular vein can be made in conscious, anaesthetized, sedated or moribund cats. Conscious cats may be held in a sitting position with the head extended on the neck while the vein is raised by applying gentle pressure over the jugular vein at the thoracic inlet. The nurse restrains the fore limbs of the cat and keeps its body pressed gently into her own body. It may help to envelop the cat in a blanket held over its back and around the base of the neck so that only the head and neck are exposed. Cat bags which have a draw string at one end may also be used to reduce the likelihood of injury to the nurse, the cat being completely enveloped in the bag with only its head and neck exposed. Sedated, anaesthetized or moribund animals are placed in lateral recumbency with the head over a small sandbag or pad, the fore limbs are stretched caudally and the uppermost jugular vein raised by applying

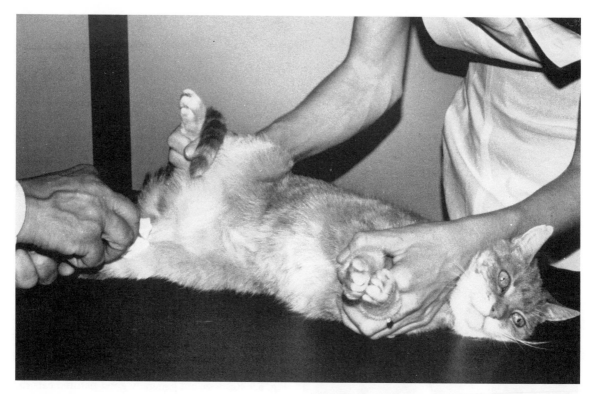

Fig. 5.10 The femoral vein is usually only used when no other small superficial veins are patent. The cat is restrained on its side and often two nurses are needed to restrain the cat in this position and to raise its vein, even when it is amenable to being held in this position. The same position is used for injection into the more distal sapheneous vein and the medial section of the recurrent tarsal vein.

thumb pressure in the jugular groove near to the thoracic inlet. For jugular venepuncture carried out to permit the intravous administration of drugs or fluids, needles should be avoided and, instead, a catheter should be introduced (see Chapter 8). Jugular venepuncture can be performed in many fully conscious cats restrained on their back over the seated nurse's lap (Fig. 5.11). Although the cat may struggle when first placed in this position most soon cease to wriggle and lie quietly while the nurse raises the jugular vein with one finger to enable venepuncture to be carried out on the distended vein.

Inhalation Induction of Anaesthesia

The fit, unsedated cat strongly resents attempts to induce anaesthesia with inhalation agents

given through a face-mask by unskilled practitioners. The skilled anaesthetist, by giving a flow of first nitrous oxide, followed by a potent anaesthetic agent (halothane, isoflurane), through a face-mask not closely applied to the cat's face can induce anaesthesia in an animal restrained in a similar manner as for the induction of anaesthesia with an intravenous agent. By speaking soothing words to the cat as the concentration of the inhaled anaesthetic is increased every third or fourth breath until the safe maximum is obtained, a very quiet, safe induction of anaesthesia is possible in some tractable animals. However, many cats resent the enforced breathing of anaesthetic agents such as halothane or isoflurane and will struggle against the restraint being employed, becoming excited and increasing the risks associated with anaesthetic induction.

For most animals the induction of anaesthesia with an inhalation agent is best carried out in an

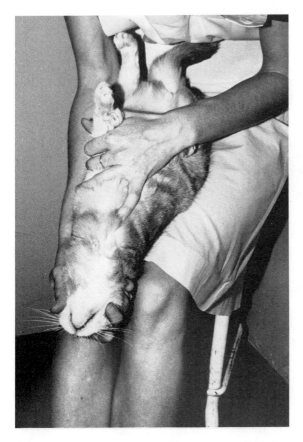

Fig. 5.11 Jugular venepuncture is often possible with the cat restrained on its back between the seated handler's thighs. Although the cat may show initial resentment at being placed in this position most soon settle, will lie quietly for some minutes and not react vigorously to venepuncture.

induction chamber (Fig. 5.12). Provided that (1) the cat can see through the walls of the chamber, and (2) that the potent inhalation agents are introduced gradually, induction of anaesthesia is quiet and uneventful. Any forcible restraint is thus avoided.

Restraint for Endotracheal Intubation

Intubation is performed under direct vision as soon as the jaw muscles are relaxed by general anaesthesia or the effects of a neuromuscular blocking agent. A skilled anaesthetist can pass

an endotracheal tube into the trachea with the unconscious cat in almost any position. However, a laryngoscope or illuminated tongue depressor is needed to expose the glottic opening and there is a critical manouvre in the use of this instrument which is best learned when the cat is held supine. This essential manouvre, which must be learned for maximum exposure of the glottis, is the necessity of *lifting* the lower jaw with the instrument in a direction parallel to the hard palate. Using the laryngoscope blade or tongue depressor as a lever to depress the tongue and to open the mouth fails to give such good exposure of the vocal cords and risks damaging the cat's incisor teeth.

The head of the supine cat is extended on the neck by placing a small sandbag under the neck, or by an assistant supporting the head with a hand placed beneath the neck, and the tongue is pulled out of the mouth, taking care not to injure it with the teeth. A standard human-type laryngoscope with an infant-sized blade, or a small tongue depressor, is introduced and the tip of the blade positioned over the dorsum of the tongue so that it rests just in front of the epiglottis. The instrument is then lifted while the upper jaw is held fixed by an assistant or by fingers of the anaesthetist's hand. This exposes the glottis, giving a good view of the vocal cords (Fig. 5.13) and by avoiding touching of the surface of the epiglottis reduces any tendency for laryngeal spasm to be provoked by the laryngoscopic exposure. The endotracheal tube may be passed, under direct vision, between the relaxed vocal cords.

In cases where regurgitation of stomach contents is a possibility, endotracheal intubation is usually performed with the cat in a prone position, its head and neck being held well above the level of the remainder of the body. Some anaesthetists prefer to intubate these cats with the cat held in a sitting position although this runs the risk of giving rise to cerebral ischaemia in hypovolaemic subjects and/or when the circulatory system is very depressed by deep anaesthesia. Maximum exposure of the glottis is again only possible when the laryngoscope or tongue depressor is used in the correct manner, avoiding contact with the dorsal surface of the epiglottis. The likelihood of using

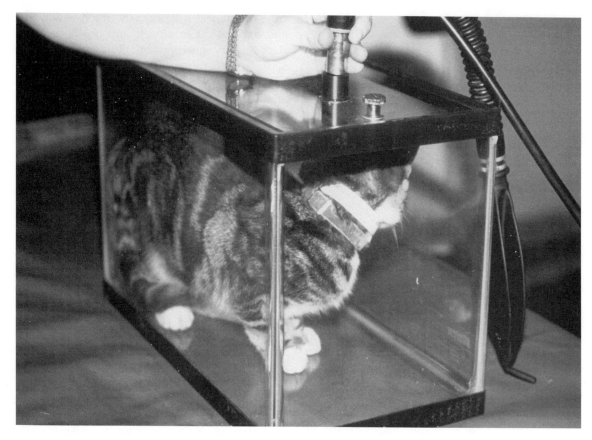

Fig. 5.12 (a) A box with transparent walls for the induction of inhalation anaesthesia. Provided the inhalation agent (volatilized in a stream of oxygen or air) is not introduced suddenly into the box in too high a concentration, cats usually show no excitement as consciousness is lost. It is most important to remove the cat from the box as soon as it becomes relaxed under the influence of the anaesthetic (b).

incorrect technique for laryngoscopy is greatest when the cat is in lateral recumbency for there is a great temptation to lever the jaws apart with the instrument used, with consequent increased risk of damage or dislodgement of teeth and failure to obtain optimal exposure of the vocal cords (see Chapter 12).

Restraint of Sedated or Anaesthetized Cats

Sedated cats cannot always be relied upon not to move at the crucial moment during radiographic and other examinations and anaesthetized cats often have to be positioned in unnatural postures. To eliminate the risk to personnel who would otherwise be needed to hold cats for radiographic procedures long, incompletely filled sandbags are very useful. By suitable twisting of the bag the sand-free portion can be applied to the cat while the filled, and therefore heavy, ends maintain restraint in the desired position (Fig. 5.14).

Capture of Feral Cats

The humane capture of feral cats can present difficulties. The most obvious technique is to use food to lure the cat into a trap-box which springs shut when the cat is inside to take the

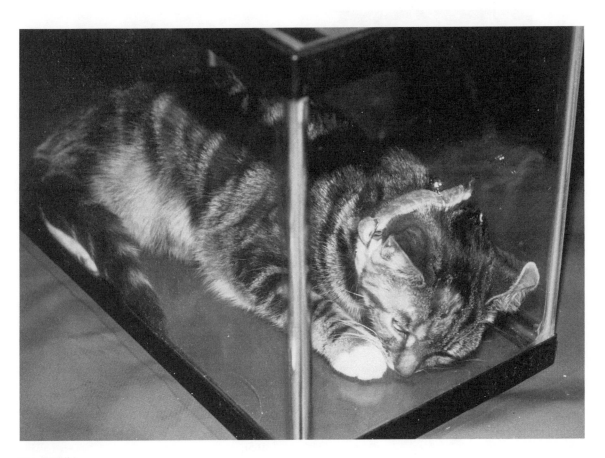

Fig. 5.12(b)

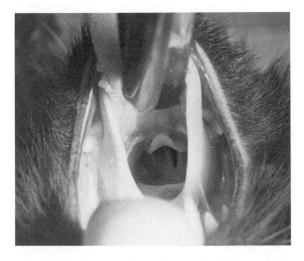

Fig. 5.13 Exposure of the larynx by lifting of the laryngoscope blade. (From Fig. 16.2 in *Veterinary Anaesthesia*, 9th edn, 1991: Hall & Clarke. By permission).

bait. However, cats are very loath to enter any form of closed container and it is most important that, as in the case of anaesthetic induction boxes, the walls of the trap are transparent. It appears that provided the cat senses that it has all round vision it feels secure enough to enter a trap of this nature. A coypu trap, as used by officers of the Royal Society for the Prevention of Cruelty to Animals (RSPCA) meets the necessary criteria for trapping cats and cats will enter them quite freely. The food bait is placed near the back wall and cats will often continue to eat, seemingly unaware (or at least apparently unconcerned) that the front of the trap has sprung closed (Jepson, 1993 personal communication).

Often it is desirable to capture a queen nursing a litter and once the queen has been captured, provided the location of the nest is known it is usually a simple matter to apprehend the individual members of the litter.

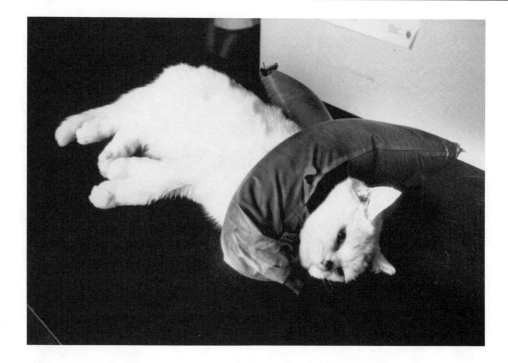

Fig. 5.14 Use of a long partially filled sand bag for restraint of the sedated cat for radiographic examination.

References

Arlet, G. & Pero, Y. (1990) Cat-scratch disease bacteria. *Nouvelle Revue Française d'Hematologie* **32**, 461–463.

Lewis, D.E. & Wallace, M.R. (1991) Treatment of adult systemic cat scratch disease with gentamycin sulfate. *West. J. Med.* **154**, 330–331.

Regnery, R.L., Anderson, B.E., Clarridge, J.E. III, Rodriguez-Barradas, M.C., Jones, D.C. & Carr, J.H. (1992a) Characterization of a novel *Rochalimaea* species, *R. henselae* sp. nov., isolated from blood of a febrile, human immunodeficiency virus-positive patient. *J. Clinic. Microbiol.* **30**, 265–274.

Regnery, R.L., Olson, J.G., Perkins, B.A. & Bibb, W. (1992b) Serological response to 'Rochalimaea henselae' antigen in suspected cat-scratch disease. *Lancet* **339**, 1443–1445.

Shinall, E.A. (1990) Cat-scratch disease: a review of the literature. *Paediat.–Dermatol.* **7**, 11–18. (Erratum **7**, 165).

Ulrich, G.G., Waecker, N.J. Jr, Meister, S.J., Peterson, T.J. & Hooper, D.G. (1992) Cat scratch disease associated with neuroretinitis in a 6-year-old girl. *Ophthalmology* **99**, 246–249.

Welch, D.F., Pickett, D.A., Slater, L.N., Steigerwalt, A.G. & Brenner, D.J. (1992) *Rochalimaea henselae* sp. nov., a cause of septicemia bacillary angiomatosis and parenchymal bacillary peliosis. *J. Clinic. Microbiol.* **30**, 275–280.

Zangwill, K.M., Hamilton, D.H., Perkins, B.A., Regnery, R.L., Plikaytis, B.D., Hadler, J.L., Cartter, M.L. & Wenger, J.D. (1993) Cat scratch disease in Connecticut: epidemiology, risk factors and evaluation of a new diagnostic test. *New England J. Med.* **329**, 8–13.

6
Pre-operative Assessment

Introduction

Evaluation of a cat's condition before anaesthesia should provide the clinician with the pertinent data to allow planning for further diagnostic evaluation, general patient care and perioperative management. It should assist in developing the best anaesthetic management for the individual concerned. This initial evaluation considers both history and physical examination. Cats are more difficult to assess in a strange environment than some other species, so in many situations the owner's comments become critical. The relevant details noted from this cursory examination will direct the clinician to further questions and tests that may be required to achieve a complete assessment.

Choices to be made in devising the best anaesthetic technique to use include which drugs to use, their precise dosage and the route of administration. Preoperative and intra-operative supportive treatment needs to be determined. The type of intra-operative monitoring best suited to the case is an important consideration at this stage. Postoperative care will be planned around both the individual's initial condition and the procedure to be carried out. Valuable time is saved and patient care improved through these preliminary deliberations. Minor adjustments to these initial plans can easily and quickly be made as required if conditions change, avoiding delay in patient progress.

Whenever possible cats should have food withheld for 8–12 h prior to anaesthesia. This precaution should reduce the chance of vomiting in the perioperative period and the associated concern of aspiration. Water is usually freely available before anaesthesia. This is especially important in the older cat

that may be very dependent on this supply to maintain fluid balance. In very young animals (less than 3 weeks) a much shorter period of starvation of 1–2 h is recommended. Kittens left with the dam almost until anaesthesia is induced are unlikely to suddenly gorge themselves just before induction. If surgery and anaesthesia are delayed, the animal should be fed rather than left without food for a prolonged period.

Healthy, Young Patients Requiring Routine Surgery

The history and physical examination will determine the group that actually fits this description. The appointment book notation, 'Castration — 1 year old cat', is not adequate to define the health of the patient and thus the reduced risk that is involved with anaesthesia of this group. Owners will assume that their cat fits this group and that no risk at all would be involved. Client communication becomes very important before the cat is admitted for surgery.

The clinician should begin the examination by taking a history in a logical manner. All relevant information warrants recording immediately. A checklist will facilitate the process. Some basic questions will relate to basic detail about the patient such as age, sex, weight, breed, past and present environment, dietary history, worming treatments and vaccination status. Anaesthesia may be influenced by the answers to these questions by association with problems encountered with a particular breed (airway in the Persian), age (young animals have undeveloped ability to eliminate parenteral agents and may have congenital cardiac anomalies) and sex (duration and postoperative differences involved in neutering). Nutritional diseases may influence the physical management of patients with related skeletal disease and significantly affect the anaesthetic management of the cat with dilated cardiomyopathy (taurine deficiency). Early clinical signs may be vague and a suspicious dietary history should make the clinician delve deeper for a positive diagnosis before proceeding with elective surgery. The combination of environment, worming and vaccination status will dictate if delay in anaesthesia is necessary to prepare the patient for the stress of the surgery.

Inquiry should be made to identify any medical problems such as previous surgery, infections, any veterinary treatment, or general malaise. Current problems are considered in more detail. When vomiting or diarrhoea is routine for their cat, the owners may not volunteer this information. Asking specifically about appetite, water intake, urination, defecation, vomiting, weight loss or gain, ambulation, behaviour and activity will be more rewarding than a general question on the animal's health. Although the owner may not be aware of the exact anaesthetic drugs administered in the past, information relating to complications associated with previous anaesthesia will provide some warning. Closer attention to mild abnormalities in preoperative haematological values and conservative choices for drug and dosage should follow. Earlier uneventful anaesthesia provides greater reassurance for safe anaesthetic management.

During the history taking, it is of value to have observed the undisturbed cat examining the strange environment. Out of his cage, the cat may begin to relax. The physical examination that follows may actually determine vital parameters that have approached the patient's normal values. Others have described physical examination technique in excellent detail (Schaer, 1989) and only a brief outline is provided here to relate to the aspects significant to anaesthesia.

Respiration should be observed from a distance for a more realistic evaluation. The physical examination should begin with pulse palpation. The femoral artery is the easiest to feel and the pulse should be regular and strong. Acceptable rates in the cat vary up to 240 beats/min, with a true resting rate of 128 ± 17 beats/min (Tilley, 1985). This information is assimilated with the cardiac examination carried out later. While the temperature is taken, the time can be used to examine the skin and hair coat. Skin turgor should be assessed to determine the state of hydration, which will influence requirements for preoperative stabilization. The obese cat is more difficult to assess in this manner for hydration. Obesity will also affect drug dose demanding the calculation of lean weight to prevent overdosing. Some grossly obese cats will not breathe well and should not be expected to do so. Plans should be made to ventilate these obese cats to avoid hypercapnia if the anaesthesia is likely to last more than 30–60 min. The temperature should always be taken and recorded on the chart; this will also ensure that the thermometer has been removed. Elevated temperatures (39.4–40.5°C) may occur in normal excited cats (Schaer, 1989). This can be reassessed following the calming effects of premedication. Fever will increase anaesthetic demands, as well as being a sign of infectious or other disease.

The examination continues from the head, moving caudally in an organized fashion. Signs of respiratory disease should be noted; if present, the implications, including potential spread of infectious disease within the clinic, as well as the effect on the patient, must be considered. Significance to the cat prior to anaesthesia includes the effect of respiratory disease on oxygenation and the effect of anaesthesia's immune suppression on the course of the disease. The mouth should be assessed for ease of opening (as this relates to intubation), mucous membrane colour (anaemia, shock, degree of cyanosis if hypoxaemia suspected), capillary refill time (greater than 1 s in hypovolemia), and apparent clear airway (loose teeth, oral lesions or masses that could result in airway obstruction). At the same time the flexibility of the neck will have been determined (influencing positioning for intubation).

The thorax demands special attention considering the impact of disease here. Evaluate the respiratory effort and sounds. Infections,

Table 6.1 American Society of Anaesthesiologists patient status assessment

ASA 1	Healthy patient — elective surgery that is not required for the patient's well being
ASA 2	Mild systemic disease, no functional limitations — routine necessary surgery that would not cause any added risk to anaesthesia
ASA 3	Marked systemic disease, definite functional limitations — some underlying disease or condition present that may increase the risk of anaesthesia and complicate the choice of anaesthestic and the postoperative care of the patient
ASA 4	Severe systemic disease that is a constant threat to life — significant problems exist in this patient that obviously affects the safety and management of anaesthesia
ASA 5	Moribund patient unlikely to survive 24 h with or without the operation

Emergency anaesthesia and surgery increases the risk and an E is added to the above category. Inexperienced anaesthetists and surgeons also increase the risk.

allergic bronchitis, pleural effusions, diaphragmatic hernia, pneumothorax and consolidation may be suspected after careful auscultation. Simultaneous pulse palpation and auscultation will determine pulse deficits and arrhythmias that will require more detailed evaluation to diagnose the extent of cardiac disease. A murmur could point towards either anaemia or an anomaly. The younger cat may present with congenital anomalies or dilated cardiomyopathy.

The remainder of the examination will have little impact on anaesthesia in the apparently healthy cat.

Laboratory Tests

When no obvious medical problems are apparent from the history and physical examination, a small number of tests may be carried out to detect subclinical problems. Blood should be drawn for haematocrit, total protein and blood urea nitrogen. These are simple, rapid tests to perform on a few drops of blood. Mild dehydration may be suspected by small increases in the values. Concern that anaemia (compromising O_2 carrying capacity) and hypoproteinaemia (reducing the dose of barbiturates) may be present can be eliminated. Renal disease should be evaluated if blood urea nitrogen (BUN) is increased, although the specificity of this test is poor. In this case fluids may be considered for a procedure where they would normally not be used.

The cat that has passed this careful scrutiny can be considered healthy and thus classified as set out by the American Society of Anaesthe-

siologists (Table 6.1) to be ASA 1 (elective surgery that is not required for the patient's well being) or ASA 2 (routine required surgery that would not cause any added risk to the anaesthesia). In studies in people the risk of mortality related to patients in these categories, undergoing anaesthesia is from 1:5000 to 1:10 000 (Lunn & Mushin, 1982; Caplan, 1992). Veterinary anaesthesia carries a greater risk and cats may be more at risk than dogs as shown in the prospective study by Clark and Hall (1990). The incidence of mortality in dogs was 1:870, while mortality in cats of the same classification had an incidence of 1:552. Veterinarians asked to respond to a questionnaire recalled a lower incidence of mortality in cats (1:1667) than dogs (1:909) related to small animal anaesthesia (Dodman & Lamb, 1992). Owners should be made aware that a risk is present, even in the healthy patient, although they should also be assured that a thorough evaluation to detect hidden disease coupled with modern anaesthesia with conscientious monitoring is carried out on each patient to reduce the chance of problems arising. The owner should be asked to sign a form with some statement relating to informed consent to perform the anaesthesia and surgery. Proper communication will be assured by this step.

Geriatric Patients

These cats may also fall into the ASA 1 or 2 classification, but, more frequently than the first group, may be determined to be ASA 3 (some underlying disease or condition present that may increase the risk of anaesthesia and complicate the choice of anaesthesia and the postoperative care of the patient). Cats over 8 years of age should be considered geriatric and assessed accordingly due to the increased incidence of some conditions in this age group. The history should include questions on activity, appetite, urination and defecation to be sure that changes perceived by the owner are not missed due to an expectation of such change with age. A healthy, 15-year-old cat can retain kitten-like activity and appetite; the 10 year-old that has become finicky and lethargic over the last year requires close attention to determine if some subclinical disease process is responsible.

The physical examination should include palpation of the thyroid glands for enlargement associated with hyperthyroidism (commonly detected in cats over 8 years and significantly influencing the anaesthetic management). The mammary glands in female cats should be checked for lumps indicating neoplasia and thus the added concern that lung metastases may have developed. Extra time is warranted in the examination of the thorax, although this is an area that should not be shortchanged in any patient.

Laboratory tests are usually more extensive in the older patient due to the increasing incidence of organ disease with age. It may be prudent to divide this group into two, in consideration of the cost/benefit ratio of laboratory testing. The first group would be the older patient classified as ASA1 or 2 according to the history and physical examination. These cats would have the basic haematology and biochemistry performed with the addition of urinalysis if over 15 years or if the BUN was increased. The possibility of chronic compensated renal disease necessitates careful evaluation in all older cats. Approximately 8% of cats over 10 years of age and 15% of cats 15 years or greater were diagnosed with renal disease in one study completed during 1990 (Lulich *et al.*, 1992). The incidence of detection of renal disease in cats increased over the entire 10 years studied. If a urine sample can be obtained before the cat is anaesthetized measurement of urine specific

gravity, to indicate the degree of concentration, is the most helpful test to differentiate prerenal from renal azotaemia. Creatinine is less influenced than BUN by extrarenal disease and more reflective of glomeruler filtration. The first sign of renal failure, however, is the inability to concentrate urine. Cats are capable of concentrating urine to a greater degree than dogs and the specific gravity may rise to greater than 1.050 during shock or dehydration. Increased BUN in the presence of urine with specific gravity less than 1.040 suggests some degree of renal disease (Lulich *et al.*, 1992).

The owner can be requested to collect the urine samples; however, going to the considerable lengths sometimes needed to extract urine from conscious cats is probably not worthwhile and preoperative urinanalysis should be abandoned in such cases. Plasma electrolyte values should be assessed to determine if special supplements are required in any fluid therapy required when concentration is affected. Although liver enzymes are commonly assessed as well in this subgroup of cats, it is highly unlikely that the results would make a significant contribution to decisions on anaesthetic management if no overt signs were apparent and no suspicions raised on clinical examination.

Geriatric cats classified as ASA 3 on history and physical examination should be evaluated more thoroughly around the abnormality suspected. Whenever there is concern that renal disease is present, from a history of anorexia, weight loss and depression, BUN, creatinine, electrolytes and acid/base status, as well as urinalysis may be performed. Suspicion of pulmonary disease dictates that chest radiographs are taken. Cardiac abnormalities are further evaluated by examination of the electrocardiogram and by radiography. Haematology and biochemistry in this subgroup is best designed to cover the entire animal due to the interaction of disease processes on different organ systems. Table 6.2 shows the tests of interest to the anaesthetist that are included in a complete blood count and biochemical profile. Expected normals are shown, although some variation may occur between laboratories. The older patient with no significant clinical disease

Table 6.2 Acceptable values for a selection of feline haematology and clinical chemistry tests (Jacobs *et al.*, 1992). Other tests that can be done provide little information in the anaesthetic management of the cat.

Haemoglobin	80–150 g l
Haematocrit	0.24–0.45%
Erythrocytes	$5.0–10.0 \times 10^6/\mu l$
Total nucleated cell count	$5.5–15.4 \times 10^3 \mu l$
Segmented neutrophils	$2.5–12.5 \times 10^3/\mu l$
Band neutrophils	$0.0–0.3 \times 10^3/\mu$
Lymphocytes	$1.5–7.0 \times 10^3/\mu$
Monocytes	$0.0–0.85 \times 10^3/\mu l$
Eosinophils	$0.0–0.75 \times 10^3/\mu l$
Basophils	$0.0–0.2 \times 10^3/\mu l$
Platelets	$190–400 \times 10^3 \mu l$
Alanine aminotransferase	10–75 U/l
Albumin	25–39 g/l
Alkaline phosphatase	0–90 U/l
Total bilirubin	0–4 µmol l
Calcium	2.23–2.90 mmol/l
Total carbon dioxide	14–26 mmol/l
Chloride	112–129 mmol/l
Creatinine	75–180 µmol/l
Glucose	3.5–9.0 mmol/l
Gamma-glutamyl transferase	0–2 U/l
Phosphorus	1.03–2.82 mmol/l
Potassium	3.7–5.8 mmol/l
Total serum protein	60–82 g/l
Sodium	150–165 mmol/l
Urea	5.0–10.0 mmol/l

may have liver function tests slightly above the listed range.

Patients with Significant Disease

This group of patients would automatically be considered at least ASA 3 or ASA 4 (significant problems exist in this patient that obviously affect the safety and management of anaesthesia). Records made at admission or preliminary examination should clearly indicate these individuals. Special tests may be required as the disease dictates, along with a complete blood cell count and biochemical profile.

The most important step following this is not to jump immediately to selection of safe anaesthetics, but to stabilize the patient so that the anaesthetics chosen are naturally safer. The final step involves recognition and preparation for any complications that might arise related to the disease or condition. Preoperative preparation is as much for the clinician as for the patient. More precise detail of decisions about anaesthetic management for patients with specific disease is covered in Chapter 13.

A number of other conditions also influence the anaesthetic management and safety of the procedure. The traumatized cat is an example of many possible management complications. This animal may be in shock, requiring aggressive fluid therapy to replace at least 50% of the deficit in advance of anaesthesia. Fluid treatment is recommended at approximately 50 ml/kg/h allowing anaesthesia to take place within 1 h of starting fluid replacement in most circumstances. Injuries (incurred by the trauma may influence the physical handling of the patient (fractured mandible relating to ability to intubate, other injuries requiring analgesia in order to restrain the cat for induction). The injuries may influence the uptake of oxygen and inhalants, and the elimination of carbon dioxide (thoracic trauma). Cats may also be admitted in a dehydrated state requiring partial correction of fluid deficits in advance of anaesthesia. The risk of anaesthesia should be lessened dramatically if patients are no greater than 5% dehydrated.

Concurrent drug therapy in all patients should be considered with respect to any interaction with anaesthetic agents. Finally the surgery or diagnostic testing that is involved in the case may compromise the anaesthetic management. The cat requiring bronchoscopy may have a more difficult recovery due to laryngeal oedema, than would be expected with other procedures. The animal requiring confining bandages may require sedation so that they accept the confinement (e.g. after skin grafting) or monitoring closely postoperatively to ensure that no discomfort arises (e.g. airway obstruction associated with a tight neck bandage). Major abdominal or thoracic surgery may be associated with bleeding that demands monitoring and fluid replacement.

The Unapproachable Cat

Every practitioner encounters a cat in this category. This cat enters the hospital in its cage and cannot be removed until anaesthetized. The owners must provide information on the animal's health, but sometimes this is unknown to them. The classification of this animal should be considered worse than the best guess. The owner should be informed that there is difficulty insuring the most appropriate anaesthetic, considering the limitations on the examination. Following restraint with reasonably safe sedative drugs, some fundamental haematology or biochemistry can be carried out before proceeding further. There may be benefit in trying to achieve sedation and control first in the excessively stressed animal. Following this a calming period is allowed for the catecholamine levels to subside which may reduce the chance of cardiac arrest due to a fatal arrhythmia. Inhalant anaesthesia, especially halothane, can enhance the chance of arrhythmias. Whenever there is doubt regarding the health of the patient and whenever emergency circumstances demand less than ideal assessment and stabilization of the patient, the cat should be given the least depressive and easiest to eliminate anaesthetics or reversible drugs with provision of careful monitoring throughout. It is worth the extra expense and manpower to approach such cases in this manner.

References

Caplan, R.A. (1992) Adverse Outcome in Anesthetic practice: What are the data? Can outcome be improved? *ASA Refresher Course* **144**.

Clarke, K.W. & Hall, L.W. (1990) A survey of anaesthesia in small animal practice: AVA/BSAVA Report. *J. Ass. Vet. Anaesth.* **17**, 4.

Dodman, N.H. & Lamb, L.A. (1992) Survey of small animal anesthetic practice in Vermont. *JAAHA* **28**, 439.

Jacobs, R.M., Lumsden, J.H. & Vernau, W. (1992) Canine and feline reference values. In: *Current Veterinary Therapy XI* (ed. R.W. Kirk & J.D. Bonagura), p. 1250. W.B. Saunders, London.

Lulich, J.P., O'Brien, T., Osborne, C.A. & Polzin, D.J. (1992) Feline renal failure: questions, answers, questions. *Comp. Cont. Ed.* **14**, 127.

Lunn, J.N. & Mushin, W.W. (1982) Mortality associated with anaesthesia. *Anaesthesia* **37**, 856.

Schaer, M. (1989) The medical history, physical examination, and physical restraint. In: *The Cat. Diseases and Clinical Management* (ed. R.G. Shearing) p. 7. Churchill Livingstone, NY.

Tilley, L.P. (1985) *Essentials of Canine and Feline Electrocardiography*, 2nd edn. p. 203. Lea & Febiger, Philadelphia.

J.C. Brearley

7
Sedation, Premedication and Analgesia

Introduction

Sedation, premedication and postoperative analgesia are related by virtue of the drugs used. Many sedatives are used for premedication and postoperative analgesia can be achieved by the pre-operative use of analgesics. Analgesics often synergize with sedative drugs to produce a more profound sedation than would be achieved by use of either class of drug alone or the theoretical summation of the sedative effects of the drugs together.

Sedation

Sedation is often required to allow stress-free handling of the animal, radiography and minor procedures to be performed. Ideally the desired result is a conscious cat that is easy to handle without excessive restraint. The drugs used should have no detrimental effects on the cardiovascular or respiratory systems and should be relatively short acting, or have specific antagonists which may be used to terminate their sedative and other actions. Unfortunately, such a drug does not exist at the moment and so compromises must be made in the choice of agent(s).

The choice of drug or combination of drugs depends on the factors listed in Table 7.1. If profound sedation is required in an animal that is suffering from cardiovascular, respiratory or metabolic disorders then consideration should be given to general anaesthesia, as support of vital systems may be best achieved when the cat is anaesthetized. The depth of sedation required

Table 7.1 Factors determining choice of drugs for sedation

Factor	Example
Temperament of the animal	Calm Handled but dislikes restraint Unhandled
Reason for sedation	Non-invasive examination Blood sampling Radiography Minor surgery under local analgesia
State of health of the animal	Healthy Minor pathology Major pathology Life-threatening condition
Depth of sedation required	Mild – behaviour modification Moderate – slightly drowsy Profound – only slight responsiveness

to allow examination of a feral cat may border on general anaesthesia and physiological monitoring of an animal under this depth of sedation should be the same as that applied to an animal given a conventional general anaesthetic. Sedative drugs alter consciousness and reactivity, diminish protective reflexes such as coughing and the response to increased blood carbon dioxide tensions, and they depress the thermoregulatory centre.

The depth of sedation achieved at varying doses of individual drugs is discussed later in

Table 7.2 Possible desirable results from premedication

Reduce stress associated with restraint and induction of anaesthesia
Reduce side-effects of anaesthetic agents, e.g. salivation
Reduce dose requirement for anaesthetic agents
Smooth induction and recovery from anaesthesia
Specific premedications for specific conditions, e.g. propanolol

---

this chapter and suggestions of drug combinations are made.

Premedication

Premedication should be considered as part of the whole anaesthetic technique. Sedation may not always be required. Often an animal is sedated for the benefit of the veterinarian rather than the animal; that is, to make the procedure more straightforward for the handler rather than the animal. This requirement from a premedicant should be questioned rather than assumed. Table 7.2 gives some of the possible desired effects of premedication. Again, as with sedation, there is no single drug which will achieve all the possible desirable effects and hence drug combinations are often used.

With some sedative premedicants (e.g. ketamine) there may be a dose-related continuum with general anaesthesia; that is, low doses will produce sedation whilst larger doses will produce general anaesthesia. Other factors which should be taken into consideration are that reactions to drugs (in particular the potentially sedative agents) may differ between sick and healthy cats. A dose which does not make any appreciable difference to a healthy cat's behaviour may provide adequate sedation in a sick one. Diazepam is particularly renowned for this effect (Seeler, 1992).

Assessment of Pain and Pain Relief

The International Association for the Study of Pain (1979) defined pain as 'an unpleasant sensory and emotional experience associated with actual or potential tissue damage, or described in terms of damage'. Inherent in this definition is that pain is a subjective emotion experienced by an individual. Although the cat is often used as an experimental model for analgesia tests in which modification of neuronal electrical activity is elicited by noxious stimuli (e.g. Tomemori *et al.*, 1981), pain is not just electrical activity in a region of the central nervous system elicited by peripheral stimulation or tissue damage. This may be one aspect but it is not the whole story.

The cat generally only vocalizes when acute trauma is being inflicted or when the animal is in acute pain when being handled (Flecknell, 1987). The tone of vocalization is often different in this case to that of protest at being handled; the pitch is higher. In the more chronic situation a cat will often shun company, secreting itself in dark, quiet corners, appetite may disappear and grooming is no longer attempted. More aggressive behaviour is displayed when the animal is disturbed, for example hissing and growling, and in severe cases the cat may pant or display open mouth breathing. The impression that if a cat is purring it might be pain free, is false. Cats in profound discomfort will often continue to purr. This is a complex, semi-automatic response to being stroked or petted. Table 7.3 gives some aspects of feline behaviour which may reflect pain. Table 7.4 gives some of the physiological parameters which may change in pain. When both behaviour and physiological parameters are taken in association, some assessment of the degree of pain or discomfort may be made. If these parameters change towards the feline normal after the administration of an analgesic then the assumption that the cat was suffering pain or discomfort may be assumed to be correct.

A more objective means of monitoring pain is to attribute a pain score. This should be the sum

Table 7.3 Feline behaviour which may reflect pain

Changes in vocalization – acoustic frequency and
  pattern
Changes in activity
Appetite
Social behaviour – towards people, grooming
Stance

Table 7.4 Physiological parameters which change
during pain

Pulse – increase
Respiratory pattern – depends on source of pain:
  generally fast and shallow
Blood pressure – increases
Hormonal parameters – generally disrupted

Table 7.5 Suggested pain scoring in cats

Behaviour and appearance	
Staring coat, unwillingness to move, unsocial	3
Staring coat, unwillingness to move, sociable	2
Staring coat, willing to move, sociable	1
Good coat, willing to move, sociable	0
Appetite	
Totally inappetant	3
Will eat strong/favourite food with encouragement	2
Will eat favourite food voluntarily, but no other	1
Eating normally	0
Vocalization	
Vocal even when not approached	3
Vocal when touched	2
Vocal when surgical site touched/moved	1
Not vocal when surgical site strongly palpated	0
Total possible score	9
Intervention score	4/5

This scoring regime is only a suggestion and does not cover
all possible aspects; grooming and other behavioural
aspects are not covered.

of the scoring of various aspects of the animal's behaviour. It allows a means of monitoring, particularly postoperatively, and provides a more objective criteria for efficacy of an analgesic or for the repeated administration of analgesic drugs. A suggested method of pain scoring is given in Table 7.5.

As many of the analgesic drugs can be given as premedication, all these drugs are considered in the second half of the chapter under their pharmacological classes.

Drugs Used for Sedation, Premedication or Analgesia

Anticholinergics – Atropine and Glycopyrrolate

These drugs antagonize acetylcholine at muscarinic sites and so block transmission at parasympathetic postganglionic nerve terminals. By this general action they decrease bronchial and vagal tone, and modify vagal reflexes. They are, therefore, used in the treatment of vagally mediated bradycardia stimulated by head, neck or ophthalmic surgery. They also decrease ocular and pulmonary secretions and are used to reduce the parasympathetic side-effects of other drugs, for example neostigmine, and the opioids. They cause some reduction in smooth muscle activity and decrease gastric secretions. Despite salivation in the cat being stimulated by nicotine, atropine is effective in reducing its secretion, by acting on central muscarinic receptors (Beleslin *et al.*, 1984).

The use of anticholinergics is controversial. The case for their use as premedicants is two pronged. First, due to the small diameter of the bronchi and bronchioles even a small amount of bronchial secretion or inhaled saliva can block the airway, leading to areas of lung collapse and so reducing the available area for gaseous exchange. The second prong is that the subcutaneous pre-operative administration of an anticholinergic is less likely to produce a severe tachycardia than the intra-operative intravenous administration in the treatment of a vagally mediated bradycardia. The intra-operative use of anticholinergics for the treatment of bradycardia necessitates adequate monitoring to detect an initial cardiac arrhythmia. All the drugs in this class take a few minutes to act and initially, in the case of atropine, the bradycardia may intensify due to this drug's central actions. The pre-operative use of these drugs generally produces a stable but higher than resting, intra-operative heart rate.

The case against the prophylactic use of anticholinergic drugs is that normal bronchial secretions are necessary for the normal functioning of the respiratory · tract and (with the exception of ketamine), salivation is rarely a problem with modern anaesthetic agents . In conscious cats, atropine produces a tachycardia which can be reduced by the concurrent administration of a β-blocker (Samonina & Hakumaki, 1983). At high heart rates myocardial oxygen consumption increases and if this situation occurs, oxygen should be administered. There is also the school of thought that drugs should not be administered unless there is a good indication and treatment of *potential* problems is not considered a good indication.

Anticholinergic drugs have been advocated for the treatment of bradycardia produced by the α2-agonists group of drugs, for example xylazine and medetomidine. However, it has been shown that although the bradycardia may be reversed, the detrimental effect of these drugs on cardiac performance is not reversed (Dunkle *et al.*, 1986).

The two commonly used drugs in this category are atropine sulphate and glycopyrronium bromide (glycopyrrolate). Atropine crosses the blood–brain barrier whereas glycopyrrolate does not. This effect results in the latter drug causing fewer visual disturbances by mydriasis than atropine. This is of importance in the cat with acute visual disturbances which is liable to panic. Likewise glycopyrrolate does not cross the placental barrier and so is probably the anticholinergic of choice for caesarian section.

A study comparing atropine and glycopyrrolate as premedicants in cats found that glycopyrrolate was effective in controlling bradycardia and salivation in 95% of the animals where atropine was effective at control-

ling salivation in 92% and bradycardia in 88% of the cats (Short *et al.*, 1983). With respect to the incidence of arrhythmias, Richards *et al.* (1989) found no difference in the incidence of atrioventricular heart block or tachycardia when the two drugs were administered to dogs.

Both drugs are effective in countering the muscarinic effects of the anticholinesterase drug neostigmine, used to antagonise the effects of the non-depolarizing muscle relaxants. In this role, however, the drugs are given just before, or with the neostigmine and not at the time of premedication.

Indications for the use of anticholinergics
Premedication prior to administration of ketamine or tiletamine.
Control of excessive salivation and bronchial secretions.
Treatment of vagally mediated bradycardia.
Concurrent premedication with opiates to prevent parasympathetic action of narcotic analgesics.

Contraindications for the use of anticholinergics
Glaucoma.
Pre-existing tachycardias.

Doses and routes of administration of anticholinergics
Atropine – 0.02–0.1 mg/kg, s/c or i/v. in an adult cat
Glycopyrronium bromide – 0.01–0.02 mg/kg i/m or i/v (Short *et al.*, 1983).

Phenothiazines

Drugs of this group are used as mild sedatives for cats. The most widely used member of the group in the UK is acepromazine maleate but other members of the group, for example chlorpromazine, promazine, propiopromazine, are used in other countries. Their suggested mechanism of action is by dopamine antagonism at excitatory receptors (Booth, 1982) . This group of drugs is characterized (with varying degrees in emphasis) by showing dose-related sedation, antimuscarinic, antiemetic and extrapyramidal effects. Chlorpromazine and acepromazine both lower seizure threshold and so

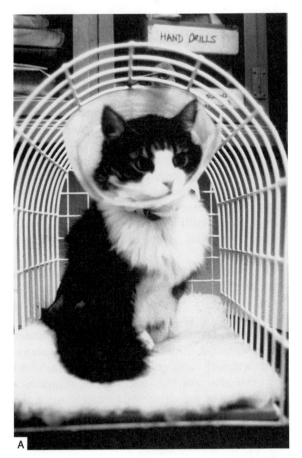 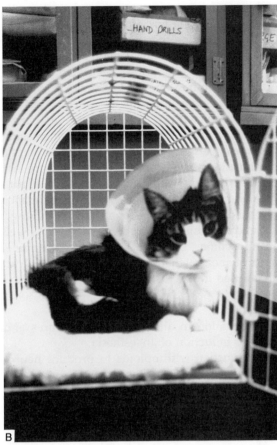

Fig. 7.1 (A) Unsedated cat. (B) Same cat 20 min after sedation with acepromazine and morphine.

these drugs should not be used in known epileptics or in premedication prior to myelography. The degree of sedation is variable and unpredictable, with some individuals showing marked sedation and others no appreciable effect for the same dose. There is a ceiling effect with no more appreciable sedation at increasing doses, but increasing undesirable side effects, for example extrapyramidal signs and duration of action.

Hypothalamic thermoregulation is directly depressed by phenothiazines. This property, coupled with the small size of cats, predisposes them to hypothermia whilst under phenothiazine sedation. The sedation produced by acepromazine is characterized by slightly decreased, but easily arousable, reactivity to external stimuli, protrusion of the third eyelid and slight hypotension. The decrease in resting blood pressure is produced principally by vasodilation and thus decreased vascular resistance. The majority of patients can compensate for this, but in fearful or hypovolaemic patients which are maintaining venous return by increasing systemic vascular resistance, the drug-induced vasodilation can be catastrophic, with orthostatic hypotension and collapse. Premedication with acepromazine does not significantly reduce the induction dose of propofol in cats (Brearley *et al.*, 1988; Geel 1991), but the dose of thiopentone required to induce anaesthesia is reduced after acepromazine by approximately one third. Acepromazine has also been used as a premedicant prior to ketamine anaesthesia in cats and similarly reduces the amount of ketamine required to produce light anaesthesia (Short, 1987a).

Useful side-effects of the phenothiazines

include their antihistamine and antiemetic actions. Thus, the use of a drug of this group for premedication may reduce the incidence of vomiting in the peri-anaesthetic period and the swelling of the extremities associated with use of Saffan (alphaxalone/alphadalone).

Acepromazine maleate is often used in combination with opiate agonists or partial agonists to increase sedation without increasing the side-effects of either drug. These neuroleptic combinations can be used in cats but are not commonly documented (Brearley, 1992). Figure 7.1A and B demonstrates the typical appearance of a cat before and after acepromazine (0.05 mg/kg) and morphine (0.1 mg/kg) sedation. As well as morphine, oxymorphone, buprenorphine, butorphanol, methadone and paravertetum can all be used in this fashion with acepromazine.

Indications
Mild sedation to allow minor procedures and prior to induction of anaesthesia.
In conjunction with opioids to produce neuro-leptanalgesia (increased sedation).

Contraindications
Hypovolaemia.
Hypotension.
Epileptiform seizure activity.

Dose and route of administration
Acepromazine 0.05–0.2 mg/kg/ i/m or i/v (s/c injection appears to be effective although absorption may be unpredictable).
Chlorpromazine 0.5-2 mg/kg orally.

Alpha-2 Agonists and Antagonists

The principal α_2-agonists used clinically in cats are xylazine and medetomidine but clonidine has been used experimentally to investigate the role of α_2-adrenoceptors in the central hypoten-sive and sedative effects of these agonists (Timmermans *et al.*, 1981). These drugs are sedatives with analgesic action having as their side-effects vomiting and bradycardia with variable degrees of hypotension. The sedative action is generally ascribed to inhibition of the locus coerulus and its ascending activating projection to the forebrain. However, other mechanisms may also be involved in producing the sedative effects of these drugs (Stenburg, 1985).

The hypotensive effects were investigated by Tsyrlin and Bravkov (1980) who observed that the sedative effects were accompanied by hypotension and increased baroreceptor reflex activity. The drugs caused no change in the decrease in baroreceptor reflex activity caused by hypothalamic stimulation, but did reduce the hypertensive and emotional responses caused by the natural stress of confrontation with a dog. Thus the increase in baroreflex activity pro-duced by clonidine was attributed to both central neuronal stimulation and sedative effects.

The effects of xylazine on cardiac function in cats was investigated by echocardiography (Dunkle *et al.*, 1986). In comparison to control (untreated) animals, animals treated with xyla-zine demonstrated a decrease in left ventricular contractility (as indicated by fractional short-ening and left ventricular wall amplitude) and heart rate after low (0.55 mg/kg) and high doses (2.2 mg/kg) of the drug. Administration of the anticholinergic glycopyrrolate minimized the bradycardia but did not influence the depressed cardiac contractility (i.e. left ventricular function values).

The emetic effect of the α_2-agonists has been investigated by Colby *et al.* (1981) using xylazine in animals in which the area postrema has been ablated and in sham operated animals. These workers concluded that the emetic effect was produced by direct stimulation of the chemor-eceptor trigger zone and they postulated that opioid-type receptors may be involved. It is considered by some clinicians that the induction of vomiting is an advantage in cats which may have been recently fed. However, in cats that may have oesophageal obstruction, an open eye globe injury or in which increases in intracranial pressure should be avoided, these drugs are contraindicated due to this very property. Vomiting appears to be more reliable or prevalent after xylazine than medetomidine (Verstegen *et al.*, 1991).

Xylazine is often used prior to general anaesthesia produced by ketamine (see Chapter 8). The effects of xylazine on the distribution

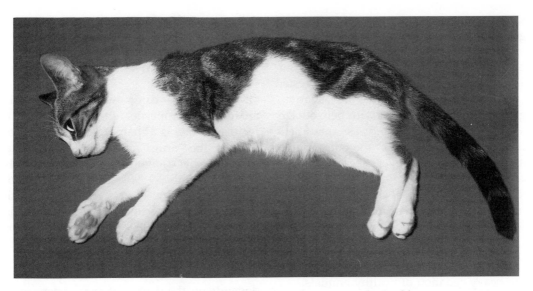

Fig. 7.2 Cat sedated with medetomidine. It appears almost anaesthetized but note open eyes.

and metabolism of intramuscularly administered ketamine in cats were investigated by Waterman (1983). Xylazine was found to prolong the duration of ketamine anaesthesia; it prolonged the half-life of ketamine and delayed the appearance of its primary metabolite.

Detomidine, an α_2-agonist more commonly used in horses, has been administered to anaesthetized cats (dose 1–30 µg/kg i/v). Hypotension and bradycardia were observed in a dose-dependent manner (Savola *et al.*, 1985). These effects were reversed by the α_2-agonist idazoxan (0.3 mg/kg i/v).

Medetomidine is a more potent α_2-agonist than xylazine. When the two drugs were compared it was found that 0.18 mg/kg medetomidine was comparable to 3 mg/kg xylazine with respect to sedation. Bradycardia was noted with both drugs (Stenburg *et al.*, 1987). The optimal dose and feasibility of various procedures under medetomidine sedation was investigated in a multicentre trial (Vähä-Vahe, 1989). Between 80 and 110 µg/kg were used and of the 678 cats treated, 85% of the animals were in 'a slight anaesthetic stage' and unable to rise (Fig 7.2). Conditions for the different procedures were deemed very satisfactory or satisfactory in 81–96%. Side-effects were limited to vomiting and this occurred in 65% of the treated animals. In combination with ketamine in 295 cats 'good'

anaesthesia was achieved which lasted 20–40 min, with a smooth recovery. Hypothermia was reported in all animals sedated with medetomidine. Similar findings were reported by Vainio (1989) with the additional observation that higher than recommended doses caused increased duration of sedation rather than increasing the depth of sedation. She also found that administration of medetomidine was initially accompanied by a slight hypertension which was followed by a longer lasting hypotension and that respiratory rates decreased but stayed within normal limits for resting animals. Vomiting occurred during the onset of sedation.

The analgesic effects of the α_2-agonists may be attributed to their stimulatory effects on pain modulation projections from the locus coeruleus to the spinal cord (Stenburg, 1989). Nociceptive reflexes were suppressed by 0.02 mg/kg medetomidine and abolished by higher doses. This proposed spinal action in the role of α_2-mediated analgesia is further supported by a study in which clonidine was found to suppress noxiously evoked spinal dorsal horn activity in spinal cord transected cats (Murata *et al.*, 1989). Benson *et al.* (1991) found that xylazine (and morphine) but not salicylate, decreased postoperative mixed venous catecholamine concentrations after onychectomy, suggesting a decreased stress response to pain if not an analgesic effect *per se*.

A review article compared xylazine and medetomidine as anaesthetic adjuncts (Tranquilli & Benson, 1992). This article suggested that both drugs were effective as sedative/ analgesic adjuncts when used with benzodiazepines or opioid agonists and as anaesthetic adjuncts when used with the dissociative agents and opioids. However, because of their marked effects on the cardiovascular system it was suggested that their use should be restricted to young healthy patients undergoing routine surgical or diagnostic procedures.

Indications
Mild to heavy sedation of healthy animals.
Sedation of animals with unknown starvation status.

Contraindications
Sedation or premedication of animals with cardiovascular or respiratory disease.
Cats with gastrointestinal obstruction.
Cats in which increases in intracranial or intraocular pressures would be detrimental (e.g. head trauma, glaucoma, open globe injuries).

Dose and route of administration
Xylazine   0.2–0.4 mg/kg i/m, for analgesia.
                1.3 mg/kg i/m or s/c for sedation lasting 30–40 min.
Medetomidine   50–150 µg/kg i/m, s/c.
                15-30 µg/kg is also effective sprayed on to buccal mucous membranes beneath the tongue (Hall, 1993, pers. comm.).
                80 µg medetomidine gives similar sedation to 3 mg/kg xylazine.

It is important to note that the α_2-agonists have very marked anaesthetic sparing effects when used with general anaesthetic agents, reported in dogs to be in the order of 50%, depending on dose (Young *et al.*, 1990). In addition, by slowing the circulation, these drugs delay the onset of effect of injected anaesthetic agents.

Alpha-2 Antagonists

Of the various drugs with α_2-adenoreceptor antagonistic properties, the only licensed drug for use in cats is atipamezole. Given intramuscularly the drug antagonizes the sedation produced by α_2-agonists in approximately 10 min (Vähä-Vahe, 1990). The administration of atipamezole alone to cats results in occasional vomiting, and defecation. Hyper-alertness is not a feature (Clarke, 1989). An atipamezole dose of 2–4 times the preceding dose of medetomidine is required to antagonize medetomidine sedation (Vähä-Vahe, 1990). The precise dose depends on the degree of antagonism required and the time elapsed since administration of medetomidine (Young & Jones, 1990).

In America, another α_2-adrenergic antagonist, yohimbine, has been used at a dose of 0.1mg/ kg, to antagonize the effects of xylazine in cats (Hsu & Lu, 1984; Jensen, 1985). Yohimbine has also been used (at 0.4 mg/kg) in combination with 4-aminopyridine (0.5 mg/kg) to arouse pethidine–acepromazine–pentobarbital, xylazine–pentobarbital or acepromazine–pentobarbital anaesthetized cats (Hatch *et al.*, 1984a,b). Yohimbine could probably be used to antagonize the effects of medetomidine. The experimental drug idazoxan has also been used to antagonize the effects of detomidine in cats (Savola *et al.*, 1985).

Doses
Atipamezole   100–600 µg/kg i/m, s/c
Yohimbine   0.1–0.4 mg/kg i/v
Idazoxan   0.3 mg/kg i/v

Benzodiazepine Agonists

The benzodiazepines diazepam and midazolam act by stimulation of the inhibitory gamma-aminobutyric acid (GABA) neurones in the central nervous system (Goeders *et al.*, 1990), producing sedation (in man), muscle relaxation and anticonvulsant effects. They have little sedative action by themselves in healthy cats and their anxiolytic properties may render a healthy cat less easy to handle (Gleed, 1987). However, they have a prime role in the premedication of cats prior to ketamine anaesthesia and in animals that may be prone to convulsions, for example cats undergoing myelography or epileptics. This class of drugs is also used to relieve postoperative restlessness in conjunction with analgesics (Hall & Clarke, 1991), as appetite stimulants (Macy & Gasper, 1985) and as anticonvulsants. They do not have any intrinsic analgesic properties, but they are particularly useful for the premedication of cats with cardiovascular or respiratory disease as classically these drugs have little influence on these systems at the recommended dose rates (0.2–1 mg/kg diazepam; Gleed, 1987). In healthy cats this is the case; however, both midazolam and diazepam have been found to decrease airway smooth muscle tone when applied on to or into the ventral medullary region of the brain in cats (Haxhiu *et al.*, 1989). This may become important in animals with increased dead space from other causes such as pneumonia.

There is increased sensitivity to the benzodiazepines in the elderly human (Fancourt & Castleden, 1986), due to altered pharmacokinetics. This has resulted in respiratory depression or arrest in this group of the population. These effects have also been seen in elderly dogs (unpublished observations). There is no reason to suppose this may not also be the case in elderly cats and so careful observation of such animals is necessary after dosing with a benzodiazepine. Metabolism is primarily hepatic and so, in common with other sedative/tranquillizers, the duration of action may be prolonged in animals with severe hepatic dysfunction.

The prime role of benzodiazepines in feline anaesthesia is as premedicant adjuncts to ketamine (see Chapter 8) because they counter the rigidity and convulsions seen with this drug. They are said not to intensify anaesthesia induced by alfentanil/etomidate or alphaxalone/alphadalone (Ittner *et al.*, 1985) but prevent the postanaesthetic excitation which occurs after these drug combinations.

Diazepam is the most widely used benzodiazepine. It is available in two formulations; either dissolved in propylene glycol (Valium, Roche) or as an emulsion with soya bean oil (Diaze-muls, Roche). The former formulation has the disadvantage that it may cause thrombophlebitis and pain on intravenous injection as well as cardiac arrhythmias and cardiovascular depression (Gleed, 1987). The more expensive Diazemuls does not have these disadvantages. Both formulations can be administered rectally, intramuscularly or intravenously. Diazepam is classified as long acting with a plasma half-life in man of 20–90 h after oral dosing (Fancourt & Castleden, 1986).

Midazolam is a short-acting water-soluble benzodiazepine which produces minimal local irritation on intramuscular or intravenous injection. Its short duration of action is due to its rapid hepatic metabolism to less active metabolites which undergo inactivation by rapid glucuronidation. Its plasma half life in man is approximately 2 h (Roche data sheet). In cats, midazolam has been mixed in the same syringe as ketamine and administered to produce sedation or light anaesthesia (Chambers & Dobson, 1989; Dobromylskyj, 1992). Chambers and Dobson (1989) used 0.2 mg/kg midazolam and 10 mg/kg ketamine, injecting this intramuscularly. After 10 min, the animals were assessed for degree of sedation, muscle relaxation and side-effects. Of the 40 cats in which this combination was used, 36 were reported as being medium or deeply sedated and muscle tone was assessed as normal or decreased on 32 occasions. Excessive salivation was noted in one cat and cyanosis was reported in one cat on three separate occasions when the combination was used. This combination was deemed to provide good sedation for minor procedures such as venepuncture, skin biopsy or radiography. Dobromylskyj (1992) combined midazolam (0.125 mg/kg) with ketamine (2.5 mg/kg), administering this intravenously after premedication with atropine and papaveretum to 20 cats presented for ovariohysterectomy. Within 60 s the animals became recumbent and would tolerate the application of a mask to allow administration of halothane in oxygen and nitrous oxide, demonstrating that this combination produced useful sedation.

Climazolam and zolazepam have been used in veterinary anaesthesia but there are no reports of their use alone in the cat. Zolazepam is available in North America and Europe in a fixed ratio combination with the dissociative agent tiletamine, for induction of anaesthesia in cats (see Chapter 8). It has the disadvantage that recovery from the combination can be excited and prolonged at the recommended dose rates (Short, 1987a).

Indications
In combination with ketamine to produce sedation.
Control of epileptiform seizures.

Contraindications
Sole agent to healthy animals.

Dose and route of administration
Diazepam 0.1–0.5 mg/kg i/v or 0.3–1.0 mg/kg i/m.
Midazolam 0.2 mg/kg i/v, i/m.

Benzodiazepine Antagonist

The benzodiazepine antagonist, flumazenil, is used in man for the reversal of benzodiazepine agonist effects. As yet, principally due to its cost, its role in veterinary medicine has not been fully explored. However, if benzodiazepines are used in a clinic it would be advisable to have flumazenil available to treat benzodiazepine overdose. In man the effects of the agonist are reversed 30–60 s after intravenous administration of the antagonist (Roche data sheet).

Flumazenil and midazolam have similar pharmocokinetic profiles making them particularly suitable partners. The antagonist has a short elimination half life of 53 min (Amrein & Hetzel, 1990), but is well tolerated at high doses so repeat administration should be safe even in the unlikely event of accumulation. In rats and mice single doses of 3000 times the clinical dose of flumazenil (0.02 mg/kg) were well tolerated (Roche data sheets). It has been used experimentally in cats to reverse mecloazepam-induced effects on spinal cord activity (Bonetti, 1982). In one dog study it was found that the agonist/antagonist ratio required to rapidly and irreversibly antagonize a 10 times preanaesthetic overdose of diazepam was 26:1 and midazolam 13:1 (Tranquilli *et al.*, 1992).

Dose rate and routes of administration
None documented for the cat.

Dissociative Agents

Ketamine and tiletamine are generally classed as anaesthetic agents rather than sedatives (see Chapter 8), but at low doses and particularly when used in combination with another sedative these dissociative agents can produce very useful sedation, particularly in cats suffering pain as they have analgesic properties. Their anaesthetic/analgesic properties may be reversed by antagonism at N-methyl-aspartate receptors (Anis *et al.*, 1983).

In this group of agents, ketamine is the most commonly used in cats. At sedative doses (5–10 mg/kg) the effects of ketamine alone on the cardiovascular system are minimal. Unlike sedation with opioids, the gag reflex and cough reflex are maintained with ketamine sedation. This is a marked advantage over the opioids, which, as well as suppressing these reflexes, can also cause vomiting. Ketamine is a good visceral analgesic. It depresses the neural response to the noxious stimulus of intra-arterial bradykinin (Tomemori *et al.*, 1981). The analgesic effect was thought to be supraspinal rather than spinal as the depressant effect disappeared following cervical cord transection at C1. However, Collins (1986) suggested that there was some spinal site of action for the analgesia produced by ketamine, but that the anaesthesia was supraspinal in origin. The difference between the two studies was that the former was in anaesthetized or decerebrate cats whilst the latter was in conscious intact animals.

Ketamine is often used by itself in cats as a sedative for procedures which do not require muscle relaxation, for example radiography and examination of intractable animals. However it can cause seizures and increased intracranial and intraocular pressure. Salivation is also a feature when the drug is used alone without anticholinergic co-administration. The duration of recovery is dose dependent, and, according to the manufacturers, prolonged recoveries are not uncommon. Care should be taken when using other drugs in combination with ketamine as the metabolism and elimination of ketamine may be altered (Waterman, 1983). Elimination of the drug depends on renal function and so the duration of action may be prolonged in cats with renal failure. Apneustic respiratory patterns occur under ketamine sedation. This may progress to respiratory arrest in some cases and so cats should be observed closely until signs of sedation are no longer apparent and the animal is again behaving normally.

Tiletamine is available in North America and Europe in a fixed ratio combination with zolazepam (see Chapter 8).

Indications
Sedation particularly of fractious animal.

Contraindications
Epileptic animals.
Raised intracranial pressure.

Dose and routes of administration
Ketamine – sedation 5–10 mg/kg i/m or i/v, 10 mg/kg orally.
– in combination, 5 mg/kg with
acepromazine 0.1 mg/kg
xylazine 1 mg/kg
medetomidine 80 mcg/kg
diazepam 0.2 mg/kg
midazolam 0.2 mg/kg.
– oral administration (20 mg/kg) to feral cats can produce useful sedation to allow handling.
– intramuscular or subcutaneous injection should be given with care due to pain on injection of the drug (see Chapter 8).

Saffan

Low doses of this alphaxalone/alphadalone mixture of steroid anaesthetic agents have been used intramuscularly for sedation and to allow minor procedures. For complete discussion of the combination see Chapter 8. It has few indications due to the volume of drug required for intramuscular injection, but doses of 4–9 mg/kg intramuscularly produce sedation of 5–15 min duration; the apparently sedated

animal can be made to struggle or convulse by external stimuli such as noise.

Opioids

Formerly, pure opioids were not given to cats because of the maniacal reaction they were said to produce (Short, 1987b). This excitation is only seen at high doses (e.g. morphine 15 mg/kg; Fertziger *et al.*, 1973) and is not a problem with clinical doses (e.g. morphine 0.1 mg/kg; Watts *et al.*, 1973). They are, without doubt, very effective analgesics, but they do cause some sedation at clinical doses.

Morphine inhibits stimulated c-fibre action potentials in dorsal horn neurones at 1–4 mg/kg i/v in anaesthetized cats. This suppression is reversed by naloxone administered into the substantia gelatinosa (SG), suggesting that opioid receptors in the SG play a role in morphine analgesia (Johnson & Duggan, 1981). Micro-injections of morphine into the dorsal horn suppressed c-fibre reflex without altering the short latency polysynaptic reflex. Injections into the ventral horn facilitated both reflexes. The dorsal horn effects were antagonized by pretreating with naltrexone, an opioid antagonist. These results support the hypothesis that the analgesic effects of morphine at the spinal cord level are mediated in the dorsal horn (Bell *et al.*, 1980). Low doses of morphine administered intrathecally had no effect on blood pressure in conscious cats (Yasuoka & Yaksh, 1983). High doses of morphine (5 mg) administered intrathecally resulted in marked elevations in blood pressure and pupil diameter following brushing of the cat's paw (Yaksh *et al.*, 1986). These different results suggest that the effects of high dose morphine may be characterized by a non-opioid receptor-mediated effect that alters the coding of sensory information in the spinal cord.

Watts *et al.* (1973) found that in cats the most effective analgesic dose of morphine was 0.1 mg/kg s/c. This dose provided good analgesia and apparent tranquillization. There was no apparent increase in analgesic or tranquillizing effects at 1 mg/kg. At 10 mg/kg maximum analgesic was evident but the animals showed toxic effects of hypermotility, ataxia, mydriasis, increased reactivity to noise and increased salivation. At 20 mg/kg convulsions have been reported (Davis & Donnelly, 1968). Hence the importance of using slightly more conservative doses in cats than those recommended in dogs.

Davis and Donnelly (1968) also reported some pharmacokinetic data for morphine and pethidine (meperidine) in cats. After morphine at 1 mg/kg s/c, they found that peak plasma values occurred at 1 h and that plasma elimination followed first-order kinetics. The plasma $t_{1/2}$ was 3.05 h. However, at this dose the drug produced mydriasis, salivation and some anxiety which were not seen after 0.1 mg/kg. The duration of effective analgesic effect was 4 h after 1 mg/kg. Pethidine was not as long acting as morphine.

The relative potencies of four opioids administered epidurally have been assessed in cats. Lofentanyl was found to be more potent than morphine which in turn was more potent then methadone and pethidine. The duration of action was morphine > lofentanyl > methadone = pethidine (Tung & Yaksh, 1982). The rank order potency of methadone and morphine was the same when the drugs were administered systemically (Ossipov et al., 1984).

In conscious, free-moving cats, the pure opiates morphine and fentanyl and the partial agonist pentazocine suppress the recovery cycles of primary responses in the second somatosensory and associative zones of the brain cortex. At larger doses, convulsive discharges on the EEG and motor excitation occur. Naloxone eliminates all these effects (Fisenko & Manula, 1980).

In North America, the dihydroxy derivative of morphine, oxymorphone, is widely used in small animals. Its has approximately 10 times the analgesic potency of morphine but has less effect on the respiratory, cardiovascular and gastrointestinal systems (Potthoff & Carithers, 1989). It has a similar duration of action to morphine (Short, 1987b). The relative potencies in cats of buprenorphine, morphine and pentazocine were assessed by Hiyama et al. (1982). Buprenorphine was found to be more potent and to have a longer duration of action than morphine and pentazocine in analgesic tests. It showed a bell-shaped response curve and its analgesic activity could be reversed by naloxone when the naloxone was administered before, but not after, the buprenorphine.

The effects of the partial opioid agonists nalbuphine, pentazocine and butorphanol were examined in the cat by Sawyer and Rech (1987). Nalbuphine was administered at doses ranging from 0.75 to 3 mg/kg i/v. These doses provided visceral analgesia for about 3 h. Some pain on injection was observed but no effects on heart or respiratory rate were noted. Pentazocine at 3 mg/kg gave consistent analgesia, which lasted approximately 6 h. Side-effects of mydriasis and anxiety were also noted. Neither heart nor respiratory rate changed from control values. There was no evidence of either nalbuphine or pentazocine giving any somatic analgesia. Butorphanol (0.8 mg/kg) increased the threshold responses to somatic stimulation, with a duration of effect of approximately 2 h. In the cat the effective analgesic dose may vary from 0.2 to 0.8 mg/kg. Visceral analgesia was noted after i/v butorphanol within this dose range, with the lowest dose producing the longest duration and greatest change from control values for visceral analgesia. There was a tendency to increased heart rate at high doses of butorphanol but only minimal sedative effects were seen. Butorphanol has good sedative properties in combination with tranquillizers (Sawyer & Rech, 1987).

Buprenorphine at 0.01 mg/kg was suggested by Taylor (1985) as an analgesic in the cat, but with the warning that it had not been widely used in the cat at that time. It is said to have a slow onset of action (30–45 min) after i/m or i/v injection (Nolan, 1989). The duration of action, on average, is about 4 h. Sedation is also seen with this drug. As with other partial opioid agonists, buprenorphine has a bell-shaped response curve. This results in less analgesia at higher dose rates and makes the drug resistant to reversal by opioid antagonists. However, buprenorphine has been used to reverse pure opioid agonists, for example fentanyl, in man (Robertson & Laing, 1980).

It is obvious that there is ample evidence that opioid analgesics can be used effectively in cats. Their use is particularly indicated in the perioperative period when some sedation may be needed. The disadvantage of these drugs is that they are not easily available in any but an injectable form.

Dose rate and routes of administration

Morphine	0.1–0.2 mg/kg s/c, i/m or i/v.
Oxymorphone	0.01 mg/kg s/c, i/m or i/v.
Pethidine (meperidine)	2–5 mg/kg i/m.
Methadone	0.1–0.2 mg/kg s/c or i/v.
Pentazocine	2 mg/kg s/c, i/m, i/v.
Buprenorphine	0.006–0.01 mg/kg s/c, i/m or i/v.
Butorphanol	0.2–0.8 mg/kg i/m.

Neuroleptanalgesia

Neuroleptanalgesia is a term used to describe the concurrent use of a tranquillizer or sedative with an opioid analgesic. The combination provides more profound sedation than would be achieved by the simple summation of the effect of either drug. The technique is used where marked sedation is required with some analgesia. The animals tend to sleep (Fig. 7.1), but are responsive to sudden stimuli, in particular noise. The classical example of this type of drug used is Small Animal Immobilon (C-Vet), in which the tranquillizer methotrime-prazine, is combined with the opiate, etorphine in a fixed ratio. This combination is *not* used in cats due to the potency of the etorphine, resulting in a tendency to maniacal behaviour.

However other combinations which may be used in the cat are:

Acepromazine (0.05 mg/kg) and morphine (0.1 mg/kg) (Brearley, 1992).
Acepromazine (0.05 mg/kg) and buprenor-phine (0.01 mg/kg).

There are few other reports of neuroleptanalgesia in cats in the literature.

Non-steroidal Anti-Inflammatory Drugs

Non-steroidal anti-inflammatory drugs (NS-AIDs) are not commonly used in cats due to the toxic effects of the more traditional ones in this species. They inhibit the formation of inflammatory mediators and have been used in the control of chronic pain. Logically, if given before surgery when tissue damage is inflicted, they probably have some role in the control of postoperative pain. The disadvantage of giving these drugs pre-operatively is that they are said to result in renal damage if hypotension occurs during anaesthesia (see Chapters 2 and 12). During hypotension blood flow to the kidney is in part maintained by the local action of prostaglandins on the renal vasculature. Inhibition of these prostaglandins by the NSAIDs results in reduced renal blood flow and possible ischaemic damage. Other effects such as that on platelet function and gastrointestinal integrity, combined with the cat's inability to metabolize these drugs rapidly, results in their high toxicity in this species. Of the drugs available in this class, aspirin (Davis & Donnelly, 1968), flunixin (Lees & Taylor, 1991; Fonda 1993), ketoprofen (Postal *et al.*, 1991), tolfenamic acid (Guelfi *et al.*, 1991) and phenylbutazone (Nolan, 1989), have doses relevant for cats in the literature. Carprofen, a recently released NSAID for use in dogs and horses, has been used experimentally in cats (Taylor, 1993, per. commun.). This drug does not appear to act by inhibition of cyclo-oxygenase or lipoxygenase (McKellar *et al.*, 1990) as do the traditional NSAIDs. The side-effects of this class of drugs generally result from inhibition of prostaglandins formation by this mechanism, so carprofen may have fewer side-effects than the other drugs. As metabolism of many of the NSAIDs is dependant on the hepatic glutathione-dependent enzyme system which is deficient in cats, slower metabolism might be expected in this species than, for example, in dogs (Hjelle & Graver, 1986). Thus the NSAIDs should be used with caution and only at recommended dose rates.

Drugs which have been reported to be contraindicated in cats are acetaminophen (paracetamol), ibuprofen, indomethacin and naproxen (Potthoff & Carithers, 1989), due to hepatotoxicity and gastrointestinal ulceration.

Dose rate and routes of administration

Aspirin   10 mg/kg every 48 h orally
                (Davis & Donnelly, 1968).
Flunixin   1 mg/kg/day (Taylor, pers.
                comm.)
Phenylbutazone 10 mg/kg daily orally (Nolan,
                1989).
Ketoprofen   2 mg/kg daily s/c injection
                (data sheet).
Tolfenamic acid 2–4 mg/kg (Guelfi *et al.*, 1991).
(Carprofen   1–4 mg/kg/day (Taylor, pers.
                comm.).)

Local Analgesia

Cats are generally considered bad candidates for local analgesic techniques. This is partly due to their nature, making additional restraint necessary, and partly due to their small size leading to inadvertent overdosage and toxicity. However, with care, there is no reason why local techniques similar to those used in the dogs cannot be used to provide intra- and postoperative analgesia as with other species. Lignocaine is the most commonly used drug and there are few reports of the clinical use of other agents specifically in the cat.

Hall and Clarke (1991) report that the maximum dose of lignocaine that can be given by infiltration before toxic signs (neurological signs, seizures and cardiovascular collapse) are seen is in the order of 10 mg/kg. This is equivalent to 20–50 mg in a cat; thus only 1–2 ml of the usual 2% solution can be used. Better local infiltration can be achieved if the solution is diluted to 1 or 0.5% but the safe volume is still small. Intravenous doses of up to 0.8 mg/kg bupivacaine were reported to have little effect on mean arterial blood pressure or heart rate in anaesthetized cats but 1.2 mg/kg caused significant cardiovascular depression (Fukuda, 1989).

Intercostal nerve block after thoracotomy has been described in dogs (Bednarski, 1989) but there are no reports of its use in cats.

Epidural analgesia is the technique which deserves most attention. This may be provided by local anaesthetic agents, α_2-agonists, ketamine or opioids. This technique has been widely reported in dogs and occasionally referred to in cats (Klide, 1971; Haskins, 1992; Trim, 1989; Hall & Clarke, 1991; Heath, 1992). Trim (1987) describes the technique in detail for the cat. Local anaesthetic solution is injected into the epidural space at the lumbosacral junction. The spinal cord ends between L7 and S3 in the cat (Habel, 1978) so care must be taken not to give a spinal injection if the subarachnoid space is penetrated. The lumbosacral space is immediately cranial to the sacrum and the needle is placed further back in the space than in the dog. The hair is clipped, the skin prepared aseptically and a small volume of lignocaine injected intradermally and subcutaneously. A 22 gauge, 4 cm spinal needle (with stilette) is inserted in the midline perpendicular to the skin to a depth of 1 cm. It is difficult to appreciate passage through the ligamentum flavum in the cat. Aspiration should be attempted and if no blood or CSF is seen a test for loss of resistance to infection should be made which indicates that the epidural space has been entered. A small volume of air above a few millilitres of saline in a test syringe can be used to avoid injecting air. Once loss of resistance is ascertained the bevel of the needle is directed cranially and the local analgesic solution is injected slowly and steadily. Speed of injection and volume can be varied slightly for different procedures. Loss of tail and anal tone should develop within 2 min after lignocaine, but 10–12 min should be allowed for full analgesia to develop. With bupivicaine about 20 min is needed for the block to develop fully (Heath, 1992). Plain lignocaine provides about 45 min analgesia but this can be extended by the addition of up to 0.1 ml of 1:1000 adrenaline to the lignocaine before injection. The cat must be restrained during recovery to prevent spinal injury.

In cats, epidural analgesia for surgery is generally combined with light general anaesthesia to provide restraint of the animal, although in some sedation may not be necessary. Epidural analgesia reduces the amount of anaesthetic agent required to maintain anaesthesia and so may be useful in very sick cats with cardiovascular instability. Analgesia is maintained into the postoperative period and if bupivicaine is used this may be as long as 6 h from the application of the block. Lignocaine, having a shorter duration of action is less useful for postoperative analgesia. The disadvantage of epidural techniques is that they require a certain amount of technical ability and even then not all blocks are successful.

Doses for epidural analgesia
Local anaesthetic agents (without adrenaline):

1 ml/5kg for a block to L1	lignocaine 2% – 20 mg/5kg bupivicaine 0.5% – 5 mg/5 kg
1 ml/3.5 kg for a block to T4	

Physical Means of Postoperative Pain Relief

Provision of warmth, appetizing food and general attention, although not strictly means of providing pain relief, will make a cat feel much better. Often cats in discomfort will cease grooming and so this should be done for the animal, as should wiping the mouth and around the eyes with damp cotton wool. Such attention will also enable the carer to notice subtle changes in the cat's progress that may not be immediately apparent to a stranger. A formalized pain scoring regime may be useful to people inexperienced in the care of sick cats. This also allows more objective criteria for the re-administration of analgesics. Instructions may be left that the veterinarian responsible for the case should be contacted when the pain score reaches a predetermined value.

Analgesia should not be denied to cats simply because the species is not fully understood. As people responsible for these animals veterinarians should be making more effort to understand the cat's metabolism and reaction to drugs to enable provision of safe and adequate analgesia. Experimental data, particularly from medical literature where the cat is often used as an experimental model, should be more closely examined by veterinarians with this in mind.

References

Amrein, R. & Hetzel, W. (1990) Pharmacology of dormicum (midazolam) and anexate (flumazenil). *Acta Anaesth. Scand. Suppl.* **92**, 6–15.

Anis, N.A., Berry, S.C., Burton, N.R. & Lodge, D. (1983) The dissociative anaesthetics, ketamine and phencyclidine, selectively reduce excitation of central mammalian neurones by *N*-methyl-aspartate. *Brit. J. Pharmacol.* **79**(2), 565–575.

Bednarski, (1989) Anesthesia and pain control. *Vet. Clin. N. Am. (SAP)* **19**, 1223–1238.

Beleslin, D.B., Krsti'c S.K. & Tomi'c-Beleslin N. (1984) Nicotinic-induced salivation in cats: effects of various drugs. *Brain Res. Bull.* **12**(5), 585–587.

Bell, J.A., Sharpe, L.G. & Berry, J.N. (1980) Depressant and excitant effects of intraspinal microinjections of morphine and methionine–enkephalin in the cat. *Brain Res.* **186**(2), 455–465.

Benson, G.J., Wheaton, L.G., Thurmon, J.C., Tranquilli, W.J., Olson, W.A., Goeders N., Bell V., Giudoz A. *et al.* (1991) Doparminergic involvement in the cocaine-induced up regulation of benzodiazepine receptors in the rat caudate nucleus. *Brain Res.* **515**(1–2), 1–8.

Bonetti, E.P. (1982) Benzodiazepine antagonist Ro 15–1788: neurological and behavioural effects. *Psychopharmacology* **78**, 8.

Booth, N.H. (1982) Psychotropic agents. In: *Veterinary Pharmacology and Therapeutics* (eds N.H. Booth & L.H. McDonald), pp. 321–345. The Iowa Press, Ames.

Brearley, J.C. (1992) Morphine and acepromazine premedication in cats: Abstract. *J. Vet. Anaesth.* **20**, 35.

Brearley, J.C., Kellagher, R.E.B. & Hall, L.W. (1988) Propofol anaesthesia in cats. *J. Small Anim. Pract.* **29**, 315–322.

Chambers, J.P. & Dobson, J.M. (1989) A midazolam and ketamine combination as a sedative in cats. *J. Ass.Vet. Anaesth.* **16**, 53–54.

Clarke, K.W. (1989) The use of atipamezole in small animals. *Proceedings: The Use of Medetomidine and Atipamezole in Small Animal Practice*, p. 17. Smith-Kline Beecham Animal Health, Norden Laboratories, Nov. 1989.

Colby, E.D., McCarthy, L.E. & Borison, H.L. (1981) Emetic action of xylazine on the chemoreceptor trigger zone for vomiting in cats. *J. Vet. Pharmacol. Ther.* **4**(2), 93–96.

Collins, J.G. (1986) Effects of ketamine on low intensity tactile sensory input are not dependent upon a spinal site of action. *Anesth. Anal.* **65**(11), 1123–1129.

Davis, L.E. and Donnelly, E.J. (1968) Analgesic drugs in the cat. *J. Am. Vet. Med. Assoc.* **53**(9), 1611–1167.

Dobromylskyj, P. (1992) A combination of midazolam with ketamine used as an intravenous induction agent in cats. *J. Vet. Anaesth.* **19**, 72–73.

Dunkle, N., Moise, N.S., Scarlett, K.J. & Short, C.E. (1986) Cardiac performance in cats after administration of xylazine or xylazine and glycopyrrolate:echocardiographic evaluations. *Am. J. Vet. Res.* **47**(10), 2212–2216.

Fancourt, G. & Castleden, M. (1986) The use of benzodiazepines with particular reference to the elderly. *Brit. J. Hosp. Med.* May 1986.

Fertziger, A.P., Stein, E.A. & Lynch, J.J. (1973) Suppression of morphine-induced mania in cats. *Psychopharmacology (Berl.)* **36**, 185–187.

Fisenko, V.P. & Manula, A.I. (1980) Action of opiate peptide and narcotic analgesics on the cerebral cortex. *Biull. Eksp. Biol. Med.* **90**(8), 175–177.

Flecknell, P.A. (1987) *Laboratory Animal Anaesthesia.* Academic Press, London.

Fonda, D. (1993) Postoperative analgesic effect of flunixin in the cat. *J. Vet. Anaesth.* **20**, 29.

Fukuda, T. (1989) Effects of intravenous bupivacaine on the renal sympathetic nerve activity in the cat. *Masui* **38**, 1554–1560.

Geel, J.K. (1991) The effect of premedication on the induction dose of propofol in dogs and cats. *J. S. Afr. Vet. Assoc.* **62**(3), 118–123.

Gleed, R.D. (1987) Tranquillisers and sedatives. In: *Principles and Practice of Veterinary Anaesthesia* (ed. C.E. Short), pp. 226, Williams and Wilkins, Baltimore.

Goeders, N., Bell., V., Guidroz, A. *et al.* (1990) Dopaminergic involvement in the cocaine-induced up regulation of benzodiazepine receptors in the rat caudate nucleus. *Brain Res.* **515**(1–2), 1–8.

Guelfi, J.F., Legeay, Y., Thomas, E. & Deleforge, J. (1991) Essai clinique effects de l'acide tolfenamique dans le traitement des coryzas du chat: resultats d'un essai comparatif. *Practique Medicale et Chirurgicale de l'Animal de Compagnie* **26**, 363–367.

Habel, R.E. (1978) *Applied Veterinary Anatomy,* 2nd edn. R.E. Habel, Ithaca, NY.

Hall, L.W. & Clarke, K.W. (1991) *Veterinary Anaesthesia,* 9th edn. Bailliere Tindall, London.

Haskins, S.C. (1992) Injectable anaesthetics In: *Opinions in Small Animal Anesthesia* (eds Haskins, S.C. & Klide A.M.) *Vet. Clin. N. Am.* **22**(2), 258.

Hatch, R.C., Zahner, J.M.and Booth, N.H. (1984a) Meperidine–acepromazine–pentobarbital anesthe-

sia in cats. Reversal by 4-aminopyridine and yohimbine. *Am. J. Vet. Res.* **45**, 2658–2662.

Hatch, R.C., Kitzman, J.V., Clark, J.D., Zahner, J.M. & Booth, N.H. (1984b) Reversal of pentobarbital anesthesia with 4-aminopyridine and yohimbine in cats pretreated with acepromazine and xylazine *Am. J. Vet. Res.* **45**, 2586–2590.

Haxhiu, M.A., van Lunteren, E., Cherniack, N.S. & Deal, E.C. (1989) Benzodiaepines acting on ventral surface of medulla cause airway dilation. *Am. J. Physiol.* **257**(4 Pt 2), R810–815.

Heath, R.B. (1992) Lumbosacral epidural management. *Vet. Clin. N. Am. (SAP)* **22**, 417–419.

Hiyama, T., Shintani, S., Tsutsui, M. & Yasuda, Y. (1982) Analgesic and narcotic antagonist effects of burprenorphine. *Nippon Yakurigaku Zasshi* **79**(3), 147–162.

Hjelle, J. & Graver, G. (1986) Acetaminophen induced toxicosis in dogs and cats *J. Am. Vet. Med. Assoc.* **188**(7), 742–746.

Hsu, W.H. & Lu, Z.X. (1984) Effect of yohimbine on xylazine-ketamine anesthesia in cats *J. Am. Vet. Med. Assoc.* **185**(8), 886–888.

International Association for the Study of Pain (1979) *Pain* **6**, 250.

Ittner, J., Kramer, A. & Erhardt, W. (1985) Comparative studies of short term anesthesia with alfentanil/etomidaate and alphaxalone/alphadalone in cats. *Tierarztl. Prax. Suppl.* **1**, 132–138.

Jensen, W.A. (1985) Yohimbine for the treatment of xylazine in the cat. *J. Am. Vet. Assoc.* **187**, 627–628.

Johnson, S.M. & Duggan, A.W. (1981) Evidence that the opiate receptors of the substantia gelatinosa contribute to the depression, by intravenous morphine, of the spinal transmission of impulses in unmyelinated primary afferents. *Brain Res.* **207**(1), 223–228.

Klide, A.M. (1971) Epidural analgesia. In: (ed. Soma L.R.). *Textbook of Veterinary Anaesthesia.* Williams and Wilkins, Baltimore.

Klide, A.M. (1992) Epidural anesthesia. *In: Opinions in Small Animal Anesthesia* (eds Haskins, S.C. and Klide, A.M.) *Vet. Clin. North America* **22**(2), 413–416.

Lees, P. & Taylor, P.M. (1991) Pharmacodynamics and pharmacokinetics of flunixin in the cat. *Br. Vet. J.* **147**, 298–305.

Macy, D.W. & Gasper, P.W. (1985) Diazepam-induced eating in anorexic cats *J. Am. Anim. Hosp. Assoc.* **21**, 17–20.

McKellar, Q.A., Pearson, T., Bogan, J.A., Galbraith, E.A., Lees, P. & Tiberghien, M.P. (1990) Pharmacokinetics, tolerance and serum thromboxane inhibition of carprofen in the dog. *J. Small Anim. Pract.* **31**, 443–448.

Murata, K., Nakagawa, I., Kumets, Y., Kitahata, L.M. & Collins, J.G. (1989) Intrathecal clonidine suppresses noxiously evolked activity of spinal wide dynamic range neurons in cats. *Anaesth. Analg.* **69**(2), 185–191.

Nolan, A.M. (1989) Analgesia. *In: BSAVA Manual of Anaesthesia for Small Animal Practice* (ed. Hilbery, A.R.) B.S.A.V.A. Cheltenham, Gloucs. p. 35.

Ossipov, M.H., Goldstein, F.J. & Malsteed, R.T. (1984) Feline analgesia following central administration of opioids. *Neuropharmacology* **23**(8), 925–929.

Postal, J. M., Autefage, A. Asimus, E., Bayle, R. & Van Gool, F. (1991) Efficacy of ketoprofen in the treatment of inflammatory and painful musculoskeletal disorders in pets. *Proceedings Congres Mondial Veterinaire Rio de Janeiro*, August, 1991.

Potthoff, A. & Carithers, R.W. (1989) Pain and analgesia in dogs and cats. *Comp. Cont. Ed. (Small Anim.)* **11**(8), 887–897.

Richards, D.L.S., Clutton, R.E. & Boyd, C., (1989) Electrocardiographic findings following intravenous glycopyrrolate to sedated dogs: a comparison with atropine *J. Ass. Vet. Anaesth.* **16**, 46–50.

Robertson, G.H. & Laing, A.W. (1980) Intravenous buprenorphine (Temgesic) use following Fentanyl analgesic anaesthesia. *Clin. Trials J.* **27**, 51–55.

Samonina, G.E. & Hakumaki, M.O. (1983) The role of the sympathetic nervous system in atropine-induced tachycardia in conscious cats. *Scand. J. Clin. Lab. Invest.* **43**(5), 389–392.

Savola, J.M., Ruskoaho, H., Puurunen, J. & Karki, N.T. (1985) Cardiovascular action of detomidine, a sedative and analgesic derivative with alpha-agonistic properties. *Eur. J. Pharmacol.* **118**(1–2), 69–76.

Sawyer, D.C. & Rech, R.H. (1987) Analgesia and behavioural effects of butorphanol, nalbuphine and pentazocine in the Cat. *J. Am. Anim. Hosp. Assoc.* **23**, 438–446.

Seeler, D.C. (1992) Anesthesia for compromised patients. *In: Veterinary Emergency and Critical Care Medicine* (eds. Murtaugh, R.J. and Kaplar, P.M.) Mosby Year Book pp. 526–535.

Short, C.E. (1987a) Dissociative anesthesia. *In: Principles and Practice of Veterinary Anesthesia* p. 163, Williams and Wilkins, Baltimore.

Short, C.E. (1987b) Pain analgesics and related medications. In: *Principles and Practices of Veterinary Anesthesia.* Williams and Wilkins, Baltimore.

Short, C.E., Martin, R. & Henry, C.W. (1983) Clinical comparison of glycopyrrolate and atropine as preanaesthetic agents in cats. *Vet. Med/Sm. Am. Clin.* **10**, 1447–1560.

Stenburg, D. (1989) Physiological role of alpha 2-adrenoceptors in the regulation of vigilance and pain: effect of medetomidine. *Acta. Vet. Scand. Suppl.* **85**, 21–28.

Stenburg, D., Salven, P. & Miettinen, M.V. (1987) Sedative action of the alpha 2-agonist medetomidine in cats. *J. Vet. Pharmacol. Ther.* **10**(4), 319–323.

Taylor, P.M. (1985) Analgesia in the dog and cat. *In Practice* Jan. 1985, 5–13.

Timmermans, P.B., Schoop, A.M., Kwa, H.Y. & Van Zwieten, P.A. (1981) Characterisation of alpha-adrenceptors participating in the central hypotensive and sedative effects of clonidine using yohimbine, rauwolscine and corynanthine. *Eur. J. Pharmacol.* **70**(1), 7–15.

Tomemori, N., Komarsu, T., Urabe, N., Seo, N., Mori, K. (1981) Activation of the supraspinal pain inhibition system by ketamine hydrochloride. *Acta. Anaesthesiol. Scand.* **25**(4), 355–359.

Tranquilli, W.J, Lemke, K.A., Williams, L.L., Ballard, G., Ko, J.C.H., Benson, G.J. & Thurmon, J.C., (1992) Flumazenil efficacy in reversing diazepam or midazolam overdose in dog. *J. Vet. Anaesth.* **19**, 65–68.

Tranquilli, W.J. & Benson, G.J. (1992) Advantages and guidelines for using alpha-2 agonists as anaesthetic adjuncts. *Vet. Clin. North Am. Small Anim. Pract.* **22**(2), 289–293.

Trim, C.M. (1989) Sedation and anesthesia. *In: Diseases of the Cat* (ed. J. Holzworth), pp. 43-67. W.B. Saunders, Philadelphia.

Tsyrlin, V.A. & Bravkov, M.F. (1980) Effects of alpha-adrenoceptor-stimulating drugs on baroreceptor reflexes in conscious cats. *Eur. J. Pharmacol.* **67**(1), 75–83.

Tung, A.S. & Yaksh, T.L. (1982) The antinociceptive effects of epidural opiates in the cat: studies of the pharmacology and the effects of lipophilicity in spinal analgesia. *Pain* **12**(4), 343–356.

Vähä-Vahe, A.T. (1989) Clinical evaluation of medetomidine, a novel sedative and analgesic drug for dogs and cats. *Acta. Vet. Scand.* **30**(3), 267–273.

Vähä-Vahe, A.T. (1990) Clinical effectiveness of atipamezole as a medetomidine antagonist in cats. *J. Small Anim. Pract.* **31**, 193–197.

Vainio, O. (1989) Introduction to the clinical pharmacology of medetomidine. *Acta. Vet. Scand. Suppl.* **85**, 85–88.

Verstegen, J., Fargetton, X., Donnay, I. & Ectors, F. (1991) An evaluation of medetomidine/ketamine and other drug combinations for anaesthesia in cats. *Vet. Record* **128**, 32–35.

Waterman, A.E. (1983) Influence of premedication with xylazine on the distribution and metabolism of intra-muscularly administered ketamine in cats. *Res. Vet. Sci.* **35**(3), 285–290.

Watts, S.J., Slocombe, R.F., Harrison, W.D. & Stewart, G.A. (1973) Assessment of analgesia and other effects of morphine and thiambutene in the mouse and cat. *Australian Vet. J.* **49**, 525–529.

Yaksh, T.L., Hary, G.J. & Onoftio, B.M. (1986) High dose of spinal morphine produce a nonopiate receptor- mediated hyperesthesia: clinical and theoretic implications. *Anesthesiology* **64**(5), 590–597.

Yasuoka, S. & Yaksh, T.L. (1983) Effects on nociscep-tive threshold and blood pressure of intrathecally administered morphine and alpha-adrenergic agonists. *Neuropharmacology* **22**(2), 309–315.

Young, L.E. & Jones, R.S., (1990) Clinical observations on medetomidine/ketamine anaesthesia and its antagonism in the cat. *J. Small Anim. Pract.* **31**, 221–224.

Young, L.E., Brearley, J.C., Richards, D.L.S., Bartram, D.H. & Jones, R.S. (1990) Medetomidine as a premedicant in dogs and its reversal by atipame-zole *J. Small Anim. Pract.* **31**, 554–559.

8
Injectable Anaesthetics

P.A. Flecknell

Introduction

A wide choice of injectable anaesthetics is available for use in the cat. Selection of the most appropriate agent requires careful consideration of a number of factors, relating both to the particular characteristics of an anaesthetic or anaesthetic combination, and the type and duration of the procedure. The experience of the anaesthetist, the temperament and state of health of the patient, and the anaesthetic and other equipment available should also influence the selection of the most appropriate injectable anaesthetic agents.

An injectable anaesthetic regimen may be selected because of its apparent simplicity of administration, requiring only a syringe and needle, but this attitude can lead to a failure to provide appropriate support for the anaesthetized patient, and in particular to a failure to intubate or supply oxygen. It is essential that injectable anaesthetic regimens are managed with care, and with appropriate attention to monitoring and supportive therapy.

A second factor in selecting a particular injectable anaesthetic regimen may be the variable temperament of some cats, and the difficulties of providing effective and humane restraint for minor manipulations such as venepuncture. Some injectable anaesthetics can be administered conveniently by the intramuscular or subcutaneous route, and anaesthesia can then be deepened once the animal has been immobilized in this way. Although this approach is convenient, and may be the most appropriate means of administering an anaesthetic to a frightened or aggressive animal, it has certain inherent problems. The dose of anaesthetic required to produce a given depth of anaesthesia will vary considerably between individual animals. Administration by intra-

venous injection allows the dose to be adjusted as anaesthesia is induced, and so provides a controlled method of administering the agent. Adminstration by the intramuscular or subcutaneous route requires administration of the total dose of anaesthetic based on recommendations in an anaesthesia text or from the manufacturer's product information sheet. Inadvertent overdosing is a possibility, with potentially serious consequences, as is underdosing requiring administration of additional drug. If anaesthetics are to be administered by intramuscular or subcutaneous injection, it is therefore important to select agents with a high therapeutic index (the ratio of the LD_{50} to the AD_{50}), hence high margin of safety, and to take especial care when anaesthetizing animals which have intercurrent illness, chronic organ dysfunction, or traumatic injuries.

The use of injectable anaesthetics has the advantage of avoiding problems associated with waste anaesthetic gases. Although the use of gas scavenging devices can reduce the magnitude of this problem, use of injectable anaesthetic regimens can eliminate it entirely.

A final general point to consider is that injectable anaesthesia should not be regarded as a total solution to all feline anaesthetic requirements, but as an integral part of an overall anaesthetic protocol. Used in this way, injectable agents can be combined with inhalational agents or local anaesthesia to produce an optimum regimen for a particular patient.

Methods of Administration

Intravenous Injection

The most convenient site for intravenous injection is the cephalic vein on the anterior aspect of the fore limb. The fur overlying the vein should be removed with scissors or with electric clippers. Most cats respond well to gentle handling, and restraint should generally be minimal (see Chapter 5). If the animal requires firm physical restraint, the stress caused by this can represent a significant hazard to the animal during induction, and in these circumstances it is often preferable to administer a potent sedative or tranquillizer and delay induction until chemical restraint has been achieved.

Venepuncture is reasonably easy in most adults using a 21 or 23 G, 1.5 cm needle. Although this approach may be found adequate if induction is free from complications, it is preferable to use either a 'Butterfly' type infusion set, or an over-the-needle catheter (Fig. 8.1). Use of a 'Butterfly' type set minimizes the risk of inadvertent extravascular placement of the needle if the cat moves its leg during venepuncture. The wings of the butterfly set enable it to be taped securely to the limb (Fig. 8.2C), and this provides a convenient route for administration of either additional anaesthetic,

fluids, or emergency drugs. If the cat is repositioned during the pre-operative or intra-operative periods, then this may result in movement of the needle through the wall of the vein. This risk is avoided by use of an indwelling flexible catheter. 'Over-the-needle' type catheters (Fig. 8.1) are most convenient for use in the cat, as they enable a relatively large diameter catheter to be placed in the vein. Most types of catheter will pass through the skin without difficulty (Fig. 8.2A,B), but occasionally resistance is encountered resulting in damage to the tip of the catheter, and this may prevent it from entering the vein. This is usually only a problem with unneutered male cats, who tend to have tougher and thicker skin than females or young neutered animals. If necessary, a small incision can be made in the skin overlying the vein using a scalpel blade, before attempting venepuncture. Subcutaneous infiltration of local anaesthetic, or prior application of EMLA cream (see below) may be required for this.

Most cats show only a minimal reaction to venepuncture, but occasionally animals will be

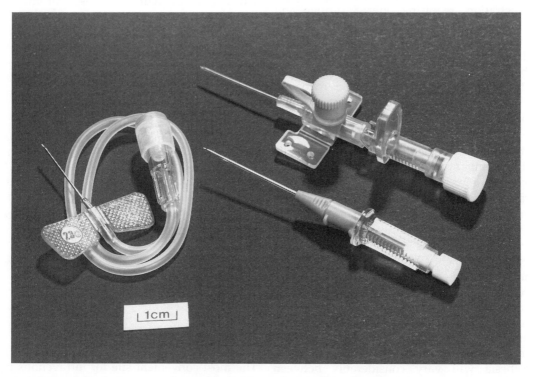

Fig. 8.1 A 'butterfly' infusion set and two types of 'over the needle' catheters.

encountered who react excessively. Problems may also be encountered when training new staff members in the technique, since repeated attempts at venepuncture may be required. Such difficulties can be overcome by prior use of local anaesthetic cream (EMLA, ASTRA). The leg is prepared for venepuncture by shaving the fur and a 2–3 mm layer of the cream is placed on the skin and covered with an occlusive dressing. After 45 min the dressing is removed, the skin wiped clean, and venepuncture carried out. Use of local anaesthetic cream provides full skin-thickness anaesthesia (Flecknell *et al.*, 1990), and prevents any reaction, either to needle puncture, or simply the touch of the needle which can be sufficient to trigger a response in frightened or 'needle-shy' individuals.

Although the cephalic vein is a convenient site for venepuncture in most animals, problems may occasionally be encountered. As alternatives (see Chapters 1 and 5), the recurrent tarsal vein can be used either on the medial aspect of the hock or more proximally where it runs across the lateral aspect of the limb. On the medial side of the limb the saphenous, or more proximally the femoral, can also be used.

In young kittens, obese animals, or animals with circulatory collapse, it may be necessary to use the jugular vein (see Chapter 5 for positioning). This is also required for longer term infusion of fluids or drugs. Reliable placement of short catheters (<5 cm) into this vein can be difficult, since they can easily be dislodged by flexion of the head and neck. However, if long enough (e.g. 6–8 cm) most types of 'over-the-needle' catheters are satisfactory and the maximum size will be governed solely by the size of the jugular vein; usually 21 or 18 G is adequate. Other suitable approaches are surgical exposure of the jugular vein and placement of a catheter after induction of anaesthesia or use of a longer catheter placed using a 'through the needle' system. Although conventional designs of 'through-the-needle' catheters can be used, these have the disadvantage of retaining the needle at the hub of the catheter, where it can damage the catheter material. A variety of designs attempt to overcome this, but the most successful provides a needle which can be split into two halves and removed after the catheter

has been successfully introduced into the blood vessel. A better alternative technique is to use a Seldinger catheter, which consists of a needle, a flexible introducer, and the catheter itself (see Chapter 10, Fig. 10.9). The needle is positioned in the vein and a flexible wire introducer passed down it and advanced into the blood vessel. The needle is then withdrawn and the catheter passed over the introducer, through the skin and into the blood vessel after which the introducer is withdrawn.

Intramuscular Injection

The same considerations with regard to physical restraint which are discussed above apply to restraint for intramuscular injection, although since the procedure is generally more rapid and needle positioning less critical, fewer problems are likely to be encountered than when attempting intravenous administration. A popular site for injection is into the muscle mass of the posterior thigh. However it has been shown that use of this site frequently results in material being injected into the fascial planes rather than into the muscle mass. Absorption is then unpredictable, some agents may not be absorbed sufficiently rapidly to produce anaesthesia, and sciatic nerve injury is a possibility. The anterior thigh provides a more suitable site and injection can be made into this muscle mass using a 1.5 cm 21 or 23 G needle. Absorption is more reliable, and inadvertent damage to large blood vessels or nerves is not a problem. Unfortunately, injection into the quadriceps seems to cause more discomfort to the animal, so it is important to use only small volumes of anaesthetic, (<1 ml in an adult cat), or to split the injection between several sites if a larger volume is required. It is also important to inject the material slowly. As an alternative to the hind-limb muscles, injection can be made into the triceps muscle on the fore limb.

Subcutaneous Administration

Subcutaneous injection, using a 23 or 21 G needle, provides a very simple, rapid and relatively painless means of administering material to the cat. Absorption is generally less

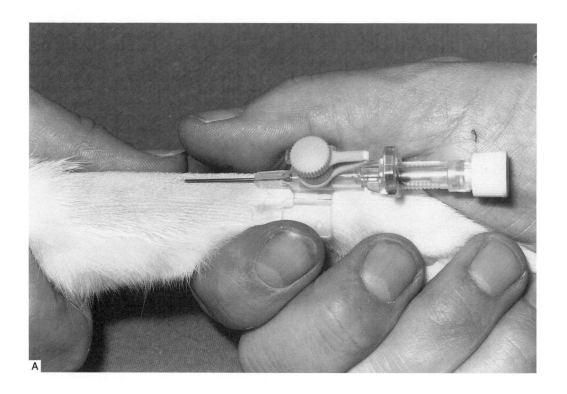

A

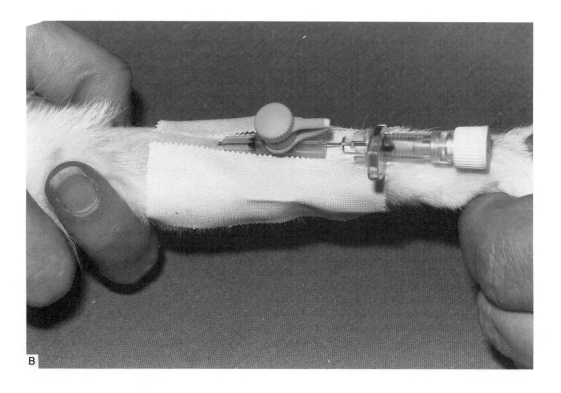

B

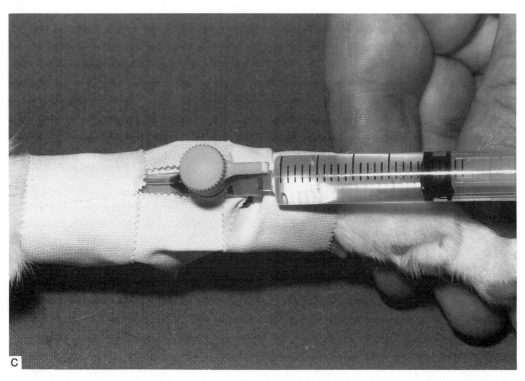

Fig. 8.2 Method of anchoring a 'winged' catheter to provide secure attachment to the limb. (A) The catheter is introduced into the cephalic vein (note the presence of blood confirming correct placement). (B) The stylette is withdrawn slightly and the catheter advanced into the vein. Two strips of tape are placed along the length of the limb anchoring the catheter wings. (C) Two further strips of tape are placed around the limb, above and below the insertion point of the catheter. The stylette is then removed.

rapid than following deep intramuscular injection, and some short-acting anaesthetics are not absorbed sufficiently rapidly for them to have a reliable effect. Irritant material should not be administered by this route, since pain and local inflammation or necrosis can occur. Animals with some degree of dehydration will have poor circulation to the skin, and drug absorption will be slow and unpredictable.

Intraperitoneal Injection

Although a number of anaesthetics can be administered by intraperitoneal injection, the less predictable absorption and risk of inadvertent injection into the viscera restrict the use of this route of injection. In an emergency, if a peripheral vein cannot be located, then intra-

peritoneal administration of anaesthetics such as pentobarbitone or ketamine combinations can be a useful means of inducing basal narcosis, especially if euthanasia is to follow.

Oral Administration

Use of this route is restricted to administration of ketamine to intractable animals (e.g. feral cats). Initial reports suggested squirting the drug at the animal's mouth using a syringe (Macy & Siwe, 1977). More controlled administration can often be achieved in caged animals by attaching a long catheter to the syringe and pushing this towards the animal's mouth. Many cats will respond by biting the catheter tip, and the drug can then be injected rapidly into the animal's mouth.

Anaesthetic Agents

Dissociative Anaesthetics

Dissociative anaesthesia is a term used to describe a state in which there is a functional and electrophysiological dissociation between the thalamoneocortical and limbic systems (White *et al.*, 1982). This functional change in the CNS is reflected in the clinical appearance of animals after they have received a dissociative anaesthetic agent. Most species develop a cataleptic state in which the eyes remain open, there is muscle rigidity, nystagmus in some species, and occasional spontaneous limb movements. In the cat, muscle rigidity with the limbs fixed in extension usually predominates. The degree of analgesia produced by these dissociative anaesthetics appears to vary considerably between animal species and man. In man, subanaesthetic doses of ketamine produce good analgesia, but in some animal species, including the cat, responses to painful stimuli persist until high doses of the agent have been administered. It appears that visceral analgesia is a particular problem, and that although responses to painful stimulus to the periphery may be abolished, animals may respond to abdominal pain (Sawyer *et al.*, 1991).

Phencyclidine and cyclohexamine were the first dissociative anaesthetics to be evaluated, but both of these agents were associated with prolonged recovery periods with psychotomimetic activity in man (Collins *et al.*, 1960). Ketamine was developed in an attempt to overcome some of the side-effects of the earlier dissociative agents (Domino *et al.*, 1965), and this agent, together with the more recently introduced agent, tiletamine, are the only dissociative anaesthetics which are currently available commercially.

Ketamine

Ketamine (2-(*O*-chlorophenyl)-2-methylamino cyclohexanone) is water soluble, and is produced commercially as a racemic mixture of two isomers. A solution of 100 mg/kg, the standard veterinary preparation, has a pH of 3.5. Lower strength solutions (10 mg/ml and 50 mg/ml) are manufactured for clinical use in man. Ketamine is metabolized extensively in the liver, producing a range of metabolites, some of which have anaesthetic activity. The pharmacokinetics of ketamine have been investigated in the cat (Baggot & Blake, 1976; Heavner & Bloedow, 1979) and the half life following intravenous administration ranges from 60 to 80 min, with a plasma clearance of 20–40 ml/min/kg. Ketamine and its metabolites are excreted via the kidneys but it has been shown that administration of diuretics does not increase the rate of elimination, and is an ineffective treatment for cases of ketamine overdose (Hanna *et al.*, 1988a,b). The duration of recovery is dose dependent, but, according to the manufacturers, prolonged recoveries are not uncommon. Care should be taken when using other drugs with ketamine as the metabolism and elimination of ketamine may be altered (e.g. xylazine, see Chapter 7). Since elimination depends upon renal function, the duration of action may be prolonged in cats with renal failure. The chronic administration of ketamine results in an increase in the activity of hepatic enzyme systems responsible for drug metabolism (Marietta *et al.*, 1976). This enzyme induction may decrease the efficacy of ketamine when given repeatedly. Ketamine has, unfortunately, become a drug of abuse in man, and care should be taken in its safe storage and disposal.

Onset of action of ketamine following intravenous or intramuscular administration is rapid but recovery can be prolonged, and is associated with ataxia, increased motor activity and increased sensitivity to external stimuli. In man, ketamine emergence reactions are associated with a range of hallucinations and mood alterations, and apparently similar effects have been reported in the cat (Wright, 1982).

Cardiovascular and respiratory systems. Ketamine has sympathomimetic effects, and causes a rise in heart rate, cardiac output and blood pressure in most species. Ketamine also has a direct negative inotropic effect on the myocardium, so that the overall effects of administration may vary depending upon the clinical state of the patient (Clanachan *et al.*, 1976; White *et al.*,

1982). In healthy, normovolaemic cats, the stimulatory action of ketamine predominates, resulting in an increase in arterial blood pressure and an increase in heart rate (Child *et al.*, 1972 (4–16 mg/kg i/v); Haskins *et al.*, 1975 (35 mg/kg i/m)). Becker and Beglinger (1982) reported that ketamine (20 mg/kg i/m) caused a slight decrease (8%) in heart rate and left ventricular pressure (16%). There was a more marked decrease (33%) in maximum rate of rise of left ventricular peak pressure (max dp/dt). The stimulatory effect of ketamine described in some studies has been interpreted as an indication for the use of this agent in hypovolaemic or traumatized animals. Studies in man suggest that in critically ill patients, the sympathomimetic action of ketamine may fail to balance its depressant effects, and a fall in blood pressure and significant cardiovascular system depression can occur in some patients (Waxman *et al.*, 1980). In addition, the concurrent use of other anaesthetic agents can block the sympathomimetic actions of ketamine, resulting in cardiovascular depression (Bidwai *et al.*, 1975). Administration of ketamine combined with acepromazine in the cat produced a fall in ventricular pressure (31%), a similar change in max dp/dt (28%) and an increase in heart rate (Becker & Beglinger, 1982). It is therefore important not to make unwarranted assumptions about cardiovascular stability during ketamine anaesthesia when using this agent in animals with compromised cardiovascular function. It is also important that effective monitoring techniques are employed to ensure that appropriate supportive therapy is provided when needed.

Ketamine causes an overall depression of respiratory function, but its effects are complex and dose dependent. At low dose rates, there is an increase in respiratory rate but production of an apneustic pattern of breathing and a decrease in tidal volume. High dose rates produce a decrease in respiratory rate, and significant hypercapnia (Child *et al.*, 1972; Evans *et al.*, 1972; Hatch *et al.*, 1973). Laryngeal cough responses and the pharyngeal swallowing reflex are reasonably well maintained during ketamine anaesthesia, but the standard good anaesthetic practice of maintaining a patent airway and providing supplemental oxygen should not be neglected. Profuse salivation frequently occurs after administration of ketamine; it may be prevented by administration of atropine. When used in healthy individuals, the degree of respiratory depression is unlikely to be significant although a number of deaths, presumed to be due to apnoea, have been reported (Clarke & Hall, 1990) when ketamine was administered following xylazine premedication.

Other body systems. Ketamine causes an increase in cerebral blood flow and a rise in intracranial pressure (Takeshita *et al.*, 1972). It is therefore inadvisable to use this agent in animals with cranial injury, since it may exacerbate intracranial haemorrhage or cerebral oedema. Ketamine has been shown to produce seizures at high doses in dogs and cats (Reid and Frank, 1972) but in man, ketamine does not induce seizures in epileptics (Celesia *et al.*, 1975), and it has been shown to reduce the seizure threshold in rodents (Myslobodsky *et al.*, 1981). Since no properly controlled studies have been undertaken in cats, it is perhaps advisable to avoid the use of ketamine in known epileptic feline patients.

Clinical use. Ketamine administered by intramuscular injection produces dose-dependent sedation and, at higher dose rates, analgesia and a cataleptic state. Low doses (5–10 mg/kg) produce sufficient restraint for minor manipulations, higher dose rates (11–33 mg/kg) produce loss of righting reflex and a degree of analgesia sufficient for minor surgery. Onset of action following subcutaneous administration is almost as rapid as following intramuscular administration. Because of the low pH of ketamine, many animals show a marked pain response following injection either by intramuscular or subcutaneous routes. This problem can be avoided by administering ketamine by intravenous injection, in which case lower dose rates (2–10 mg/kg) are sufficient to produce equivalent effects. As discussed earlier, there is some disagreement concerning the degree of analgesia produced by ketamine alone. At dose rates in excess of 20 mg/kg, most animals are unresponsive to surgical procedures such as a skin incision, but

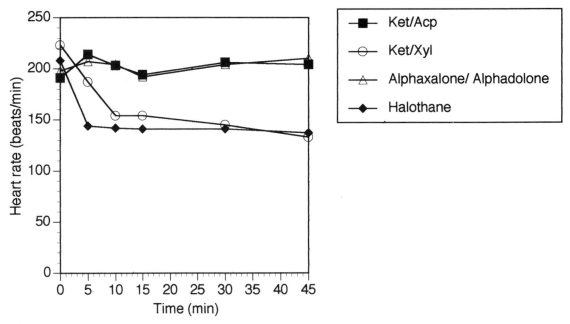

Fig. 8.3 Effects on heart rate of several anaesthetics in the cat. Ketamine 20 mg/kg, acepromazine 0.11 mg/kg, i/m (■) *; ketamine 10 mg/kg, xylazine 1 mg/kg i/m (○)[+]; alphaxalone/alphadolone, 12 mg/kg i/v (Δ) #; halothane (0.9–1.5%) (◆)**. Data derived from * Ingwersen *et al.*, 1988; [+] Allen *et al.*, 1986; # Dyson *et al.*, 1987; ** Ingwersen *et al.*, 1988.

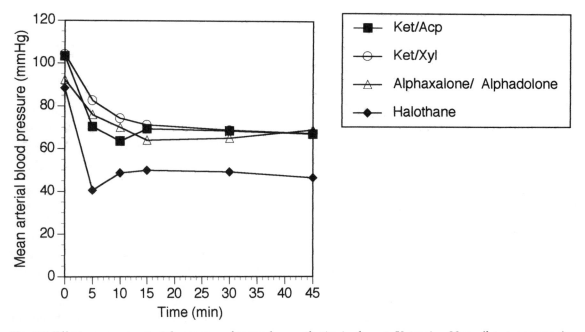

Fig. 8.4 Effects on mean arterial pressure of several anaesthetics in the cat. Ketamine 20 mg/kg, acepromazine 0.11 mg/kg i/m (■) *; ketamine 10 mg/kg, xylazine 1 mg/kg i/m (○)[+]; alphaxalone/alphadolone, 12 mg/kg i/v (Δ) #; halothane (0.9–1.5%) (◆) **. Data derived from * Ingwersen *et al.*, 1988; [+] Allen *et al.*, 1986; # Dyson *et al.*, 1987; ** Ingwersen *et al.*, 1988.

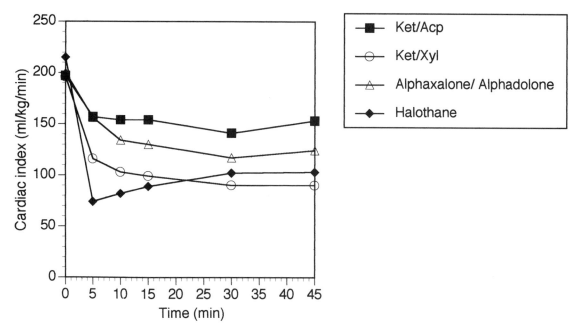

Fig. 8.5 Effects on cardiac index of several anaesthetics in the cat. Ketamine 20 mg/kg, acepromazine 0.11 mg/kg i/m (■) *; ketamine 10 mg/kg, xylazine 1 mg/kg i/m (○)[+]; alphaxalone/alphadolone, 12 mg/kg i/v (Δ) #; halothane (0.9–1.5%) (◆)**. Data derived from * Ingwersen *et al.*, 1988; [+]Allen *et al.*, 1986; # Dyson *et al.*, 1987; ** Ingwersen *et al.*, 1988.

may respond with movements or even vocalizations if abdominal procedures are undertaken. In any event, the muscle rigidity associated with the use of ketamine as the sole anaesthetic agent makes it unsuitable for major surgery and it is recommended that when used alone it be used only for minor procedures, not involving penetration of a body cavity.

Ketamine combinations
In an attempt to overcome the disadvantage of using ketamine as the sole anaesthetic agent, a variety of combinations of ketamine with sedatives and tranquillizers have been evaluated. The most widely used of these has been ketamine in combination with xylazine, but acepromazine, diazepam, midazolam and, most recently, medetomidine, have also been used as adjuncts to ketamine anaesthesia.

Ketamine/xylazine. When xylazine is combined with ketamine (0.5–1.0 mg/kg xylazine s/c or i/m; 20 mg/kg ketamine i/m) the combination provides approximately 30 min of surgical anaesthesia, with good muscle relaxation and sufficient analgesia to undertake a range of operative procedures (Cullen & Jones, 1977). The combination of ketamine and xylazine can be premixed and administered as a single injection, but it is preferable to administer xylazine first, followed by ketamine 10–15 min later, since a relatively high proportion of cats vomit after administration of xylazine. Vomiting has not been associated with any untoward sequelae, and is regarded by some anaesthetists as an advantage, since it ensures that the stomach is empty prior to the onset of general anaesthesia and the loss of the pharyngeal and laryngeal reflexes. Atropine (0.3 mg total dose in adult cats) is usually included in this regimen to minimize the salivary and bronchial secretions associated with ketamine anaesthesia. Atropine also prevents any bradycardia caused by xylazine, but correction of the bradycardia does not necessarily improve cardiac performance (see Chapter 7).

Recovery from ketamine/xylazine anaesthesia is generally satisfactory, but can be very

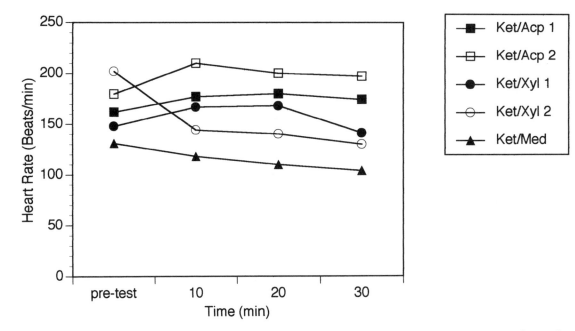

Fig. 8.6 Effects on heart rate of ketamine in combination with acepromazine, xylazine or medetomidine. Ketamine 10 mg/kg, acepromazine 1 mg/kg (■) *; ketamine 29 mg/kg, acepromazine 0.29 mg/kg (❑) #; ketamine 10 mg/kg, xylazine 1 mg/kg (●) *; ketamine 21 mg/kg, xylazine 2.0 mg/kg (○) #; ketamine 7.5 mg/kg, medetomidine 80 μg/kg (▲) *. Data derived from * Verstegen *et al.*, 1991, and # Sanford & Colby, 1982.

prolonged, especially if the cat becomes hypothermic (Cullen & Jones, 1977). Recovery times can be shortened dramatically by administration of the α_2-adrenoceptor antagonist, atipamezole, (see Chapters 3 and 7).

Although ketamine/xylazine has been widely used in feline anaesthesia, it is important to recognize that it has significant depressant effects on the cardiovascular and respiratory systems. Ketamine (10 mg/kg) and xylazine (1 mg/kg) caused a 50% fall in cardiac output, bradycardia, and a prolonged fall in systemic arterial pressure (Figs 8.3–8.5), although blood gas parameters remained stable and within normal limits (Allen *et al.*, 1986). A similar fall in arterial pressure and bradycardia was reported by Sanford and Colby (1982), following administration of a higher dose of ketamine (30–35 mg/kg) (Figs 8.6–8.7), and these authors also reported a marked fall in respiratory rate, accompanied by moderate hypoxia and a small rise in carbon dioxide tensions. Administration of a deliberate overdose of 50 mg/kg ketamine and 1–2 mg/kg xylazine (Arnbjerg, 1979) caused

more marked hypoxia (pO_2 57–88 mmHg), but no hypercapnia (pCO_2 31–42 mmHg). Respiratory rates were markedly depressed (4–14 /min) and after an initial small increase, heart rate fell progressively for the remainder of the period of anaesthesia and sedation.

A notable feature of several of these studies was the very prolonged period of hypotension and sustained decrease in heart rate, which persisted even when the cats were showing signs of recovery from anaesthesia. In addition, two authors (Arnbjerg, 1979; Colby & Sandford, 1981) recorded periods of apnoea during anaesthesia. It is clear, therefore, that the sympathomimetic effects of ketamine do not offset xylazine's hypotensive effects, and although no cats died in these studies, it would seem sensible to avoid the use of this combination in hypovolaemic animals or in cats with cardiovascular or respiratory system injury or disease. The use of xylazine in association with ketamine may be associated with an increased anaesthetic mortality which may have been related to a failure to monitor the animals

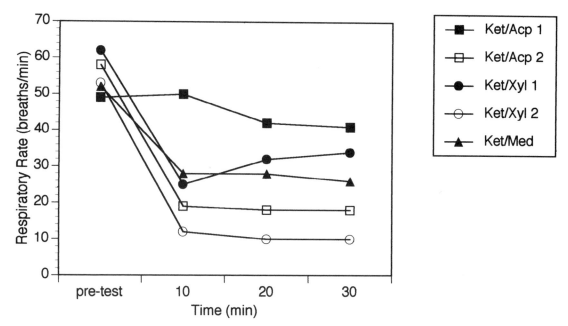

Fig. 8.7 Effects on respiratory rate of ketamine in combination with acepromazine, xylazine or medetomidine. Ketamine 10 mg/kg, acepromazine 1 mg/kg (■) *; ketamine 29 mg/kg, acepromazine 0.29 mg/kg (❑) #; ketamine 10 mg/kg, xylazine 1 mg/kg (●) *; ketamine 21 mg/kg, xylazine 2.0 mg/kg (○) #; ketamine 7.5 mg/kg, medetomidine 80 μg/kg (▲) *. Data derived from * Verstegen *et al.*, 1991, and # Sanford & Colby, 1982.

adequately during the recovery period (Clarke & Hall, 1990).

Ketamine/medetomidine. As an alternative to xylazine, the more recently introduced α_2-agonist, medetomidine, has been evaluated as an adjunct to ketamine anaesthesia (Verstegen *et al.*, 1989, 1990, 1991a; Young & Jones, 1990). The additional analgesia provided by medetomidine enabled a reduction in the dose of ketamine required for surgical anaesthesia (Table 8.1). In two studies of the use of this agent in a range of surgical procedures, medetomidine (80 μg/kg i/m) and ketamine (5 or 7 mg/kg i/m) provided satisfactory anaesthesia with good analgesia (Verstegen *et al.*, 1990; Young & Jones, 1990). When used at these dose rates, a mild to moderate bradycardia was produced (Verstegen *et al.*, 1991a; Fig. 8.6), but higher dose rates (80 μ/kg medetomidine/10 mg/kg ketamine) caused a mild tachycardia. Respiratory rate was depressed (Fig. 8.7), but apnoeic periods were only noted in animals receiving the highest dose rate of ketamine (10 mg/kg). No data are

available concerning the cardiovascular effects of this combination except for measurements of heart rate. Similarly, studies of the effect of this combination on the respiratory system have not included blood gas analysis or measurement of tidal volume. Given the similar modes of action of xylazine and medetomidine, it seems reasonable to assume that medetomidine/ketamine will cause moderate hypotension.

ANTAGONISM OF MEDETOMIDINE/XYLAZINE. A significant advantage of both ketamine/xylazine and ketamine/medetomidine in comparison to other ketamine combinations, is that the anaesthetic effects can be partially antagonized with α_2-antagonists such as yohimbine or atipamezole (see Chapter 7). Atipamezole appears to be a particularly suitable antagonist, and is largely free from undesirable side-effects (Vähä-Vahe, 1990). Data obtained in cats anaesthetized with chloralose, followed by administration of medetomidine, demonstrated that the cardiovascular depressant effects of medetomidine could be reversed using atipamezole (Savola, 1989). Comparative

Table 8.1 Injectable anaesthetics in the cat. Dose rates, duration of action and approximate time to recovery in non-premedicated animals. Note that concurrent use of other agents can prolong recovery or reduce the dosage required

Anaesthetic	Dose rate	Route of injection	Approx. duration of anaesthesia	Approx. recovery time (standing/walking)
Alphaxalone/	9–12 mg/kg	i/v	10–15 min	45–120 min
alphadolone	18 mg/kg	i/m		
Chloralose	70 mg/kg	i/p	3–12 h	Non-recovery only
	60 mg/kg	i/v		
Fentanyl/	0.02 mg/kg	i/m	–	5 h
metomidate	20 mg/kg	i/m		
Ketamine	11–33 mg/kg	i/m	30–45 min	3–4 h
Ketamine/	20 mg/kg	i/m	20–30 min	3–4 h
acepromazine	0.11 mg/kg	i/m		
Ketamine/	7 mg/kg	i/m	30–40 min	3–4 h
medetomidine	80 μg/kg	i/m		
Ketamine/	10 mg/kg	i/m	20–30 min	3–4 h
midazolam	0.2 mg/kg	i/m		
Ketamine/	15 mg/kg	i/m	20–30 min	3–4 h
promazine	1.12 mg/kg	i/m		
Ketamine/	22 mg/kg	i/m	20–30 min	3–4 h
xylazine	1.1 mg/kg	i/m		
Methohexitone	5–11 mg/kg	i/v	5–6 min	60–90 min
Pentobarbitone	20–30 mg/kg	i/v	60–90 min	4–8 h
Propanidid	8–16 mg/kg	i/v	4–6 min	20–30 min
Propofol	5–8 mg/kg	i/v	3–6 min	30 min
Thiamylal	12–18 mg/kg	i/v	10–15 min	1–2 h
Thiopentone	20–30 mg/kg	i/v	5–10 min	1–2 h
Tiletamine/	7.5 mg/kg	i/m	20–40 min	
zolezepam	7.5 mg/kg	i/m		
Urethane	750 mg/kg	i/v	6-8 h	Non-recovery only
	1500 mg/kg	i/p		

studies of a number of antagonists (Verstegen *et al.*, 1991b) indicated that atipamezole (200 μg/kg i/m) was most effective in countering the bradycardia and anaesthesia produced by ketamine/medetomidine. Although some residual effects of ketamine remain, normal posture and consciousness are resumed within a few minutes of administration of the antagonist.

Ketamine/acepromazine. Ketamine (30 mg/kg) combined with acepromazine (0.3 mg/kg) (Sanford & Colby, 1982) has been advocated as a suitable combination for providing surgical anaesthesia. As with other combinations, addition of a tranquillizer reduces the muscle rigidity associated with ketamine alone and appears to produce unconsciousness and a

state more resembling conventional general anaesthesia, although the eyes remain open with a dilated pupil. This combination produces a degree of cardiovascular depression comparable to that induced by ketamine/xylazine (Figs 8.3–8.6) (Sanford & Colby, 1982; Becker & Beglinger, 1982; Ingwerson *et al.*, 1988). Although respiratory rate was also depressed (Fig 8.7), periods of apnoea appear less frequent and severe, and blood gas parameters were relatively unaffected (Sanford & Colby, 1982). The depressant effects of ketamine/acepromazine are dose dependent, and lower dose rates of this combination (ketamine 10 mg/kg, acepromazine 0.1 mg/kg) have less effect on the cardiovascular and respiratory systems. However, at this lower dose rate, the degree of muscle relaxation and analgesia produced by ketamine/acepromazine is generally less than that seen when ketamine/xylazine or ketamine/medetomidine are administered, (Verstegen *et al.*, 1991a). The use of an intermediate dose rate (ketamine 20 mg/kg, acepromazine 0.1 mg/kg) is advisable, and results may be improved by pre-anaesthetic administration of an opioid such as butorphanol (0.4 mg/kg s/c) to increase the degree of intra-operative analgesia (Tranquilli *et al.*, 1988).

Ketamine/promazine. A similar combination of ketamine and the phenothiazine tranquillizer promazine has also been evaluated. This combination has been produced as a commercial preparation in North America, incorporating an anticholinergic, aminopentamide (Christie & Buyniski, 1977). As with other combinations, surgical anaesthesia with good muscle relaxation was claimed to be produced, although some degree of cardiovascular and respiratory depression was also noted (Buyniski & Christie, 1977).

Ketamine/midazolam. Ketamine (10 mg/kg i/m) and midazolam (0.2 mg/kg i/m) administered as a single, pre-mixed injection produced heavy sedation in cats with good muscle relaxation (Chambers & Dobson, 1989). Higher dose rates (ketamine 15–25 mg/kg) and midazolam (1.0 mg/kg) i/m, provides a sufficient plane of anaesthesia for abdominal surgery (Cruz-Madorran, pers. commun.). Ketamine (2.5 mg/kg i/v) and midazolam (0.125 mg/kg i/v) after premedication with papaveretum (0.4 mg/kg) provided a depth of anaesthesia sufficient to allow endotracheal intubation (Dobromylskyj, 1992).

Tiletamine

Tiletamine (2-(ethylamino)-2-(2-thenyl)cyclohexanone) is a dissociative anaesthetic agent related to ketamine. It produces immobilization and typical dissociative anaesthesia, with extensor rigidity and an apneustic respiratory pattern. As with ketamine, the eyes remain open, and the palpebral and laryngeal and pharyngeal reflexes are maintained (Calderwood *et al.*, 1971). Administration of tiletamine (11 mg/kg i/m)

produced a moderate respiratory acidosis, but with no significant effects on arterial oxygen tensions. Heart rate and blood pressure showed a gradual decline, although there was considerable individual variation in response. Recovery was characterized by periods of hyperresponsiveness to external stimuli (Calderwood *et al.*, 1971). Cats receiving tiletamine have also been reported to have temperament changes during the recovery period (Massopust *et al.*, 1973).

Tiletamine/zolezepam. Tiletamine is rarely used as the sole immobilizing agent in cats, and is more frequently administered in combination with zolezepam, a benzodiazepine (Telazol, 50 mg/kg tiletamine plus 50 mg/kg zolezepam/ml, Parke Davis). Administration of this combination to cats (6–16 mg/kg i/m of Telazol, equivalent to 3–8 mg/kg tiletamine and 3–8 mg/kg of zolezepam) produced light to medium planes of anaesthesia (duration approximately 60 min), with a reasonable degree of muscle relaxation. Most animals salivated profusely, but this could be controlled by concurrent administration of atropine (Ward *et al.*, 1974). The degree of analgesia after administration of tiletamine (5.5 mg/kg) and zolezepam (5.5 mg/kg) (11 mg/kg i/m of Telazol) has been reported as satisfactory, but some animals still responded to stimulation of the perineum and scrotum (Bree *et al.*, 1976). The degree of muscle relaxation in comparison to ketamine/medetomidine and ketamine/xylazine was considered poor (Verstegen *et al.*, 1991a), but tiletamine/zolezepam (7.5 mg/kg, 7.5 mg/kg) did not cause significant changes in heart rate. As with tiletamine administered alone, tiletamine/zolazepam produces respiratory depression (Verstegen *et al.*, 1991a). Pain may be noted on injection and although recovery is reasonably rapid (2–3 h), there may be periods of excitement.

Barbiturates

Several barbiturates are currently available for clinical use: thiopentone, thiamylal, methohexitone and pentobarbitone, although the last is now most widely used as a euthanasia agent. All of the barbiturates produce hypnosis (sleep) at moderate doses, but because of their poor analgesic effects, relatively high doses are required to produce surgical anaesthesia. At these high doses, cardiovascular and respiratory depression are often pronounced.

Pentobarbitone

Pentobarbitone is widely available as an aqueous solution, under a variety of trade names. Most commercial preparations intended for anaesthetic use contain 60 mg/ml pentobarbitone. Relatively few studies of the effects of this anaesthetic have been undertaken in cats, and much of our information concerning the action of this agent is by extrapolation from other species. In most species, pentobarbitone produces an initial fall in cardiac output and systemic arterial pressure, and tachycardia. Blood pressure may return to normal later in the course of anaesthesia, but cardiac output remains depressed (Priano *et al.*, 1969). Respiration is usually depressed, and animals may frequently become hypercapnic. In the cat, pentobarbitone produces marked hypotension and tachycardia after intravenous administration (Child *et al.*, 1972), accompanied by respiratory depression and occasionally apnoea.

Pentobarbitone (20–30 mg/kg i/v) produces 30–90 min of light to moderate surgical anaesthesia. In order to avoid involuntary excitement during induction, half of the calculated dose should be administered rapidly, followed by the remainder more slowly, to effect. Pentobarbitone has a relatively slow onset of action, so that administration of the remaining dose should generally take around 5–6 min. Too rapid injection is frequently associated with apnoea and severe cardiovascular depression. Alternative routes of administration (intraperitoneal, oral, intrathoracic and subcutaneous) have been described but these are generally unsatisfactory and not recommended (Clifford & Soma, 1969). Pentobarbitone has a narrow safety margin in the cat, as in other species, and dose rates of 72 mg/kg have been reported to be lethal (Clifford & Soma, 1969). Recovery can be very prolonged, especially if the animal is allowed to become hypothermic, and may be associated with excitement. Cats may remain ataxic and sedated for 8–24 h, particularly if tranquillizers have been administered as pre-anaesthetic

medication. In other species, pentobarbitone anaesthesia may be prolonged by 40–50% if glucose is administered during anaesthesia (Lamson *et al.*, 1951).

Methohexitone

Methohexitone is supplied as a dry powder, which can be reconstituted with either water or saline for intravenous injection. Effects on the cardiovascular system appear variable in the cat. When administered to animals during nitrous oxide administration, animals developed transient marked hypotension, which rapidly recovered as anaesthesia lightened (Skovsted *et al.*, 1970). In studies in conscious cats, all of the dose rates used (3, 6, 12, and 24 mg/kg i/v) produced rapid loss of consciousness, and most animals developed a tachycardia. Effects on blood pressure were variable, with both hypotension and hypertension occurring in different individuals (Child *et al.*, 1972). Respiratory depression and a short period of apnoea on induction are commonly observed.

Methohexitone (5–10 mg/kg) produces short duration anaesthesia in cats, with recovery commencing within 4–5 min of intravenous administration and most cats are able to stand after 30 min. Unfortunately, recovery is frequently associated with considerable involuntary excitement and incoordination, although use of sedatives or tranquillizers can reduce the severity of these reactions. Methohexitone is best administered to cats as a 0.5% solution, and is effective only when administered intravenously. Recovery is associated both with redistribution and metabolism of the compound. Anaesthesia can be prolonged by incremental doses of methohexitone without unduly prolonging recovery (Lees, 1991), provided no more than three or four increments are administered (Flecknell, personal experience).

Thiopentone

Thiopentone is unstable in aqueous solution and when exposed to air. Commercial preparations are supplied as dry powder, mixed with sodium carbonate, in sealed ampoules or bottles. The powder is mixed with either sterile water or saline shortly before injection.

Unused solution may be stored for up to 7–10 days at room temperature, but storage at 4°C will further minimize decomposition. Solutions become cloudy, and may form crystals as they break down. After intravenous administration thiopentone rapidly crosses the blood–brain barrier to induce anaesthesia. Redistribution to other tissues occurs rapidly, and this largely accounts for the prompt recovery of consciousness.

Administration of thiopentone produces a mild hypotension in healthy cats (Child *et al.*, 1972; Middleton *et al.*, 1982), and a mild tachycardia (Figs 8.8 and 8.9). Respiratory depression and transient apnoea may be observed on induction with thiopentone, but blood gas changes are generally minimal (Middleton *et al.*, 1982).

Thiopentone has a rapid onset of action following intravenous administration, and the rapid injection of a low dose (5–6 mg/kg) produces a short period of anaesthesia. More gradual administration of higher dose rates (20–30 mg/kg) produces 10–15 min anaesthesia. Thiopentone forms an alkaline solution which is highly irritant to tissues, and inadvertent extravascular administration causes tissue necrosis (see Chapter 12). To minimize these possible effects, a 1.25% solution should be used in cats. If extravascular administration occurs, the area should be infiltrated with a solution of 1 ml of lignocaine 2% in 4 ml Normal saline (Trim, 1987). Recovery is largely as a result of redistribution to body fat, and although anaesthesia can be extended by administration of incremental doses it has been shown in other species that recovery will then be very prolonged (Wyngaarden *et al.*, 1947; Glen, 1980).

Thiamylal
Thiamylal is marketed as a dry preparation, mixed with sodium carbonate. After reconstitution with distilled water the solution, like thiopentone, is highly alkaline. Thiamylal is very similar to thiopentone in its actions in other species, but no detailed studies of its physiological effects in the cat appear to have been undertaken. It is a slightly more potent anaesthetic agent that thiopentone, and is reported to

have less cumulative effects in the dog (Wyngaarden *et al.*, 1947). It has been widely used as an induction agent in the cat, at doses of 12–18 mg/kg i/v, when it produces 10–15 min anaesthesia.

Alphaxalone/Alphadolone

Steroids were first shown to have anaesthetic properties in animals in the 1940s and hydroxydione was used as an induction agent in man for a number of years, but was abandoned because of some undesirable properties, notably slow induction and a high incidence of thrombophlebitis (Sutton, 1972). Alphaxalone and alphadolone were developed in an effort to overcome the problems associated with earlier steroid anaesthetics. These two anaesthetics are combined in the commercial preparation 'Saffan' (Coopers Pitman-Moore) together with a solubilizing agent, Cremophor EL (polyoxyethylated castor oil). Alphaxalone and alphadolone differ slightly in their anaesthetic potency, but dose rates of the commercial preparation are conventionally reported as milligrams per kilogram of total steroid.

Initial evaluation of alphaxolone/alphadolone in laboratory animals (Child *et al.*, 1971) showed that following intravenous administration it produced rapid onset anaesthesia followed by rapid recovery. Repeated administration of the agent to mice had minimal cumulative effects, and this was also demonstrated in the cat and subsequently in other species. Some cumulative effect does occur, however, since although cats which received a continuous infusion of alphaxalone/alphadolone (0.24 mg/kg/min i/v) for 2 or 4 h recovered rapidly, cats infused for 6 h had prolonged recoveries, and one of the three animals in this study died (Child *et al.*, 1971).

Alphaxolone/alphadolone was shown to have a high therapeutic index and to be non-irritant following intravenous injection. These steroid compounds appear to have no significant endocrine effects (Child *et al.*, 1972).

Cardiovascular and respiratory system. Initial studies in a small number of cats (*n*=3) showed that low doses of alphaxalone/alphadolone

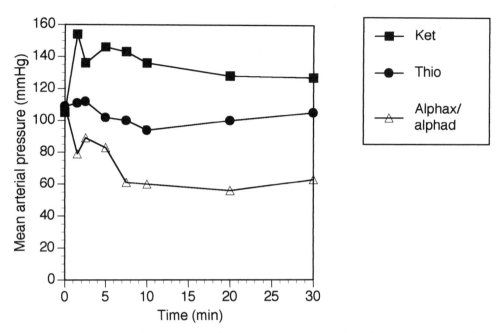

Fig. 8.8 Effects of intravenous administration of ketamine (6.6 mg/kg) (■), thiopentone (20 mg/kg) (●) and alphaxalone/alphadolone (9 mg/kg) (Δ) on mean arterial blood pressure in the cat. Data from Middleton *et al.*, 1982.

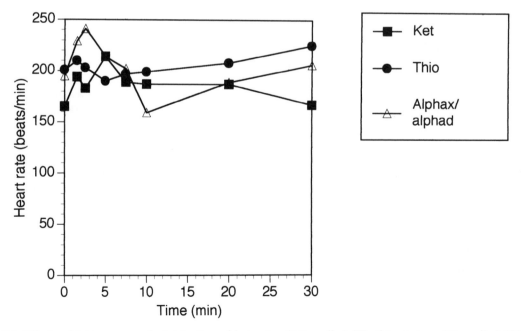

Fig. 8.9 Effects of intravenous administration of ketamine (6.6 mg/kg) (■), thiopentone (20 mg/kg) (●) and alphaxalone/alphadolone (9 mg/kg) (Δ) on heart rate in the cat. Data from Middleton *et al.*, 1982.

(1.2 mg/kg i/v) produced a small fall in mean arterial blood pressure (−18 mmHg) immediately following injection, which was followed by a small rise above the pre-anaesthetic level (+9 mmHg) (Child *et al.*, 1971). More extensive studies confirmed these findings, and also showed that higher dose rates (19.2 mg/kg) caused an immediate profound hypotension (−50% of base-line) (Child *et al.*, 1972). Blood pressure then rose slightly, but subsequently fell to produce a marked hypotension. In comparison with other injectable anaesthetics, alphaxalone/alphadolone had a greater margin of safety than barbiturates and propanidid, and produced less respiratory depression than these agents (Child *et al.*, 1972). Subsequent detailed studies by Middleton *et al.* (1982) and Dyson *et al.* (1987) confirmed that alphaxalone/alphadolone at higher dose rates (9 mg/kg i/v and 12 mg/kg i/v respectively) produced significant cardiopulmonary depression (Figs 8.3, 8.4, 8.8, 8.9). Most studies indicate that alphaxalone/alphadolone produces an initial fall in arterial pressure, and a marked tachycardia, but the magnitude of the hypotension varies considerably (Haskins *et al.*, 1975; Sapthavichaikul *et al.*, 1975; Middleton *et al.*, 1982; Dyson *et al.*, 1987). Hypotension is caused both by peripheral vasodilation (Gordh, 1972) and by a fall in cardiac output (Dyson *et al.*, 1987). It is worth noting, however, that even at high dose rates, no animals died as a result of cardiac depression in any of these studies, indicating that alphaxalone/alphadolone probably has a high margin of safety in healthy cats. It therefore seems likely that although administration of the clinically recommended dose rate of this anaesthetic (up to 9 mg/kg i/v) will result in a significant degree of hypotension, this appears to be well tolerated by healthy cats, and to cause no significant clinical problems in normal individuals.

Respiratory rate has been reported to either increase (Middleton *et al.*, 1982) or decrease (Dyson *et al.*, 1987), but even in animals which showed a fall in respiratory rate, blood gas parameters showed no significant changes. Occasional transient apnoea has been noted following induction of anaesthesia with alphaxalone/alphadolone.

Clinical use. Alphaxalone/alphadolone was first reported as a suitable anaesthetic for clinical use in the cat by Hall (1972), and following its introduction it has been widely used in the UK and elsewhere. Initial reports of its use in clinical practice indicated that alphaxalone/alphadolone produced safe and effective anaesthesia (Evans *et al.*, 1972). The duration of anaesthesia is dose dependant, dose rates of 3 mg/kg i/v produce 2–3 min of anaesthesia, whilst doses of 9–12 mg/kg produce 10–15 min of anaesthesia. Given the individual variation in dose responses which may be encountered, it is advisable to administer 2–3 mg/kg of anaesthetic by rapid injection, assess the effects in the individual patient, and then administer a proportion of the remaining dose as required. Anaesthesia may be prolonged by incremental administration of the agent (2–3 mg/kg as required), or maintained by a continuous infusion of 0.2–0.25 mg/kg/min. The agent is non-irritant, and inadvertent extravascular injection does not appear to be associated with any adverse effects.

Administration by intramuscular injection (9 mg/kg) provides light sedation suitable for radiography or other minor procedures. Higher dose rates (12–18 mg/kg) produce light to medium planes of anaesthesia, which may be suitable for surgical procedures. It should be noted that the volume of drug required (1–1.5 ml/kg) could entail administration of 3–4 ml into the quadriceps of an adult cat. Failure to achieve deep intramuscular injection and inadvertent injection into the facial planes almost certainly accounts for the variable results encountered when administering alphaxalone/alphadolone by this route. If high doses are to be administered, it is advisable to use several sites of injection, or alternatively administer a low dose, and to give the remaining drug intravenously once the cat has become sedated.

Recovery from anaesthesia is usually rapid, but may be associated with excitement and muscle tremors and occasional opisthotonos (Dodman, 1980; Chapter 12). These responses are usually mild, and their occurrence can be minimized by providing a quiet recovery area.

Although alphaxalone/alphadolone produces satisfactory anaesthesia, the inclusion of Cremophor EL in the commercial formulation results in a number of adverse reactions (see Chapter 12). Cremophor produces histamine release in the cat, causing hyperaemia and oedema of the pinnae, facial oedema, oedema of the paws, and occasional more severe reactions involving laryngeal oedema and possible bronchospasm (Stogdale, 1978; Dodman, 1980; Middleton *et al.*, 1982). Although histamine release would be expected to produce hypotension, injection of Cremophor alone in cats caused a rise in blood pressure and a tachycardia (Child *et al.*, 1972). The hypertension was attributed by these authors to the irritant effects of injection and pain associated with its administration. Alphaxalone/alphadolone administration does not cause a fall in total peripheral resistance (Sapthavichaikul *et al.*, 1975), despite a reduction in sympathetic tone and the presumed likely effects of histamine release. It seems reasonable to conclude, therefore, that the major problem likely to be encountered in cats associated with Cremophor induced histamine release is not a profound hypotension, but complications associated with laryngeal oedema or adverse effects on pulmonary function. Treatment of severe adverse reactions should consist of administration of antihistamines or other agents designed to reduce laryngeal oedema (e.g. corticosteroids), together with intubation and administration of oxygen, assisted ventilation if necessary, and general supportive therapy (see Chapter 12). In some cases of severe laryngeal oedema, tracheostomy may be required (Stogdale, 1978). In man, adrenaline is used for the treatment of histamine release, but its use for this purpose in the cat does not appear to have been documented. Despite these well-documented side-effects, alphaxolone/alphadolone has proven particularly safe in comparison with other anaesthetic regimen (Clarke & Hall, 1990).

Propofol

Propofol (2,6 di-isopropylphenol, Rapinovet, Coopers Animal Health; Diprivan, ICI) is an anaesthetic agent which is unrelated to the barbiturates, steroids, imadazoles or eugenols. Propofol, referred to as disoprofol or ICI 35 868 in early studies of its properties, is one of a series of alkyl phenols found to have anaesthetic properties in animals (James & Glen, 1980). Because of the poor water-solubility of these compounds, propofol was initially formulated with the solubilizing agent Cremophor EL (polyoxyethylated castor oil). For a variety of reasons this formulation was deemed unsatisfactory, and an alternative formulation of 1% propofol in an aqueous solution of 10% soyabean oil, 2.25% glycerol and 1.25% purified egg phosphatide was produced. This emulsion formulation has virtually identical anaesthetic effects to the Chremophor formulation (Glen & Hunter, 1984), and has been marketed commercially.

Initial evaluation of propofol in a range of laboratory species (including the cat) showed that intravenous administration of this compound produced rapid onset anaesthesia, with a sleep time similar to thiopentone (Glen, 1980). In contrast to thiopentone, mice regained co-ordination more rapidly following propofol administration, and this rapid and smooth recovery has been noted in the majority of species studied subsequently. Evaluation of the EEG changes produced by propofol in the rat indicated profound depression of cerebral activity at anaesthetic dose rates, but that this depression in activity reversed rapidly (Glen, 1980). Propofol has been shown to have no anticonvulsant properties (Glen *et al.*, 1985). The emulsion formulation of propofol does not cause histamine release in the dog and minipig, unlike the Cremophor formulation (Glen & Hunter, 1984).

The pharmacokinetics of propofol have been investigated in a number of species, including the cat (Adam *et al.*, 1980). Its anaesthetic effects have been shown to correlate closely with plasma concentration, hence the main factor determining the duration of action in a particular species is the pharmacokinetic profile. It has also been shown that no changes in effect or pharmacokinetics occur on continued or repeated administration of propofol (Adam *et al.*, 1980); therefore sleep times are not prolonged following repeated dosing (Glen, 1980). Propofol has a large initial volume of distribution which exceeds blood volume, and which is considered to include the well-perfused organs such as brain. After intravenous administration rapid redistribution to other, less well-perfused, tissues occurs, resulting in a rapid fall in blood and brain concentrations. Metabolic clearance is also rapid, with an elimination half life of 55 min in cats (Adam *et al.*, 1980). This pharmacokinetic profile explains the rapid onset of action and recovery following its administration. There are also important practical implications. To be effective, propofol must be given by rapid intravenous injection, otherwise the rapid redistribution will prevent anaesthetic concentrations being achieved in the brain.

Propofol is metabolized in the liver, and is believed also to undergo metabolism in extra-hepatic sites (Matot *et al.*, 1993). In the cat, considerable first pass extraction of propofol occurs in the lung (61%) (Matot *et al.*, 1993). It is uncertain whether all of the propofol is released back into the circulation, or if some lung metabolism of the compound occurs. Prior administration of fentanyl significantly reduced the first pass extraction of propofol (39% cf. 61%).

In man, no differences in the clearance of propofol in patients with hepatic or renal disease have been found, suggesting that this anaesthetic can be used safely in these groups of patients (Sebel & Lowdon, 1989). Both the volume of distribution of propofol, and its clearance have been shown to be lower in elderly human patients in comparison with young adults, and clinical experience has confirmed that lower dose rates of propofol are required in elderly patients (Dundee *et al.*, 1986; Kirkpatrick *et al.*, 1988). Similar data for the cat have not been obtained, but it seems reasonable to extrapolate from these findings in man, and suggest that elderly or geriatric cats may require a lower dose of this anaesthetic.

Cardiovascular and respiratory effects. The cardio-vascular effects of propofol have been studied in a range of animal species. In most species, induction with propofol produces a moderate fall in systolic blood pressure, and a small fall in cardiac output. Data are limited in the cat; Weaver and Raptopoulos (1990) reported no significant changes following induction of anaesthesia but no pre-anaesthetic measure-

ments were made. Since both blood pressure and heart rate increased with time, when anaesthesia was maintained with halothane, the authors of this study believed that heart rate and blood pressure may have been reduced on induction of anaesthesia. Continuous infusion of propofol is associated with a moderate degree of hypotension. The effects of propofol on the cardiovascular system in man and other species have been reviewed by Sebel and Lowdon (1989).

Propofol causes significant respiratory depression in most species, but no detailed studies have been carried out in the cat. Administration of a lethal dose to the cat produced respiratory arrest before cardiac arrest (Glen, 1980). A small number of cats develop transient apnoea on induction of anaesthesia with propofol (Morgan & Legge, 1989). Most species either show a reduction in respiratory rate (Glen, 1980), or little change in rate but a fall in arterial oxygen tension, suggesting a fall in tidal volume (Watkins *et al.*, 1987). It is therefore advisable to provide supplemental oxygen.

Other body systems. Few data have been obtained directly in the cat, but studies in other animal species and man indicate that propofol has no clinically significant effect on adrenal steroido-genesis (Newman *et al.*, 1987) although *in vitro* effects have been demonstrated (Lambert *et al.*, 1986). Propofol is believed to have no significant effects on hepatic (Robinson & Patterson, 1985) or renal function (Stark *et al.*, 1985), nor on platelet function or blood coagulation (Sear *et al.*, 1985). In man, propofol causes a fall in intraocular pressure (Vanacker *et al.*, 1987), but no data are available for its effects in the cat or other animal species.

Clinical use. Propofol administered by intrave-nous injection (5.0–8.0 mg/kg) to unpremedi-cated cats produces rapid onset anaesthesia, with smooth induction. Administration of low dose rates (5.0 mg/kg) produces fewer depres-sant effects on respiration, but requires earlier supplementation with incremental propofol or other anaesthetic agents. The pain on injection of propofol which has been reported in man does not appear to be a significant problem in the cat (Brearley *et al.*, 1988; Weaver & Raptopoulos, 1990). No adverse sequelae were reported when propofol was accidentally injected perivascularly (Morgan & Legge, 1989). Endotracheal intubation is easy to achieve with the aid of either topical application of lignocaine to the larynx or neuromuscular blockade with suxamethonium (Brearley *et al.*, 1988).

Surgical anaesthesia in cats which have received no pre-anaesthetic medication has a duration of 3–6 min (Morgan & Legge, 1989), and full recovery occurs within approximately 30 min. The quality of recovery is generally excellent, with no excitement associated with emergence from anaesthesia. Some animals may retch or sneeze during recovery, and some animals may paw at their mouths (Brearley *et al.*, 1988). Anaesthesia can be supplemented with incremental doses (2 mg/kg every 5 min) or by a continuous infusion of approximately 0.5 mg/kg/min (Brearley *et al.*, 1988). Prior administration of acepromazine and other tranquillizers prolongs recovery times, but the effects on induction dose are variable (Brearley *et al.*, 1988; Morgan & Legge, 1989; Weaver & Raptopoulos, 1990; Geel, 1991). This variation in result is almost certainly due to the difference in propofol dose rate used in these studies. Morgan and Legge (1989), using a dose of 8.0 mg/kg in unpremedicated cats, reported a reduction in induction dose to 6.0 mg/kg after administration of a tranquillizer or sedative. Weaver and Raptopoulos (1990), and Brearley *et al.* (1988) using dose rates of 5.0 mg/kg and 6.8 mg/kg respectively, in unpremedicated cats, reported no significant reduction in dose after premedication.

Imidazole Derivatives

Etomidate and metomidate
Etomidate and metomidate produce short periods of hypnosis (sleep) following intravenous administration, but have little or no analgesic action (Janssen *et al.*, 1975). Etomidate has been shown to cause very little cardiovascular depression in animals and man (Nagel *et al.*, 1979, Kissin *et al.*, 1983; see also Chapter 11).

There is little cumulative effect following repeated administration or continuous infusion of this agent. Prolonged infusion has been associated with suppression of adrenocortical function in man and similar effects have been demonstrated in the dog (Kruse-Elliott *et al.*, 1987).

Metomidate (20 mg/kg) combined with the opioid analgesic fentanyl (0.02 mg/kg) and administered intramuscularly produced safe and effective anaesthesia in cats (Symoens & Van Gestel, 1974), although recovery was prolonged (5 h) (Erhardt *et al.*, 1978).

Propanidid

Propanidid is a eugenol derivative which produces short duration anaesthesia. It has been little used in the cat and is no longer available commercially in the UK. Dose rates of 8–16 mg/kg i/v produced light anaesthesia in cats but this anaesthetic was reported to have a narrow range of safety (Child *et al.*, 1972).

Opioid Combinations

Perhaps because of longstanding misconceptions concerning the cat's responses to opioids, few trials of neuroleptanalgesic combinations have been undertaken in this species. All aspects of opioid use in cats are described in Chapter 7. The combination of fentanyl (0.025 mg/kg) and droperidol (0.8 mg/kg) (Thalamonal, Janssen) administered intramuscularly was reported to produce good analgesia and immobilization in cats, although animals responded to noise (Sovijarvi & Sainio, 1972), and two animals developed excitement. Other reports claimed satisfactory results (Love, 1970), but it seems likely that unless an appropriate dose of tranquillizer is administered, the high doses of opioids used in neuroleptanalgesic combinations may cause excitement in some animals.

Fentanyl (0.025 mg/kg, i/m) combined with metomidate (25 mg/kg, i/m) was reported to produce surgical anaesthesia in cats (Erhardt *et al.*, 1978). The animals developed marked respiratory depression, accompanied by hypercapnia. Blood pressure was slightly reduced, as was heart rate, but cardiac output did not fall significantly. The respiratory depression could be reversed rapidly by administration of the opioid antagonist levallorphan.

Drugs for Research Applications

A number of other anaesthetic agents are used for specific research applications in the cat, notably chloral hydrate, chloralose, and urethane. Chloralose produces long duration anaesthesia with relatively little effect on the cardiovascular system. The degree of analgesia produced is variable, and induction can be slow and accompanied by excitement. It is usually preferable to induce anaesthesia with a short-acting injectable agent (e.g. propofol) or a volatile anaesthetic, and then administer chloralose. Urethane produces long duration surgical anaesthesia in cats. Both agents are associated with very prolonged recovery periods and i/p administration of urethane can produce peritoneal irritation. Urethane can also cause haemolysis and is carcinogenic. Because of these side-effects, these agents should not be used for procedures from which the cats are intended to recover.

Total Intravenous Anaesthesia

The technique of total intravenous anaesthesia has increased in popularity in human anaesthetic practice, due primarily to the introduction of anaesthetic agents which can be infused for prolonged periods without resulting in excessively long recovery periods. The majority of older anaesthetic agents such as thiopentone or pentobarbitone have marked cumulative effects when administered as repeated incremental injections or by continuous infusion. Newer agents such as etomidate, alphaxalone/alphadolone and propofol can all be infused continuously for prolonged periods without unduly prolonging recovery times. Since all three of these anaesthetics have relatively poor analgesic properties in man, regimens for total intravenous anaesthesia for human clinical use frequently include one of the new potent μ-opioids such as fentanyl, alfentanil or sufentanil. In the

cat, propofol and alphaxalone/alphadolone alone can provide sufficient depth of anaesthesia for surgery, so it is generally not necessary to provide supplemental analgesia with opioids. Although opioids have not been used extensively in the cat, because of early misconceptions concerning this species' responses to morphine, short-acting agents such as alfentanil and fentanyl can be used in the cat to provide intraoperative analgesia and reduce the requirement for other anaesthetics (see below).

The administration of anaesthetics by continuous intravenous infusion has not been widely used in cats but incremental injection of agents to maintain anaesthesia is frequently employed. Although this simple approach requires no investment in new equipment, it has several disadvantages. The most obvious is that administration of increments of anaesthetic will lead to major fluctuations in the depth of anaesthesia. The animal will vary between an inadequate depth of anaesthesia to one which is too deep, and which may be associated with undesirable side-effects. A second problem concerns the constant attention that must be given to monitoring depth of anaesthesia and injecting additional drug whenever necessary. This can be a considerable inconvenience, particularly if the anaesthetist is also required to assist with any surgical procedure. These problems can be reduced by administering the anaesthetic by continuous infusion, and a variety of systems can be devised to achieve this.

Methods of administration
The simplest approach is to use a burette, with a roller clamp to control the fluid drip rate. Although this may be useful in an emergency when prolonged sedation is required, the drip rate is difficult to control and will vary over time because of gradual movement of the roller clamp, changes in the height of the fluid column and changes in venous pressure. Partial occlusion of the infusion cannula will also markedly affect the rate of infusion (Glen, 1988). If this type of apparatus is to be used, then it is preferable to select a paediatric burette (see Fig. 10.15), which provides a drip rate of 60 drops/ml to enable the infusion rate to be controlled more accurately. It is also advisable

to consider the use of a simple controller to provide an improved method of adjusting the drip rate. At their simplest, drip rate controllers consist of disposable devices. Alternatively, an electronic drip rate controller can be used, which monitors the drip rate via a sensor clamped onto the drip chamber of the infusion set. These devices vary the drip rate by altering the diameter of a section of the infusion set tubing, and maintain reasonably stable infusion rates, although partial occlusion of the intravenous cannula can result in under-infusion. Most electronic drip rate controllers are fitted with alarms that will alert the anaesthetist to changes in the infusion rate.

If total intravenous anaesthesia is to be used on a routine basis, then it is preferable to use some type of infusion pump. Although roller pumps can be used, the most practicable designs for veterinary anaesthesia are motorized syringe drivers. A large number of these are available from different manufacturers and when contemplating purchase, the following features should be assessed:

1. The ability of the pump to accept syringes of a wide range of sizes, from a number of different manufacturers.
2. A wide range of infusion rates (μl/h–ml/min) and the capability of changing infusion rates in small steps. This enables the infusion pump to be used for anaesthetic purposes, for the infusion of small volumes of emergency drugs, and the infusion of large volumes of solution for fluid therapy.
3. An occlusion alarm.
4. A 'syringe empty' alarm.
5. Battery backup if operated by mains electricity, and 'power failure' alarm.
6. Small size and weight.
7. Robust and easy to clean.
8. Computer interface for computer-assisted infusion profiles.

It is also helpful if the controls of the pump are simple to master, and the apparatus can be set up quickly and easily. Finding a pump that meets all of these criteria is difficult, particularly at a realistic price, but rapid developments are being made in this field. In general, pumps designed for clinical use in man have the full range of safety features (3–5), but may be limited in the sizes of syringes they will accept. Pumps designed for use in a research environment are generally much more versatile in their ability to handle different syringe sizes, but may lack desirable safety features.

Infusion techniques

When using a continuous infusion system, initial adjustments to the infusion rate will be required. Ideally, the infusion rate would be based upon the known pharmacodynamics of the anaesthetic agent or agents used. In practice, even when 'utilization rates' of the agent have been published, individual animals may vary considerably in their requirements. If the pharmacokinetics of the anaesthetic are known, then the infusion rates can be calculated from the volume of distribution and the rate constants (Mather, 1983; Bentley, 1985). The volume of distribution is the theoretical space in the body available to contain the drug.

Those unfamiliar with pharmacokinetics may find a simple analogy helpful. If you have a bath-tub full of water, and want to obtain a particular concentration of dye in the water, then the amount of dye you need to add is equal to the volume of water multiplied by the target concentration. If the bath taps are running, and the plug is out, then the situation is more complicated. Now, to maintain a target concentration, you will need to keep adding dye to the bath. If the dye is added at a constant rate, eventually a situation will be reached where the rate of removal of dye from the bath will equal the rate at which it is being added. This is known as a steady state.

The same considerations apply to intravenous drug infusions. If drug is infused at a constant rate, its concentration will stabilize when the rate of removal from the plasma is equal to the rate of infusion. So that in the steady state, when drug is being added at the same rate as it is being removed:

$$\text{Maintenance dose} = \text{Clearance} \times \text{Plasma concentration}$$

Unfortunately, the pharmacokinetics of many anaesthetics are better described by more complex models than a single bath-tub, or single compartment. Usually one compartment is characterized by rapid distribution and rapid elimination, and is often thought to represent the blood and well-perfused tissues, other compartments usually have slower equilibration and elimination times. The drug will therefore have a rapid half life, and one or more slower half lives, which are calculated from the fall in plasma concentration of the drug after administration of a single i/v dose. The half life of a compound is the time taken for its plasma concentration to fall by 50%.

Attaining a steady state rapidly is not easily achieved. If drug is infused at a constant rate, it will require 4–5 half lives to achieve a steady state. The alternative is to administer an initial loading dose, followed by a constant infusion. The problem with this technique is that if the pharmacokinetics of the drug are better described by a multicompartment system, then the plasma concentration will fall rapidly as redistribution to other compartments occurs. If more drug is given rapidly to compensate, the plasma concentration may reach dangerously high levels. An estimation of the loading dose required to attain rapidly a steady plasma concentration can be made from the maintenance infusion rate and the half life of the drug (Norwich, 1977):

$$\text{Loading dose} = \text{Maintenance rate} \times \text{Half life}/0.693$$

With drugs modelled using multicompartment systems, the slow half life is used for this calculation. As already mentioned, this can result in high initial plasma concentrations. For example, the loading dose needed if propofol was to be administered at 0.2 mg/kg/min would be 15 mg/kg. A safer approach might be to multiply the maintenance rate by the half life of the drug. This would take longer to achieve a steady plasma concentration, but would reduce the chance of overdose. An alternative approach is to use two sequential infusions, an initial rapid one, followed by a slower maintenance rate, with the rates determined by the drug clearance and half life (Wagner, 1974). More complex infusion regimens involving variable rate infusions have also been proposed, and these have become more readily applicable with the introduction of computer-controlled infusion pumps (Schuttler et al., 1983). Of course, with all of these techniques, it is preferable to monitor the plasma concentration of drug, since the half lives and volumes of distribution can show considerable variation in different individuals.

If pharmacokinetic data are not available, experience may have been gained in maintaining anaesthesia with a particular anaesthetic using incremental doses of the drug. An infusion rate can then be calculated from an estimate of the quantity of anaesthetic which would be required for maintenance of anaesthesia using incremental injections. For example, following a standard induction dose of propofol (7 mg/kg) most cats require increments of about 30–40% of this dose every 10–15 min. This provides a basic rate of 0.14–0.28 mg/kg/min, which can then be adjusted after assessment of the depth of anaesthesia. This calculation is in good agreement with the reported utilization rate of propofol (0.19 mg/kg/min; Glen, 1980), but is lower than the rates used by Brearley et al. (1988) to maintain surgical anaesthesia (0.51 mg/kg/min). It is important to appreciate that despite the initial induction dose, which acts as a loading dose, this technique will not achieve steady state very rapidly, and regular adjustments to the rate of infusion may be needed for about 2–3 half lives of the drug (about 2–3 h). As a further complication, during prolonged periods of anaesthesia, the infusion rates of most anaesthetics can be reduced by approximately 25–50% after 2–3 h infusion, since some accumulation of anaesthetic occurs, even with short-acting agents such as propofol or alphaxalone/alphadolone. Despite these problems, as practical experience is gained, stable anaesthesia can be achieved rapidly using an induction dose followed by an infusion which is varied according to the clinical assessment of anaesthetic depth. The results will be a more stable plane of anaesthesia, without the wide changes in anaesthetic depth associated with intermittent injections.

Neuromuscular Blocking Agents

Although neuromucular blocking agents are not anaesthetics they are included in this chapter as the methods used for their administration are similar to those used for the injectable anaesthetic agents. Neuromuscular blocking agents are not often used in the cat as the small muscle mass does not interfere with surgical access as in other, larger species. However, there are a few specific indications for their use in cats. As in any species, whenever neuromuscular blocking agents are used it is essential that the cat is fully anaesthetized and that artificial ventilation is used. Neuromuscular blockade when conscious is reported to be extremely unpleasant and surgery under these conditions is obviously quite unacceptable. As neuromuscular blocking agents affect all skeletal muscles the respiratory muscles are paralysed and artificial ventilation is essential for survival of the patient.

The short-acting, depolarizing agent suxamethonium is sometimes used to facilitate intubation and completely removes any chance of laryngeal spasm. Reynolds and Keates (1988) found that 0.2 mg/kg was sufficient to produce complete laryngeal relaxation providing excellent conditions for intubation. Suxamethonium stimulates the receptors before blocking them and muscular spasm of all skeletal muscles preceeds relaxation. Suxamethonium is rapidly broken down by plasma cholinesterases and, at 0.2 mg/kg, provides only 3–5 min of relaxation. IPPV using a close fitting face mask is efficient in the cat and a few breathes of 100% oxygen after the muscle spasms have abated will oxygenate the cat sufficiently to allow time for unhurried intubation.

As reversal of suxamethonium-induced relaxation is dependent upon its breakdown in the body by plasma pseudocholinesterase, paralysis is markedly prolonged if these enzymes are suppressed. Organophosphorus insecticides inhibit pseudocholinesterase activity and are widely used in flea control in domestic cats. If a cat has been wearing a flea collar or has recently been treated with any organophosphorus 'spot' flea treatment such as

fenthion (Tiguvon; Bayer) suxamethonium should not be used, as prolonged paralysis may result.

Non-depolarizing, longer-acting relaxants such as vecuronium, atracurium and pancuronium can be used as components of balanced anaesthesia, but the technique is not commonly used in the cat for clinical purposes. There are a number of reports of the effect of these agents under experimental conditions and most agents are similar in their duration and effect as in the dog (see below). The older agents such as pancuronium require reversal with an anticholinesterase, usually neostigimine or edrophonium, to ensure return of full muscle function. The newer neuromuscular blocking agents are broken down in the body and, in particular, atracurium is subject to Hoffmann degradation and often requires no antagonism. If cholinesterase antagonism is required neostigmine should be given with or slightly preceeded by an anticholinesterase such as atropine or glycopyrrolate to block the muscarinic effects. This is usually not required with edrophonium (Baird *et al.*, 1982). Muscular paralysis is best monitored by train-of-four technique (see Chapter 10) so that both further doses of relaxant and cholinesterase antagonism are given appropriately.

Atracurium and vecuronium are probably the most suitable agents for use in the cat. Their effect is slightly potentiated by volatile anaesthetic agents and a single dose of 0.1 mg/kg of either agent used during clinical volatile agent anaesthesia generally gives around 15 min of relaxation although vecuronium has been reported to be four times as potent as atracurium in the cat under experimental conditions (Sutherland *et al.*, 1983). Recovery after atracurium was also slightly slower than after vecuronium in this study. Vecuronium (0.1 mg/kg, initial dose) has been used successfully for eye surgery in cats (see Chapter 12) with incremental doses of 0.05 mg/kg given at 15–20 min intervals to prolong relaxation if necessary. It is rarely necessary to antagonize its effect 20 min after the last dose. Ilkiw *et al.* (1990) used 0.1 mg/kg atracurium as an initial dose followed by an infusion of 4 µg/kg/min to maintain 90–95% depression of T1 (train of four monitoring) in a group of cats undergoing surgery. Doses of both atracurium and vecuronium used under experimental conditions vary enormously but 0.25 mg/kg atracurium produced 29 min neuromuscular blockade which was readily antagonized by neostigmine (Meistelman & Lienhart, 1985). Smaller doses of atracurium provide a shorter period of relaxation and Sutherland *et al.* (1983) reported that those in the order of 0.1 mg/kg gave 15–23 min. Vecuronium 0.25–0.05 mg/kg produced 13–16 min blockade (Sutherland *et al.*, 1983). Hepatic failure slows elimination of vecuronium but renal failure has little effect (Bencini *et al.* 1985a,b). Atracurium elimination is little affected by either renal or hepatic failure (Neill & Chapple, 1982). Vecuronium and atracurium have been used safely in the presence of other drugs and a comprehensive investigation with atracurium demonstrated little change in its activity with a wide range of anaesthetic drugs (Chapple *et al.*, 1983). Gentamycin, however, potentiates the effect of most non-depolarizing neuromuscular blockers (Potter *et al.*, 1980).

References

Adam, H.K., Glen, J.B. & Hoyle, P.A. (1980) Pharmacokinetics in laboratory animals of ICI 35 868, a new I.V. anaesthetic agent. *Brit. J. Anaesth.* **52**, 743–746.

Allen, D.G., Dyson, D.H., Pascoe, P.M. & O'Grady, M.R. (1986) Evaluation of a xylazine–ketamine hydrochloride combination in the cat. *Can. J. Vet. Res.* **50**, 23–26.

Arnbjerg, J. (1979) Clinical manifestations of overdose of ketamine–xylazine in the cat. *Nord. Vet.* **31**, 155–161.

Baggot, J.D. & Blake, J.W. (1976) Disposition kinetics of ketamine in the domestic cat. *Arch. Inte. Pharmacodyn.* **220**, 115–124.

Baird, W.L., Bowman, W.C. & Kerr, W.J. (1982) Some action of Org NC45 and of edrophonium in the anaesthetized cat and in man. *Brit. J. Anaesth.* **54**, 375–385.

Becker, M. & Beglinger, R. (1982) Ketamine and myocardial contractility in the cat. *J.A.V.A.* **10**, 232–236.

Bencini, A.F., Scaf, A.H., Agoston, S., Houwertjes,

M.C. & Kersten, U.W (1985a) Disposition of vecuronium in the cat. *Brit. J. Anaesth.* **57**, 782–788.

Bencini, A.F., Houwertjes, M.C. & Agoston, S. (1985b) Effects of hepatic uptake of vecuronium bromide and its putative metabolites on their neuromuscular blocking actions in the cat. *Brit. J. Anaesth.* **57**, 789–795.

Bentley, J. (1985) Pharmacokinetic approach. *In: Acute Pain* (ed. G. Smith & B.G. Covino), pp. 42–67. Butterworths, London.

Bidwai, A.R., Stanley, T.H., Graves, C.L., Kawamura, R. & Sentker, C.R. (1975) The effects of ketamine on cardiovascular dynamics during halothane and enflurane anesthesia. *Anesth. Analg.* **54**, 588–592.

Brearley, J.C., Kellagher, R.E.B. & Hall, L.W. (1988) Propofol anaesthesia in cats. *J. Small Anim. Pract.* **29**, 315–322.

Bree, M.M., Park, J.S., Short, C.E., Beck, C.C. & Moser, J.H. (1976) Effects of chloramphenicol on Tilazol (CI-744) anesthesia in cats. *Vet. Med./Small Anim. Clin.* **71**, 764–771.

Buyniski, J.P. & Christie, G.J. (1977) Ketaset Plus – a new combination anesthetic for cats. 2-Pharmacologic aspects. *Vet. Med./Small Anim. Clin.* **72**, 559–567.

Calderwood, H.W., Klide, A.M., Cohn, B.B. & Soma, L.R. (1971) Cardiorespiratory effects of tiletamine in cats. *Am. J. Vet. Res.* **32**, 1511–1515.

Celesia, G.G., Chen, R-C. & Bamborth, B.J. (1975) Effects of ketamine in epilepsy. *Neurology* **25**, 169–172.

Chambers, J.P. & Dobson, J.M. (1989) A midazolam and ketamine combination as a sedative in cats. *J.A.V.A.* **16**, 53–54.

Chapple D.J., Clark J.S. & Hughes R. (1983) Interaction between atracurium and drugs used in anaesthesia. *Brit. J. Anaesth.* **55** (Supp 1), 175S–22S.

Child, K.J., Currie, J.P., Davis, B., Dodds, M.G., Pearce, D.R. & Twissell, D.J. (1971) The pharmacological properties in animals of CT 1341 – a new steroid anaesthetic agent. *Brit. J. Anaesth.* **43**, 2–13.

Child, D.J., Davis, B., Dodds, M.G. & Twissell, D.J. (1972) Anaesthetic, cardiovascular and respiratory effects of a new steroidal agent CT 1341: a comparison with other intravenous anaesthetic drugs in the unrestrained cat. *Brit. J. Pharmacol.* **46**, 189–200.

Christie, G.J. & Buyniski, J.P. (1977) Ketaset Plus – a new combination anesthetic for cats (1-clinical aspects). *Vet. Med./Small Anim. Clin.* **72**, 383–386.

Clanachan, A.S., McGrath, J.C. & MacKenzie, J.E. (1976) Cardiovascular effects of ketamine in the pithed rat, rabbit and cat. *Brit. J. Anaesth.* **48**, 935–939.

Clarke, K.W. & Hall, L.W. (1990) A survey of anaesthesia in small animal practice. *AVA/BSAVA Report* **17**, 4–10.

Clifford, D.H. & Soma, L.R. (1969) Feline anesthesia. *Fed. Proc.* **28**(4), 1479–1499.

Colby, E.D. & Sanford, T.D. (1981) Blood pressure and heart and respiratory rates of cats under ketamine/xylazine, ketamine/acepromazine anesthesia. *Feline Pract.* **11**, 19–24.

Colby, E.D. & Sanford, T.D. (1982) Feline blood gas values during anesthesia induced by ketamine/acepromazine and ketamine/xylazine. *Feline Pract.* **12**, 23–26.

Collins, V.J., Gorospe, C.A. & Rovenstine, E.A. (1960). Intravenous nonbarbiturate, nonnarcotic analgesics: preliminary studies. 1. cyclohexylamines. *Anesth. Analg.* **39**, 302–306.

Cullen, L.K. & Jones, R.S. (1977) Clinical observations on xylazine/ketamine anaesthesia in the cat. *Vet. Rec.* **101**, 115–116.

Dobromylskyj, P. (1992) A combination of midazolam with ketamine used as an intravenous induction agent in cats. *J. Vet. Anaesth.* **19**, 72–73.

Dodman, N.H. (1980) Complications of Saffan anaesthesia in cats. *Vet. Rec.* **107**, 481–483.

Domino, E.F., Chodoff, P. & Corseen, G. (1965) Pharmacologic effects of CI-581, a new dissociative anesthetic, in man. *Clin. Pharm. Ther.* **6**, 279–291.

Dundee, J.W., Robinson, F.P., McCollum, J.S.C. & Patterson, C.C. (1986) Sensitivity to propofol in the elderly. *Anaesthesia* **41**, 482–485.

Dyson, D.H., Allen, D.G., Ingwersen, W., Pascoe, P.J. & O'Grady, M. (1987) Effects of Saffan on cardiopulmonary function in healthy cats. *Can. J. Vet. Res.* **51**, 236–239.

Erhardt, W., Fritsch, R., Christ, K., Sprenzinger, P. & Blumel, G. (1978) Anaesthesia with fentanylmetomidate in the cat and its effects on respiration and circulation. *J. Small Anim. Pract.* **19**, 401–407.

Evans, J.M., Aspinal, K.W. & Hendy, P.G. (1972) Clinical evaluation in cats of a new anaesthetic CT 1341. *J. Small Anim. Pract.* **13**, 479–486.

Flecknell, P.A., Liles, J.H. & Williamson, H.A. (1990) The use of lignocaine–prilocaine local anaesthetic cream for pain-free venepuncture in laboratory animals. *Lab. Anim.* **24**, 142–146.

Geel, J.K. (1991) The effect of premedication on the induction dose of propofol in dogs and cats. *J. S. Afr. Vet. Assoc.* **62**, 118–123.

Glen, J.B. (1980) Animal studies of the anaesthetic activity of ICI 35 868. *Brit. J. Anaesth.* **52**, 731–741.

Glen, J.B. (1988) Comparative aspects of equipment for the intravenous infusion of anaesthetic agents. *J.A.V.A.* **15**, 65–79.

Glen, J.B. & Hunter, S.C. (1984) Pharmacology of an emulsion formulation of ICI 35 868. *Brit. J. Anaesth.* **56**, 617–626.

Glen, J.B., Hunter, S.C., Blackburn, T.P. & Wood, P. (1985) Interaction studies and other investigations of the pharmacology of propofol ('Diprivan'). *Postgrad. Med. J.* **61**, (Suppl.3), 7–14.

Gordh, T. (1972) The effect of althesin on the heart *in situ* in the cat. *Postgrad. Med. J.* **6**, 31–33.

Hall, L.W. (1972) Althesin in the larger animal. *Postgrad. Med. J.* **6**, 55–58.

Hanna, R.M., Borchard, R.E. & Schmidt, S.L. (1988a) Effect of diuretics on ketamine and sulfanilate elimination in cats. *J. Vet. Pharmacol. Ther.* **11**, 121–129.

Hanna, R.M., Borchard, R.E. & Schmidt, S.L. (1988b) Pharmacokinetics of ketamine HC1 and metabolite I in the cat: a comparison of i.v., i.m., and rectal administration. *J. Vet. Pharmacol. Ther.* **11**, 84–93.

Haskins, S.C., Peiffer, R.L. & Stowe, C.M. (1975) A clinical comparison of CT1341, ketamine, and xylazine in cats. *Am. J. Vet. Res.* **36**, 1537–1543.

Hatch, R.G., Clark, J.D., Jernigan, A.D. & Tracy, C.H. (1988) Searching for a safe, effective antagonist to Telazol overdose. *Veterinary Medicine* 112–117.

Heavner, J.E. & Bloedow, D.C. (1979). Ketamine pharmacokinetics in domestic cats. *Vet. Anaesthetics* **6**(2) 16–19.

Ilkiw J.E., Forsyth S.F., Hill T. & Gregory C.R. (1990) Atracurium administration, as an infusion to induce neuromuscular blockade in clinically normal and temporarily immune suppressed cats. *J. Am. Vet. Med. Ass.* **197**, 1153–1156.

Ingwersen, W., Allen, D.G., Dyson, D.H., Pascoe, P.J. & O'Grady, M.R. (1988a) Cardiopulmonary effects of a halothane/oxygen combination in healthy cats. *Can. J. Vet. Res.* **52**, 386–391.

Ingwersen, W., Allen, D.G., Dyson, D.H., Pascoe, P.J. & O'Grady, M.R. (1988b) Cardiopulmonary effects of a ketamine hydrochloride/acepromazine combination in healthy cats. *Can. J. Vet. Res.* **52**, 1–4.

James, R. & Glen, J.B. (1980) Synthesis, biological evaluation and preliminary structure – activity considerations of a series of alkylphenols as intravenous anaesthetic agents. *J. Med. Chem.* **23**, 1350.

Janssen, P.A.J., Niemegeers, C.J.E. & Marsboom, R.P.H. (1975) Etomidate, a potent non-barbiturate hypnotic. Intravenous etomidate in mice, rats, guinea pigs, rabbits and dogs. *Arch. Int. Pharmacodyn.* **214**, 92–132.

Kirkpatrick, T., Cockshott, I.D., Douglas, E.J. &

Nimmo, W.S. (1988) Pharmacokinetics of propofol (Diprivan) in elderly patients. *Brit. J. Anaesth.* **60**, 146–150.

Kissin, I., Motomura, S., Aultman, D.F. & Reves, J.G. (1983) Inotropic and anesthetic potencies of etomidate and thiopental in dogs. *Anesth. Analg.* **62**, 961–965.

Kruse-Elliott, K.T., Swanson, C.R. & Aucoin, D.P. (1987) Effects of etomidate on adrenocortical function in canine surgical patients. *Am. J. Vet. Res.* **48**, 1098–1100.

Lambert, A., Frost, J., Mitchell, R. & Robertson, W.R. (1986) On the assessment of the *in vitro* biopotency and site(s) of action of drugs affecting adrenal steroidogenesis. *Ann. Clin. Biochem.* **23**, 225–229.

Lamson, P.D., Greig, M.E. & Hobday, C.J. (1951) Modification of barbiturate anesthesia by glucose, intermediary metabolites and certain other substances. *J. Exp. Pharmacol. Ther.* **103**, 460–470.

Lees, P. (1991) The injectable anaesthetics. *In: Veterinary Applied Pharmacology and Therapeutics, 5th edn* (ed. G.C. Brander, D.M. Pugh, R.J. Bywater & W.L. Jenkins), pp. 358–359. Bailliere Tindall, London.

Love, J.A. (1970) Use of fentanyl and droperidol in guinea pigs, lemmings, ground squirrels, and cats. *J. Am. Vet. Med. Ass.* **157**, 675–677.

Macy, D.W. & Siwe, S.T. (1977) The use of ketamine as an oral anesthetic in cats. *Feline Pract.* **1**, 44–46.

Marietta, M.P., White, P.F., Pudwill, C.R., Way, W.L. & Trevor, A.J. (1976) Biodisposition of ketamine in the rat: self-induction of metabolism. *J. Pharmacol. Exp. Ther.* **196**, 536–544.

Massopust Jr, L.C., Wolin, L.R. & Albin, M.S. (1973) The effects of a new phencyclidine derivative on the electroencephalographic and behavioral responses in the cat. *Tower International Technomedical J. Life Sci.* **3**, 1–10.

Mather, L.E. (1983) Pharmacokinetic and pharmacodynamic factors influencing the choice, dose and route of administration of opiates for acute pain. *Clinics Anaesthesiol.* **1**(1), 17–40.

Matot, I., Neely, C.F., Ray, M.D., Katz, R.Y. & Neufield, G.R. (1993) Pulmonary uptake of propofol in cats, effect of fentanyl and halothane. *Anesthesiology*, **78**, 1157–1165.

Meistelman, C. and Lienhart, A. (1985) Pharmacologie experimentale du dibesylate d'atracurium. *Ann. Fr. Anesth. Reanim.* **4**, 461–464.

Middleton, D.J., Ilkiw, J.E. & Watson, A.D.J. (1982) Physiological effects of thiopentone, ketamine and CT 1341 in cats. *Res. Vet. Sci.* **32**, 157–162.

Morgan, D.W.T. & Legge, K. (1989) Clinical evalua-tion of propofol as an intravenous anaesthetic agent in cats and dogs. *Vet. Rec.* **124**, 31–33.

Myslobodsky, M.S., Golovchinsky, V. & Mintz, M. (1981) Ketamine: convulsant or anti-convulsant? *Pharmacol. Biochem. Behav.* **14**, 27–33.

Nagel, M.L., Muir, W.W. & Nguyen, K. (1979) Comparison of the cardiopulmonary effects of etomidate and thiamylal in dogs. *Am. J. Vet. Res.* **40**, 193–196.

Neill, E.A. & Chapple D.J. (1982) Metabolic studies in the cat with atracurium: a neuromuscular blocking agent designed for non-enzymic inactivation at physiological pH. *Xenobiotica*, **12**, 203–210.

Newman, L.H., McDonald, J.C., Wallace, P.G.M. & Ledingham, I.McA. (1987) Propofol infusion for sedation in intensive care. *Anaesthesia* **42**, 929–937.

Norwich, K.H. (1977) *Molecular Dynamics in Biosystems. The Kinetics of Tracers in Intact Organisms.* Pergamon, New York.

Potter J.M., Edeson R.O., Cambell R.J. & Forbes A.M. (1980) *Anaesth Intensive Care*, **8**, 20–25.

Priano, L.L., Traber, D.L. & Wilson, R.D. (1969) Barbiturate anesthesia: an abnormal physiologic situation. *J. Pharmacol. Exp. Ther.*, **165**, 126–135.

Reid, J.S. & Frank, R.J. (1972) Prevention of undesirable side reactions of ketamine anesthesia in cats. *JAAHA* **8**, 115–119.

Reynolds W.T. & Keates H.L. (1988) Dosage of suxamethonium for endotracheal intubation in the cat. *Aust. Vet. Pract.* **18**, 66–67.

Robinson, F.P. & Patterson, C.C. (1985) Changes in liver function tests after propofol ('Diprivan'). *Postgrad. Med. J.* **61**, 160–161.

Sanford, T.D. & Colby, E.D. (1982) Feline anesthesia induced by ketamine/acepromazine and ketamine/xylazine. *Feline Pract.* **12**, 16–24.

Sapthavichaikul, S., Wisborg, K. and Skovsted, P. (1975) The effects of althesin on arterial pressure, pulse rate preganglionic sympathetic activity and barostatic reflexes in cats. *Can. Anaesth. Soc. J.* **22**, 587–600.

Savola, J-M. (1989) Cardiovascular actions of medetomidine and their reversal by atipamezole. *Acta Vet. Scand.* **85**, 39–47.

Sawyer, D.C., Rech, R.H. & Durham, R.A. (1991) Does ketamine provide adequate visceral analgesia when used alone or in combination with acepromazine, diazepam, or butorphanol in cats? *Proceedings of the 4th International Congress of Veterinary Anaesthesia*, p. 381. Special suppl. to *J. Vet. Anaesth.* Hall, L.W. (ed).

Schuttler, J., Schwilden, H. & Stoekel, H. (1983) Pharmacokinetics as applied to total intravenous anaesthesia. Practical implications. *Anaesthesia* (Suppl.) **38**, 53–56.

Sear, J.W., Uppington, J. & Kay, N.H. (1985) Haematological and biochemical changes during anaesthesia with propofol ('Diprivan'). *Postgrad. Med. J.* **61**, 165–168.

Sebel, P.S. & Lowdon, J.D. (1989) Propofol: a new intravenous anesthetic. *Medical Intelligence Article* **71**, 260–277.

Skovsted, P., Price, M.L. & Price, H.L. (1970) The effects of short-acting barbiturates on arterial pressure, preganglionic sympathetic activity and barostatic reflexes. *Anesthesiology* **33**, 10–18.

Sovijarvi, A.R.A. & Sainio, K. (1972) Neuroleptanalgesia and the function of the auditory cortex in the cat. *Anesthesiology* **37**, 406–412.

Stark, R.D., Binks, S.M., Dutka, V.N., O'Connor, K.M., Arnstein, M.J.A. & Glen, J.B. (1985) A review of the safety and tolerance of propofol ('Diprivan'). *Postgrad. Med. J.* **61**, 152–156.

Stogdale, L. (1978) Laryngeal oedema due to Saffan in a cat. *Vet. Rec.* **102**, 283–284.

Sutherland, G.A., Squire I.B., Gibb A.J. & Marshall I.G. (1983) Neuromuscular blocking and autonomic effects of vecuronium and atracurium in the anaesthetized cat. *Brit. J. Anaesth.* **55**, 1119–1126.

Sutton, J.A. (1972) A brief history of steroid anaesthesia before althesin (CT1341). *Postgrad. Med. J.* **8**, 9–13.

Symoens, J. & Van Gestel, J. (1974) Anaesthesia with metomidate and fentanyl in cats. *Tijdschr. Diergeneesk.* **99**, 427–432.

Takeshita, H., Okuda, Y. & Sari, A. (1972) The effects of ketamine on cerebral circulation and metabolism in man. *Anesthesiology* **36**, 69–75.

Tranquilli, W.J., Thurmon, J.C., Speiser, J.R., Benson, G.J. & Olson, W.A. (1988) Butorphanol as a preanesthetic in cats: its effects on two common intramuscular regimens. *Vet. Med.* **83**, 848–854.

Trim, C.M. (1987) Sedation and Anaesthesia. *In: Diseases of the Cat: Medicine and Surgery*, Vol.1, (ed. J. Holzorth), pp. 43–67. Saunders, Philadelphia.

Vähä-Vahe, A.T. (1990) Clinical effectiveness of atipamezole as a medetomidine antagonist in cats. *J. Small Anim. Pract.* **31**, 193–197.

Vanacker, B., Dekegel, D., Dionys, J., Garcia, R., Van Eeckhoutte, L., Dralants, G. & Van de Walle, J.

(1987) Changes in intraocular pressure associated with the administration of propofol. *Brit. J. Anaesth.* **59**, 1514–1517.

Verstegen, J., Fargetton, X. & Ectors, F. (1989) Medetomidine/ketamine anaesthesia in cats. *Acta Vet. Scand.* **85**, 117–123.

Verstegen, J., Fargetton, X., Donnay, I. & Ectors, F. (1990) Comparison of the clinical utility of medetomidine/ketamine and xylazine/ketamine combinations for the ovariectomy of cats. *Vet. Rec.* **127**, 424–426.

Verstegen, J., Fargetton, X., Donnay, I. & Ectors, F. (1991a) An evaluation of medetomidine/ketamine and other drug combinations for anaesthesia in cats. *Vet. Rec.* **128**, 32–35.

Verstegen, J., Fargetton, X., Zanker, S., Donnay, I. & Ectors, F. (1991b) Antagonistic activities of atipamezole, 4-aminopyridine and yohimbine against medetomidine/ketamine-induced anaesthesia in cats. *Vet. Rec.* **128**, 57–60.

Wagner, J.G. (1974) A safe method for rapidly achieving plasma concentration plateaus. *Clin. Pharmacol. Ther.* **16**, 691–700.

Ward, G.S., Johnsen, D.O. & Roberts, C.R. (1974) The use of CI 744 as an anesthetic for laboratory animals. *Lab. Anim. Sci.* **24**, 737–742.

Watkins, S.B., Hall, L.W. & Clarke, K.W. (1987) Propofol as an intravenous anaesthetic agent in dogs. *Vet. Rec.* **14**, 326–329.

Waxman, K., Shoemaker, W.C. & Lippmann, M. (1980) Cardiovascular effects of anesthetic induction with ketamine. *Anesth. Analg.* **59**, 355–358.

Weaver, B.M.Q. & Raptopoulos, D. (1990) Induction of anaesthesia in dogs and cats with propofol. *Vet. Rec.* **126**, 617–620.

White, P.F., Way, W.L. & Trevor, A.J. (1982) Ketamine – its pharmacology and therapeutic uses. *Anesthesiology* **56**, 119–136.

Wright, M. (1982) Pharmacologic effects of ketamine and its use in veterinary medicine. *J. Am. Vet. Med. Assoc.* **180**, 1462–1471.

Wyngaarden, J.B., Woods, L.A. & Seevers, M.H. (1947) The cumulative action of certain thiobarbiturates in dogs. *Fed. Proc.* **6**, 388–389.

Young, L.E. & Jones, R.S. (1990) Medetomidine/ketamine anaesthesia and its antagonism by atipamezole. *J. Small Anim. Pract.* **31**, 221–224.

9
Inhalation Anaesthesia

E.P. Steffey

Introduction

Inhalation anaesthesia is one of the preferred techniques for producing general anaesthesia because the depth of anaesthesia can be altered rapidly and predictably. If the level of general anaesthesia is insufficient the inspired concentration of the anaesthetic agent can be increased and, conversely, if the depth of anaesthesia becomes excessive, the inspired concentration can be decreased and surplus anaesthetic eliminated by enforced lung ventilation. However, while the major advantage of inhalation anaesthesia relates to ease of control of anaesthetic depth, other advantages exist. For example, an anaesthetic delivery apparatus is usually used to administer inhaled anaesthetic agents and this includes a source of oxygen and a patient breathing circuit that in turn usually includes an endotracheal tube and a compliant gas reservoir. These components contribute significantly to the ease of physiological support (i.e. oxygenation and lung ventilation) of the anaesthetized cat and thereby help to minimize morbidity and mortality. In addition, inhalation anaesthetics in delivered gas and breath samples can now be readily measured. Measurement of inhalation anaesthetic concentration enhances the precision and safety of management beyond the extent commonly possible with injectable anaesthetic agents.

This chapter discusses the clinical pharmacology and techniques of use of inhalation anaesthetics with particular focus on the anaesthetic management of cats. Unfortunately, little information is available from direct studies in cats so that data from a variety of species are conservatively summarized with the justification that the scientific basis for the use of these drugs applies across species lines.

Inhaled anaesthetics can be classified according to their clinical use (Table 9.1). Group 1 includes agents like chloroform and cyclopropane that are no longer used in clinical circumstances. They have long been discarded for use with feline patients because they cause liver failure (chloroform) or are explosive (cyclopropane) and are of historical interest only. They will, therefore, not be discussed further. However, diethyl ether, which was widely used in years past for anaesthetizing cats, has a reputation for safety even in unskilled hands. Accordingly, it is an agent that has value in those parts of the world where facilities are limited and newer drugs are not available or affordable. Unfortunately, diethyl ether is flammable and this characteristic negates its use in the environment of the modern operating room which includes electro-

Table 9.1 Inhalation anaesthetic agents

Group 1 – Agents of historical interest
  Chloroform
  Cyclopropane
  Diethyl ether
  Fluroxene
  Trichlorethylene

Group 2 – Agents in current clinical use for animals
  Major use
    Halothane
    Isoflurane
  Minor use
    Enflurane
    Methoxyflurane
    Nitrous oxide
Group 3 – New agents
  Desflurane
  Sevoflurane

Table 9.2 Some chemical and physical properties of modern inhalation anaesthetics (Eger, 1985a)

Property	Enflurane	Halothane	Isoflurane	Methoxyflurane	Nitrous oxide
Tradename	Ethrane	Fluothane	Aerrane	Metofane	N_2O

Formula	Cl F F
	  | | |
	H–C–C–O–C–H
	  | | |
	  F F F
		Br F
		  | |
		H–C–C–F
		  | |
		  Cl F
			F Cl F
			  | | |
			F–C–C–O–C–H
			  | | |
			  F H F
				Cl F H
				  | | |
				H–C–C–O–C–H
				  | | |
				  Cl F H
					O⟨N‖N

Vapour pressure (mmHg at 20°C)	172	244	240	23	Gas at room temperature
Vapour concentration (% saturated at 20°C)	23	32	32	3	100
Preservative	Not needed	Required	Required	Not needed	Not needed

Stability in
  sodalime
  UV light
	
	Stable
	Stable
		
		Decomposes
		Decomposes
			
			Stable
			Stable
				
				Decomposes
				Decomposes
					
					Stable
					Stable

Reacts with metal	No	Yes	No	Yes	No

Solubility*
  Blood/gas
  Oil/gas
  Rubber/gas
	
	2.0
	96
	74
		
		2.5
		224
		120
			
			1.4
			91
			62
				
				15
				970
				630
					
					0.5
					1.4
					1.2

* Partition coefficients for human blood and olive oil at 37°C and rubber at room temperature.

cautery and a variety of electronic monitoring devices.

The focus in this chapter is on Group 2 agents; the five anaesthetic agents in current use (Table 9.1). Although halothane and isoflurane are most widely used, nitrous oxide, methoxyflurane and enflurane retain varying degrees of clinical importance. There will also be brief discussion of a third group consisting of two new agents. One of these new agents, desflurane, has recently been released in the United States for clinical use in human patients while the other, sevoflurane, is undergoing laboratory and clinical testing for medical use. Although these agents have no immediate importance in feline anaesthesia both of them have potential for at least focused use in the management of feline patients.

Characteristics of Inhalation Anaesthetics

The molecular structure of inhalation anaesthetics and their physical properties are important determinants of their actions and in part dictate the safety of their administration.

Chemical Characteristics

An in-depth analysis of the impact of agent chemical structure and physical properties on clinical practice is beyond the scope of this chapter. Brief focus on aspects of Tables 9.2 and 9.3 is, however, justified.

The systematic search for new and improved

Table 9.3 Chemical and physical properties of two new inhalation anaesthetics (Steffey, 1992)

Property	Desflurane	Sevoflurane
Tradename	Suprane (I653)	–
Formula	F H F | | | F–C–C–O–C–H | | | F F F	F | H F–C–F | | F–C–O–C–H | | H F–C–F | F
Vapour pressure (mmHg @ 20°C)	664	160
Vapour concentration (% saturated @ 20°C)	87	21
Stability in sodalime	Stable	Decomposes
Solubility*		
Blood/gas	0.42	0.60
Oil/gas	18.7	53.4

* Partition coefficient for human blood and olive oil at 37°C.

inhalation anaesthetics is focused on structure–activity relationships (e.g. organic vs. inorganic compounds). Predictions that a halogenated (fluorine, chlorine, bromine) structure would provide non-flammability and molecular stability encouraged the development of halothane. In clinical circumstances, however, the concurrent presence of halothane and catecholamines increases the incidence of cardiac arrhythmias in feline patients (Muir *et al.*, 1959). An ether linkage in the molecule favours a reduction in the incidence of cardiac arrhythmias. Consequently this chemical structure is a predominant characteristic of all agents developed or proposed for clinical use since the introduction of halothane in 1956.

Despite its many favourable characteristics and improvements over earlier anaesthetics, including improved chemical stability, halothane is susceptible to decomposition. For this reason halothane is stored in dark bottles and a very small amount of preservative (thymol) is added to the commercial preparation. Thymol, being much less volatile than halothane, collects within halothane vaporizers

and causes them to malfunction. The substitution of fluorine for chlorine or bromine in the anaesthetic molecule makes the molecule more stable, adding to shelf life and negating the need for additives. Unfortunately, the fluoride ion is toxic to some tissues (e.g. kidneys). This is of substantial concern if the parent compound (e.g. methoxyflurane) is not resistant to metabolism by the patient.

Physical Properties

The physical properties of inhalation anaesthetics can be conveniently divided into two general categories; those that determine the means by which the agents are administered and those that help determine their kinetics in the body. Use of this information is helpful in clinically manipulating anaesthetic induction and recovery and in facilitating changes in anaesthetic levels in a timely fashion.

Vapour pressure

A variety of physical properties determine the means by which inhalation anaesthetics are administered. These include characteristics such as molecular weight, boiling point, liquid density, vapour density and vapour pressure. Of these the vapour pressure is the most important property on which the clinician should focus.

Nitrous oxide is a gas at ambient conditions and is stored under pressure in cylinders as a liquid. The other modern inhaled anaesthetics are commercially available as volatile liquids. The molecules of these liquids are in constant motion and some of them at the surface of the liquid reach a velocity sufficient to escape from the liquid and become a vapour molecule in the gas phase. This process is dynamic and an equilibrium is established when the number of molecules leaving the liquid equals the number of molecules returning to the liquid. The gas molecules exert a force or pressure that is measurable. The partial pressure (units of measure are mmHg or kPa) that the vapour exerts when the liquid and vapour phases are in equilibrium is known as the vapour pressure. Thus, the vapour pressure of an anaesthetic is a measure of its ability to evaporate; that is, it is a measure of the tendency for molecules to leave the liquid state and enter the gaseous (vapour) form. Vapour pressure is unique for each volatile agent (Tables 9.2 and 9.3) and is directly related to liquid temperature. If the temperature of the liquid is increased more molecules escape the liquid phase and enter the gaseous state. The greater the number of molecules in the vapour phase the greater the vapour pressure becomes. The vapour pressure is a measure of the maximal concentration of inhaled anaesthetic deliverable for a given condition (Tables 9.2 and 9.3). This can easily be determined by relating the vapour pressure to ambient pressure. For example, in the case of halothane, a maximal concentration of 32% is possible under normal conditions; that is, $244/760 \times 100 = 32.0\%$, where 760 mmHg is the barometric pressure at sea level.

The vapour pressure of a volatile drug must at least be sufficient to provide enough molecules in the vapour state to produce anaesthesia at ambient conditions. Other variables being constant, the greater the vapour pressure the greater the concentration of the drug deliver-

able to the patient. Therefore, for example, from Table 9.2, halothane is more volatile than methoxyflurane under similar conditions.

Solubility of gases
Anaesthetic gases and vapours dissolve in liquids and solids. The amount of gas dissolving depends on the gas itself, the partial pressure of the gas, the nature of the solvent and the temperature. This relationship is described by Henry's Law, $V = S \times P$, where V is the volume of gas, P is the partial pressure of gas and S is the solubility coefficient for the gas in the solvent at a given temperature. With inhalation anaesthetics solubility is most commonly expressed as a partition coefficient. Other expressions of solubility include the Bunsen and Ostwald solubility coefficients (Eger, 1974). The partition coefficient describes the capacity per unit volume of one solvent relative to the second solvent (e.g. blood and gas phases) for a given anaesthetic at a specific temperature when the anaesthetic is in equilibrium between the two phases (i.e. the partial pressure of the gas is the same in the two phases and there is no further net movement of gas molecules). Temperature plays an important role in the magnitude of agent dissolved in a solvent such as blood. As the temperature decreases, the solubility of an anaesthetic increases. Because of this it is important to compare partition coefficients at similar temperatures; in the case of anaesthetics partition coefficients are commonly described for a temperature of 37°C (normal *human* body temperature).

It is important to recall that anaesthetic gases like respiratory gases (oxygen and carbon dioxide) move down partial pressure gradients; that is, pass from a medium in which there is a higher partial pressure to one of a lower partial pressure. At equilibrium the partial pressure of the gases in the two phases are the same and there is no further net movement but, as explained above, the concentration in the two phases is different. Thus the partition coefficient describes the concentration ratio of the anaesthetic in the two different solvents. Two solubility characteristics are of particular importance in selecting appropriate inhaled agents for feline anaesthesia: the blood/ gas and oil/gas solubilities (Tables 9.2 and 9.3).

Blood/gas partition coefficient. The blood/gas solubility is a measure of the speed of anaesthetic induction, recovery and change of anaesthetic levels. The reasoning behind this is as follows. Consider anaesthetic X with a blood/ gas partition coefficient of 15. This value indicates that anaesthetic X is 15 times more soluble in blood than in gas despite an equal partial pressure in the two phases at equilibrium. Alternatively, consider anaesthetic Y with a partition coefficient of 1.4. This indicates that anaesthetic Y is only 1.4 times as soluble in blood as it is in air. Comparing the partition coefficient of anaesthetic X with that of anaesthetic Y indicates that anaesthetic X is much more soluble in blood than anaesthetic Y (nearly 11 times more soluble; 15/1.4). From this, and assuming other things are equal, anaesthetic X will require a longer time of administration to attain a required level in the body (as for example for induction of anaesthesia) than anaesthetic Y. Also elimination (and therefore recovery from anaesthesia) will be prolonged with anaesthetic X vs. anaesthetic Y. Further data to support this concept that low blood solubility is desired for rapid anaesthetic induction and recovery are presented in a later section entitled 'Uptake and Distribution'.

Oil/gas partition coefficient. The oil/gas partition coefficient is another solubility characteristic of clinical importance. This partition coefficient describes the ratio of concentrations of an anaesthetic in oil (olive oil is the standard) and gas phases at equilibrium. The oil/gas partition coefficient correlates inversely with anaesthetic potency and describes the capacity of lipids for the anaesthetic.

Other partition coefficients. Solubility factors for tissues and other media like rubber are also important. Readers are directed elsewhere (Eger 1974, 1985a, 1990; Lowe and Ernst, 1981) for further information.

Anaesthetic Dose: The Minimum Alveolar Concentration (MAC)

The minimum alveolar concentration (MAC) of an inhaled anaesthetic measured at sea level (one atmosphere, 760 mmHg or approximately 108.6 kPa) that just prevents gross purposeful movement in response to a supramaximal noxious stimulus was first described by Merkel and Eger in 1963. Since then MAC has become the standard by which all inhaled anaesthetics are compared and is a major index of anaesthetic potency. Anaesthetic potency of an inhaled anaesthetic is inversely related to MAC (i.e. potency = 1/MAC). From the information presented above it also follows that MAC is inversely related to the oil/gas partition coefficient. Thus a very potent anaesthetic has a low MAC value and an agent of low potency has a high MAC value.

MAC is defined in terms of a percentage of one atmosphere and, therefore, represents an anaesthetic partial pressure (i.e. $P_x = C/100 \times P_b$, where P_x stands for the partial pressure of the anaesthetic in a gas mixture, C is the anaesthetic concentration in volumes % and P_b is the ambient or total pressure of the gas mixture). Although the concentration at MAC may vary

Table 9.4 The minimum alveolar concentration of inhalation anaesthetics*

Agent	Cat	Dog	Human
Methoxyflurane	0.23	0.23	0.16
Halothane	0.81–1.14**	0.87	0.77
Enflurane	2.37‡	2.20	1.68
Isoflurane	1.63	1.28	1.15
Diethyl ether	2.10	3.04	1.92
Sevoflurane*	2.58	2.36	1.71
Desflurane*	NA	7.20	4.58
Cyclopropane	19.7	15.9	9.20
Nitrous oxide	255	188–222	105

* Data are listed in order of increasing MAC for cats and, except where indicated by superscript, are taken from a review by Cullen (1986).
** Steffey, 1992.
† Webb, 1987.
‡ Drummond *et al.*, 1983.
NA = not available.

depending on ambient conditions, for example altitude, the anaesthetic partial pressure at MAC would be the same in pressurized environments or at high elevations. A second point deserving emphasis is that the alveolar concentration, *not* inspired or delivered (as for example from a vaporizer) concentration is used because after sufficient time for equilibrium (minutes) alveolar partial pressure represents arterial and brain anaesthetic partial pressures. Although admittedly data from arterial blood anaesthetic partial pressure would be an even more precise reflection of brain tissue anaesthetic partial pressure, alveolar gas (end-tidal gas) is more easily and more rapidly sampled and analysed.

The MAC values for inhaled anaesthetics determined for cats are given in Table 9.4; values for dogs and humans are also given for comparison. In animals MAC is measured under laboratory conditions whereas surgical patients were studied to obtain values for humans. Subjects are anaesthetized only with the anaesthetic agent of interest and that anaesthetic is delivered in oxygen. So that the requirement for anaesthesia is not altered, no other drugs are administered and it is important to maintain body temperature and other physiological conditions normal and stable. Factors that influence anaesthetic requirement (increase or decrease) are reviewed elsewhere (Eger, 1974; Cullen, 1986). The standard noxious stimulus applied in the study of dogs and cats is a tail clamp but with humans response to a surgical skin incision is taken as the standard stimulus. Other details of MAC determination are given elsewhere (Eger, 1974; Steffey *et al.*, 1974a; Steffey & Howland, 1977; Cullen, 1986). The MAC value is derived as the alveolar concentration of anaesthetic midway between that which allows, and that which prevents, purposeful movement. Anaesthetic dose can then be expressed as multiples of MAC such as 1.2 MAC, 1.5 MAC, etc.; that is, an alveolar dose 20% and 50% respectively greater than MAC. It must always be remembered that MAC corresponds to the median anaesthetic dose (the AD_{50}); the dose at which 50% of the animals are anaesthetized (no response to stimulus) and 50% are not. The AD_{95} (95% anaesthetized) requires an increase in alveolar dose of about

20–40%; that is, 1.2–1.4 MAC. Surgical levels of inhaled anaesthetics in the absence of usual injectable preanaesthetic and/or anaesthetic induction drugs are most likely in the range of 1.4–1.8 MAC.

The values for MAC determined in healthy cats differ among inhalation anaesthetics (Table 9.4). As noted, methoxyflurane is the most potent drug (i.e. has the lowest MAC and the highest oil/gas partition coefficient, Tables 9.4 and 9.2) and nitrous oxide is the least potent. In healthy otherwise unmedicated cats, nitrous oxide administered by itself is unable to produce general anaesthesia under ambient conditions (Venes *et al.*, 1971; Steffey *et al.*, 1974a). Because the anaesthetic properties of inhalation agents are additive, nitrous oxide is usually administered along with a volatile agent in oxygen to achieve the desired anaesthetic level. It is noticeable also that except for nitrous oxide, the potency of a given inhaled anaesthetic agent does not differ greatly between cats, dogs and humans. In animals the anaesthetic potency of nitrous oxide is only about one half that reported for humans (Steffey *et al.*, 1974a; Eger, 1985a).

Pharmacological Characteristics

In one way or another inhalation anaesthetics influence all body systems and organs. Their influence may be general, that is a resultant action may be common to all agents. Some actions are not associated with all agents but are a special or prominent feature of one or a number of agents. Undesirable actions or side-effects provide focus for the development of new agents and/or anaesthetic techniques. The difference in actions and, in particular undesirable actions, between anaesthetic agents form the basis for selecting one agent rather than another for a particular patient and/or procedure.

Specific actions of inhaled anaesthetics in cats have not been widely studied. Accordingly, the following review of the actions and toxicity of the inhaled anaesthetics draws from results of studies of many species as presented in recent reviews (Eger, 1985a, 1990; Short, 1987; Stoelting, 1987; Baden & Rice, 1990; Hall & Clarke, 1991; Haskins & Klide, 1992). When specific data from cats are available this information is included and, in particular, the properties of halothane and isoflurane are emphasized. Halothane is available at modest cost, has a proven record of safety and there is the largest body of practical experience with it. Isoflurane has become the inhalation agent most widely used in North America for human patients and has attained or is attaining a similar status in other regions of the world. It is increasingly replacing the use of halothane in cats, especially critically ill individuals. Its popularity for widespread use is presently limited only by its cost. Since most cats are allowed to breathe spontaneously during general anaesthesia (vs. controlled mechanical ventilation) this condition will be reflected in the data used to describe the actions of the anaesthetic agents.

It is important to recognize that there are many variables that commonly accompany the anaesthetic management of patients under clinical conditions. They influence the pharmacologic effects of anaesthetics and may cause individuals to respond differently from those studied under standardized conditions. In the majority of cases the most profound modifications are on circulatory function. The variables include mechanical ventilation, noxious stimulation, duration of anaesthesia and coexisting drugs. Mechanical intermittent positive pressure ventilation (IPPV) is often used to overcome the respiratory depressant properties of the anaesthetic and normalize P_aCO_2. This may depress circulation by either a direct mechanical action (i.e. intermittent elevation of intrathoracic pressure and reduction in venous return) or by an indirect pharmacological action (e.g. normalization of P_aCO_2 reduces the impact of sympathetic nervous system stimulation resulting from CO_2 accumulation). Mechanical ventilation associated reductions in cardiac output, stroke volume and arterial blood pressure may be considerable in cats (Grandy *et al.*, 1989). Confounding variables in addition to mechanical ventilation of the lung and variations in arterial carbon dioxide partial pressure include duration of anaesthesia, surgical stimulation,

physical status of the patient and concurrent medication.

Surgery and other forms of noxious stimulation tend to decrease the depressant action of light and moderate surgical levels of halothane and other volatile anaesthetics on circulation and respiration. For example, under similar conditions of anaesthetic dose, P_aO_2 and P_aCO_2, arterial blood pressure is greater during noxious stimulation than in its absence. The mechanism presumably relates to stress and associated sympathetic nervous system activation. The magnitude of effect (e.g. increase in blood pressure with stimulation) decreases with increasing anaesthetic depth (Roizen *et al.*, 1981).

Volatile Agents of Frequent Use

Halothane
Halothane was first prepared in 1952 and introduced into veterinary clinical practice in 1956 (Hall, 1957). It is a potent inhalation anaesthetic that produces relatively rapid anaesthetic induction and recovery.

Effects on respiration. Halothane depresses respiration in a dose-dependent manner (Fig. 9.1). Minute ventilation is depressed, initially because the volume of each breath (tidal volume) is decreased (Nagi *et al.*, 1965). As anaesthetic depth is increased breathing rate also decreases (Nishino & Honda, 1980). In otherwise unmedicated healthy dogs the alveolar halothane concentration that is associated with complete respiratory arrest is 2.9 MAC (Regan & Eger, 1967). Results of recent studies by Grandy *et al.* (1989) suggest that halothane is more of a respiratory depressant in cats than dogs and therefore may produce respiratory arrest at a MAC multiple less than that found for dogs. Halothane depresses chemoreceptor activity in cats and as a result decreases ventilatory responses to both hypoxia and hypercapnia (Nagi *et al.*, 1965; Davies *et al.*, 1982).

When administered initially at high concentration to awake unmedicated cats halothane may stimulate laryngospasm. This response is

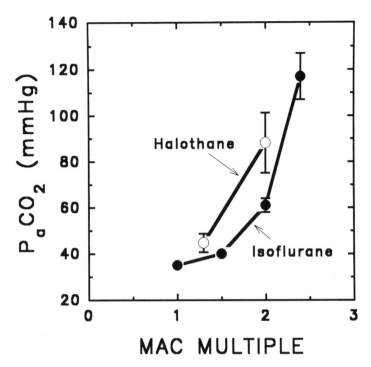

Fig. 9.1 Respiratory response to increase of halothane and isoflurane MAC. Arterial carbon dioxide tension (P_aCO_2) in cats anaesthetized with halothane and isoflurane (Steffey & Howland, 1977; Grandy *et al.*, 1989).

not unlike that reportedly associated with diethyl ether (Rex, 1973). A patent airway is essential for the safe conduct of general anaesthesia so that laryngospasm and associated airway narrowing or closure presents a potential life-threatening hazard. However, halothane seems to cause bronchodilation and decreased airway resistance. This action may make it a useful agent in the anaesthetic management of patients with reactive airway disease.

Effects on circulation. Halothane depresses circulatory system function (Eger, *et al.*, 1970; Steffey *et al.*, 1974b; Stoelting, 1987; Ingwersen *et al.*, 1988a,b; Grandy *et al.*, 1989). In studies of cats Ingwersen and co-workers showed that cardiac output, stroke volume and arterial blood pressure were lower under halothane anaesthesia than the values obtained from the animals while they were awake. Further decrease in arterial blood pressure usually accompanies increasing dose of halothane (Fig. 9.2) because cardiac output decreases further. The reduction

in cardiac output is caused by direct depression of the myocardium (Brown & Crout, 1971) and a resultant decrease in stroke volume (Grandy *et al.*, 1989). Heart rate is little changed (Fig. 9.3) over a range of clinical anaesthetic doses and, therefore, unlike arterial blood pressure is an unreliable indicator of anaesthetic depth (Grandy *et al.*, 1989).

Halothane may increase the automaticity of the heart with resultant spontaneous arrhythmias (Muir *et al.*, 1959; Purchase, 1966) especially at light levels of anaesthesia (see Chapter 12). There is some evidence that deeper levels of halothane decrease this incidence (Purchase, 1966; Muir *et al.*, 1988) but this has not been a consistent finding in dogs (Metz & Maze, 1985). Halothane is especially noted for its likelihood to predispose the heart to premature ventricular extrasystoles in the presence of catecholamines (Stoelting, 1987). In this regard it is the most potent of contemporary inhaled anaesthetics.

The cardiovascular effects of halothane change with duration of anaesthesia. Though not studied in cats, time-related increases in

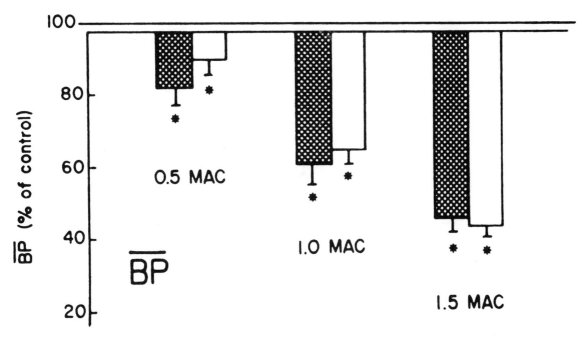

Fig. 9.2 The decrease in mean arterial blood pressure (expressed as % of control) during halothane (hatched bars) and isoflurane (open bars) anaesthesia. During both the control and anaesthetic study periods, the cats breathed an inspired gas mixutre of 75% N_2O balance oxygen. Three alveolar doses of halothane and isoflurane were studied as indicated above (adapted with permission from Todd & Drummond, 1984).

arterial blood pressure, stroke volume and cardiac output are consistently reported from studies of dogs (Steffey *et al.*, 1987a), horses (Steffey *et al.*, 1987b) and humans (Eger *et al.*, 1970).

Prior or concurrent drug therapy may also influence cardiovascular function during halothane (or anaesthesia produced by other inhaled anaesthetics). This may occur as a result of the coexisting drug(s) altering anaesthetic requirement (i.e. increasing or decreasing MAC) (Cullen, 1986; Eger, 1990). If this goes unrecognized and the drug decreases the anaesthetic requirement for halothane the anaesthetic depth realized may be excessive for the clinical circumstances and cardiovascular function further compromised. Coexisting drugs (e.g. premedication and injectable anaesthetic induction agents) may also have an influence by virtue of their own specific cardiovascular actions, for example sympathomimetic and parasympathomimetic drugs.

Effects on the liver. Halothane, like most of the inhaled anaesthetics directly depresses hepatic function. This effect may be further exaggerated by the decrease in hepatic blood flow that usually accompanies halothane anaesthesia (Stoelting, 1987). Results of a study in dogs (Reilly *et al.*, 1985) suggests that halothane inhibits the drug-metabolizing capacity of the liver. Such an effect, along with alterations in regional blood flow that commonly accompany general anaesthesia, may profoundly influence the extent and/or duration of action of concurrently administered injectable drugs. Prolonged or increased plasma concentrations of some drugs may increase their likelihood of causing toxicity, especially if the patient is already critically ill.

In humans halothane anaesthesia is occasionally associated with liver damage (centrilobular necrosis) especially after repeated administration (Baden & Rice, 1990). Hypoxic conditions may influence the likelihood of developing halothane associated hepatic dysfunction.

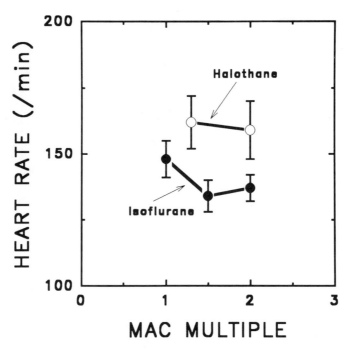

Fig. 9.3 Heart rate in cats anaesthetized with halothane and isoflurane administered in oxygen (Steffey & Howland, 1977; Grandy *et al.*, 1989).

Information on any similar condition in cats is not available but, if it occurs, its incidence is rare.

Effects on the central nervous system. Halothane causes generalized central nervous system depression. Deep levels of anaesthesia cause electrical electroencephalographic (EEG) silence. Halothane is a direct cerebral vasodilator and depresses autoregulation of cerebral blood flow (Todd & Drummond, 1984; Stoelting, 1987; Drummond & Shapiro, 1990). It is the most potent of the contemporary volatile anaesthetics in causing a dose-dependent increase in cerebral blood flow. An increase in intracranial pressure parallels the increase in cerebral blood flow making halothane a less desirable anaesthetic for cats with pre-existing space occupying intracranial lesions and/or elevations in cerebrospinal fluid pressure. Alveolar hyperventila-tion to reduce P_aCO_2 to about 30 mmHg will reduce the effect of halothane on intracranial pressure.

Effects on the kidney and its function. Halothane does not have a direct nephrotoxic effect but, like other volatile anaesthetics, it decreases urine flow and electrolyte excretion. These changes are secondary to reductions in renal blood flow and glomerular filtration rate as a result of more direct anaesthetic effects on circulatory, sympathetic nervous and endocrine systems. The degree of antidiuresis is anaes-thetic dose related and is influenced by other factors usually included in patient management such as intravenous fluid administration and the magnitude of hypotension. In most healthy cats anaesthetic effects on the kidneys are transient and normal function is rapidly restored after discontinuing the anaesthetic.

Other effects. Malignant hyperthermia (MH) is a potentially life-threatening pharmacogenetic myopathy most commonly reported in susceptible swine and human patients (Hall *et al.*, 1966, 1972; Woolf *et al.*, 1970; Stoelting, 1987). The cat is also a potential victim (deJong *et al.*, 1974; Deuster *et al.*, 1985; Bellah *et al.*, 1989) (see Chapter 12). The syndrome is characterized by a rapid rise in body temperature that, if not treated quickly, causes death. It is initiated by a variety of drugs and anaesthetic techniques. Halothane is considered the most potent 'triggering' agent relative to other inhalation anaesthetics.

Biotransformation. Inhaled anaesthetics are not inert but are biodegraded to varying degrees, particularly by the liver. The major importance of biotransformation of inhaled anaesthetics is not related to recovery from anaesthesia but to the possible production of metabolites that are toxic to the liver, kidney or other organs.

Most of the halothane taken up by the body during the course of anaesthesia is exhaled unchanged; however, a portion is metabolized. Indeed, halothane is the second most biodegraded agent among the contemporary inhaled anaesthetics (Table 9.5). The major metabolites in humans and rats is trifluoroacetic acid which is eliminated in urine. Other urinary metabolites include small amounts of Cl^-, Br^- and F^- (Baden & Rice, 1990).

Isoflurane
Isoflurane is one of the newest inhalation anaesthetics. It was first synthesized in 1965 and began widespread clinical use for human patients in 1981. It is possibly currently the most widely used volatile anaesthetic agent for humans and its use for cats continues to increase.

Effects on respiration. Isoflurane depresses ventilation (Fig. 9.1) and causes hypercapnia in a dose related manner (Steffey & Howland, 1977). Respiratory frequency remains relatively constant in the cat from 1.0 MAC to 2.0 MAC isoflurane, then as the apnoeic concentration is approached it rapidly decreases. The constancy of respiratory frequency accompanying a dose-related increase in P_aCO_2 implies that tidal alveolar ventilation decreases with increasing isoflurane dose. The alveolar concentration that causes apnoea has been reported as 2.4 MAC – a value similar to that reported by Steffey and Howland (1977) for isoflurane anaesthetized dogs (2.5 MAC).

Effects on circulation. Isoflurane causes a dose-related decrease in arterial blood pressure (Fig. 9.2). The magnitude of effect is similar to that accompanying halothane anaesthesia. Also like halothane, isoflurane depresses cardiac contractility and decreases stroke volume. However, although data from cats are lacking, studies in a variety of other species indicate that in contrast to results with halothane, cardiac output is better maintained with isoflurane and affords a wider margin of patient safety. Presuming these results apply equally to cats, isoflurane

Table 9.5 Metabolism of inhalation anaesthetics in humans

Anaesthetic	Anaesthetic recovered as metabolites (%)	Reference
Methoxyflurane	50	Holaday *et al.*, 1970
Halothane	20–25	Rehder *et al.*,1967
Enflurane	2.4	Chase *et al.*, 1971
Isoflurane	0.17	Holaday *et al.*, 1975
Sevoflurane	Similar to enflurane	Baden & Rice, 1990; Holaday & Smith, 1981
Desflurane	Likely less than isoflurane	Baden & Rice, 1990
Nitrous oxide	0.004	Hong *et al.*, 1980

would be generally preferred in cats with cardiovascular instability.

Heart rate tends to remain relatively constant over a range of isoflurane doses and heart rhythm is generally little affected by isoflurane (Fig. 9.3). Unlike halothane, isoflurane does not sensitize the myocardium to epinephrine-related premature ventricular contractions in cats (Bednarski & Majors, 1986) (Chapter 12) or other species (Eger, 1984, 1985a).

Effects on the central nervous system. Isoflurane, unlike its isomer enflurane, does not cause convulsions. However, intermittent high voltage EEG activity (hypersynchrony) has been reported to accompany isoflurane anaesthesia (Kavan & Julien, 1974).

Isoflurane at doses less than 1.2 MAC causes no change in cerebral blood flow, but at doses greater than 1.2 MAC cerebral blood flow is increased – though less so than with halothane. Autoregulation of cerebral blood flow in response to changes in arterial blood pressure is preserved during isoflurane anaesthesia. As with halothane, intracranial pressure is increased as a result of cerebrovascular vasodilatation but because these effects are more limited with isoflurane the changes in intracranial pressure with isoflurane are less than with halothane or enflurane. In addition, the changes that do occur can be controlled by hyperventilation because the cerebral circulation remains responsive to changes in P_aCO_2 (Eger, 1984).

Effects on the liver. As with halothane, blood flow to the liver is reduced as isoflurane dose is increased. Results of tests of hepatic cell integrity and function show no or minimal changes associated with isoflurane anaesthesia and any changes are rapidly reversed with recovery from anaesthesia.

Effects on the kidney. As with other volatile anaesthetics renal blood flow, glomerular filtration rate and urinary flow decrease during isoflurane anaesthesia. The changes are rapidly reversed on recovery from anaesthesia.

Biotransformation. Holaday *et al.* (1975) found that in humans less than 0.2% of the isoflurane taken up by the body is metabolized (Table 9.5). Degradation produces fluoride ion but the amount generated is far below the level of clinical significance (Eger, 1985b; Baden & Rice, 1990). Similar data for cats are not available but based on clinical experience there is no reason to believe cats substantially deviate from biotransformation characteristics found in humans.

Methoxyflurane

Methoxyflurane was first synthesized in 1958 and introduced clinically a few years thereafter. It is a potent anaesthetic and excellent analgesic. Its low vapour pressure limits its delivered concentration to a 3% maximum under usual operating room conditions at sea level.

Effects on respiration. Methoxyflurane, like halothane, depresses ventilation in cats (Nagi *et al.*, 1965). As a result P_aCO_2 increases in a methoxyflurane dose-related manner. Results of studies in dogs indicate that methoxyflurane is at least as potent a respiratory depressant as halothane (Steffey, Farver & Wolinger, 1984). Compared to values while animals are awake both tidal volume and respiratory frequency are decreased at light anaesthetic levels and respiratory frequency decreases further as anaesthetic dose is increased.

Effects on circulation. Methoxyflurane progressively depresses arterial blood pressure and cardiac output as anaesthetic dose is increased (Steffey *et al.*, 1984a). The magnitude of effect in dogs is at least equal to that noted with halothane. That the reduction in cardiac output stems largely from a depressant action on myocardial contractility (Brown and Crout 1971). The myocardium is sensitized to the arrhythmogenic potential of catecholamines but the effect is less than that associated with halothane.

Effects on the central nervous system. Methoxyflurane is a general central nervous system depressant. Cerebral blood vessels are dilated by methoxyflurane resulting in increased cerebral blood flow and increased intracranial pressure.

Effects on the liver. As with other inhaled anaesthetics methoxyflurane reversibly depresses liver function. Although hepatic necrosis has been reported in human patients following methoxyflurane anaesthesia, it is considered to be an agent with low potential for hepatotoxicity. Despite a probably low incidence of hepatotoxicity it is best to avoid methoxyflurane in feline patients suspected or known to have liver disease.

Effects on the kidney. Methoxyflurane reduces renal blood flow, glomerular filtration rate and urine flow. In humans and some strains of rats, methoxyflurane causes high output renal failure unresponsive to vasopressin. This results from the biotransformation of methoxyflurane and the release of fluoride ion which in turn causes direct damage to the renal tubules. For this reason the use of methoxyflurane in humans has been discontinued. In dogs, renal injury has been reported when methoxyflurane was used in combination with tetracycline antibiotics (Pedersoli, 1977) and flunixin (Matthews *et al.*, 1990).

Biotransformation. Methoxyflurane is metabolized to a greater extent than other contemporary volatile anaesthetics (Table 9.5). Free fluoride ion and oxalic acid are important endproducts because they can cause renal damage. Readers are referred elsewhere (Holaday *et al.*, 1970; Stoelting, 1987; Baden & Rice, 1990) for a more complete review of the subject.

Other comments. The use of methoxyflurane for anaesthetic management of cats is becoming increasingly limited. Because of its high blood and tissue solubility and nephrotoxic potential it has been eliminated from clinical use with human patients. These circumstances along with limited clear advantages in veterinary patients will almost certainly ultimately force its withdrawal from the market.

Volatile Agents of Infrequent Use

Enflurane

Enflurane was first synthesized in 1963 and released for general clinical use for human patients in North America in 1972. It is an anaesthetic with rapid induction and recovery characteristics.

Effects of respiration. Enflurane is a potent respiratory system depressant. The degree of hypoventilation and magnitude of P_aCO_2 is dose dependent and at least in dogs exceeds that caused by other contemporary volatile anaesthetics at equipotent doses (Klide, 1976; Steffey & Howland, 1978).

Effect on circulation. As with other volatile anaesthetics arterial blood pressure decreases as alveolar dose of enflurane increases (Skovsted & Price, 1972). In this regard its magnitude of effect is similar to other agents. It profoundly depresses myocardial contractility and in turn cardiac output. These effects are at least as severe or greater than those caused by other agents (Iwatsuki *et al.*, 1970; Brown & Crout, 1971). Heart rate and rhythm are stable with enflurane and it only mildly sensitizes the myocardium to catecholamines.

Effect on central nervous system. Normally as the depth of anaesthesia is increased with inhalation agents the electrical activity of the cerebral cortex as demonstrated by EEG recording is slowed. Deep levels of anaesthesia cause electrical silence. Enflurane's effects differ from the other volatile agents in that the usual EEG pattern may be interrupted at moderate to deep anaesthetic levels by high voltage, fast frequency patterns. During these periods isolated muscle twitches or frank tonic–clonic convulsive episodes may occur (Joas *et al.*, 1971; Julien & Kavan, 1972; Bassell *et al.*, 1982). The onset of these effects can be hastened by excessive hyperventilation. Enflurane is not, therefore, to be recommended for use in cats prone to seizures. The other effects of enflurane on the central nervous system are similar to those of halothane; that is, cerebrovascular dilation, increased cerebral blood flow and increased intracranial pressure.

Effect on the liver. Liver blood flow is reduced in proportion to the reduction in cardiac output. Hepatic necrosis has seldom been reported in humans anaesthetized with this agent.

Effect on the kidney. Enflurane, like halothane, causes reduced renal blood flow, glomerular filtration rate and urine volume. The magnitude of effect is similar to that caused by an equipotent level of halothane anaesthesia. Enflurane is metabolized (Table 9.5) and free fluoride ion is released in the process. The amount of fluoride released is small, however, and except in unusual circumstances like prolonged anaesthesia, not likely to reach levels of magnitude that are nephrotoxic. Nevertheless, use of enflurane in patients with known or suspected renal damage is best avoided.

Biotransformation. As noted above a small quantity of enflurane is biodegraded in the liver (Table 9.5).

Diethyl ether

Diethyl ether (ether) is one of the oldest inhalation anaesthetic agents and is probably the safest volatile anaesthetic available in terms of its influence on respiratory and circulatory function. It has good analgesic properties and respiratory function is spared over a range of clinical doses. The profound dose-related hypercapnia noted with other volatile agents is not associated with ether at low to moderate anaesthetizing doses. Spontaneous respiration remains adequate even at deep levels of anaesthesia. Although it directly depresses myocardial contractility this action in the intact animal is opposed by sympathetic stimulation (Millar et al., 1970) so that cardiac output and arterial blood pressure are usually little changed from normal. Ether does not sensitize the heart to catecholamines.

The agent is seldom used in modern operating rooms because it has a propensity to increase salivary and respiratory system secretions but especially because it is flammable at clinical doses. The disadvantages of ether can be minimized by use of parasympatholytic agents like atropine (vs. secretions), delivery in well-ventilated areas, use of closed circuit anaesthetic delivery equipment and/or an environment free of electrical sparks. Consequently, its use in some environments especially if anaesthesia is to be administered by inexperienced personnel should not be discounted.

New and Potentially Useful Volatile Anaesthetics

Desflurane

Desflurane is a new inhalation anaesthetic recently released in the United States and elsewhere for general clinical use in humans. It was previously referred to as I-653. As noted in Table 9.3 it has a high vapour pressure and therefore requires a newly designed, special temperature-controlled, pressurized vaporizer to deliver the agent to patients in a predictable fashion. According to Eger (1992) induction and recovery are the most rapid of the volatile anaesthetics. It is a dose-related respiratory and circulatory depressant. Data to date suggest the effects are similar to those of isoflurane (Warltier & Pagel, 1992).

Desflurane has the lowest rate of biodegradation of the contemporary volatile anaesthetics (Koblin, 1992) and results to date have not indicated any toxicity associated with its use. Other aspects of its use for small veterinary patients have recently been reviewed by Steffey (1992). For at least the first few years of introduction to clinical practice desflurane will be expensive to use. Because its effects on vital organ function are similar to those of isoflurane there are no obvious advantages for most feline patients seen in general practice. Accordingly its use for feline anaesthesia will probably be slow to develop.

Sevoflurane

The characteristics of sevoflurane were first described in 1975. With the possible exception of a higher heart rate with sevoflurane, its circulatory and respiratory actions are qualitatively and quantitatively similar to those for isoflurane. Like isoflurane, sevoflurane does not appear to increase the arrhythmogenicity of the heart to catecholamines. Sevoflurane is unstable and degrades in the presence of soda lime, a commonly used carbon dioxide absorber in anaesthetic delivery circuits. Dehalogenation of sevoflurane (and a transient increase in serum fluoride) occurs *in vivo* to about the same extent as with isoflurane. Nephrotoxicity is not expected and a chance for hepatotoxicity lies somewhere between that with isoflurane and halothane.

Sevoflurane is not likely to compete with existing volatile anaesthetics for use in the anaesthetic management of cats for at least the foreseeable future. For a further review of its actions see Steffey (1992).

Nitrous Oxide – The Gaseous Anaesthetic

Nitrous oxide (N_2O) has a long history and has formed the basis for more techniques of general anaesthesia than any other inhalation anaesthetic. As noted in Table 9.2, N_2O is relatively insoluble in blood and therefore its onset of action and the patient's recovery from its effects are rapid. Nitrous oxide is not a potent anaesthetic (Table 9.4). According to Eger (1985) in humans its MAC is 105%. Thus N_2O will not anaesthetize a fit, healthy individual because to avoid hypoxemia 75% is the highest concentration that can be given with safety. The value of N_2O in clinical practice is as an anaesthetic adjuvant, accompanying other inhaled or injectable drugs in the anaesthetic management of the patient. In humans, for each percent of N_2O administered the amount of the accompanying more potent volatile anaesthetic can be reduced by about 1% (i.e. 50% N_2O reduces the MAC of the more potent volatile agent by about 50%). Smaller doses of the potent volatile anaesthetic results in less circulatory and respiratory depression.

The N_2O MAC for cats is more than double that for humans, thus it is an even less potent anaesthetic in cats (Venes *et al.*, 1971; Steffey *et al.*, 1974a). The advantages of its use in cats while qualitatively similar to those considered for human patients are quantitatively smaller and, therefore, its use in cats is more equivocal.

Nitrous oxide's relative insolubility in plasma is responsible for a rapid onset in action. Although it does not have the potency to produce anaesthesia it may be used to speed induction of anaesthesia as a result of its own central nervous system effects and by augmenting the uptake of a concurrently administered more potent volatile anaesthetic such as halothane. This slight and short lived (minutes) augmentation of a second gas by N_2O is referred to as the 'second gas effect' (Eger, 1985).

Nitrous oxide is frequently considered for use because the effects on circulation and respiration in the absence of hypoxemia are comparatively small. Nitrous oxide depresses myocardial function directly but its sympathetic stimulating properties counteract some of the direct depressing actions by the volatile anaesthetics (Fukunaga & Epstein, 1973; Steffey *et al.*, 1974b; Steffey & Eger, 1984b; Eger, 1985).

Nitrous oxide has little or no effect on the liver and kidneys. Although there is evidence of N_2O-induced interference with production of red and white blood cells by bone marrow, risk to cats under most clinical circumstances is virtually non-existent.

Nitrous oxide is rapidly and mainly eliminated in the exhaled breath. The extent of biotransformation mainly by intestinal flora is very small (Eger, 1985).

The high partial pressure of N_2O required to ensure sufficient clinical value and its low blood gas partition coefficient accounts for a number of precautions. For example, N_2O exchanges with nitrogen (80% of air) when a cat (breathing air) is given a gas mixture containing N_2O. Because N_2O is 34 times more soluble in blood compared to nitrogen, a great deal more N_2O is available for exchange; that is, there is not a one for one exchange of N_2O and nitrogen. Consequently, N_2O will enter air-containing spaces such as loops of intestine at a faster rate than nitrogen leaves with a resultant net increase in volume of the space. Considerable bowel distension can thereby result in pain and risk of bowel rupture or other complications. A pneumothorax will likewise increase in volume and compromise ventilation. The large increases in volume (or pressure in spaces of low compliance) accompanying N_2O influx into the gas pocket is usually undesirable and a relative contraindication for its use in certain conditions (e.g. intestinal obstruction, pneumothorax).

Because of the large volumes of N_2O stored in the body during anaesthesia and the associated consideration for differential movement of N_2O and nitrogen, a deficiency in blood oxygenation may occur at the end of anaesthesia if air is abruptly substituted for N_2O. The rapid outpouring of N_2O into the alveoli results in a transient, marked decrease in alveolar oxygen tension with a resultant decrease in arterial oxygen tension. This is commonly known as diffusion hypoxia (Fink, 1955) and is discussed in greater depth later in this chapter.

There is increased availability and use of equipment in the operating room to monitor expired carbon dioxide (capnometry). In most cases infrared detectors are used but with this technology N_2O interferes with the accurate recording of carbon dioxide and must be accounted for. A more complete summary of advantages and disadvantages of N_2O use is given by Eger (1985) and a summary of advantages and disadvantages of all the commonly used inhalation anaesthetics in cats is given in Table 9.6.

Anaesthetic Delivery

In its simplest form the administration of inhalation anaesthetics requires a carrier gas

Table 9.6 Advantages and disadvantages of inhalation anaesthetics in cats

Agent	Advantages	Disadvantages
Diethyl ether	Inexpensive Little circulatory or respiratory depression	Flammable Airway secretions
Enflurane	Rapid induction and recovery	Seizure activity Circulatory and respiratory depression Expensive
Halothane	Inexpensive Potent	Cardiac depression and arrhythmias Metabolites Potential for hepatic necrosis Slow intake and elimination
Isoflurane	Rapid induction and recovery Less circulatory depression Limited metabolism	Respiratory depression Expensive
Methoxyflurane	Most potent Analgesia in low doses	Very slow induction and recovery Extensively metabolized Renal toxicity potential

Nitrous oxide	Analgesia
	Rapid induction and recovery
	Little circulatory or respiratory
	  depression
		Low potency
		Limits inspired O_2
		Expansion of closed gas spaces
		Diffusion hypoxia
		Interference with CO_2 measurement
		High fresh gas flow rate – wasteful,
		  polluting

that must include oxygen, a source of anaesthetic and a patient breathing circuit. Consequently, placing the patient in a closed air-filled chamber containing a cotton pledget saturated with liquid anaesthetic (such as diethyl ether) will serve to induce general anaesthesia. It is more common and appropriate in contemporary veterinary practice to use specialized equipment in an effort to provide safe, controlled delivery of inhalation anaesthetics and oxygen. This equipment includes a gas delivery system (frequently referred to as the 'anaesthetic machine') and a patient breathing system. Because this equipment greatly influences the safety of the anaesthetic technique more extensive reviews of the subject may be desired by some readers. In this regard there are a number of sources that can be recommended (Dorsch &

Dorsch, 1984; Short, 1987; White & Calkins, 1989; Andrews, 1990; Hall & Clarke, 1991).

The anaesthetic machine
An understanding of the function of the components of an anaesthetic machine is necessary in order to avoid complications. The outward appearance of the anaesthetic machine varies widely but the essential components are the same. These include: a source of oxygen and if desired N_2O, the means to control and measure the delivery of these gases, and a means to control volatilization of liquid anaesthetic and measure its delivery. A variety of safety devices can also be added to the basic equipment. A schematic diagram of a basic anaesthetic delivery device is given in Fig. 9.4.

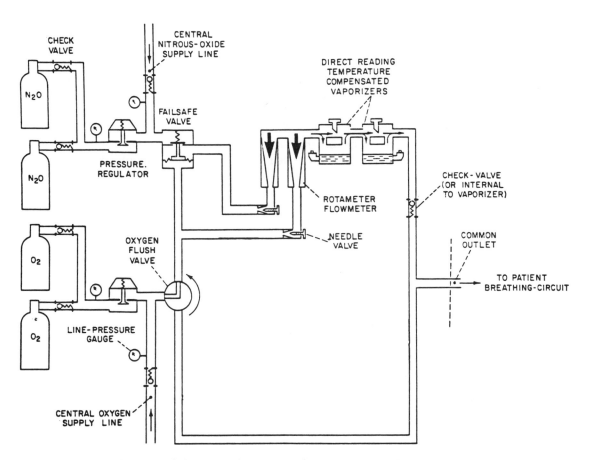

Fig. 9.4 Schematic diagram of the internal circuitry of a generic anaesthetic machine. The common outlet directs the total fresh gas flow to the patient breathing system. Reprinted with permission (Stoelting & Miller, 1987).

Gas source and metering

Oxygen (and N_2O) enters the circuit from cylinders attached to the machine or from a central service supply. The central service supply most commonly draws from large cylinders of compressed gas. In very large practice circumstances, as for example in some university-based practices, liquid oxygen sources may be more economical. In recent years oxygen concentrating devices (Steffey *et al.*, 1984b; Swar, 1987) and oxygen generators (Hall *et al.*, 1986) have also been used.

The cylinder and pipeline gas is compressed to a high pressure (e.g. at full cylinder capacity oxygen is at $2000\,lb/in^2$ or 138 atmospheres). Consequently the cylinders should be handled carefully to minimize risk of explosion. Nitrous oxide is stored in the cylinder as a liquid at about $750\,lb/in^2$ (as long as liquid remains).

Cylinder pressure is determined by a pressure gauge with the sampling port positioned just downstream of the gas source attachment to the anaesthetic machine.

Pressure-reducing valves or regulators reduce the pressure of the gas to a constant working line pressure of about $50\,lb/in^2$ regardless of the gas source. Check valves are within the circuit to prevent transfilling of cylinders from other cylinder or central pipeline sources. The flow of each gas is monitored and controlled via needle valves and rotameters (flow meters). The gas is then directed to either a patient breathing circuit directly or to a vaporizer positioned upstream of the patient breathing circuit.

Vaporizers

For circumstances requiring brief periods of general anaesthesia older volatile anaesthetics (e.g. ether) were frequently administered by simple methods. The liquid anaesthetic was poured on the floor or on a gauze lying on the floor of an anaesthetic chamber which contained the cat. This was an adaptation of a technique often used in the past for human patients commonly referred to as the 'open drop' technique. With it, inspired concentrations were often erratic and might span the extremes of anaesthetic overdose to concentrations insufficient for anaesthesia. After induction anaesthesia could be prolonged by having the animal

breath from a mask attached to an anaesthetic gas source so that the anaesthetic was vaporized by air or oxygen drawn over the surface of the liquid.

The standard in contemporary practice, especially for the use of the potent volatile anaesthetics, is to deliver anaesthetics under more controlled and precise conditions. This is accomplished by use of a vaporizer and the precision or controllability of the delivered anaesthetic concentration is dependent on its degree of sophistication. The vaporizer may be positioned within the circuitry of the gas delivery system (i.e. upstream and outside of the patient breathing circuit, known as a vaporizer out of circuit (VOC) arrangement) or within the patient breathing circuit (vaporizer in circuit, VIC) as illustrated in Fig. 9.5.

The positioning of the vaporizer in part determines the requirement for a simple, inexpensive and usually non-calibrated vaporizer (in circuit) or permits use of a complex, relatively expensive, precision, calibrated vaporizer (out of circuit). Each vaporizer position has associated advantages and disadvantages (Dorsch & Dorsch, 1984). In general, except perhaps for ether and methoxyflurane, potent volatile anaesthetics are best and most safely delivered to feline patients from precision vaporizers positioned outside the breathing circuit (Fig. 9.5).

The precision or calibrated vaporizers can be conveniently classified as either (1) measured flow or bubble-through vaporizers (an example is the copper kettle style), or (2) variable bypass. Further description of these types is beyond the scope of this summary and the reader is directed elsewhere for further information (Short, 1987; White & Calkins, 1989; Andrews, 1990; Hall & Clarke, 1991). Suffice it to say that most circuits used in feline practice incorporate the variable bypass type vaporizer (Fig. 9.6). These vaporizers are designed and calibrated for a specific inhalation anaesthetic agent. They are designed to maintain anaesthetic delivery constant by compensating for moderate changes in liquid anaesthetic temperature.

Vaporizer output is also not influenced substantially by a range of commonly used fresh gas (i.e. oxygen) flow rate until very low

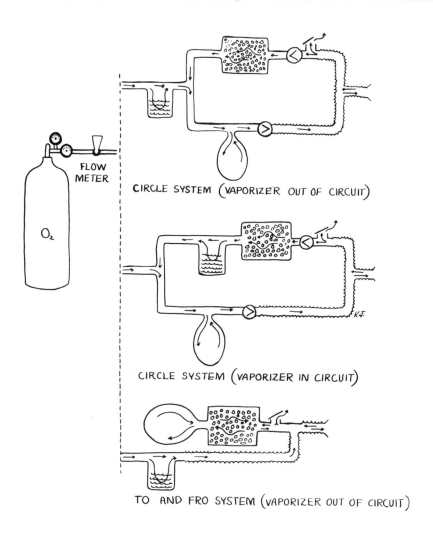

CIRCLE SYSTEM (VAPORIZER OUT OF CIRCUIT)

CIRCLE SYSTEM (VAPORIZER IN CIRCUIT)

TO AND FRO SYSTEM (VAPORIZER OUT OF CIRCUIT)

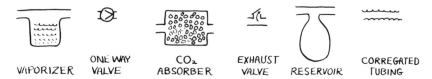

VAPORIZER   ONE WAY VALVE   CO₂ ABSORBER   EXHAUST VALVE   RESERVOIR   CORREGATED TUBING

Fig. 9.5 Schematic diagram of circle and to-and-fro patient breathing system showing different vaporizer positioning relative to the systems. Reprinted with permission (Steffey, 1982).

flowrates (i.e. $\pm$ 250 ml/min) are used. Effects from gas back pressure as might be transmitted to the vaporizer during positive pressure ventilation is also minimized in these advanced design vaporizers. Agent specificity for a vaporizer is based largely on the uniqueness of

agent vapour pressure. In the case of halothane and isoflurane, their vapour pressures at conditions of usual use are quite close (Table 9.2). Consequently the concentration dial settings on a precision vaporizer specific for one of these anaesthetics will be accurate for the other agent

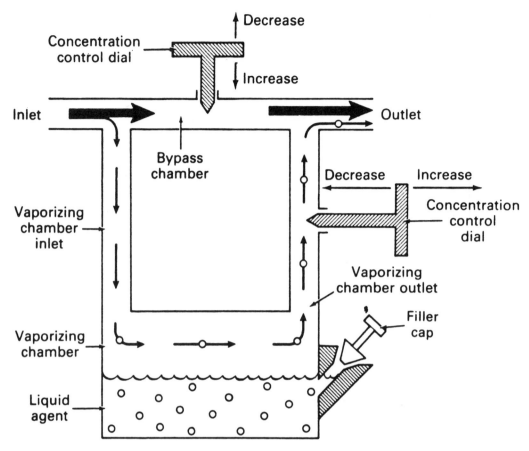

Fig. 9.6 Generic variable bypass agent, specific, precision vaporizer. Reprinted with permission (Andrews, 1989).

(Steffey *et al.*, 1983). Deliberate cross agent use is not to be encouraged, however, since this may result in use of the 'wrong' agent or delivery of the two agents simultaneously and perhaps the sum in overdose concentration.

The patient breathing system
Gases leave the anaesthetic machine via a common outlet and enter a patient breathing system (circuit). The function of the breathing system is to deliver anaesthetic gases and oxygen from the anaesthetic machine to the patient's lungs and remove expired carbon dioxide. It is an assembly of tubes and other components through which or from which the patient breathes. Although this equipment has traditionally been referred to as a circuit, the term 'system' is now in favour since not all systems conduct gases in a circuitous route.

Breathing systems can add considerable resistance to inhalation, decrease alveolar ventilation by adding equipment related ventilatory dead space and increase the animal's work of breathing. Because of the cat's small tidal volume and finite mechanical breathing capabilities, any or all of these equipment hazards are of particular concern. For example, a healthy 2-kg cat has an inspired breath volume of about 20 ml. About one-third of this is normally respiratory dead space leaving no more than about 14 ml of gas reaching the alveoli. Consequently, even a few millilitres of added equipment dead space will markedly increase the volume of exhaled gas (i.e. gas high in carbon dioxide and low in oxygen) that is rebreathed. This rebreathed gas in turn causes an increase in P_aCO_2 and the cat needs to increase breathing efforts to ensure adequate exchange of respiratory gases. Alternatively, breathing system components such as connectors, unidirectional valves and tubing can add considerable resistance to breathing and again either increase the

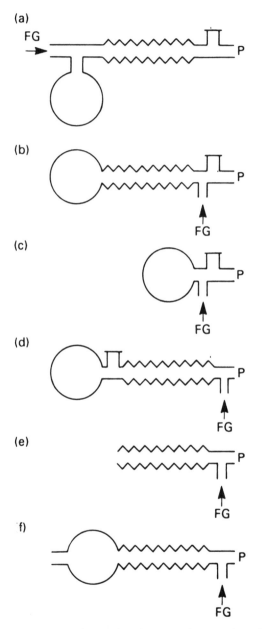

(a)

FG

P

(b)

P

FG

(c)

P

FG

(d)

P

FG

(e)

P

FG

f)

P

FG

Fig. 9.7 The Mapleson classification of patient breathing system. FG, fresh gas flow; P, patient. The patient connection is made to attach to mask or an endotracheal tube connector. Note: e is the T-piece system and f the modified T-piece system. From Hall and Clarke (1991) with permission.

animal's metabolic work of breathing or result in hypoxemia and/or hypercapnia. Anaesthetic breathing systems are frequently classified according to their components and whether or not there is intentional rebreathing of exhaled gas. An in-depth analysis and review of breathing systems is not appropriate here. Other sources for this information are available (Dorsch & Dorsch, 1984; Short, 1987; White & Calkins, 1989; Andrews, 1990; Hall & Clarke, 1991). Instead the focus will be on those systems of prominent use in feline anaesthesia and include both non-rebreathing and rebreathing systems. Advantages and disadvantages of these systems for small companion animals including cats have recently been reviewed (Haskins & Klide, 1992).

Anaesthetic gases are usually delivered to cats through a non-rebreathing system composed of wide bore gas conducting tubing and a gas reservoir bag. They use a unidirectional (exhaust) valve and/or high fresh gas flow rates to minimize resistance to breathing and prevent rebreathing of exhaled gases. Since gases are not rebreathed the composition of the inspired gas closely approximates that delivered by the anaesthetic machine. Non-rebreathing systems include many different component designs (Dorsch & Dorsch, 1984; White & Calkins, 1989; Andrews, 1990; Hall & Clarke, 1991) but all fall within the general categories originally classified by Mapleson (1989) (Fig. 9.7). Systems using high fresh gas flow as opposed to unidirectional valves are favoured for feline anaesthesia. These include modifications of the Ayre's T-piece (Fig. 9.8) and the Bain coaxial (Fig. 9.9) systems (Manley & McDonell; 1979a,b).

Total fresh gas (i.e. oxygen or oxygen plus N_2O) flow rates of 2–3 times the cat's minute ventilation are recommended for either design to prevent rebreathing during spontaneous ventilation. This means a minimal total gas delivery to the system of 300–500 ml/kg/min is necessary. These systems can be used with mechanical ventilation and because of improved ventilatory efficiency under these conditions flow rates of 200–300 ml/kg/min are satisfactory.

The Bain system (Fig. 9.9) is a coaxial version

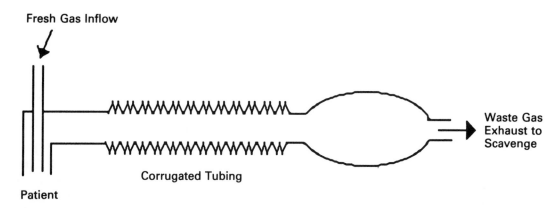

Fresh Gas Inflow

Corrugated Tubing

Patient

Waste Gas Exhaust to Scavenge

Fig. 9.8 The Jackson-Rees modification of the T-piece patient breathing system consists of the addition of a rebreathing bag with an opening for gas exhaust and a directed fresh gas inlet. The directed fresh gas flow port being positioned at the connection of the endotracheal tube minimizes dead space and chance for rebreathing expired gas. This modification, along with its lack of moving parts (e.g. valve), makes this system highly desirable for very small patients.

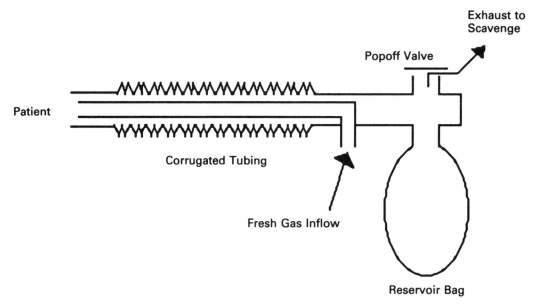

Exhaust to Scavenge

Popoff Valve

Patient

Corrugated Tubing

Fresh Gas Inflow

Reservoir Bag

Fig. 9.9 The Bain system is a coaxial (note fresh gas delivery tube within corrugated [exhaust] tube). It is a modification of the Mapleson D circuit (Fig. 9.7). This system, along with the Jackson-Rees modification of the T-piece (Fig. 9.8), is highly desirable for very small patients.

of the T-piece in which the fresh gas inflow enters through a narrow tube within the corrugated expired limb. In recent years an expiratory valve is frequently positioned at the distal end of the system making it a modification of the Mapleson D system (Fig. 9.7). An advantage of the Bain system is the warming of fresh inhaled gases by the surrounding exhaled gases in the corrugated tubing. Scavenging of waste anaesthetic gases is easily accomplished with either of the two commonly used non-rebreathing systems.

A variety of non-rebreathing systems have been described that use valves to minimize the likelihood of rebreathing of expired gases. Like other non-rebreathing systems discussed above, use of a continuous fresh gas supply and a reservoir bag is incorporated in the system to supply peak inspiratory flow rate and to facilitate mechanical ventilation by hand. Use of a valve or valves, however, permits reduction in fresh gas inflow compared to non-valve systems and therefore is more economical than other non-rebreathing systems, although with the low flow rates necessary for cats economic considerations are of minor importance. The valve systems generally are classified under the Mapleson (A–D) system (Fig. 9.7) and are explained in greater detail elsewhere (White & Calkins, 1989; Andrews, 1990; Hall & Clarke, 1991).

Rebreathing systems provide for partial or complete rebreathing of exhaled gases. This is acceptable because valves direct exhaled gases through an absorber that removes carbon dioxide. Two styles of rebreathing systems are available, the circle and the to-and-fro systems (Fig. 9.5). The circle system is the most commonly used of the two types. It is so named because the path of gas flow within the system is unidirectional and in a circular path. The to-and-fro system includes a carbon dioxide absorber circuit positioned between an endotracheal tube and a reservoir bag. The gases moving to and from the patient flow through this equipment in a to-and-fro pattern; that is, in a back and forth or bidirectional pattern (Dordsch & Dorsch, 1984; Short, 1987; Hall & Clarke, 1991). Because of the gas flow pattern in the to-and-fro system respiratory dead space increases with duration of anaesthesia as an increasing amount of the carbon dioxide absorbent is consumed. This along with other concerns make the to-and-fro system less than desirable for routine use with the feline patient.

Compared to non-rebreathing systems, and as a result of rebreathing, these systems conserve respiratory moisture and body heat better, factors of particular concern in very small patients like cats. They also diminish operating room anaesthetic gas pollution and risk of fires and pollution with older flammable agents (e.g.

ether). Despite these benefits, however, valves and carbon dioxide absorbers increase resistance to respiration. Greater equipment bulk decreases portability and increases mechanical dead space which in turn increases the chance for rebreathing carbon dioxide laden gas. Rebreathing systems are also more complex in their construction compared to non-rebreathing systems thereby increasing purchase cost and the opportunity for malfunction. Consequently rebreathing systems are less frequently used than non-rebreathing systems in the anaesthetic management of cats.

The amount of rebreathing in these systems is largely determined by the flow rate of fresh gas delivered to the system from the anaesthetic machine. The lower limit of theoretical safety is dictated by the metabolic oxygen requirement of the patient per minute: that is, $10 \times$ weight in $kg^{0.75}$ which is equivalent to 6–9 ml/kg/min (Brody, 1945) for the anaesthetized cat. At this level of oxygen inflow, the system would be referred to as a closed system; that is, the inflow of fresh gas from the anaesthetic machine equals the uptake of all the gases by the patient and there is total rebreathing of exhaled gases (minus of course the carbon dioxide which is removed by the carbon dioxide absorber). Although this mode of use of a rebreathing system has distinct advantages for managing larger animals, its routine use for a domestic cat patient would be impractical and possibly dangerous. For example, based on the above information, a 2-kg domestic shorthair cat presented for an anaesthesia on an elective basis has an estimated metabolic oxygen requirement of about 16 ml/min. This magnitude of oxygen inflow from the anaesthetic machine to a typical adult human circle breathing system would be far below the range of accuracy of the flow meter incorporated in most anaesthetic machines and consequently inspired oxygen and anaesthetic concentrations would be unpredictable. Furthermore, because of the low fresh gas inflow and the relatively large internal gas volume of the breathing system, significant rebreathing would almost certainly occur with resultant hypercapnia. These and other reasons usually make selection of this technique an unwise decision for a feline patient.

If it is determined that a circle system is desirable for specific use with a feline patient at least some of the disadvantages can be minimized by selecting a human paediatric circle system where the components are small and compact in arrangement. Alternatively a relatively high fresh gas inflow rate can be used (i.e. 200–300 ml/kg of body weight, making it a 'low-flow' system) and mechanical ventilation. Interestingly the high cost of the newer volatile anaesthetics is leading some medical paediatric anaesthesiologists to advocate return to the circle absorber systems with modifications suitable for the very small patients.

When N_2O is used as part of the anaesthetic management scheme not only is the total gas flow important but also the flow rate of oxygen in proportion to N_2O. The maximal amount of N_2O delivered is based on the inflow rate of oxygen which in turn should exceed the animal's metabolic requirements by a good safety margin and for most domestic cats 100 ml/kg/min of oxygen is appropriate. With a total fresh gas flow (oxygen plus N_2O) of 200–300 ml/kg/min (the low-flow set-up) this results in an inspired N_2O concentration of 50–67%.

Scavenging Equipment

Gases escaping from the anaesthetic circuit contaminate the operating room atmosphere to varying degrees with trace amounts of inhalation anaesthetic. There is considerable controversy about possible health hazards to personnel exposed to these exhaust gases and vapours. Numerous investigations to determine the effects of chronic low level anaesthetic exposure, in particular, congenital birth defects and carcinogenicity have been carried out and an updated review of this subject appears elsewhere (Baden & Rice, 1990). Results of some animal studies indicate that inhalation anaesthetics have the potential for creating undesirable effects in humans. Consequently it is recommended that, to avoid possible litigation, anaesthetic scavenging equipment be a component of the anaesthetic delivery machinery. Waste inhalation anaesthetic agents can be collected from the patient breathing system pop-off valve and removed from the operating room environment (Manley & McDonell, 1980; Dorsch & Dorsch, 1984; Short, 1987; Hall & Clarke, 1991).

Masks, Endotracheal Tubes and Closed Containers

Face masks and endotracheal tubes are common examples of airway equipment used to interface the patient with the breathing circuit. Masks enable the anaesthetist to administer anaesthetic gases and/or oxygen to the patient without introducing any tubes into the trachea. Masks are used to supplement the inspired breath with oxygen prior to anaesthetic induction (by inhalation or intravenous routes), to induce general anaesthesia with inhalation agents and, in some circumstances, to maintain general anaesthesia. The mask should closely conform to the patient's face and the connector to the breathing circuit. When the mask is properly selected and applied, dead space ventilation and, therefore, rebreathing of expired gas is minimized. Moreover, unlike the use of endotracheal tubes, use of a face mask is not associated with potential laryngeal damage which can give rise to oedema of the mucous membranes resulting in severe respiratory obstruction in small cats due to the small dimensions of the larynx (see Chapter 12).

There are anecdotal reports that the smallest available laryngeal mask airway, the 'LMA', designed for use in humans (Brain, 1983), has been found to be suitable for medium- to large-sized cats and, if these reports are confirmed, the use of the LMA should provide a safe way of providing a gas-tight seal with the cat's airway without the possibility of laryngeal damage. However, it is probable that the LMA is currently too expensive for veterinary use.

Anaesthetic induction and/or pre-anaesthetic oxygenation can be facilitated with the use of an airtight chamber in which the patient is placed. Ideally the chamber should be close in size to that of the patient, allow for exhaust gas scavenge and provide a clear view of the

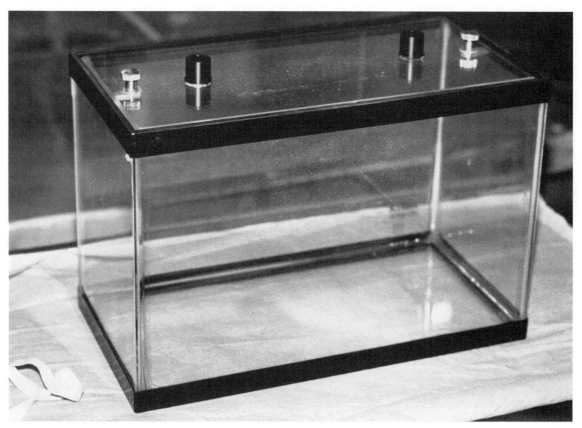

Fig. 9.10 Anaesthetic chamber for vicious or unmanageable cats.

patient (Fig. 9.10) (see Chapter 5). Maintenance of inhalation anaesthesia is most commonly facilitated via the use of tracheal intubation. In uncomplicated circumstances this means a tracheal tube is inserted via the mouth through the larynx into the trachea so that anaesthetic gases are conveyed directly from the breathing system into the trachea. The tube may include a cuff near its distal end to produce a leak-free tracheal seal or it may be cuffless (Fig. 9.11).

There are a variety of cuffed and cuffless endotracheal tubes manufactured for use with human paediatric patients that are applied to veterinary circumstances. The Cole style (Fig. 9.11) endotracheal tube is a cuffless variety sometimes used for feline patients in which maximal tube lumen diameter and a tracheal seal is highly desired (Short, 1987). However, a better solution for providing a less laryngeal damaging airtight seal is to pack the pharynx and fauces with gauze around an ordinary cuffless tube of the maximum bore that can be passed atraumatically through the larynx (see Chapter 12). A 4.0- or 4.5-mm (internal diameter) tube is satisfactory for a 2–3 kg cat. Regardless of the tube style, it should be long enough to just pass into the trachea beyond the larynx (the tip should not extend beyond the level of the thoracic inlet). To minimize dead space the tracheal tube connector ideally should be level with the incisor teeth.

Anaesthesia Ventilators

A ventilator can be substituted for the breathing bag of the circle system, the Bain system and the modified Ayres T-piece system. Use of a

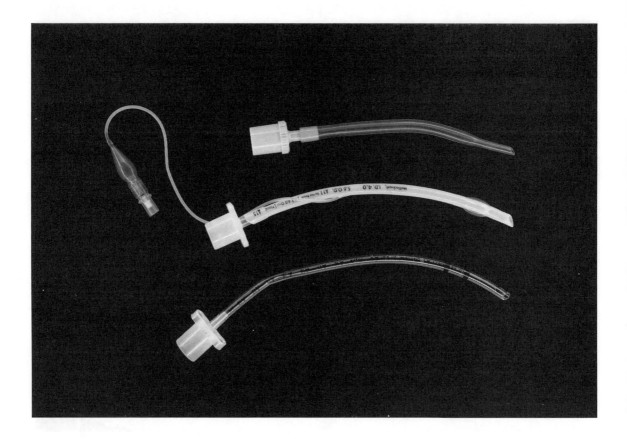

Fig. 9.11 Three styles of tracheal tubes for cats: from top to bottom, the Cole, and the straight styles without and with a low volume, high pressure cuff. The cuff is intended to seal the airway and maximize the quality of inspired gas and minimize the chance for aspiration of foreign matter. The Cole tube attempts to accomplish a similar situation via its flared or shoulder design. The smaller base portion of the tube is intended to be entirely within the trachea. Tube sizes of 3–5.5 mm (internal diameter, tracheal portion) are usual for adult cats.

ventilator during anaesthesia to assist or control ventilation allows the anaesthetist to attend to other matters essential to the care of the patient. When human paediatric ventilators or specially designed animal ventilators are not available, the cat's lungs may be ventilated using a ventilator designed for use in adult human patients provided excess tidal gas is allowed to escape around the endotracheal tube and out of the larynx during the inspiratory phase of the respiratory cycle.

If no ventilator is available the cat's lungs are easy to ventilate manually. The most suitable circuits for this purpose are the Jackson Rees modified Ayre's T-piece or the unmodified Bain coaxial circuit.

Uptake and Elimination of Inhalation Anaesthetics

General anaesthesia results from the delivery of an anaesthetic drug to, and interaction with, an effective site of action in the central nervous system. Inhalation anaesthetics are unique among anaesthetic drugs because the respiratory tract is used as the means of entry into the body. Special characteristics associated with this mode of drug delivery are the focus of this section and form the fundamental knowledge necessary for skilful control of general inhalation anaesthesia.

The characterization of this form of drug delivery, commonly referred to as the uptake and distribution of inhaled anaesthetics, has been most actively investigated by Eger (1974). It is not the purpose of this chapter to provide an exhaustive review of these principles. This is readily available elsewhere (Mapleson, 1989; Eger, 1990, 1992). However, brief emphasis of some clinically important points is warranted.

The aim in administering an inhalation anaesthetic is to achieve and maintain a critical partial pressure or 'tension' of anaesthetic in the brain. This is accomplished by manipulating the anaesthetic tension in the patient breathing system. Anaesthetic agents, like respiratory gases (e.g. oxygen), move down pressure gradients from regions of higher tension to those of lower tension until equilibrium between compartments is established. Thus, by controlling the tension of the agent 'upstream' in the flow pattern of anaesthetics a gradient is established and the anaesthetic dose reaching

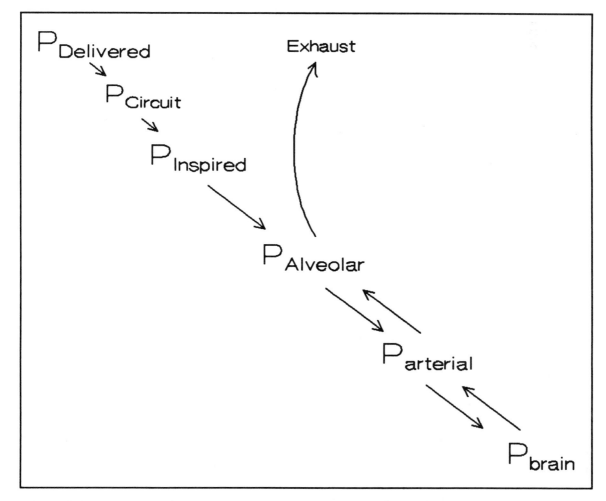

Fig. 9.12 The flow pattern of inhaled anaesthetic agents during anaesthetic induction and recovery. When referring to the gas phase the partial pressure and concentration are directly related; that is Anaesthetic partial pressure/Total pressure × 100 = concentration (vol %). $P_{Delivered}$ is the tension in the fresh gas delivered to the breathing circuit from the vaporizer.

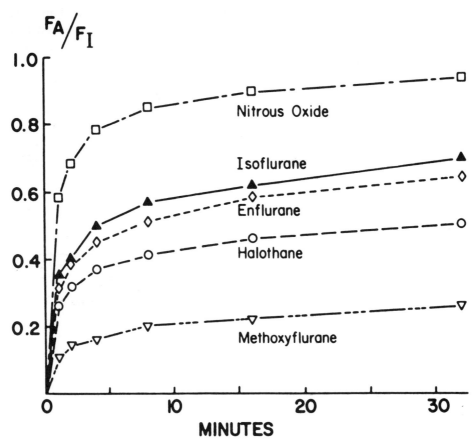

Fig. 9.13 The rise in alveolar (F_A) anaesthetic concentration toward the inspired (F_I) concentration with time. The rise is most rapid with the least soluble agent (N_2O) and slowest with the most soluble (methoxyflurane). From Eger (1985) with permission.

the site of action in the brain is controlled (Fig. 9.12).

At this point it is important to stress that it is the partial pressure of the anaesthetic at its site of action that is important in any understanding of concepts of uptake and distribution and anaesthetic dose (i.e. MAC). Although it is common to define the clinical dose of an inhalation anaesthetic (e.g. vaporizer dial setting, inspired, MAC) in terms of concentration (i.e. volumes %) this is not necessarily representative of the concentration in the brain. This is because in a gaseous phase the partial pressure of the anaesthetic equals the fractional concentration of the gas in question multiplied by the total ambient gas pressure (Fig. 9.13).

The actual quantity of anaesthetic vapour contained in a liquid or tissue phase, however,

depends both on partial pressure and its solubility in the particular phase (i.e. its partition coefficient). Consequently, at equilibrium the partial pressure in all phases should be equal while the concentration will vary. For example, if alveolar gas containing halothane is equilibrated with blood, the blood will contain 2.3 times the amount of halothane in the alveolar gas phase despite an equal tension in both phases and no further net uptake of halothane by blood. The significance of anaesthetic agent solubility to principles of uptake and distribution is important and needs further illustration.

The brain and other body tissues equilibrate with the partial pressure of anaesthetic delivered to them by arterial blood (P_a) (Fig. 9.12). The arterial blood in turn equilibrates with the alveolar gas tension (P_A). Therefore the task of achieving a tension of anaesthetic in brain (P_{brain}) is dependent on developing an appropriate P_A. The P_A thus serves as a mirror of the P_{brain} and is the reason the alveolar concentration is used as an index of anaesthetic dose (i.e. MAC) and, as discussed below, is a reflexion of the rate of induction and recovery from anaesthesia.

Anaesthetic Uptake: Factors that Determine the P_A of Anaesthetic

The alveolar anaesthetic tension is a balance between anaesthetic input (i.e. delivery to the alveoli) and uptake (removal by the blood) from the lungs. A rapid rise in P_A of anaesthetic is associated with a rapid anaesthetic induction or change in anaesthetic level. Conditions are summarized in Table 9.7.

Delivery to alveoli

Delivery of anaesthetic to alveoli depends on the inspired anaesthetic concentration and magnitude of alveolar ventilation. Increasing either or both increases the rate of rise of the P_A; that is, other things considered equal the speed of anaesthetic induction or change in anaesthetic level. The inspired concentration in turn has a number of variables controlling it. A major factor is the breathing system in use. Since in the case of feline anaesthesia a non-rebreathing system or a relatively high fresh gas inflow into a rebreathing circuit ('low flow system') are

Table 9.7 Factors related to a rapid change in alveolar anaesthetic tension

---

Increased alveolar delivery
Increased inspired anaesthetic concentration
   Increased vaporizer dial setting
   Increased fresh gas inflow
   Decreased gas volume of patient breathing circuit
Increased alveolar ventilation
   Increased minute ventilation
   Decreased dead space ventilation
Decreased removal from the alveoli
   Decreased blood solubility of anaesthetic
   Decreased cardiac output
   Decreased alveolar–venous anaesthetic gradient

---

used there is usually not a clinically important difference between the delivered and inspired concentrations (partial pressure). Accordingly, under usual clinical conditions of feline anaesthesia, inspired anaesthetic concentration is largely related only to vaporizer dial setting.

Alveolar ventilation is altered by changes in anaesthetic level (decreased level equals increased ventilation), mechanical ventilation (increased ventilation) or changes in dead space ventilation (increased dead space equals decreased alveolar ventilation).

The alveolar concentration can also be influenced by administering potent volatile anaesthetics like halothane with N_2O. Very early in the administration of, for example, 70% N_2O (during the period of large volume uptake) the rate of rise of the alveolar concentration of concurrently administered halothane is increased. This is commonly referred to as the 'second gas effect' and knowledge of this phenomenon is sometimes used clinically to speed anaesthetic induction (Eger, 1974).

Uptake by the blood

Anaesthetic uptake from the lung by blood is the product of three factors: anaesthetic solubility, the cardiac output and the difference in anaesthetic partial pressure or tension in alveolar gas and venous blood.

The solubility of inhaled anaesthetics in blood and tissues is characterized by partition coefficients (Tables 9.2 and 9.3). Based on their blood/gas partition coefficient, inhalation anaesthetics range from highly soluble (e.g. methoxyflurane), to poorly soluble (e.g. N_2O, desflurane). Agents such as halothane and isoflurane are intermediary.

A highly soluble anaesthetic is associated with a prolonged anaesthetic induction time because a large amount of anaesthetic must be dissolved in the blood before equilibrium is reached with the gas phase. In this case the blood acts like a large sink into which the anaesthetic is poured with little output to the brain (until blood solubility limits are approached). Accordingly the rate of rise of the alveolar concentration is slow (Fig. 9.13) as the $P_{anaesthetic}$ in all tissues approaches that in the alveoli. On the other hand, only a small amount of a poorly soluble anaesthetic would have to be dissolved in blood before equilibrium is reached. Thus, the poorly soluble agent has a faster rise in P_A and is, therefore, associated with a more rapid (compared to the soluble agent) rate of anaesthetic induction and/or change in anaesthetic depth. Figure 9.13 summarizes and compares the rate of rise of all of the contemporary inhalation anaesthetics (Eger, 1985). The characteristics of the two newest volatile anaesthetics are compared in Fig. 9.14 (Eger, 1992).

The influence of cardiac output on the rate of rise of the alveolar concentration (P_A) is straight forward. The greater the output the more blood passes through the lungs and therefore the more blood the alveolar anaes-

thetic is exposed to. This condition then, like an increase in agent solubility, lowers the alveolar tension of the anaesthetic by creating a large pharmacologically inactive reservoir.

An increased cardiac output might be expected clinically in association with patient excitement. Conversely, a reduced cardiac output would accompany shock and be expected to increase the rate of rise of P_A of anaesthetic and make an anaesthetic induction with a high inspired anaesthetic more risky. Cardiac output and anaesthetic solubility probably account for much of the clinically important uptake considerations in feline patients.

Alveolar to venous anaesthetic tension difference results from tissue uptake of anaesthetic. Once the tissues no longer take up anaesthetic

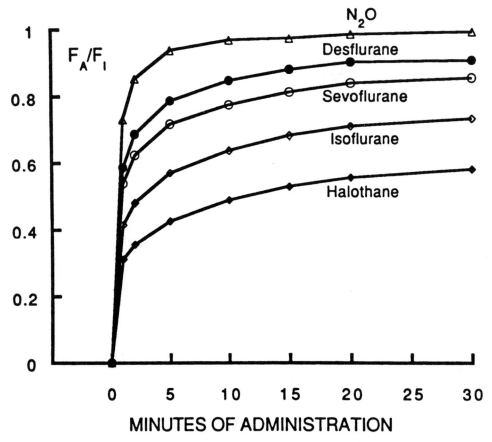

Fig. 9.14 The rise in alveolar (F_A) anaesthetic concentration toward the inspired (F_I) concentration with time. This differs from Fig. 9.13 by the absence of the curve for methoxyflurane and the addition of curves for the two new volatile anaesthetics desflurane and sevoflurane. Data to construct these curves were derived from humans. From Eger (1992) with permission.

there would no longer be any uptake of agent by arterial blood (i.e. the venous blood returning to the lungs would contain as much as when it left the lungs). The clinical importance of this gradient relates heavily to duration of anaesthesia (less influence with time) and agent partition coefficient (less influence of gradient with reduced solubility).

There are other factors that can further influence the magnitude of arterial to venous anaesthetic partial pressure gradient. They include loss of anaesthetic into closed gas spaces and metabolism. These influences are of lesser degree, however, and further discussion on these matters is considered beyond the scope of this chapter. The reader is referred elsewhere (Eger, 1974, 1990) for additional information.

Anaesthetic Recovery

Recovery from anaesthesia is related to the fall in P_A and therefore the brain tension of the anaesthetic. The rate of recovery from anaesthesia is dependent largely on the rate of fall of P_A of anaesthetic (concentration). (An exception may be associated with methoxyflurane whereby, clinically, metabolism may play as important role as elimination via the lungs.) In many respects recovery from inhalation anaesthesia is the inverse of induction of anaesthesia (Fig. 9.15). Many factors that regulate the fall of P_A of anaesthetic are identical to those governing the rate of rise; that is, alveolar ventilation, anaesthetic agent solubility (partition coefficient) and cardiac output.

When anaesthetic is no longer a component of

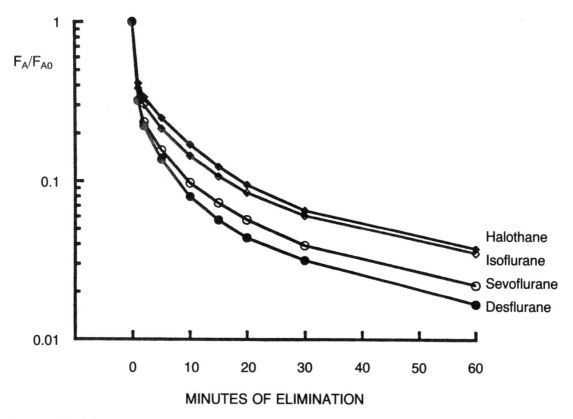

Fig. 9.15 The fall in alveolar (F_A) concentration relative to the last alveolar concentration found during anaesthesia (F_AO). The newest, most insoluble, volatile anaesthetic desflurane is eliminated in humans more rapidly than the other contemporary potent anaesthetics. Not shown is information for methoxyflurane – if present, the curve for methoxyflurane would appear above that for halothane. From Eger (1992) with permission.

the inspired breath the alveolar anaesthetic tension decreases rapidly. This establishes an anaesthetic tension gradient between alveoli and the venous blood causing anaesthetic loss from blood into the alveoli. The magnitude of impact is related again to solubility; a more soluble agent (e.g. methoxyflurane) leaves the blood at a slower rate (i.e. prolonged recovery) compared to the more insoluble agent (e.g. isoflurane).

The duration of anaesthesia also influences anaesthetic recovery. Because a greater reserve of a highly soluble agent like methoxyflurane exists in the body following a prolonged anaesthetic its P_A is slower to fall compared to an agent such as isoflurane.

Metabolism of some anaesthetics (e.g. methoxyflurane) may be an important determinant of the rate of fall of the P_A of anaesthetic especially following prolonged exposure (e.g. 4 h or more). In this regard any effect by metabolism would be expected (Eger, 1990) to be less with halothane and virtually non-existent with isoflurane (Table 9.5).

A special consideration occurs during recovery from an anaesthetic technique that includes N_2O; that is, a potential for hypoxemia (Eger, 1985, 1990). In the case of a cat recovering from anaesthesia a large volume of N_2O enters the lung from the blood. This early rapid inflow of N_2O dilutes other gases that are in the lung. If at this time the cat is breathing air as opposed to oxygen the further dilution of alveolar oxygen from levels found in ambient air may cause what Fink (1955) called diffusion anoxia (more appropriately referred to today as diffusion hypoxia). The effect on reducing arterial oxygenation is small and is short-lived (i.e. minutes) in healthy cats. Consequently any danger to these animals is probably small. However, in cats with, for example, lung disease, the danger added by even brief periods of further arterial oxygen desaturation via diffusion hypoxia may be substantial and life threatening. Since the major effect is in the first few moments after discontinuing N_2O, the condition can be prevented by administering oxygen at the conclusion of N_2O administration rather than immediately allowing the patient to breathe ambient air.

Practical Points

Anaesthetic Induction

Induction of anaesthesia is accomplished either by administering an injectable anaesthetic (intravenous or intramuscular) or by inhalation of an appropriate mixture of anaesthetic and oxygen. The administration of the inhalation anaesthetic may be via a mask or an induction box depending upon the nature of the patient and other circumstances pertinent at the time. If the patient is manageable either by its nature or as a result of pre-anaesthetic medication, induction by mask rather than via box is usually preferred because this technique provides better direct care to the patient. In the case of fractious cats use of an induction chamber may be more desirable (see Chapter 5). The actual dose of inhalation anaesthetic administered depends upon many variables including the agent itself. Suffice is to say that the dose of anaesthetic administered at this stage of anaesthetic management exceeds the maintenance dose and may be in the range of 4–5 times the MAC for the agent in an otherwise healthy unmedicated cat. This magnitude of delivery is frequently selected to overcome delays in anaesthetic induction imposed by such things as the solubility of the agent in blood. A rapid induction is usually desirable to reduce excitement of the cat that may be dangerous to both the animal and personnel. A rapid induction also facilitates timely patient airway management. On the other hand, a physiologically compromised patient is most likely better served by a more cautious and delayed anaesthetic induction. Under these circumstances the patient is administered oxygen via a face mask connected to a non-rebreathing system. The modified Ayre's T-piece and the Bain coaxial circuits are most commonly used. After a period of breathing oxygen the inhaled anaesthetic agent(s) is added to the inspired gas in gradually (e.g. every 5–10 breaths) increasing concentration. The magnitude of stepwise concentration increase is dependent on the patient's physical status. Because of its low partition coefficient isoflurane is frequently a good choice despite its somewhat higher cost. Reduced incidence of cardiac arrhythmias compared to, for example, halothane are an added advantage; it may be administered with or without N_2O. In relation to a rapid anaesthetic induction the use of N_2O is less important with isoflurane than if halothane, or even more so methoxyflurane, was selected as the primary volatile agent of choice.

A pre-anaesthetic fast of food and liquid is recommended for the elective surgical patient because vomiting sometimes occurs during induction of general anaesthesia (see Chapter 6). Attempts early in the course of anaesthesia to place an endotracheal tube frequently contributes to an increased frequency of vomiting. The anaesthetist should also be on the alert for warning signs of vomiting (e.g. frequent swallowing, retching). Vomiting can sometimes be avoided if preliminary signs are recognized and corrective action taken (see Chapter 12).

Orotracheal intubation should be considered for most cats receiving general inhalation anaesthesia. On the other hand, some procedures requiring only very short periods of inhalation anaesthesia (minutes) in healthy cats can be safely performed via mask without undue hazard to the patient.

Intubation of the trachea using direct laryngoscopy in anaesthetized patients is the usual technique. Rarely intubation via a tracheostomy site is necessary. Equipment and supplies necessary to perform the procedure properly include a size range of endotracheal tubes bracketing the size considered ideal for the patient in question (e.g. 3–5 mm), sterile lubricant to facilitate atraumatic tube placement, a laryngoscope and gauze or tape to secure the tube in place after intubation. If a cuffed tracheal tube is chosen its cuff is checked for air leaks before anaesthetic induction. Selection of the appropriate tracheal tube diameter and length is critical in cats due to the relative small size of their airway. Too large a tube ensures unnecessary trauma with potential for airway problems after tracheal tube extubation. Likewise a tube too long increases the risk of having the distal end of the tube entering one or the other of the mainstem bronchi and resulting in ventilation of only one lung. Resistance to breathing is an

important consideration associated with the small size of tubes and connectors necessary for cats. Intubation is performed in the cat only after an adequate level of general anaesthesia is attained (Rex, 1971) or after the administration of a neuromuscular blocking drug (Hall & Clarke, 1991). To attempt to intubate an inadequately anaesthetized or relaxed cat increases the risk of laryngospasm, failed or traumatic intubation, regurgitation of gastric contents, and/or injury to personnel from an aroused and/or angry animal (see Chapter 12). Intubation is usually performed with a laryngoscope to provide a clear view of the larynx. With the cat's head held in extension, and the lower jaw lifted with the laryngoscope blade, the endotracheal tube is passed through the mouth into the glottis under direct vision. A few drops of local anaesthetic (e.g. 0.1–0.2 ml 2% lignocaine) applied by swab or aerosol to the laryngeal area also helps minimize laryngeal spasm. Common causes of failure to intubate the patient frequently related to inadequate visualization of the glottic opening. Details of positioning for and hazards of intubation are described in more detail in Chapters 5 and 12 respectively.

Following tracheal intubation anaesthetic depth is adjusted to suit the prevailing circumstances and monitoring aids are applied to the patient. The lightest level of anaesthesia compatible with patient safety and good operating conditions is then maintained. The actual dose of anaesthetic administered corresponds to the degree of reflex response to surgical stimulation. It is varied throughout the operative period according to need of the moment and in anticipation of the needs associated with the anaesthetic recovery period.

If IPPV is deemed necessary (see Chapters 8, 10, 11 and 12), whether manual or mechanical ventilation is used, care should be taken not to overventilate as this is a potential hazard in such a small patient. If no carbon dioxide monitoring is available a non-rebreathing system should be used and the cat's lungs should be inflated 10–15 times per minute so that, visually, the chest appears to move the same amount or slightly more than if the cat were breathing spontaneously. As IPPV reduces cardiac output by decreasing venous return as a result of the positive pressure in the thorax, the inspiratory to expiratory ratio should be kept low and inspiratory flow rate relatively high. This results in long expiratory pauses to maintain a low mean thoracic pressure and allow as much venous return as possible.

Recovery from inhalation anaesthesia is usually routine and uneventful. The administration of anaesthetic drugs is discontinued and the animal allowed to recover under direct supervision in a warm, quiet environment. The rate of recovery from anaesthesia is related to the rate of fall of the alveolar concentration of anaesthetic as previously discussed. Removal of the endotracheal tube from the trachea (extubation) is usually accomplished when the cat is just beginning to arouse and swallowing is evident. To extubate too early risks patient hypoventilation or worse airway obstruction. Conversely, to delay extubation risks hyper-responsive airway reflexes, laryngospasm, retching and/or vomiting (see Chapter 12).

References

Andrews, J.J. (1989) Anesthesia systems. In: Clinical Anesthesia (ed. P.G. Barash, B.F. Cullen & R.K. Stoelting), p. 505. J.B. Lippincott, Philadelphia.

Andrews, J.J. (1990) Inhaled anesthetic delivery systems. In: Anesthesia, 3rd edn (ed. R.D. Miller), p. 171. Churchill Livingstone, New York.

Baden, J.M. & Rice, S.A. (1990) Metabolism and toxicity. In: Anesthesia, 3rd edn (ed. R.D. Miller), p. 135, Churchill Livingstone, New York.

Bassell, G.M., Cullen, B.F., Fairchild, M.D. & Kusske, J.A. (1982) Electroencephalographic and behavioral effects of enflurane and halothane anaesthesia in cats. Brit. J. Anaesth. 54, 659–665.

Bednarski, R.M. & Majors, L.J. (1986) Ketamine and arrhythmogenic dose of epinephrine in cats anesthetized with halothane and isoflurane. Am. J. Vet. Res. 47, 2122–2126.

Bellah, J.R., Robertson, S.A., Buergelt, C.D. & McGavin, A.D. (1989) Suspected malignant hyperthermia after halothane anesthesia in a cat. Vet. Surg. 18, 483–488.

Brain, A.I.J. (1983) The laryngeal mask – a new concept in airway management. Brit. J. Anaesth. 55, 801–805.

Brody, S. (1945) Bioenergetics and Growth. Reinhold, New York.

Brown, B.R. & Crout, J.R. (1971) A comparative study of the effects of five general anesthetics on myocontractility: I. Isometric conditions. Anesthesiology 34, 236–245..

Chase, R.E., Holaday, D.A., Fiserova-Bergerova, V. Saidman, L.J. & Mack, F.E. (1971) The biotransformation of ethrane in man. Anesthesiology 35, 262–267.

Cullen, D.J. (1986) Anesthetic depth and MAC. In: Anesthesia, 2nd edn (ed. R.D. Miller), p. 553. Churchill Livingstone, New York.

Davies, R.O., Edwards, M.W., Jr & Lahiri, S. (1982) Halothane depresses the response of carotid body chemoreceptors to hypoxia and hypercapnia in the cat. Anesthesiology 57, 153–159.

deJong, R.H., Heavner, J.E. & Amory, D.W. (1974) Malignant hyperpyrexia in the cat. Anesthesiology 41, 608–609.

Deuster, P.A., Bockman, E.L. & Muldoon, S.M. (1985) In vitro responses of cat skeletal muscle to halothane and caffeine. J. Appl. Physiol. 58, 521–528.

Dorsch, J.A. & Dorsch, S.E. (1984) Understanding Anesthesia Equipment; Construction, Care and Complications, 2nd edn. Williams & Wilkins, Baltimore.

Drummond, J.C. & Shapiro, H.M. (1990) Cerebral physiology. In: Anesthesia, 3rd edn (ed. R.D. Miller), p. 621. Churchill Livingstone, New York.

Drummond, J.C., Todd, M.M. & Shapiro, H.M. (1983) Minimal alveolar concentrations for halothane enflurane, and isoflurane in the cat. J. Am. Vet. Med. Assoc. 182, 1099–1101.

Eger, E.I. (1984) The pharmacology of isoflurane. Brit. J. Anaesth. 56S, S71.

Eger, E.I., II (1974) Anesthetic Uptake and Action. Williams & Wilkins, Baltimore.

Eger, E, I., II (1985a) Isoflurane – a Compendium and Reference, 2nd edn. Anaquest, Madison.

Eger, E.I., II (1985b) Nitrous Oxide/N₂O. Elsevier, New York.

Eger, E.I., II (1990) Uptake and distribution. In: Anesthesia, 3rd edn (ed. R.D. Miller), p. 85. Churchill Livingstone, New York.

Eger, E.I., II (1992) Desflurane animal and human pharmacology: aspects of kinetics, safety, and MAC. Anesth. Analg. 75, S3–S9.

Eger, E.I., Smith, N.T., Stoelting, R.K., Cullen, D.J., Kadis, L.B. & Whitcher, C.E. (1970) Cardiovascular effects of halothane in man. Anesthesiology 32, 396–409.

Fink, B.R. (1955) Diffusion anoxia. *Anesthesiology* **16**, 511–519.

Fukunaga, A.F. & Epstein, R.M. (1973) Sympathetic excitation during nitrous–oxide–halothane anesthesia in the cat. *Anesthesiology* **39**, 23–36.

Grandy, J.L., Hodgson, D.S., Dunlop, C.I., Curtis, C.R. & Heath, R.B. (1989) Cardiopulmonary effects of halothane anesthesia in cats. *Am. J. Vet. Res.* **50**, 1729–1732.

Hall, L.W. (1957) Bromochlorotrifluoroethane (Fluothane); a new volatile anaesthetic agent. *Vet. Rec.* **69**, 615–618.

Hall, L.W. & Clarke, K.W. (1991) *Veterinary Anaesthesia*, 9th edn. Baillière Tindall, London.

Hall, L.W., Woolf, N., Bradley, J.W.P. & Jolly, D.W. (1966) Unusual reaction to suxamethonium chloride. *Brit. Med. J.* **ii**, 1305.

Hall, L.W., Trim, C.M. & Woolf, N. (1972) Further studies of porcine malignant hyperthermia. *Brit. Med. J.* **ii**, 145–148.

Hall, L.W., Kellagher, R.E.B. & Fleet, T. (1986) A portable oxygen generator. *Anaesthesia* **41**, 516–518.

Haskins, S.C. & Klide, A.M. (eds) (1992) Opinions in small animal anesthesia. *Veterinary Clinics of North America Small Animal Practice* **22**, 381–411.

Holaday, D.A. & Smith, F.R. (1981) Clinical characteristics and biotransformation of sevoflurane in healthy human volunteers. *Anesthesiology* **54**, 100–106.

Holaday, D.A., Rudofsky, S. & Treuhoft, R.S. (1970) Metabolic degradation of methoxyflurane in man. *Anesthesiology* **33**, 579–593.

Holaday, D.A., Fiserova-Bergerova, V., Latto, I.P. & Zumbiel, M.A. (1975) Resistance of isoflurane to biotransformation in man. *Anesthesiology* **43**, 325–332.

Hong, K., Trudell, J.R., O'Neil, J.R. & Cohen, E.N. (1980) Metabolism of nitrous oxide by human and rat intestinal contents. *Anesthesiology* **52**, 16–19.

Ingwersen, W., Allen, D.G., Dyson, D.H., Black, W.D., Goldberg, M.T. & Valliant, A.E. (1988a) Cardiopulmonary effects of a halothane/oxygen combination in hypovolemic cats. *Can. J. Vet. Res.* **52**, 428–434.

Ingwersen, W., Allen, D.G., Dyson, D.H., Pascoe, P.J. & O'Grady, M.R. (1988b) Cardiopulmonary effects of a halothane/oxygen combination in healthy cats. *Can. J. Vet. Res.* **52**, 386–392.

Iwatsuki, N., Shimosato, S. & Etsten, B.E. (1970) The effects of changes in time interval of stimulation on mechanics of isolated heart muscle and its response to Ethrane. *Anesthesiology* **32**, 11–16.

Joas, T.A., Stevens, W.C. & Eger, E.I. (1971) Electro-encephalographic seizure activity in dogs during anaesthesia: studies with Ethrane, fluroxene, halothane, chloroform, divinyl ether, diethyl ether, methoxyflurane, cyclopropane and forane. *Brit. J. Anaesth.* **43**, 739–745.

Julien, R.M. & Kavan, E.M. (1972) Electrographic studies of a new volatile anesthetic agent: enflurane (Ethrane). *J. Pharmacol. Exp. Ther.* **183**, 393–403.

Kavan, E.M. & Julien, R.M. (1974) Central nervous systems' effects of isoflurane (forane). *Can. Anaesth. Soc. J.* **21**, 390–402.

Klide, A.M. (1976) Cardiovascular effects of enflurane and isoflurane in the dog. *Am. J. Vet. Res.* **37**, 127–131.

Koblin, D.D. (1992) Characteristics and implications of desflurane metabolism and toxicity. *Anesth. Analg.* **75**, S10–S16.

Lowe, H.J. & Ernst, E.A. (1981) *The Quantitative Practice of Anesthesia; Use of Closed Circuit.* Williams & Wilkins, Baltimore.

Manley, S.V. & McDonell, W.N. (1979a) A new circuit for small animal anesthesia: the Bain coaxial circuit. *J. Am. Anim. Hosp. Assoc.* **15**, 61–66.

Manley, S.V. & McDonell, W.N. (1979b) Clinical evaluation of the Bain breathing circuit in small animal anesthesia. *J. Am. Anim. Hosp. Assoc.* **15**, 67–72.

Manley, S.V. & McDonell, W.F. (1980) Recommendations for reduction of anesthetic gas pollution. *J. Am. Vet. Med. Assoc.* **176**, 519–524.

Mapleson, W.W. (1989) Pharmacokinetics of inhalational anaesthetics. In: *General Anaesthesia*, 5th edn (ed. J.F. Nunn, J.E. Utting, & B.R. Brown, Jr), p. 44. Butterworths, London.

Matthews, K.A., Doherty, T., Dyson, D.H., Wilcock, B. & Valliant, A. (1990) Nephrotoxicity in dogs associated with methoxyflurane anesthesia and flunixin meglumine analgesia. *Can. Vet. J.* **31**, 766–771.

Merkel, G. & Eger, E.I. II (1963) A comparative study of halothane and halopropane anaesthesia. *Anesthesiology* **24**, 346–357.

Metz, S. & Maze, M. (1985) Halothane concentration does not alter the threshold for epinephrine-induced arrhythmias in dogs. *Anesthesiology* **62**, 470–475.

Millar, R.A., Warden, J.C., Cooperman, L.H. & Price, H.L. (1970) Further studies of sympathetic actions of anaesthetics in intact and spinal animals. *Brit. J. Anaesth.* **42**, 366–378.

Muir, B.J., Hall, L.W. & Littlewort, M.C.G. (1959) Cardiac irregularities in cats under halothane anaesthesia. *Brit. J. Anaesth.* **1**, 488–489.

Muir, W.W., III, Hubbell, J.A.E. & Flaherty, S. (1988) Increasing halothane concentration abolishes anesthesia-associated arrhythmias in cats and dogs. *J. Am. Vet. Med. Assoc.* **192**, 1730–1735.

Nagi, S.H., Katz, R.L. & Fahrie, S. (1965) Respiratory effects of trichloroethylene halothane and methoxyflurane in the cat. *J. Pharmacol. Exp. Ther.* **148**, 123–130.

Nishino, T. & Honda, Y. (1980) Changes in the respiration pattern induced by halothane in the cat. *Brit. J. Anaesth.* **52**, 1191–1197.

Pedersoli, W.M. (1977) Blood serum inorganic ionic fluoride tetracycline and methoxyflurane anesthesia in dogs. *J. Am. Anim. Hosp. Assoc.* **13**, 242–246.

Purchase, I.F. (1966) Cardiac arrhythmias occurring during halothane anaesthesia in cats. *Brit. J. Anaesth.* **38**, 13–22.

Regan, M.J. & Eger, E.I. (1967) Effect of hypothermia in dogs on anesthetizing and apneic doses of inhalation agents. Determination of the anesthetic index (apnea/MAC). *Anesthesiology* **28**, 689–700.

Rehder, K., Forbes, J., Alter, H., Hessler, O. & Stier, A. (1967) Halothane biotransformation in man: a quantitative study. *Anesthesiology* **28**, 711–715.

Reilly, C.S., Wood, A.J.J., Koshakji, R.P. & Wood, M. (1985) The effect of halothane on drug disposition: contribution of changes in intrinsic drug metabolizing capacity and hepatic blood flow. *Anesthesiology* **63**, 70–76.

Rex, M.A.E. (1971) Laryngospasm and respiratory changes in the cat produced by mechanical stimulation of the pharynx and respiratory tract: problems of intubation in the cat. *Brit. J. Anaesth.* **43**, 54–57.

Rex, M.A.E. (1973) Laryngeal activity during the induction of anaesthesia in the cat. *Aust. Vet. J.* **49**, 365–368.

Roizen, M.F., Horrigan, R.W. & Frazer, B.M. (1981) Anesthetic doses blocking adrenergic (stress) and cardiovascular responses to incision – MAC BAR. *Anesthesiology* **54**, 390–398.

Short, C. E., ed (1987) *Principles and Practice of Veterinary Anesthesia.* Williams & Wilkins, Baltimore.

Skovsted, P. & Price, H.L. (1972) The effect of ethrane on arterial pressure, preganglionic sympathetic activity and barostatic reflexes. *Anesthesiology* **36**, 257–262.

Steffey, E.P. (1982) Inhalation anesthesia. *In: Equine Medicine and Surgery* (ed. R. Mansmann, E. McAllister & P. Pratt), p. 262. American Veterinary Publication, Santa Barbara.

Steffey, E.P. (1992) Other new and potentially useful inhalational anesthetics. *Veterinary Clinics of North America: Small Animal Practice* **22**, 335–340.

Steffey, E.P. & Eger, E.I. (1984) Nitrous oxide in veterinary practice and animal research. *In: Nitrous Oxide/N$_2$O* (ed. E.I. Eger II), p. 305. Elsevier, New York.

Steffey, E.P. & Howland, D., Jr (1977) Isoflurane potency in the dog and cat. *Am. J. Vet. Res.* **38**, 1833–1836.

Steffey, E.P. & Howland, D., Jr (1978) Potency of enflurane in dogs: comparison with halothane and isoflurane. *Am. J. Vet. Res.* **39**, 673–677.

Steffey, E.P., Gillespie, J.R., Berry, J.D., Eger, E.I. & Munson, E.S. (1974a) Anesthetic potency (MAC) of nitrous oxide in the dog, cat and stumptail Monkey. *J. Appl. Physiol.* **36**, 530–532.

Steffey, E.P., Gillespie, J.R., Berry, J.D., Eger, E.I. & Rhode, E.A. (1974b) Circulatory effects of halothane and halothane–nitrous oxide anesthesia in the dog: controlled ventilation. *Am. J. Vet. Res.* **35**, 1289–1293.

Steffey, E.P., Woliner, M.J. & Howland, D. (1983) Accuracy of isoflurane delivery by halothane-specific vaporizers. *Am. J. Vet. Res.* **44**, 1071–1078.

Steffey, E.P., Farver, T.B. & Woliner, M.J. (1984a) Circulatory and respiratory effects of methoxyflurane in dogs: comparison of halothane. *Am. J. Vet. Res.* **45**, 2574–2579.

Steffey, E.P., Hodgson, D.S. & Kupershoek, C. (1984b) Monitoring oxygen concentrating devices. *J. Am. Vet. Med. Assoc.* **184**, 626.

Steffey, E.P., Farver, T.B. & Woliner, M.J. (1987a) Cardiopulmonary function during 7 h of constant-dose halothane and methoxyflurane. *J. Appl. Physiol.* **63**, 1351–1359.

Steffey, E.P., Kelly, A.B. & Woliner, M.J. (1987b) Time-related responses of spontaneously breathing, laterally recumbent horses to prolonged anesthesia with halothane. *Am. J. Vet. Res.* **48**, 952–957.

Stoelting, R.K. (1987) *Pharmacology and Physiology in Anesthetic Practice.* J.B. Lippincott, Philadelphia.

Stoelting, R.K. & Miller, R.D. (1987) *Basics of Anesthesia,* 2nd edn. Churchill Livingstone, New York.

Swar, B.B. (1987) Oxygen concentrators. *Can. J. Anaesth.* **34**, 538–539.

Todd, M.M. & Drummond, J.C. (1984) A comparison of the cerebrovascular and metabolic effects of halothane and isoflurane in the cat. *Anesthesiology* **60**, 276–283.

Venes, J.L., Collins, W.F. & Taub, A. (1971) Nitrous oxide: an anesthetic for experiments in cats. *Am. J. Physiol.* **220**, 2028–2031.

Warltier, D.C. & Pagel, P.S. (1992) Cardiovascular and

respiratory actions of desflurane: is desflurane different from isoflurane? *Anesth. Analg.* **75**, S17–S31.

Webb, A.I. & McMurphy, R.M. (1987) Effect of anticholinergic preanesthetic medicaments on the requirements of halothane for anesthesia in the cat. *Am. J. Vet. Res.* **48**, 1733–1736.

White, D.C. & Calkins, J. (1989) Anaesthetic machines and breathing systems. *In: General Anaesthesia*, 5th edn (ed. J.F. Nunn, J.E. Utting & B.R. Brown), p. 428. Butterworths, London.

Woolf, N., Hall, L.W., Thorne, C., Down, M. & Walker, R.G. (1970) Serum creatine–phosphokinase levels in pigs reacting abnormally to halogenated anaesthetics. *Brit. Med. J.* **iii**, 386–387.

C.M. Trim

10
Monitoring the Anaesthetized Cat

Introduction

Adequate pre-anaesthetic evaluation to guide appropriate choice of anaesthetic agents and perioperative management is essential to a successful outcome from anaesthesia. Intraoperative monitoring cannot fully compensate for inadequate preparation for anaesthesia. However, even when planning is adequate, pharmacological and physiological responses to anaesthetic agents vary in individual cats and the surgical procedure may impose adverse effects such as interference with breathing, impaired venous return to the heart, or unexpected blood loss. All anaesthetized cats should receive basic monitoring care to provide early warning of adverse physiological trends, to guide treatment, and to prevent complications developing. Use of available equipment should not be restricted to cats considered to be high risk. Monitoring should not cease at the completion of the surgical procedure but be continued during recovery until the cat resumes its pre-anaesthetic status. Data from surveys of deaths and adverse reactions during anaesthesia in veterinary practice in Great Britain from 1976 to 1978 and from 1984 to 1986 identified cats dying both during anaesthesia and during recovery from anaesthesia (Clarke & Hall, 1990). The authors concluded that monitoring was essential from the time the anaesthetic drugs were given until recovery to full consciousness.

The standard of care is changing as more monitors become available, and many are now cost effective for the general practitioner. Monitors that produce an audible beep with heart beat and breathing are commonly used. Cats are prone to develop hypothermia during anaesthesia and, since measurement of temperature is simple, this is easy to detect early. Equipment is now available for easy measurement of blood pressure in cats and this has proved to be a valuable aid to anaesthesia with halothane and isoflurane. Pulse oximetry is a method of detecting hypoxia by placing a sensor on the cat's tongue and is a valuable monitor when the cat is breathing air during anaesthesia produced by injectable drugs.

This chapter provides comprehensive information not only on monitoring techniques that can be used in general veterinary practice, but also techniques used in teaching and research.

Depth of Anaesthesia

Traditionally, depth of anaesthesia is partitioned into stages and further into planes. Although this classification scheme was originally developed with diethyl ether anaesthesia, it still has some relevance for all the inhalation anaesthetics. Anaesthesia progresses from the conscious state to Stage I (voluntary excitement), through Stage II (involuntary excitement), and then to Stage III or general anaesthesia. Stage III is subdivided into four planes; plane 1 or light anaesthesia, plane 2 or medium anaesthesia, plane 3 or deep anaesthesia, and plane 4, which is overdosage. Usually, induction of anaesthesia with an injectable agent allows a rapid transition from consciousness to Stage III, plane 1 or 2. Stages I and II may be observed only when induction of anaesthesia occurs slowly. Signs differentiating planes in Stage III are less clear when opioid analgesia is included in the anaesthetic technique.

Monitoring depth of anaesthesia begins with observation of the degree of muscle relaxation

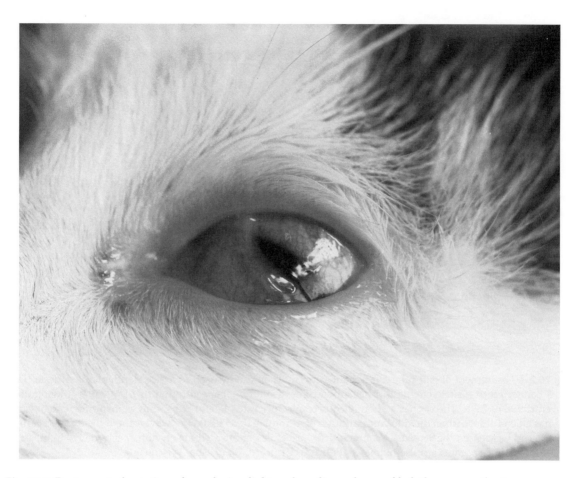

Fig. 10.1 Rostroventral rotation of eye during light and medium planes of halothane anaesthesia.

and the strength of certain reflexes. Changes in these parameters occur as the depth of anaesthesia increases and may be consistent for a given anaesthetic agent or combination of agents; these responses vary considerably according to which agent has been administered. Methoxyflurane causes good muscle relaxation during light anaesthesia whereas ketamine increases muscle tone. Therefore, the degree of relaxation that is present during ketamine anaesthesia depends largely on the properties of the sedative drug used in conjunction with ketamine. Relaxation of the jaw may be helpful when titrating injectable anaesthetic agents during induction of anaesthesia, but this response cannot be used reliably to assess the depth of anaesthesia.

Rotation of the eye is relatively consistent during anaesthesia with thiobarbiturate, propofol, halothane and isoflurane. During light anaesthesia, the eye is central in the socket with little sclera showing. As anaesthesia deepens, the eye rotates, usually rostroventrally, so that the iris is partially obscured and the sclera is easily visible during medium plane anaesthesia (Fig. 10.1). With further deepening of anaesthesia, the extraocular muscles relax fully and the eye returns to a central position. Light and deep anaesthesia are differentiated by the palpebral reflex; during light anaesthesia the palpebral reflex should be fairly brisk whereas in deep anaesthesia the palpebral reflex is absent. In contrast, the eye is positioned centrally, and the palpebral reflex is brisk, after induction of anaesthesia with ketamine.

Pupil size is less reliable in the cat than it is in the dog. Atropine premedication does not usually result in full dilation. In general,

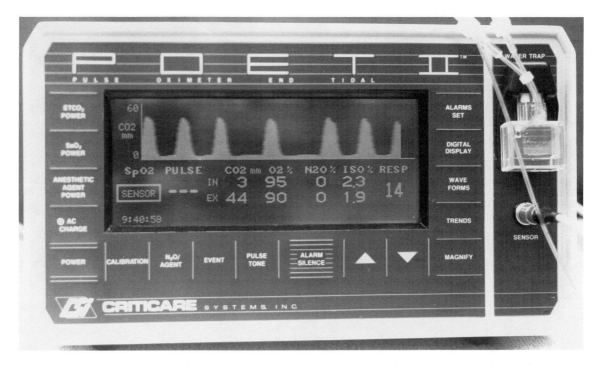

Fig. 10.2 Measurement of end-tidal anaesthetic concentration can be used to assess depth of anaesthesia. This cat is connected to a circle circuit and has an end-tidal isoflurane concentration of 1.9% with an inspiratory concentration of 2.3%. The cat has a spontaneous respiratory rate of 14 breaths/min, is inspiring 95% oxygen, and has an end-tidal carbon dioxide concentration of 44 mmHg (5.85 kPa). The waveform of the exhaled carbon dioxide can be seen on the screen. This model uses principles of infrared absorption spectrometry to measure gases. It also incorporates a pulse oximeter (POET II, Criticare, Waukesha, Wisconsin).

pupillary dilation occurs during deep anaesthesia, after ketamine administration, and if the depth of anaesthesia decreases substantially in response to surgical manipulation.

The pedal reflex, withdrawal of the limb in response to pressure on the nail bed or pinching between the toes, should be absent during anaesthesia with barbiturate, propofol, or inhalation agents. The corneal reflex is a blink elicited by touching the cornea. The corneal reflex is unreliable for assessing depth of anaesthesia and may, in fact, be present after cardiac arrest. The whisker reflex, twitching of the whiskers in response to pinching the pinna, may be of use when titrating pentobarbitone during induction of anaesthesia.

Computerized analysis of the electroencephalogram has been developed as a means of assessing directly the depth or adequacy of anaesthesia (Schwilden, 1989) and has even been used to drive the infusion of an intravenous anaesthetic (Schwilden *et al.*, 1987). Although this technique is under investigation in horses (Otto & Short, 1991; Johnson *et al.*, 1993) and dogs (Moore *et al.*, 1992), it has not yet been reported in cats.

End-tidal Inhalation Agent Concentration

Measurement of the concentration of anaesthetic agent in the patient provides an estimate of the depth of inhalation anaesthesia. A close correlation with blood concentration is obtained from the non-invasive technique of measuring the concentration of the agent in alveolar gas at the end of exhalation (end-tidal concentration). The equipment required for this measurement is expensive for general practice but is particularly useful for quantitating and controlling the depth of anaesthesia in cats used in research investigations. An adaptor is connected to the endotracheal tube that either contains a special

Table 10.1 Isoflurane causes dose-dependent decreases in arterial blood pressure and tidal volume in cats. (Adapted from Steffey & Howland (1977) with permission.)

Measurement	Depth of anaesthesia		
	1.0 MAC Light	1.5 MAC Medium	2.0 MAC Deep
Heart rate (beats/min)	148 ± 7	134 ± 6	137 ± 5
Mean arterial pressure (mmHg)	85 ± 9	61 ± 3	53 ± 3
Respiratory rate (breaths/ min)	36 ± 5	27 ± 2	28 ± 2
P_aCO_2 (kPa) (mm Hg)	4.7 ± 0.3 35 ± 2	5.3 ± 0.3 40 ± 2	8.1 ± 0.4 61 ± 3

Data are mean ± standard error.

Table 10.3 Combined cardiovascular values for medium and deep halothane anaesthesia in cats during spontaneous versus controlled ventilation. (Adapted from Grandy *et al.*, 1989, with permission.)

Variable	Spontaneous ventilation	Controlled ventilation
Heart rate (beats/min)	168 ± 34	152 ± 25
Systolic arterial pressure (mmHg)	99 ± 15	85 ± 21*
Diastolic arterial pressure (mmHg)	62 ± 12	56 ± 17
Mean arterial pressure (mmHg)	74 ± 13	66 ± 18*
Cardiac output (ml/kg/min)	108 ± 41	89 ± 24*

Data are expressed as mean ± standard deviation.
* Significantly different from spontaneous ventilation ($P < 0.05$).

Table 10.2 Average values for heart rate, arterial blood pressure, and arterial carbon dioxide tension (P_aCO_2) after 10 min of anaesthesia

Anaesthetic agent	Heart rate (beats/min)	Mean arterial pressure (mmHg)	P_aCO_2 (kPa / mmHg)	Reference
Thiopentone	199	94	4.26 / 32	Middleton *et al.*, 1982
Ketamine	200	125	5.32 / 40	Haskins *et al.*, 1975
	187	137	3.99 / 30	Middleton *et al.*, 1982
Alphaxalone / alphadalone	170	105	4.66 / 35	Haskins *et al.*, 1975
	159	63	3.59 / 27	Middleton *et al.*, 1982

sensor or has a side arm that allows aspiration of a continuous flow of gas. The concentration of the anaesthetic gas then is measured at a distance from the patient (Fig. 10.2). The relevance of the measured concentration depends on the potency of the anaesthetic agent, the type and quantity of injectable drugs administered as part of the anaesthetic protocol, and the physical status of the patient. The potency of the agent is defined as the minimum alveolar concentration (MAC) that will prevent a response to a standard painful stimulus in 50% of cats (see Chapter 9). This concentration differs between agents and between species of animals.

The MAC values in cats for halothane, isoflurane, and enflurane are 1.1–1.2%, 1.6%, and 2.4%, respectively (Steffey & Howland, 1977; Drummond *et al.*, 1983) (Table 9.4). An end-tidal concentration of 1.2–1.5 times MAC should ensure an adequate depth of anaesthesia for surgery in most cats. However, a variety of factors in clinical patients may necessitate adjustment of the vaporizer to deliver a lower concentration, such as when a portion of anaesthesia has been produced by preanaesthetic and induction agents. Cats that are very young or old, and those with central nervous system depression, metabolic acidosis

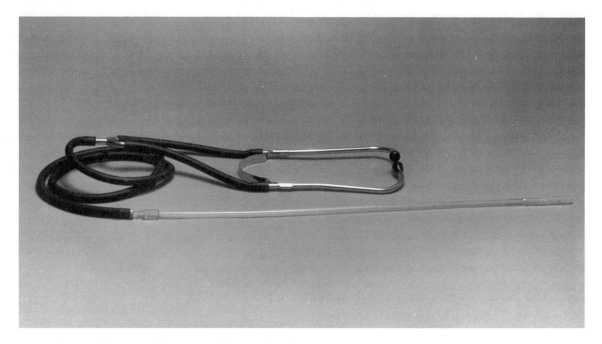

Fig. 10.3 Oesophageal stethoscope and binaural stethoscope earpiece.

or severe hemorrhage, also have a decreased anaesthetic requirement compared with healthy young adult cats.

Evaluation of Cardiovascular Function

The peripheral arterial pulse rate and strength, mucous membrane colour, and capillary refill time should be monitored at 5-min intervals, or more frequently when the patient's condition is unstable. The femoral artery is the easiest artery to palpate, but access may be limited during an operation. The lingual artery, easily palpable in dogs, is not always palpable in cats. If an emergency arises during laparotomy, the surgeon can palpate the aorta or a mesenteric artery to confirm the existence of a pulse. Although palpation of the pulse may give some indication of the animal's blood pressure, it is possible to misinterpret a low pressure as being adequate. Pink mucous membrane colour is desirable. Pale mucous membrane colour may be the result of drug-induced vasocontriction or poor periph-

eral perfusion. Capillary refill time should be less than 2 s.

Heart Rate

The heart rate in most normal conscious cats is 120 beats/min or greater and usually not over 240 beats/min (Harpster, 1986). Average heart rates during anaesthesia will be influenced by the anaesthetic agents and the presence or absence of an anticholinergic drug (Tables 10.1–10.3).

Heart rate is easily counted using an oesophageal stethoscope. An oesophageal stethoscope consists of a plastic tube with an air-filled bulb at the end (Fig. 10.3). The stethoscope should first be held alongside the cat to determine the distance from the mouth to the level of the heart. The stethoscope then is inserted into the cat's mouth, dorsal to the endotracheal tube, and passed down the oesophagus this distance until the bulb is level with the heart. The cardiac sounds heard through an oesophageal stethoscope are from vibrations and pressure changes caused by myocardial contractions and movement of blood in the heart and great vessels. Single

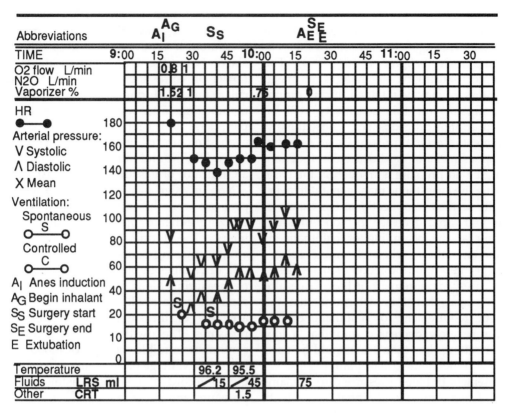

Fig. 10.4 Monitoring arterial blood pressure is a useful guide to anaesthetic management. Note that the blood pressure in this cat anaesthetized with halothane decreased without significant change in heart rate.

earpieces can be worn by the surgeon, who can then listen to the heart and surrounding noise at the same time. Alternatively, the oesophageal stethoscope can be connected to a small amplifying box (several models are commercially available) so that the heart beat can be heard by everyone in the operating room. The sounds of air entering and leaving the lungs usually can be heard, allowing respiratory rate to be monitored. A disadvantage of this equipment is that the heart beat can be heard clearly even though cardiac output or peripheral perfusion may have decreased to a critically low level. The results of a study in dogs indicate that the systemic blood pressure and cardiac output decrease to an unacceptable level long before there is a decrease in loudness of the heart beat (Waelchli-Suter *et al.*, 1986). The authors concluded that size of the stethoscope and adjustment of the volume dial must be considered. To improve sensitivity, the largest oesophageal

stethoscope should be used so that the oesophagus surrounds the stethoscope tubing in a sleeve-like manner. In addition, the volume gain on the amplifier should initially be set at the lowest clearly audible volume. Then if the intensity of the cardiac sounds decreases, the patient's condition should be assessed rather than changing the volume setting (Waelchli-Suter *et al.*, 1986).

Other monitors that supply heart rate are the electrocardiogram (ECG), pulse oximeters and blood pressure monitoring devices.

Arterial Blood Pressure Measurement

Monitoring of heart rate alone provides insufficient information about the status of the animal's cardiovascular system. Heart rate may not change in response to a decrease in arterial pressure during inhalation anaesthesia because the sensitivity of the baroreceptor reflex is significantly depressed (Sellgren *et al.*, 1992) (Fig. 10.4). Similarly, changes in heart rate are unpredictable during methohexitone or thiopentone anaesthesia (Sellgren *et al.*, 1992). The baroreceptor sensitivity to changes in mean arterial pressure may be retained during propofol anaesthesia, but this sensitivity will be decreased at high drug dosages. Consequently, measurement of arterial pressure is an essential part of assessment of cardiovascular function. Declining blood pressure is frequently the basis for altering the anaesthetic management to avert potentially serious complications. For example, an early and rapid decrease in blood pressure may occur at the beginning of halothane or isoflurane anaesthesia when tiletamine–zolazepam has been used for induction of anaesthesia. In these cases, measurement of blood pressure allows the anaesthetist to determine that the anaesthetic requirement for halothane or isoflurane is severely decreased and that a low vaporizer setting (less than 1%) should be used initially with tiletamine–zolazepam.

Measurement of blood pressure during maintenance of anaesthesia with inhalation agents provides additional information about the depth of anaesthesia. As a general rule, arterial pressure decreases progressively with increasing depth of anaesthesia (Table 10.1). Not only is cardiovascular collapse less likely to occur at lighter planes of anaesthesia, but cardiovascular depression associated with deep anaesthesia may be avoided in old or sick cats, minimizing compromise of hepatic, splanchnic, and renal blood flows.

The mean arterial blood pressure in conscious cats exceeds 100 mmHg. Average values for arterial pressure during anaesthesia with different agents are given in Tables 10.1–10.3. Cardiac output and mean arterial pressure are lower during controlled ventilation compared with spontaneous breathing because venous return to the heart is diminished during inspiration due to the increase in intrathoracic pressure. During anaesthesia, the mean pressure should be maintained above 65–70 mmHg to provide the best physiological conditions for the anaesthetized cat. When only systolic and diastolic pressures are recorded, mean pressure can be calculated using the formula: 0.33 (systolic pressure – diastolic pressure) + diastolic pressure. When only the systolic pressure is measured, it is advisable to keep this pressure above 80 mmHg with appropriate treatment. Lower pressures increase the risk of cardiovascular failure during anaesthesia and organ malfunction after anaesthesia. Adequacy of peripheral perfusion should be assessed by evaluating arterial pressure together with capillary refill time and mucous membrane colour as an indicator of vasodilation or constriction.

Non-invasive measurement of arterial blood pressure can be achieved with equipment utilizing either doppler ultrasound or oscillometry. The former technique produces an audible pulsing sound, allowing ready detection of changes in blood pressure. This method of measuring blood pressure is more cumbersome than the oscillometric technique and the accuracy of measurements decreases at low pressures. The oscillometric technique has no continuous audible monitor of blood flow, but has the advantage of automatically generating a digital record of systolic, diastolic, and mean pressures and pulse rate.

Doppler ultrasound technique

A thin flat transducer containing two crystals is placed on the skin over an artery. One of the crystals emits ultrasound signals which are reflected back to the second crystal by a moving structure such as the artery wall (Stegall *et al.*, 1968). The reflected ultrasound is at a different frequency and mixing of the frequencies is converted to an audible pulsing sound. The pitch of the sound is proportional to the velocity of the reflective surface and the volume of the sound is proportional to the area of the moving reflective surface. The probe usually is placed over the metacarpal (Fig. 10.5) or metatarsal arteries on the plantar surface of the fore and hind limbs, although the tibial or coccygeal arteries also can be used. A special contact gel should be applied to the concave surface of the transducer and the transducer positioned on the skin to give the loudest signal (a whooshing noise) before the transducer is secured to the limb with tape. An inflatable cuff then is placed around the limb proximal to the transducer (Fig. 10.6). The cuff bladder should extend at least

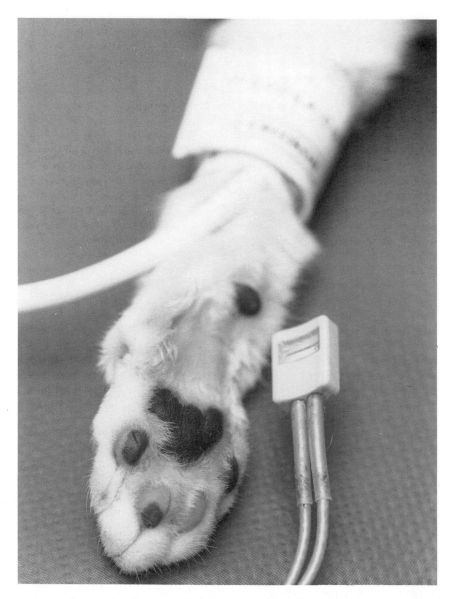

Fig. 10.5 The metacarpal artery is a frequent site for measurement of blood pressure using doppler ultrasound. Gel is placed on the concave surface of the probe before placement on the skin over the artery. The probe is held in position with tape.

halfway around the limb, on the side of the artery, and the width of the cuff must be between 40 and 60% of the circumference of the limb. Cuffs used for human newborns and infants are the appropriate sizes for cats. The cuff should fit snugly and should be positioned over the muscular part of the leg; placement of the cuff over the carpus or hock will result in an erroneously high pressure reading.

To record the pressure, the screw next to the pressure bulb is tightened and the bulb squeezed to inflate the cuff. Once the pressure in the cuff exceeds the systolic pressure, there will be no arterial wall motion and no sound. The screw then is loosened partially to slowly deflate the cuff. The systolic pressure is that pressure on the aneroid manometer at which the first pulse sounds are heard. Sometimes a soft

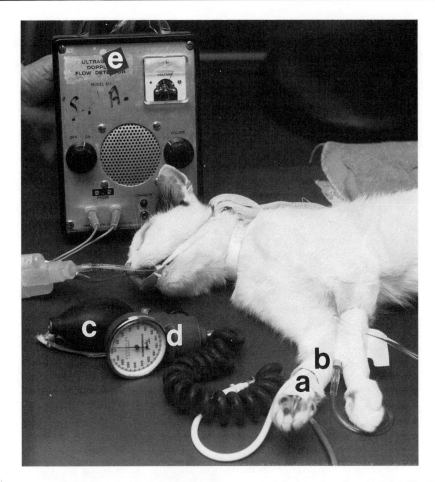

Fig. 10.6 Non-invasive measurement of arterial blood pressure using doppler ultrasound: a, Probe placed over a peripheral artery; b, inflatable cuff; c, bulb for inflating the cuff; d, manometer for reading pressure; e, unit produces audible sound of blood flow (Pediatric flat probe with Model 811, Parks Electronics, Aloha, Oregon).

tapping noise is heard just before true systolic pressure; this may lead to an erroneous estimation of systolic pressure. When the cuff is deflated to a pressure between systolic and diastolic pressure, the artery wall opens and closes at least once with each cardiac cycle. These movements generate signals proportional to the velocity of the arterial wall and blood flow. Because the artery opens more abruptly than it closes, there are two sounds. The cuff then is deflated until the pressure in the cuff approaches the diastolic pressure, at which time separation of the sounds becomes more obvious until sounds of adjacent cardiac cycles merge. The change in sounds indicative of the diastolic pressure can be heard in some but not all cats. Sometimes accuracy of assessing the diastolic pressure is confused by the presence of muffled sound 10–15 mmHg higher than the true diastolic pressure. A cuff that is taped too loosely will result in an erroneously high reading and a cuff that is too wide will result in an erroneously low pressure. In one investigation of measurement of systolic arterial pressure in cats comparing the doppler ultrasonic method with direct arterial catheterization of the femoral artery, it was determined that the indirect frequently underestimated the systolic pressure (Grandy *et al.*, 1992). Using a blood pressure monitoring cuff with a width that was 37% the limb circumference placed half way between the elbow and the carpus, a useful calibration adjustment was: femoral systolic pressure = doppler systolic pressure + 14 mmHg.

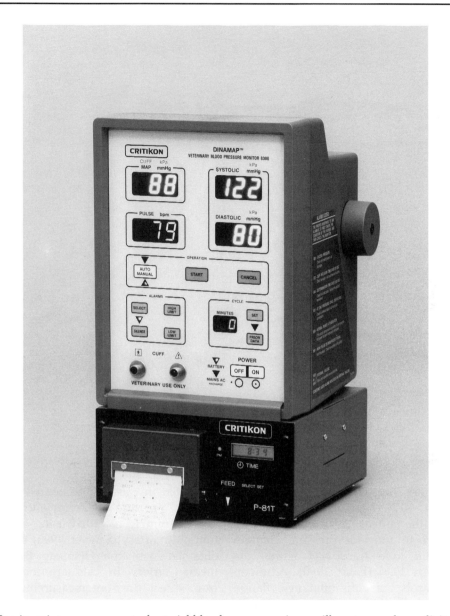

Fig. 10.7 Non-invasive measurement of arterial blood pressure using oscillometry produces digital display of systolic, diastolic, and mean arterial pressures, and pulse rate (Dinamap Veterinary Monitor 8300, Criticon, Tampa, Florida).

The doppler probe also can be used to obtain an estimate of peripheral blood flow during emergency resuscitation. Within seconds, the probe can be placed on the ventral surface of the tongue over the lingual artery, or beneath the third eyelid next to the malar artery where it courses over the medial border of the orbit. The sounds of peripheral blood flow can be used to assess the effectiveness of cardiac massage and treatment.

Oscillometric technique
In the automated oscillometric technique using the Dinamap (*d*evice for *i*ndirect *n*oninvasive *a*utomatic *m*ean *a*rterial *p*ressure; Criticon,

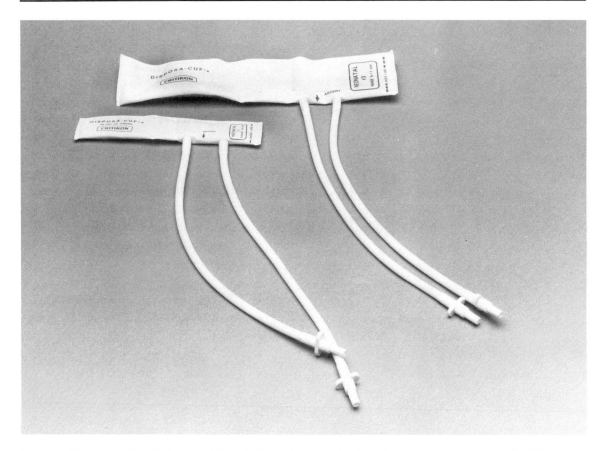

Fig. 10.8 Two sizes of cuffs (neonatal Nos 1, 3) used to measure blood pressure in cats using the Dinamap.

Tampa, Florida) the cuff and sensor are combined (Fig. 10.7). The cuff has two tubes, one to inflate the cuff using an electric pump and the other to transmit pressure changes within the cuff to a transducer within the instrument (Fig. 10.8) (Lake, 1990). A microprocessor controls the cuff inflation–deflation sequence. The cuff is inflated to exceed systolic pressure and then is deflated slowly one step each time that it detects two pulsations of relatively equal amplitude (Sawyer *et al.*, 1991). Recording two matching pulses helps to increase accuracy by eliminating artefacts caused by movement. The degree of inflation is maintained until successive comparative beats occur. Consequently, if the cat is moving, the time for measurement may be prolonged. The averaged pairs of data are analysed electronically to determine the systolic, mean, and diastolic pressures, and pulse rate.

Six sites for placement of the cuff have been evaluated in cats and compared to a range of systolic pressure measurements between 90 and 120 mmHg recorded using direct cannulation of an artery (Sawyer, 1992). Measurements obtained with the Dinamap 8300 from the median artery in cats are indistinguishable from direct pressure measurements. Diastolic pressures recorded from the brachial, carpal, anterior tibial, popliteal, and coccygeal arteries are significantly different from direct measurements, with the greatest differences recorded from the popliteal artery and the tail (Sawyer, 1992). To measure blood pressure, the cuff should be placed with the 'artery arrow' over the medial surface of the cat's fore limb between the elbow and the carpus or, in cats weighing less than 1.8 kg, proximal to the elbow (Sawyer, 1992). Clipping of hair is not necessary unless it is matted. The width of the cuff should be between 40 and 60% of the limb circumference.

Direct measurement of arterial pressure

Direct measurement of pressure allows rapid and accurate monitoring of pressures during low flow states and generates a pressure waveform that provides additional information on myocardial performance and peripheral vascular resistance.

The femoral artery is the easiest artery to catheterize percutaneously. The dorsal pedal artery on the dorsomedial aspect of the tarsus, often used in dogs, may be used in some cats. One approach for catheterization of the femoral artery is to position the hindquarters of the cat in a lateral position with the underneath limb extended, so that the skin overlying the artery is tensed. The upper limb is flexed and held out of the way. The area over the femoral artery is then clipped and the skin prepared as for a surgical procedure. A 22-gauge over-the-needle type

catheter should be used. A 20-gauge hypodermic needle can be used to make a nick in the skin to avoid damage to the tip of the catheter. Starting about two-thirds of the way down the length of the femur, the catheter is inserted through the skin nick at an angle of 20–30° to the skin using a steady, slow advancement. When blood flashes into the needle hub, the angle of the catheter is decreased to about 10° and the needle is advanced a few millimetres before threading the catheter into the artery using a gentle back and forth twisting motion. After capping the catheter and flushing it with heparinized saline, the catheter should be secured to the skin with a suture. It may be advisable to label the catheter to ensure that it is not mistaken for a venous catheter. Although tubing containing heparinized saline may be connected directly to the catheter, insertion of a

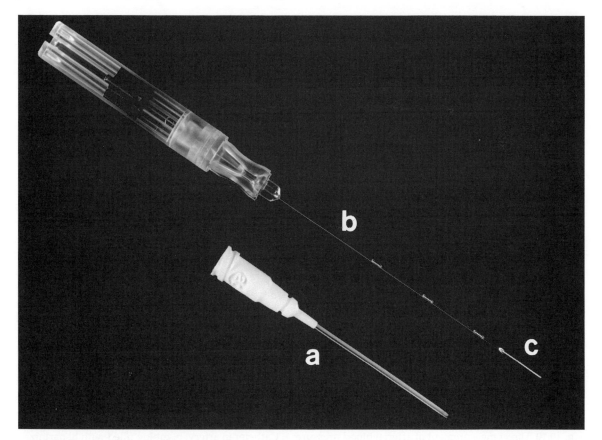

Fig. 10.9 Catheter for arterial catheterization has been disassembled to show the catheter (a), the needle (b) and the flexible wire stilette (c) that has been advanced beyond the tip of the needle (Arrow International Inc. Reading, Pennsylvania).

needle through a catheter cap introduces less risk of dislodging by producing less drag on the catheter and by facilitating disconnection whenever the cat is moved.

The easiest catheters to use are those that employ the Seldinger technique (Arrow International Inc., Reading, Pennsylvania) (Fig. 10.9). This technique involves insertion of a thin flexible wire into the artery. This wire serves as a guide for the catheter during its advancement. The technique of catheterization is similar to that just described except that, after flashback of blood in the catheter has been observed, gentle pressure is applied to the plunger to see if the guidewire will advance. If resistance is felt, the tip of the needle must be repositioned otherwise the wire will kink. After the wire is advanced to its depth inside the artery, the catheter is advanced into the artery, the needle and wire are removed and the catheter is capped, flushed and secured to the skin. Introducer sets that include needle, catheter, and flexible guide wire as separate entities also are available from several manufacturers. Some catheters are available in Vialon® (Insyte, Deseret Medical Inc., Becton Dickinson and Company, Sandy, Utah) which is smooth and flexible and causes significantly less peeling back of the catheter tip, kinking or thrombophlebitis than Teflon® (Gaukroger *et al.*, 1988).

Chronic vascular catheters are used in research animals and involve surgical exposure of the vessel, catheterization, and tunnelling of tubing subcutaneously to an exit site that the animal cannot reach. The site of skin penetration is at risk for infection and any external tubing

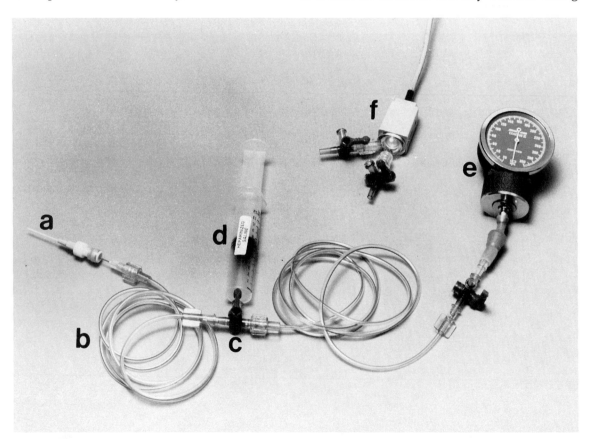

Fig. 10.10 Direct measurement of arterial blood pressure: a, Catheter in artery; b, tubing filled with heparinized saline; c, three-way stopcock; d, syringe filled with heparinized saline; e, aneroid manometer. An electrical pressure transducer (f) connected to an oscilloscope (not shown) may be used instead of the aneroid manometer.

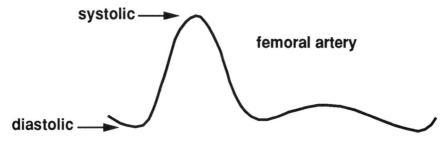

Fig. 10.11. Drawing of a blood pressure waveform. Systolic and diastolic pressures are indicated.

may be damaged by the animal. The subcutaneously implanted vascular port, frequently used in research animals for venous blood collection and drug administration, also can be used for chronic arterial blood pressure measurement (Dalton, 1985).

A simple and cheap device for measuring mean arterial pressure is the aneroid manometer. The assembly of connecting tubing and manometer are shown in Fig. 10.10. The middle three-way stopcock is turned so that heparinized saline can be flushed from the syringe into tubing and a 22-gauge needle. The three-way stopcock then is turned to connect the syringe with the manometer and the plunger depressed so that saline enters the tubing until the pressure on the manometer reads 100 mmHg. After inserting the needle through the cap of the arterial catheter, the three-way stopcock is turned to connect the manometer to the artery. Pressurizing the tubing first will minimize back flow of blood after connection to the artery. The air–saline interface in the tubing must be placed at heart level for accurate pressure measurement. Heart level is the sternum or thoracic inlet when the cat is lying on its side and axilla when on its back. The position of the manometer itself is not important and it can be placed on the table or suspended vertically. The mean arterial pressure can be read from the manometer after allowing 30–60 s for equilibration of pressures within the tubing.

More convenient than an aneroid manometer is an electrical transducer that will provide a continuous waveform display on an oscilloscope from which systolic and diastolic pressures can be measured (Figs. 10.10 & 10.11). The transducer first must be opened to air for zero calibration and then positioned at heart level for accurate measurement of pressure. Many monitors provide a digital record of systolic, diastolic, and mean pressures, and heart rate. The pressure pulse may be altered by a variety of factors. A large catheter may almost occlude the artery mechanically, which will magnify the amplitude of the pulse. An air bubble within the tubing will diminish the pulse amplitude.

Pressure should be applied to the puncture site for several minutes after the catheter is removed to prevent haematoma formation. Complications, including infection, following multiple attempts at catheterization and large haematoma formation are possible but have not been reported in small animal veterinary patients. Ligation of the femoral artery after a cut-down technique does not cause circulatory embarrassment due to extensive collateral circulation (Burrows, 1973).

Electrocardiogram

The beep of the ECG can be used simply for immediate recognition of heart rate and rhythm. Since arrhythmias may develop even in healthy cats, it is advisable to connect the ECG to all patients undergoing surgery and/or inhalation anaesthesia. A lead that provides adequate P waves and analysis of the QRS configuration is necessary for accurate arrhythmia detection. Sinus arrythmia is usually absent when atropine has been used for premedication but will return in about 1.5 h when the effect of atropine wanes. Commonly occurring arrhythmias are premature atrial beats, supraventricular and ventricular premature contractions, and second degree atrioventricular heart block. When the arrhythmia results in a weak or absent pulse because of insufficient time for ventricular filling, cardiac output and blood pressure are decreased. Premature ventricular contractions may be serious because of their association with life-threatening ventricular arrhythmias such as ventricular tachycardia and fibrillation.

Accurate analysis of the arrhythmia coupled with a basic knowledge of the pharmacological effects of the anaesthetic agents are essential for determination of the appropriate treatment. For example, the early stages of ketamine–halothane anaesthesia may be accompanied by premature ventricular contractions. Frequently these are caused by the interaction of hypercarbia from hypoventilation and sensitization of the heart by halothane, and are abolished by controlled ventilation. Subsequent lightening of anaesthesia by decreasing halothane administration may relieve the respiratory depression such that arrhythmias do not reappear at the resumption of spontaneous ventilation. Alterna-

Table 10.4 Methods for monitoring respiratory rate, tidal volume, and oxygenation

Equipment	Measurement	Comment
Visual observation of chest excursion or movement of reservoir bag in the anaesthetic circuit	Respiratory rate and subjective evaluation of depth of breathing	
Observation of mucous membrane colour	Estimate of oxygenation	Cyanosis is not always detectable
Oesophageal stethoscope with stethoscope earpiece(s) or audible monitor	Respiratory rate	Must observe chest excursion for adequacy of depth of breathing
Circumferential belt around the chest connected to monitor that beeps	Respiratory rate	No estimation of depth of breathing
Sensor connected to the endotracheal tube and produces beep	Respiratory rate	Not all models are sensitive for very low volume movement
Respirometer connected to the endotracheal tube	Tidal volume	May be inaccurate for small volumes when placed within the anaesthetic breathing circuit
Pulse oximetry	Haemoglobin oxygen saturation	Useful, but does not evaluate tissue oxygen delivery
Capnography: sensor or aspiration port inserted between endotracheal tube and anaesthetic circuit	End-tidal carbon dioxide concentration and respiratory rate	False negatives possible
Blood gas analysis of arterial blood	P_aCO_2 and P_aO_2	Invasive
Mechanical ventilator	Rate, tidal volume, and inspiratory : expiratory time ratio are preset	Cat must be checked for thoracic expansion

tively, excessively light anaesthesia also can be responsible for induction of the same arrhythmia due to catecholamine release and the appropriate treatment is to deepen anaesthesia.

Cardiac Output

Three methods for cardiac output determination in cats have been compared (Dyson *et al.*, 1985). The thermodilution method involves injection of 1–2 ml 5% dextrose in water (18–20°C) into the right atrium and the cardiac output is computed from the temperature change detected by a thermistor in the pulmonary artery. The Fick technique, using oxygen consumption and differences in arteriovenous oxygen content, was more inconsistent than the thermodilution technique and echocardiography was not reliable (Dyson *et al.*, 1985). Others have used the dye dilution technique involving injection of a bolus of indocyanine green into the right atrium and withdrawal of blood from a femoral artery through a photo-electrical cuvette densitometer where the concentration of dye is measured (Grandy *et al.*, 1989). The cardiac output is computed from the area under the dye-dilution curve.

Evaluation of Respiratory Function

Respiratory Rate, Depth, and Character

Respiratory rates of 43 ± 7 breaths/min have been recorded in normal conscious cats (McKiernan & Johnson, 1992). Monitoring the respiratory rate can provide important information to the anaesthetist, as a slow rate usually indicates hypoventilation and may be a sign of excessive depth of anaesthesia. An exception is halothane anaesthesia in which increased depth of anaesthesia is usually accompanied by an increased respiratory rate.

Rate of breathing can be counted from visual observation of movement of the chest or abdominal wall or the reservoir bag on the anaesthetic circuit. Several types of equipment

are available to monitor respiratory rate and provide beeps or respiratory sounds, and may include an audible warning device for low respiratory rate (Table 10.4). Some pieces of equipment attach to the oesophageal stethoscope and are sufficiently sensitive to detect and amplify breath sounds as well as heart sounds. Other models require attachment of a short adaptor containing a heat sensor to the endotracheal tube to detect exhalation (Fig. 10.12). Yet another monitor detects chest movements from a strap that has been secured around the thorax.

Hypoventilation (ventilation inadequate to remove carbon dioxide) is more frequently due to shallow breathing than to a decrease in rate of breathing. In one study of cats anaesthetized with halothane, increasing the depth of anaesthesia from 1.3 MAC to 2.0 MAC produced no change in respiratory rates, which were 51 ± 24 breaths/min and 57 ± 25 breaths/min respectively, but a substantial increase in arterial carbon dioxide tension (P_aCO_2) from 6.0 ± 1.5 kPa (45 ± 11 mmHg) to 11.7 ± 4.9 kPa (88 ± 37 mmHg) (Grandy *et al.*, 1989). Tachypnoea with halothane anaesthesia and with increasing depth of anaesthesia similarly has been observed in clinical patients and investigated in research animals. In one group of cats, deepening anaesthesia by increasing the inspired concentration of halothane from 1.2 to 3% resulted in an increase in respiratory rate from 33 to 57 breaths/min, an increase in P_aCO_2, and a decrease in mean arterial pressure (Mazzarelli *et al.*, 1979). Data from another investigation support the hypothesis that the increase in respiratory frequency is due to action of halothane in the brainstem (Berkenbosch *et al.*, 1982).

Consequently, the depth of breathing should be evaluated regularly in addition to counting the rate. An approximate estimate of depth of breathing can be made by observing thoracic and abdominal movements. Volume meters, such as the Wright's respirometer, can be inserted in the anaesthetic circuit for measurement of tidal volume and minute ventilation in dogs. These meters are not sufficiently sensitive to measure the tidal volumes of small cats but may be satisfactory if connected directly to the

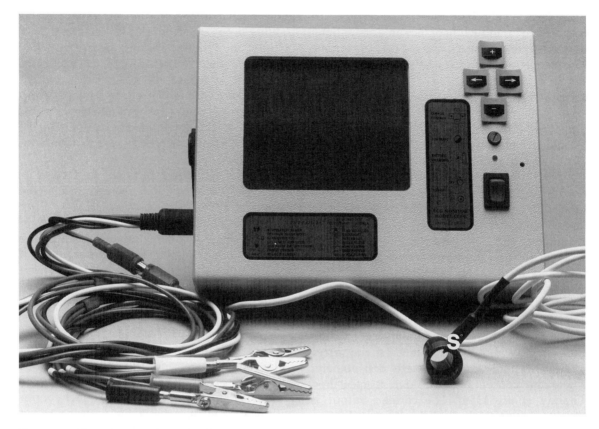

Fig. 10.12 This monitor displays ECG, heart rate, and respiratory rate (EC-60, Silogic Design Limited, Stewartstown, Pennsylvania). s, Respiratory sensor within an adaptor to be connected to the endotracheal tube.

endotracheal tube in larger cats. The tidal volume of a cat is usually less than 50 ml.

Some anaesthetic agents, notably ketamine, produce a characteristic pattern of breathing called apneustic breathing whereby the cat inhales and continues to hold inspiration for several seconds before exhaling.

Mucous Membrane Colour

Common signs of hypoxaemia are dark purple blood at the operative site and cyanotic mucous membranes. However, it should not be assumed that cyanosis will always develop with hypoxaemia. Cyanosis may not be observed in hypoxaemic, anaemic cats because of insufficient reduced haemoglobin (5 g/dl). In contrast, mucous membranes may appear cyanotic due to peripheral vasoconstriction even when arterial oxygen tension (P_aO_2) is adequate. For example,

cats heavily sedated with xylazine may have grey–white mucous membranes and adequate P_aO_2. Interpretation of mucous membrane colour also can be difficult during surgery when the cat is covered by blue or green drapes, and with different types of lighting.

Capnometry

Capnometry offers a non-invasive method of evaluating ventilation by measuring the carbon dioxide concentration in alveolar (end-tidal) gas at the end of exhalation ($ETCO_2$) (Fig. 10.2). This is accomplished either by placing an in-line sensor directly in the breathing system with a special adaptor close to the patient or by connecting an adaptor with a side arm to the endotracheal tube from which a continuous stream of gas is aspirated at a rate of 50, 150, or 250 ml/min. The gas flow must be low with

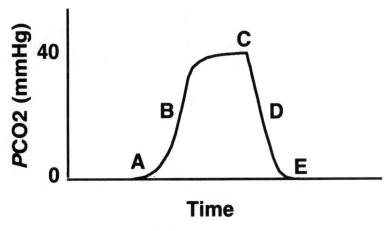

Fig. 10.13 Capnogram waveform. C, End-tidal CO_2.

small patients to avoid diluting the patient's tidal breath with fresh gas, producing a falsely low ETCO$_2$. Aspirated air must be returned to the anaesthetic circuit or scavenger to avoid pollution of the operating room with anaesthetic gases.

The characteristic waveform of the capnogram is shown in Fig. 10.13. At the beginning of expiration (A), gas is cleared from the anatomic dead space and should contain little CO_2. The expiratory upstroke (B) is a mixture of residual deadspace gas and alveolar gas. A prolonged upstroke may be caused by sampling tubing that is too wide or due to an obstruction in the endotracheal tube. The highest value of the expiratory plateau (C) is the ETCO$_2$ and this is the best reflection of the alveolar PCO_2. During controlled ventilation this plateau is longer and almost horizontal. Bumps and dips in the plateau can be caused by spontaneous respiratory efforts during controlled ventilation, cardiogenic oscillations, and compressions of the chest and lungs. As the patient begins to inspire there is a sharp downstroke (D) back to baseline. The inspiratory baseline (E) should be zero. An elevated baseline is indicative of CO_2 rebreathing, perhaps from excessive apparatus dead space, incompetent expiratory valve in a circle circuit, exhausted sodalime, or a disassembled Bain circuit.

The ETCO$_2$ can be used as an estimate of P_aCO_2 (Table 10.5). Under ideal conditions these

Table 10.5 Causes of increased and decreased end-tidal CO_2

High ETCO$_2$	Low ETCO$_2$
Hypoventilation	Hyperventilation
Rebreathing	Increased P_aCO_2– ETCO$_2$ gradient
Increased CO_2 production: Malignant hyperthermia Laparoscopy with CO_2 insufflation	Decreased CO_2 delivery: Cardiac output decreased Decreased CO_2 production: Hypothermia Sampling line leak

values are identical; however, in general, the ETCO$_2$ is lower than the P_aCO_2 by at least 0.7 kPa (5 mmHg). When ETCO$_2$ is increased, P_aCO_2 is increased; when ETCO$_2$ is normal, P_aCO_2 may be normal or increased. The gradient between ETCO$_2$ and P_aCO_2 is increased by ventilation and perfusion mismatch and this gradient has been found to increase with increased duration of anaesthesia in other veterinary species. A sudden decrease in end-tidal CO_2 may be serious and the patient should be immediately checked for cardiac arrest, airway obstruction, or disconnection of the anaesthetic circuit.

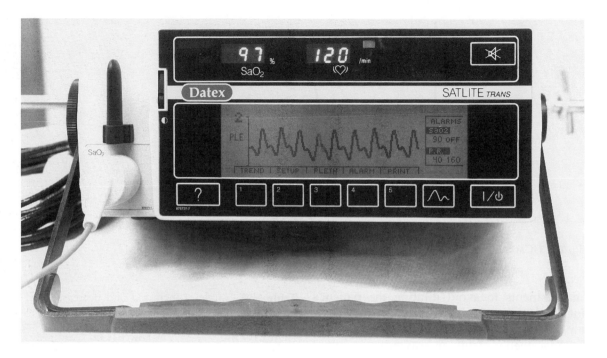

Fig. 10.14 A pulse oximeter continuously measures blood oxygen saturation and pulse rate when the sensor (not shown) is attached to the tongue (Datex, Instrumentarium Corp., Helsinki, Finland).

Pulse Oximetry

Observation of mucous membrane colour is an unreliable method of detecting hypoxaemia, and a cat's tongue may remain pink even after cardiac arrest. Pulse oximetry is a non-invasive method of continuously measuring haemoglobin oxygen saturation and is an appropriate and useful monitor for veterinary practice (Fig. 10.14). A monitor for detection of decreased arterial oxygen saturation is especially useful in anaesthetized cats breathing room air or during recovery from anaesthesia. Measurement is based on the fact that oxygenated haemoglobin absorbs light differently from deoxygenated haemoglobin (Tremper & Barker, 1990). When the sensor is clipped to the tongue or toe, light in the red and infrared wavelengths emitted on one side of the sensor is transmitted through the tissue and detected on the other side. The oximeter assumes only pulsatile absorbance is that of arterial blood. When there is a small absorbance signal from a weak pulse, the signal is amplified until it can be interpreted by the pulse oximeter. However, extraneous 'noise'

also will be picked up and, therefore, the pulse rate on the pulse oximeter must first be checked for accuracy when a low saturation is detected.

A haemoglobin saturation exceeding 96% is desirable. When an animal is breathing oxygen, wide fluctuations in P_aO_2 can occur even though oxygen saturation is 98%. Arterial hypoxaemia is defined as a P_aO_2 of 8.0 kPa (60 mmHg); venous blood has a PO_2 of 5.3 kPa (40 mmHg). The approximate equivalent saturations at normal pH are easily remembered from the following sequence:

PO_2 (mmHg)	40	50	60
O_2 saturation (%)	70	80	90

It is important to remember that the presence of adequate haemoglobin oxygen saturation does not infer adequate peripheral perfusion nor does it estimate oxygen delivery to tissues. Studies in human patients indicate that the pulse oximeter can accurately detect saturation when tissue blood flow has decreased to 5% of normal. Haemoglobin concentration also plays a large part in maintaining adequate oxygen delivery to the tissues.

Blood Gas Analysis

Definitive information about the adequacy of ventilation is obtained from analysis of P_aCO_2 and P_aO_2 in samples of arterial blood. Blood must be collected anaerobically (no air bubbles) into a heparinized syringe or capillary tube, sealed, and submerged in iced water, if not analysed immediately. Polypropylene or glass syringes may be used (Evers *et al.*, 1972). Heparin, 1000 IU/ml, should be drawn into the syringe, the plunger withdrawn to coat the inside of the barrel with heparin, and the excess expelled from the syringe leaving only the space in the nozzle filled. Excess heparin left in the syringe will alter the results by decreasing the PCO_2 and bicarbonate measurements. Blood is usually collected from the femoral artery using a 25-gauge needle inserted percutaneously in the opposite direction to blood flow. Blood should be withdrawn into the syringe over three respiratory cycles and without aspirating air bubbles. When the needle is removed, digital pressure must be applied to the artery for about 3 min to prevent formation of a haematoma. The syringe should be sealed immediately with a cap or by introducing the needle tip into a rubber stopper and then rotated to mix the blood with heparin. The patient's temperature is needed for correction of pHa and P_aO_2. Published normal values for conscious cats are given in Table 10.6 (Middleton *et al.*, 1981). Normal values for PO_2 decrease with increasing altitude.

Table 10.6 pH and blood gas analysis of arterial and venous blood in awake cats. (Modified from Middleton *et al.*, 1981, with permission.)

Parameter	Arterial blood	Venous blood
pHa	7.344 ± 0.104	7.300 ± 0.087
P_aCO_2 (kPa)	4.47 ± 0.94	5.56 ± 1.21
(mmHg)	33.6 ± 7.1	41.8 ± 9.12
P_aO_2 (kPa)	13.7 ± 2.0	5.2 ± 1.5
(mmHg)	103 ± 15	39 ± 11
HCO_3 (mmol/l)	17.5 ± 3.0	19.4 ± 4.0
TCO_2 (mmol/l)	18.4 ± 3.9	20.1 ± 4.2
Base excess (mmol/l)	−6.4 ± 5.0	−5.7 ± 4.6

A technique for collection of blood for blood gas analysis from a cut claw has been described (Solter *et al.*, 1988). Strict attention must be paid to preventing venous contamination of the sample if accurate results are to be obtained. With the cat gently restrained, the paw from which the sample is to be collected is warmed to 42–45°C for 10 min. The foot is elevated approximately 10 cm above the sternum during the warming and collection procedure to decrease venous back flow. The claw is cut back to the vascular bed using sharp nail trimmers and a quick cutting motion. The first drop of blood is blotted away and blood is then collected into a capillary tube. A metal bead may be added to the tube for mixing and, when all air is eliminated from the tube, the ends are sealed with clay. Blood samples that cannot be collected within 90 s should be discarded. With this technique, paired measurements of PCO_2 and PO_2 with samples from the femoral artery do not differ significantly, although the capillary blood has a significantly higher pH (Solter *et al.*, 1988).

An increase in P_aCO_2 of up to 1.3 kPa (5–10 mmHg) is considered mild respiratory acidosis, an increase of 1.3–2.6 kPa (10–20 mmHg) a moderate respiratory acidosis, and an increase greater than 2.7 kPa (20 mmHg) a severe respiratory acidosis. A decrease in P_aCO_2 is due to hyperventilation. Hyperventilation to a P_aCO_2 less than 2.7 kPa (20 mmHg) may cause cerebral hypoxia due to decreased cerebral blood flow from removal of the vasodilating influence of CO_2 on cerebral vasculature.

Monitoring Fluid and Acid–Base Balance

Fluid Administration

For most healthy cats, an adequate fluid infusion rate of balanced electrolyte solution during anaesthesia for surgery is 10 ml/kg/h. This can be administered using either a bag or bottle with a standard paediatric infusion set

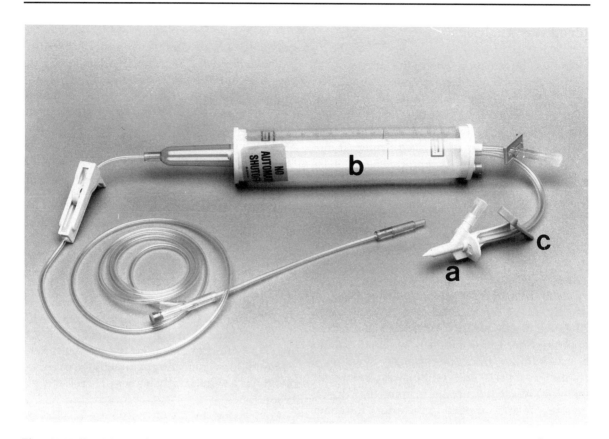

Fig. 10.15 Precision volume intravenous infusion set with a 150-ml calibrated burette (Soluset®, Abbott Laboratories, Chicago, Illinois). Adaptor (a) is inserted into the bag or bottle of fluid from which the infusion set is primed and then the required volume is withdrawn into the burette (b), after which clamp (c) is attached to prevent any further fluid administration. The remainder of this unit is a regular infusion set delivering 60 drops/ml fluid.

delivering 60 drops/ml solution using the calculation:

$$\frac{\text{Bodyweight (kg)} \times \text{Infusion rate (ml/h)} \times 60\ \text{(drops/ml)}}{60\ \text{(min/h)}}$$

$$= \text{drops/min}$$

Example: 3 kg cat to be given 10 ml/kg/h
= 3 × 10
= 30 drops/min

For small cats, an hour's worth of fluid can be drawn into a syringe and given over 1 h in 0.25–0.5 ml increments at intervals. This is a practical technique when small volumes of 5% dextrose in water are given to supplement maintenance fluids in paediatric cats and cats with diabetes or liver disease. There are several devices available to control the rate of infusion of fluids. These range from a sterile graduated cylinder (burette) incorporated into the infusion set (Fig. 10.15) to a pump that regulates flow by counting drops (Fig. 10.16). A drop counter is of particular value in exercising tight control over administration of potent vasoactive drugs such as dopamine and dobutamine.

Although cats may not be more susceptible to the adverse effects of overtransfusion than any other species (Bjorling & Rawlings, 1983), their small size makes it easy to administer too much fluid inadvertently. No increase in central venous pressure (CVP) or extravascular lung water was measured in healthy cats anaesthetized with halothane and infused with 90 ml/kg/h of lactated Ringer's solution (Bjorling &

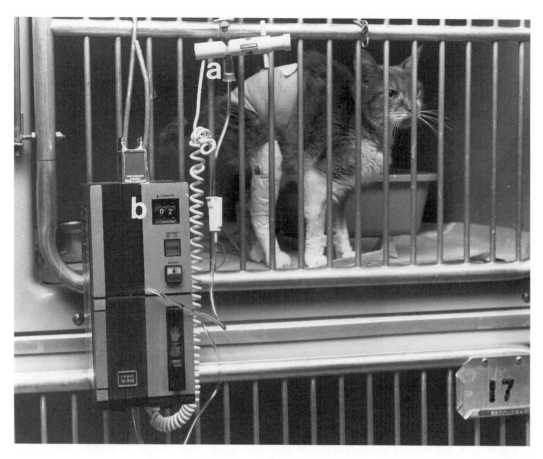

Fig. 10.16 Precise control of fluid infusion can be obtained with this pump which counts (a) and regulates the number of drops of fluid delivered per minute to a preset value (b) (IVAC® Corporation, San Diego, California).

Rawlings, 1983), nor was there a significant increase in CVP in cats anaesthetized with ketamine subjected to haemorrhage followed by 70 ml/kg/h (Boothe *et al.*, 1985). In contrast, cats given lactated Ringer's solution at either 225 ml/kg/h or 140 ml/kg/h developed unacceptably high CVP and evidence of pulmonary oedema (Bjorling & Rawlings, 1983; Boothe *et al.*, 1985).

Central Venous Pressure

Central venous pressure (CVP) measures the pressure in the right atrium and is indicative of blood volume. Normal values in cats are between 0 and 4 cmH$_2$O. Values less than these should be considered hypovolaemia and values over 8 cmH$_2$O indicate hypervolaemia. Measurement of CVP is of most use in the monitoring of

volume and rate of administration of intravenous fluids during treatment of hypovolaemia before induction of anaesthesia. This measurement may be necessary to identify the extent of fluid therapy required because vasoconstriction in the conscious cat may maintain blood pressure within normal limits despite hypovolaemia and decreased cardiac output. Without treatment, anaesthetic drugs may cause vasodilation and a dramatic decrease in blood pressure.

The jugular vein catheter (e.g. Delmed I-Cath®, Venocath®) that has been installed for fluid therapy in sick cats can also be used in the measurement of CVP provided that it has been advanced until the tip is within the thorax in the right atrium or in the cranial vena cava. A plastic manometer graduated in centimetres is used for measurement of CVP. The manometer

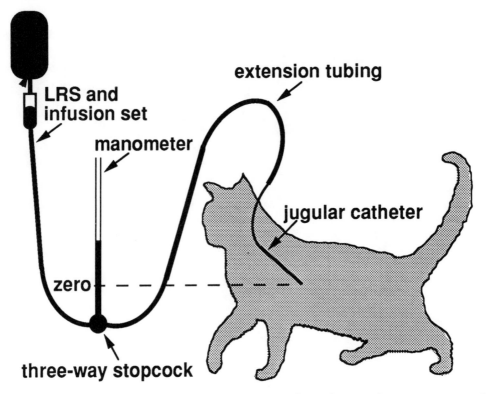

Fig. 10.17 Central venous pressure measurement using a jugular catheter and a manometer graduated in centimetres.

is filled with lactated Ringer's solution and then connected to the jugular catheter (Fig. 10.17). The fluid level in the manometer falls as the pressure of the column of fluid equalizes with the pressure in the venous system. Oscillations can be observed in the fluid meniscus from changes in intrathoracic pressure during breathing. The zero graduation on the manometer should correspond with the right atrium (spine, sternum, or thoracic inlet when the cat is in lateral recumbency and axilla when the cat is in dorsal or sternal recumbency) before the fluid height is measured.

Blood Loss

The mean blood volume of cats is 56 ml/kg bodyweight (Breznock & Strack, 1982a), which is less on a per weight basis than in dogs. Cats with normovolemia and adequate haematocrit before anaesthesia should be able to tolerate up to a 20% loss of circulating blood volume before a blood transfusion is necessary. This is provided that large volumes of crystalloid solution are infused (e.g. 2.5 times the volume of blood lost) with lactated Ringer's solution. Because mean arterial pressure changes very little until there is a 25% decrease in cardiac output, it is vital that fluids be administered early and not reserved until cardiovascular deterioration becomes obvious (Fig. 10.18). The volume of blood lost can be determined by weighing gauze swabs or estimating the number of swabs used times the volume of blood needed to saturate a swab (1 g = 1 ml). The packed cell volume and total protein measurements are not often useful in determining how much blood has been lost. The packed cell volume will be reduced when large volumes of crystalloid are infused and yet the packed cell volume changes little with acute severe haemorrhage. Anaesthesia alone also substantially decreases the packed cell volume; this has been reported after intravenous or intramuscular ketamine, intravenous alphaxalone–alphadalone (Saffan®) (Frankel & Hawkey, 1980) or pentobarbitone

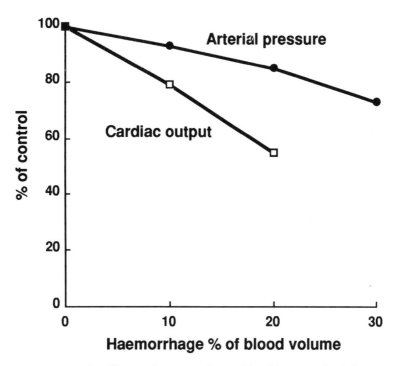

Fig. 10.18 Accurate assessment of cardiovascular status during blood loss may be difficult when arterial blood pressure is within acceptable limits. This graph of the cardiovascular effects of graded haemorrhage in dogs anaesthetized with pentobarbitone illustrates an early significant decrease in cardiac output. Data from Hinshaw *et al.*, 1961.

(Breznock & Strack, 1982b), and with halothane (Steffey *et al.*, 1976). Mean packed cell volumes for 8-week old, 18-week old, and adult cats are given as 31, 35, and 38%, respectively (Earle *et al.*, 1990). However, a wide range of packed cell volume is considered normal and, therefore, it is important to measure packed cell volume and total protein in every cat before sedation and anaesthesia for surgery.

Metabolic Status

Measurements of metabolic status in the form of bicarbonate (HCO_3) and base excess/deficit can be obtained from the relationship between pH and $PaCO_2$. Bicarbonate concentration is influenced by both respiratory and metabolic mechanisms and is of questionable value for estimating metabolic status in anaesthetized patients that may be hypoventilating. Base excess/deficit is a measure of the total buffering power of the blood and is independent of P_aCO_2. This determination requires the haemo-

globin concentration for complete accuracy. Either arterial or venous blood can be used for evaluation of base excess/deficit. Cats normally have a mild metabolic acidosis (Fink & Schoolman, 1963; Middleton *et al.*, 1981; Solter *et al.*, 1988); values for conscious cats are given in Table 10.6 (Middleton *et al.*, 1981). Mild, moderate, and severe metabolic acidosis will be reflected in an increase in the base deficit of 5, 10, and 15 mmol/l, respectively. More detail on the pathophysiology of acid–base disorders is available elsewhere (Orsini, 1989).

Temperature

Anaesthesia severely reduces normal temperature homeostasis of the body by depressing hypothalamic activity and preventing heat production by increased muscle activity and heat conservation or loss through changes in circulation to the skin. It is thus important that temperature is monitored so that artificial control can replace the natural homeostasis. This is particularly important in the cat, which, as a result of its small size and high body surface area to volume ratio, is particularly susceptible to heat loss.

Hypothermia develops easily in cats and often results in a slow recovery from anaesthesia. It is particularly likely to occur when the room is cold or when a large area of the body is prepared for surgery using cold fluids or alcohol. The degree of hypothermia does not appear to be related to the anaesthetic agents used (Haskins, 1981). Hypothermia may result in increased mortality and morbidity as in man. Paediatric and geriatric patients are less well able to thermoregulate and are at particular risk of developing hypothermia. Once a cat's body temperature has decreased it may be difficult to return it to normal until the animal begins to recover from anaesthesia. Therefore, it is advisable to make every effort to prevent any decrease in body temperature and to continue monitoring temperature during recovery, until it returns to normal or at least shows an upward trend.

Hyperthermia may occasionally occur in cats. An increase in temperature during anaesthesia may be due to excessive application of heat, pyrexia of bacterial or viral origin, malignant hyperthermia syndrome, or may occur for no apparent reason. Overheating may develop when the cat has a heavy hair coat and is anaesthetized lying on a warm water pad and covered with drapes in a warm room. Hyperthermia may also develop in active cats during recovery from ketamine or tiletamine anaesthesia. Malignant hyperthermia syndrome (MH) has rarely been reported in cats (de Jong et al., 1974; Bellah et al., 1989).

Hyperthermia requires immediate and aggressive therapy and is difficult to detect unless temperature is monitored. It is relatively straightforward to measure temperature continuously throughout anaesthesia and in the early recovery period. Several models of electrical thermometers and temperature probes are available. Rectal or intrathoracic oesophageal temperatures are usually more accurate reflections of core temperature than oral temperature.

Neuromuscular Blockade

When monitoring a paralysed cat, the anaesthetist's objectives should be to provide sufficient anaesthetic agent to prevent awareness, to avoid overdosage from excessive administration of anaesthetic agent, and to obtain information on the degree of neuromuscular blockade in order to manage redosing and reversal of the muscle relaxant correctly.

Because neuromuscular blocking drugs provide no analgesia, an important part of monitoring the paralysed patient is ensuring that the patient is unconscious and analgesic without inducing anaesthetic overdose. Delaying administration of the paralysing agent until the cat is stabilized at a suitable depth of anaesthesia is likely to ensure adequate anaesthesia in the individual patient. When inhalation anaesthesia is used and a gas analyser is available, an adequate depth of anaesthesia can be maintained by adjusting the vaporizer setting to achieve an appropriate end-tidal concentration; usually 1.2–1.5 MAC. This concentration may need to be adjusted, depending on the nature and quantity of other anaesthetic drugs given to the patient. Because nitrous oxide has such a low potency in cats, nitrous oxide alone will not produce unconsciousness or analgesia unless the cat is extremely ill.

If signs of autonomic system stimulation are observed, such as an increase in heart rate or when the heart rate and blood pressure are higher than expected for the anaesthetic regime used, the cat may not be sufficiently anaesthetized. Other signs that are indicative of a light plane of anaesthesia or lack of analgesia include salivation, small tongue twitches, and respiratory movements before the neuromuscular blockade is expected to fade.

There is a consistent sequence in which groups of muscles become paralysed after administration of a neuromuscular blocking agent. This sequence can be utilized in monitoring the degree of paralysis. The muscles of facial expression, jaw and tail are paralysed first, followed in sequence by neck and limb muscles, swallowing, abdominal muscles, intercostal

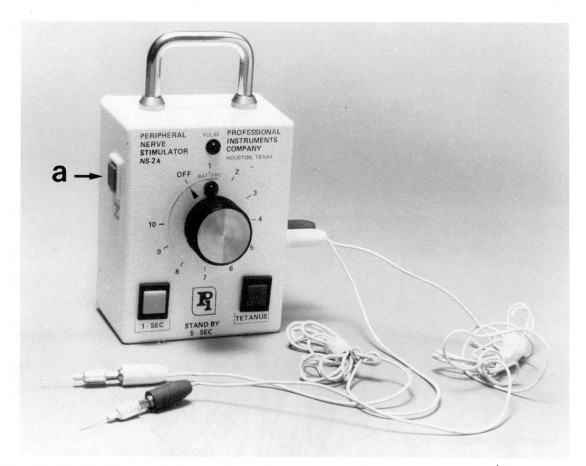

Fig. 10.19 Peripheral nerve stimulator used to evaluate neuromuscular transmission. a, Train-of-four button.

muscles, and finally the diaphragm. This sequence is reversed as the agent is detoxified or chemically reversed, with function of the respiratory muscles returning first. Because only 20% of receptors need to be available for the respiratory muscles to begin to function, as spontaneous respiratory movements resume, the cat may be unable to protect its airway (swallowing and lifting the head may not be present). Thus, the true signs of successful reversal are the return of the palpebral reflex and rotation of the eye in the orbit into a rostroventral position. Only then should anaesthetic administration cease and the cat be allowed to recover from anaesthesia.

Peripheral Nerve Stimulation

Neuromuscular transmission can be evaluated using a peripheral nerve stimulator (Fig. 10.19).

The information obtained using this device permits the anaesthetist to identify the need for additional neuromuscular blocking agent before increased muscle tone becomes apparent to the surgeon. This also allows the anaesthetist to avoid giving incremental doses of neuromuscular blocking agent that might result in excessive use of drug and make reversal at the end of the procedure difficult or prolonged. The peripheral nerve stimulator also can be used during reversal of non-depolarizing blockade to guide the administration of reversal agents. When a cat is slow to breathe or awaken after anaesthesia in which a neuromuscular blocker has been used, the nerve stimulator can be used to rule out persistent curarization. Although a person experienced with neuromuscular blocking agents may feel comfortable managing a paralysed patient without a peripheral nerve stimulator, the information provided by the

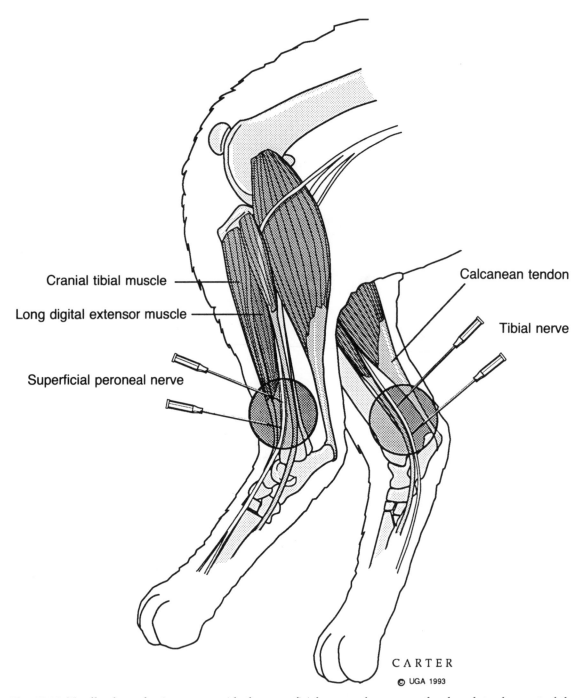

Cranial tibial muscle

Long digital extensor muscle

Superficial peroneal nerve

Calcanean tendon

Tibial nerve

CARTER
© UGA 1993

Fig. 10.20 Needle electrodes in contact with the superficial peroneal nerve on the dorsolateral aspect of the hind limb, lateral to the long digital extensor muscle and proximal to the lateral malleolus of the tibia. The tibial nerve is situated cranial to the common calcanean tendon and proximal to the medial malleolus of the tibia. The circles indicate the most superficial locations of the nerves.

stimulator greatly assists in deciding when to adjust anaesthetic administration and the timing and dosages of the reversal agent. Without a nerve stimulator not *all* paralysed patients will be managed in the best possible way.

The electrodes of the peripheral nerve stimulator must be placed over a peripheral nerve in the fore or hind limb. Twenty-five gauge needles with metal hubs are convenient and the tip of the needles, about half an inch apart, can be inserted through the skin near the nerve (Fig. 10.20). The needles should not penetrate muscle fascia as this may stimulate the muscle directly and give a false impression of neuromuscular function. The nerve stimulator is turned on to deliver a supramaximal electrical stimulus to the nerve which results in a paw twitch. Each electrical stimulus lasts less than 0.2 ms. For clinical purposes, the strength of the electrical current should simply be increased until maximum movement of the cat's foot can be seen. For research purposes, the magnitude of the twitch can be measured using a force-displace-ment transducer attached to the limb and the force of flexion recorded (Ilkiw *et al.*, 1990). An alternative method of quantifying the motor response is by measurement of the compound action potential (EMG) resulting from nerve stimulation. Specific EMG monitors are available for recording evaluations of neuromuscular transmission.

When a neuromuscular blocking agent is administered, the decrease in contraction force during supramaximal stimulation indicates the degree of blockade. The most useful stimulation pattern for monitoring the stage of non-depolarizing blockade is the train-of-four stimulation (TOF). Pressing the TOF button on the stimulator will trigger delivery of four supramaximal stimuli at intervals of 0.5 s. In a non-paralysed patient, each stimulus will be followed by a strong contraction of equal strength (Fig. 10.21). The amplitude of the fourth response in relation to the first gives the train-of-four ratio. During non-depolarizing blockade this ratio is reduced and is approxi-

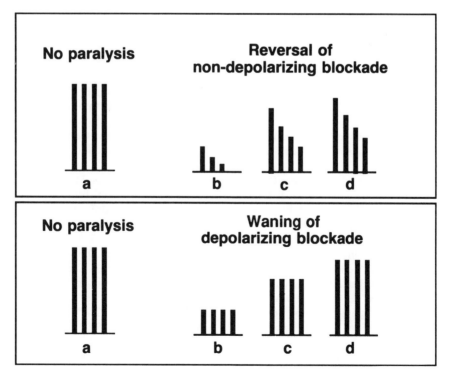

Fig. 10.21 Characteristic responses to train-of-four stimulation of a peripheral nerve before (a) administration of a neuromuscular blocking agent and during recovery from blockade (b sequentially through d and finally to a). Each vertical bar represents the strength of contraction of the stimulated muscle.

mately inversely proportional to the degree of block. The TOF ratio begins to decrease when approximately 75% of the receptors are blocked. The response to the fourth stimulus disappears (TOF ratio = 0) when the height of the first response is about 25% of the preblockade value.

During depolarizing block with suxamethonium (succinylcholine), all contraction strengths are equal (Fig. 10.21). A decrease in the TOF ratio during suxamethonium paralysis indicates that phase II or dual block exists.

Approximately 2 min after administration of a non-depolarizing agent such as pancuronium or atracurium, paralysis ensues and no contraction should be seen in response to any of the stimuli. As the effect of the agent wanes or when reversal with neostigmine, pyridostigmine, or edrophonium is initiated, muscle contraction will not be observed with all four stimuli (Fig. 10.21). With time, the TOF ratio increases until maximal contraction is observed with all four stimuli. During reversal of blockade, a TOF ratio of 0.8 equates with the animal being able to lift its head as well as having adequate respiratory function.

References

Bellah, J.R., Robertson, S.A., Buergelt, C.D. & McGavin, A.D. (1989) Suspected malignant hyperthermia after halothane anesthesia in a cat. *Vet. Surg.* **18**, 483–488.

Berkenbosch, A., de Goede, J., Olievier, C.N., & Quanjer, P.H. (1982) Sites of action of halothane on respiratory pattern and ventilatory response to CO_2 in cats. *Anesthesiology* **57**, 389–398.

Bjorling, D.E. & Rawlings, C.A. (1983) Relationship of intravenous administration of Ringer's lactate solution to pulmonary edema in halothane-anesthetized cats. *Am. J. Vet. Res.* **44**, 1000–1006.

Boothe, H.W., Clark, D.R. & Merton, D.A. (1985) Cardiovascular effects of rapid infusion of crystalloid in the hypovolaemic cat. *J. Small Anim. Pract.* **26**, 477–489.

Breznock, E.M. & Strack, D. (1982a) Blood volume of nonsplenectomized and splenectomized cats before and after acute hemorrhage. *Am. J. Vet. Res.* **43**, 1811–1814.

Breznock, E.M. & Strack, D. (1982b) Effects of the spleen, epinephrine, and splenectomy on determination of blood volume in cats. *Am. J. Vet. Res.* **43**, 2062–2066.

Burrows, C.F. (1973) Techniques and complications of intravenous and intraarterial catheterization in dogs and cats. *J. Am. Vet. Med. Assoc.* **163**, 1357–1363.

Clarke, K.W. & Hall, L.W. (1990) A survey of anaesthesia in small animal practice: AVA/BSAVA report. *J. Ass. Vet. Anaesth.* **17**, 4–10.

Dalton, M.J. (1985) The vascular port: A subcutaneously implanted drug delivery depot. *Lab. Animal* **14**, 21–30.

de Jong, R.H., Heavner, J.E. & Amory, D.W. (1974) Malignant hyperpyrexia in the cat. *Anesthesiology* **41**, 608–609.

Drummond, J.C., Todd, M.M. & Shapiro, H.M. (1983) Minimal alveolar concentrations for halothane, enflurane, and isoflurane in the cat. *Am. J. Vet. Res.* **182**, 1099–1101.

Dyson, D.H., Allen, D.G. & McDonell, W.N. (1985) Comparison of three methods for cardiac output determination in cats. *Am. J. Vet. Res.* **46**, 2546–2552.

Earle, K.E., Smith, P.M., Gillott, W.M. & Poore, D.W. (1990) Haematology of the weanling, juvenile and adult cat. *J. Small Anim. Pract.* **31**, 225–228.

Evers, W., Racz, G.B. & Levy, A.A. (1972) A comparative study of plastic (polypropylene) and glass syringes in blood-gas analysis. *Anesth. Analg.* **51**, 92–97.

Fink, B.R. & Schoolman, A. (1963) Arterial blood acid–base balance in unrestrained waking cats. *Proc. Soc. exp. Biol. Med.* **112**, 328–330.

Frankel, T. & Hawkey, C.M. (1980) Haematological changes during sedation in cats. *Vet. Rec.* **107**, 512–513.

Gaukroger, P.B., Roberts, J.G. & Manners, T. A. (1988) Infusion thrombophlebitis: A prospective comparison of 645 Vialon® and Teflon® cannulae in anaesthetic and postoperative use. *Anaesth. Intens. Care* **16**, 265–271.

Grandy, J.L., Hodgson, D.S., Dunlop, C.I., Curtis, C.R. & Heath, R.B. (1989) Cardiopulmonary effects of halothane anesthesia in cats. *Am. J. Vet. Res.* **5**, 1729–1732.

Grandy, J.L., Dunlop, C.I., Hodgson, D.S., Curtis, C.R. & Chapman, P.L. (1992) Evaluation of the Doppler ultrasonic method of measuring systolic arterial blood pressure in cats. *Am. J. Vet. Res.* **53**, 1166–1169.

Harpster, N.K. (1986) The cardiovascular system. *In: Diseases of the Cat* (ed. J. Holzworth), pp. 820–933. W.B. Saunders, Philadelphia.

Haskins, S.C. (1981) Hypothermia and its prevention during general anesthesia in cats. *Am. J. Vet. Res.* **42**, 856–861.

Haskins, S.C., Peiffer, R.L. & Stowe, C.M. (1975) A clinical comparison of CT1341, ketamine, and xylazine in cats. *Am. J. Vet. Res.* **36**, 1537–1542.

Hinshaw, D.B., Peterson, M., Huse, W.M., Stafford C.E. & Joergenson E.J. (1961) Regional blood flow in hemorrhagic shock. *Am J. Surg.* **102**, 224–230.

Ilkiw, J.E., Forsyth, S.F., Hill, T. & Gregory, C.R. (1990) Atracurium administration, as an infusion, to induce neuromuscular blockade in clinically normal and temporarily immune-suppressed cats. *J. Am. Vet. Med. Assoc.* **197**, 1153–1156.

Johnson C.B., Young S.S. & Taylor P.M. (1993) Spectral analysis of the equine electroencephalogram during halothane anaesthesia. *Res Vet Sci* (in press).

Lake, C.L. (1990) Monitoring of arterial pressure. *In: Clinical Monitoring* (ed. C.L. Lake), pp. 115–146. W.B. Saunders, Philadelphia.

Mazzarelli, M.S., Haberer, J.P., Jaspar, N. & Miserocchi, G. (1979) Mechanism of halothane-induced tachypnea in cats. *Anesthesiology* **51**, 522–527.

McKiernan, B.C. and Johnson, L.R. (1992) Clinical pulmonary function testing in dogs and cats. *Vet. Clinics N. Am.: Small Anim. Pract.* **22**, 1087–1099.

Middleton, D.J., Ilkiw, J.E. & Watson, A.D.J. (1981) Arterial and venous blood gas tensions in clinically healthy cats. *Am. J. Vet. Res.* **42**, 1609–1611.

Middleton, D.J., Ilkiw, J.E. & Watson, A.D.J. (1982) Physiological effects of thiopentone, ketamine and CT1341 in cats. *Res. Vet. Sci.* **32**, 157–162.

Moore, M.P., Greene S.A. & Keegan, R.D. (1992) A method for assessing noxious stimuli in anesthetized dogs. *In: Animal Pain* (ed. C.E. Short & A. van Poznak), pp. 429–436. Churchill Livingstone, New York.

Orsini, J.A. (1989) Pathophysiology, diagnosis, and treatment of clinical acid–base disorders. *Compend. Cont. Educ.* **11**, 593–604.

Otto, K. & Short, C.E. (1991) Electroencephalographic power spectrum analysis as a monitor of anesthetic depth in horses. *Vet. Surg.* **20**, 362–371.

Sawyer, D.C. (1992) Indirect blood pressure measurements in dogs, cats, and horses: Correlation with direct arterial pressures and site of measurement. *Proc XXVII World Small Animal Veterinary Association Congress*, Rome, Italy pp. 93–98.

Sawyer, D.C., Brown, M., Striler, E.L., Durham, R.A., Langham, M.A. & Rech, R.H. (1991) Comparison of direct and indirect blood pressure measurement in anesthetized dogs. *Lab. Anim . Sci.* **41**, 134–138.

Schwilden, H. (1989) Use of the median EEG frequency and pharmacokinetics in determining depth of anaesthesia. *Bailliere's Clinical Anaesthesiology* **3**, 603–622.

Schwilden, H., Schüttler, J. & Stoeckel, H. (1987) Closed loop feedback control of methohexital anaesthesia by quantitative EEG analysis in humans. *Anesthesiology* **67**, 341–347.

Sellgren, J., Biber, B., Henriksson, B.-Å., Martner, J. & Pontén, J. (1992) The effects of propofol, methohexitone and isoflurane on the baroreceptor reflex in the cat. *Acta Anaesthesiol. Scand.* **36**, 784–790.

Solter, P.F., Haskins, S.C. & Patz, J.D. (1988) Comparison of PO_2, PCO_2, and pH in blood collected from the femoral artery and a cut claw of cats. *Am. J. Vet. Res.* **49**, 1882–1883.

Steffey, E.P. & Howland Jr, D. (1977) Isoflurane potency in the dog and cat. *Am. J. Vet. Res.* **38**, 1833–1836.

Steffey, E.P., Gillespie, J.R., Berry, J.D., Eger, E.I. II & Schalm, O.W. (1976) Effect of halothane and halothane–nitrous oxide on hematocrit and plasma protein concentration in dog and monkey. *Am. J. Vet. Res.* **37**, 959–962.

Stegall, H.F., Kardon, M.B. & Kemmerer, W.T. (1968) Indirect measurement of arterial blood pressure by Doppler ultrasonic sphygmomanometry. *J. Appl. Physiol.* **25**, 793–798.

Tremper, K.K. & Barker, S.J. (1990) Monitoring of oxygen. *In: Clinical Monitoring* (ed. C.L. Lake), pp. 283–313. W.B. Saunders, Philadelphia.

Waelchli-Suter, C.M., McDonell, W.N., Pascoe, P.J. & Douthwaite, S. (1986) Evaluation of an esophageal stethoscope as an early predictor of serious cardiovascular insufficiency in the dog. *Vet. Surg.* **15**, 453–457.

J.E. Ilkiw

11
Anaesthesia and Disease

Introduction

Anaesthesia in people is considered to be reasonably safe with a mortality of approximately 1 in 10 000 (0.01%) in ASA categories 1 and 2, increasing to approximately 0.46% in ASA categories 3, 4 and 5 (Marx *et al.*, 1973). Very little information is available concerning morbidity and mortality in veterinary practice. One study, conducted in veterinary practice in Great Britain, reported a mortality of 1 in 552 (0.18%) in healthy cats (ASA categories 1 and 2) and 1 in 30 (3.33%) in sick cats (ASA categories 3,4 and 5) (Clarke & Hall, 1990). It is obvious from these figures that, while the overall standard of anaesthetic practice in small animals needs to be raised, much improvement is required in the anaesthetic management of cats with systemic disease.

When anaesthetizing animals with systemic diseases, it is important to take into consideration the disease process when selecting anaesthetic drugs. It is also important to understand the pathophysiology of the disease in order best to prepare the patient prior to anaesthesia and to handle effectively complications which arise during anaesthesia or in the postanaesthetic period. The effects of anaesthetic drugs on various body systems, in both health and disease, are considered elsewhere in this book (see Chapter 4). This chapter describes the pre-, post- and anaesthetic management of four important diseases whose incidence is greater in cats than in other species; hyperthyroidism, urethral obstruction, idiopathic hepatic lipidosis and hypertrophic cardiomyopathy.

Hyperthyroidism

Naturally occurring hyperthyroidism has become the most common endocrine disorder of middle-aged to old cats and is one of the most frequently diagnosed disorders in small animal practice (Peterson & Randolph, 1989). The disorder results from excessive circulating concentrations of thyroid hormones, thyroxine (T_4) and triiodothyronine (T_3). Actions of thyroid hormones are generally stimulatory and their effects far-ranging. Thyroid hormones regulate metabolic processes from heat production to carbohydrate, protein and lipid metabolism in virtually all body tissues. The increased energy metabolism and heat production cause the increased appetite, weight loss, muscle wasting, weakness, heat intolerance and slightly elevated body temperature characteristic of hyperthyroidism. Thyroid hormones also appear to interact with the central nervous system. The increased overall sympathetic drive causes the hyperexcitability or nervousness, behavioural changes, tremor and tachycardia characteristic of hyperthyroidism (Peterson, 1984).

Thyrotoxic cats require anaesthesia primarily for elective surgical management of hyperthyroidism, but occasionally they require anaesthetic management as an emergency for problems unrelated to hyperthyroidism.

Clinical Signs and Laboratory Findings Relevant to Anaesthetic Management

Hyperthyroidism is a multisystemic disease and thus most cats have clinical signs which reflect dysfunction of many organ systems (see Chapter 4). From an anaesthetist's viewpoint, cardiovascular, respiratory, gastrointestinal and hepatic systems may all be seriously affected (Peterson, 1981). In one study of 131 hyperthyroid cats, weight loss, polyphagia, hyperactivity and tachycardia were the most common clinical signs and were found in 98, 81, 76 and 66% of affected cats, respectively. Polydypsia/polyuria, vomiting, cardiac murmur, muscle weakness, congestive heart failure and dyspnoea were found in 60, 55, 53, 25, 12 and 11% of affected cats, respectively (Peterson *et al.*, 1983).

Weight loss may affect the pharmacokinetics of some anaesthetic agents by changing the volume of distribution, and together with excessive shedding of hair, will make these cats more susceptible to hypothermia under anaesthesia.

The restless, apprehensive state induced by hyperthyroidism can cause cats to be difficult to handle and to become aggressive if restrained. Some cats with hyperthyroidism tend to become unable to cope with stressful conditions. Respiratory distress, weakness and development of cardiac arrhythmias may follow stress such as forced restraint (Peterson & Randolph, 1989). Muscle weakness, if present, may predispose to hypoventilation under anaesthesia and the increased arterial carbon dioxide tension that results from this may predispose to arrhythmias.

Renal blood flow, glomerular filtration rate and tubular reabsorptive and secretory capacities are increased in people with hyperthyroidism and in animals given large doses of thyroid hormone (Vaamonde & Michael, 1981). Despite these alterations, electrolyte balance and serum electrolyte concentrations are usually normal. Polyuria and polydipsia may be prominent signs and studies in thyrotoxic people usually reveal impaired concentrating ability probably due to increased renal blood flow and the resultant decline in intramedullary solute concentration. In cats with hyperthyroidism, renal dysfunction is relatively common, with 42% of affected cats being azotaemic (Feldman & Nelson, 1987). Following successful management of hyperthyroidism, 18% of these cats still appeared to have renal insufficiency (Feldman & Nelson, 1987). In fact, the increased renal blood flow associated with untreated hyperthyroidism may be beneficial in maintaining sustainable

renal function (and delaying the clinical and biochemical consequences of severe renal failure) in some cats with chronic renal failure (Peterson & Ferguson, 1989). Deterioration of renal function with clinical signs of renal failure has been reported after correction of the hyperthyroid state in some cats with normal or slightly increased values for blood urea nitrogen (BUN) and creatinine prior to treatment (Peterson & Randolph, 1989). Maintenance of renal blood flow during anaesthetic management of hyperthyroid cats is therefore very important in order to avoid postanaesthetic renal dysfunction or failure. Hyperthyroid cats may be unable to concentrate urine even in the face of clinical dehydration. This may be important in the hyperthyroid cat presented for emergency anaesthesia.

Dyspnoea, panting and hyperventilation have been reported in some cats with hyperthyroidism, often associated with some form of stress (Peterson & Randolph, 1989). Alterations in respiratory function reported in people with hyperthyroidism include decreased vital capacity, decreased pulmonary compliance and increased minute respiratory volume (Ingbar & Woeber, 1981). These abnormalities in respiratory function probably result from a combination of respiratory muscle weakness and increased carbon dioxide production. Ventilatory responses to hypoxaemia or hypercapnia are increased in hyperthyroidism (Massey *et al.*, 1967). Respiratory depression induced by anaesthetic drugs is common under general anaesthesia and control of ventilation in hyperthyroid cats is advisable. Dyspnoea in cats with congestive heart failure may be caused by pulmonary oedema and/or pleural effusion. If pleural effusion is extensive, thoracocentesis is advisable prior to induction of anaesthesia.

Cardiovascular signs, including tachycardia, systolic murmurs, gallop rhythm, dyspnoea, cardiomegaly and congestive heart failure, are common in cats with hyperthyroidism. A recent study has reported that 80% of hyperthyroid cats are hypertensive (Kobayashi *et al.*, 1990). Electrocardiographic changes include tachycardia, increased R-wave amplitude in lead II, atrial and ventricular arrhythmias and intraventricular conduction disturbances (Fig. 11.1).

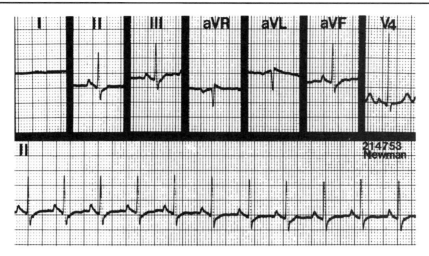

Fig. 11.1 Electrocardiogram from a cat with hyperthyroidism showing increased QRS voltage indicative of left ventricular enlargement.

Catecholamine-dependent mechanisms may influence the development of many ECG disturbances. Studies suggest that thyroid hormones increase cardiac responsiveness to circulating catecholamines by increasing the number of receptors (McConnaughey *et al.*, 1979) or the affinity (Bilezikian *et al.*, 1979) of cardiac β-adrenergic receptors. Also, thyroid hormones have positive chronotropic properties and directly increase heart rate, even in the absence of autonomic interventions (Cairoli & Crout, 1967). Over a period of time, most cats with hyperthyroidism will develop a hypertrophic cardiomyopathy with hypertrophy of the left ventricular free wall and ventricular septum. Echocardiographic changes include left ventricular dilation, left ventricular hypertrophy and hypercontractility (Bond, 1988). Hypertrophy may arise from the hypermetabolic state which increases cardiac demands for tissue perfusion (Cohen 1974) or it could occur from direct effects of thyroid hormones which increase oxygen consumption and protein synthesis in cardiac tissue (Skeleton *et al.*, 1970). Intraventricular conduction disturbances could be caused by inflammatory or infiltratory lesions in the myocardium. In both people and rats, foci of necrosis, round cell infiltration and replacement fibrosis have been reported in the thyrotoxic myocardium (Weller *et al.*, 1932). These cardiac changes predispose to arrhythmias or cardiac arrest during anaesthesia.

Haematocrit and mean corpuscular volume were increased in 45% of hyperthyroid cats in one study (Peterson *et al.*, 1983). These changes appear to result from direct effects of thyroid hormones on erythroid marrow and an increased production of erythropoietin (Peterson, 1984).

The most common serum biochemical abnormalities in one study included high activities for alkaline phosphatase, lactate dehydrogenase, aspartate aminotransaminase and alanine aminotransaminase with increases in at least one of these enzymes in 97% of cats (Peterson *et al.*, 1983). Histologic examination of the liver reveals only modest and non-specific changes, including centrilobular fatty infiltration and mild hepatic necrosis or degeneration (Peterson & Randolph, 1989). Hepatic dysfunction may be due, in part, to localized hypoxia as splanchnic bed oxygen consumption is increased while blood flow is essentially unchanged (Feldman & Nelson, 1987). Avoidance of hypoxaemia and maintenance of liver blood flow are thus important anaesthetic considerations.

Pre-anaesthetic Assessment and Preparation of the Patient

Thyrotoxic cats are often considered poor anaesthetic risks because they tend to be elderly, cachectic, fragile animals with organ system dysfunction (Feldman & Nelson, 1987).

Preparation is important in the hyperthyroid cat as anaesthesia can induce serious complications such as ventricular arrhythmias, or even sudden death (Peterson, 1984). Of 85 hyperthyroid cats treated surgically at one centre, 10% died either intra-operatively or immediately postoperatively. Six of these eight cats had not been rendered euthyroid with antithyroid drugs preoperatively (Peterson *et al.*, 1984). In another series undergoing thyroidectomy, 4 out of 44 (9.1%) cats died due to anaesthetic complications, whilst another 2 died in the immediate postoperative period (Feldman & Nelson, 1987). Thus pre-anaesthetic, anaesthetic and postanaesthetic management of these cats can significantly affect mortality and morbidity.

The most important preparation for cats undergoing elective thyroidectomy, is to render them euthyroid by the administration of methimazole or propylthiouracil. These drugs are actively concentrated in the thyroid gland, where they inhibit the synthesis of thyroid hormones. A 3-year evaluation found methimazole to be better tolerated and safer than propylthiouracil in cats and this drug is now considered the antithyroid drug of choice for both pre-operative and long-term medical management of feline hyperthyroidism (Peterson *et al.*, 1988). Initially, methimazole should be administered at a dose of 10–15 mg/day, depending on the severity of the disease. This dosage ensures that serum T_4 concentrations will decrease to normal or low values within 2–3 weeks of starting treatment in most cats. Cats should be rechecked every 2–3 weeks and blood collected for measurement of serum T_4 concentration and complete blood and platelet counts. Surgery can be performed once serum T_4 concentration has decreased to normal or low (usually within 2–4 weeks). Surgical risks in cats with subnormal circulating T_4 concentrations do not appear to be increased, probably because normal T_3 concentrations are maintained in these cats. The last dose of methimazole should be administered on the morning of surgery (Peterson & Randolph, 1989). Once cats are rendered euthyroid, cardiovascular signs associated with hyperthyroidism are significantly reduced or eliminated.

Since hyperthyroidism is a multisystemic disease in which cardiovascular, respiratory, renal and liver functions may all be seriously compromised, it is important that the clinical examination, laboratory data and other diagnostic tests accurately define the involvement of these body systems. Full haematological and biochemical examination, an electrocardiogram and serum thyroid hormone measurement are essential in all cases. Cats with cardiac abnormalities on auscultation or ECG, should have further cardiac investigation, which may include thoracic radiography and echocardiography. Even the thyrotoxic cat without obvious cardiac disease may benefit from complete cardiac evaluation, including ECG, radiographs and echocardiography, to exclude subclinical cardiac problems (Feldman & Nelson, 1987). Management of cardiac problems before or at the same time as management of the thyroid problem may prevent serious complications (Feldman & Nelson, 1987).

If pleural effusion is severe, thoracocentesis should be carried out and diuretics (frusemide, 1 mg/kg BID or TID) should be administered to aid in removal of oedema or effusion. If the cat has hypertrophy with increased contractility, sinus or atrial tachycardia and pulmonary oedema, management should include cage rest and administration of propranolol, as well as a diuretic (Gompf, 1991). When propranolol is used, an oral dose of 2.5–5.0 mg BID or TID is adjusted to maintain heart rate at less than 120 beats/min. If the cat has evidence of cardiac dilation with poor contractility and pleural effusion, propranolol should not be given, but administration of digoxin and captopril may prove beneficial (Peterson *et al.*, 1988).

If anaesthesia is required without time to render the patient euthyroid and the cat does not have heart failure with poor contractility, the peripheral manifestations of hyperthyroidism can be dramatically improved within a few days of initiation of therapy with propranolol. The chronotropic and inotropic manifestations of excess hormone secretion are decreased and left ventricular efficiency is enhanced. Cardiac output is reduced but oxygen consumption remains unchanged (Stehling & Roizen, 1989). In addition, treatment with a β-adrenergic blocking drug helps prevent the arrhythmias that commonly develop during the anaesthetic period in untreated cats with hyperthyroidism (Peterson & Ferguson, 1989).

Anaesthetic and Intra-operative Management

If the cat has been rendered euthyroid, the risks of anaesthesia are reduced and many drugs can be tolerated if cardiac involvement is minimal. The safest approach is to sedate the cat to avoid excitement and sympathetic nervous system stimulation, choose less arrhythmogenic anaesthetic drugs, monitor the patient closely and be prepared to treat arrhythmias should they arise.

Cats are generally premedicated with a μ-agonist opioid, such as oxymorphone (0.05 mg/kg or methadone 0.2 mg/kg subcutaneously). Although sedation is slight, analgesia is pronounced and cats will tolerate intravenous (i/v) catheterization with very minimal restraint. Acepromazine (0.05 mg/kg subcutaneously) has been recommended as a useful premedicant in these cats because it decreases the incidence of epinephrine-induced arrhythmias in the presence of thiobarbiturates and inhalation agents (Muir *et al.*, 1975) although sedation is often unreliable in cats. However, acepromazine (0.1 mg/kg), in combination with an opioid such as oxymorphone (0.1 mg/kg), has been reported to provide excellent restraining conditions in these often excitable cats (Mason & Atkins, 1991). Xylazine, which increases myocardial sensitivity to arrhythmic effects of catecholamines (Muir *et al.*, 1975), should be avoided. It is usually suggested that anticholinergics such as atropine should be omitted because they induce sinus tachycardia and enhance anaesthetic-induced arrhythmias. Glycopyrrolate (0.01 mg/kg subcutaneously) can be used since it has minimal effects on cardiac rate and rhythm (Short & Miller, 1978).

Intravenous induction is generally preferred to mask or chamber induction so that struggling and thus catecholamine release are minimized. In cats without heart failure, thiobarbiturates (thiopentone sodium, ≤10 mg/kg or thiamylal sodium, ≤10 mg/kg) are considered suitable agents because they provide a smooth induction without catecholamine release (Joyce *et al.*,

1983). Diazepam (0.5 mg/kg) can be administered in combination with thiobarbiturates, to decrease the dose of thiobarbiturate and slightly prolong the duration of action. Another often quoted advantage of barbiturates is their antithyroid activity, presumably related to their thiocarbamate structure which induces an immediate dose-related impairment of thyroid activity (Wase & Foster, 1956). Intraperitoneal thiopentone (40 mg/kg) was reported to cause 80% impairment of thyroid activity, which required 6–7 days for full recovery (Wase & Foster, 1956). Thiobarbiturates are also arrhythmogenic (Hayashi *et al.*, 1989) and should be avoided in patients with pre-existing arrhythmias.

In the UK the steroid mixture Saffan has been widely used to induce anaesthesia (see Chapter 8). Small doses of Saffan (up to 2 mg/kg) do not cause significant arterial hypotension and although not devoid of anaphylactoid side-effects (see Chapter 12), its use has not been associated with any increased mortality in hyperthyroid cats with heart failure or arrhythmias (Editor, pers. commum.). There is anecdotal evidence that propofol has also been used quite safely and satisfactorily. Both Saffan and propofol will produce a smooth, rapid induction of anaesthesia when administered intravenously to a properly handled cat (Editor, Pers. commum.).

At Davis, in cats with heart failure or arrhythmias, anaesthesia is induced with etomidate (1 mg/kg) and diazepam (0.5 mg/kg). Etomidate has minimal effects on cardiovascular and respiratory function (Nagel *et al.*, 1979) and, in combination with diazepam, provides a smooth, rapid induction. Etomidate blocks cortisol production for 2–3 h following administration (Kruse-Elliott *et al.*, 1987); however, this is not generally a problem provided it is used only for induction of anaesthesia. The dissociatives ketamine and tiletamine should be avoided because they stimulate the sympathetic nervous system (Wong & Jenkins, 1974).

All cats should be intubated and anaesthesia maintained with inhalant agents. The vocal cords should be sprayed with lignocaine to aid intubation and attenuate catecholamine release. The tip of the orotracheal tube should extend beyond the surgical site to prevent obstruction during retraction and dissection. The goals during maintenance of anaesthesia are to avoid administration of drugs which sensitize the heart to catecholamines and to provide a depth of anaesthesia which prevents exaggerated responses to surgical stimulation. Isoflurane is the preferred inhalant for these reasons, as well as because liver blood flow is better preserved (Gelman *et al.*, 1984). Since cats under inhalants alone respond to surgical stimulation with increases in heart rate and arterial blood pressure, nitrous oxide can be added to provide greater stability. Although nitrous oxide is reported to cause sympathetic stimulation, it is not contraindicated in thyrotoxic people (Stoelting *et al.*, 1988). The possibility of organ toxicity due to altered or accelerated drug metabolism in the presence of hyperthyroidism must be considered. Exposure of triiodothyronine-treated rats to halothane, enflurane or isoflurane resulted in hepatic centrilobular necrosis in 92, 24 and 28% of animals, respectively (Berman *et al.*, 1983). Despite the clinical impression of increased anaesthetic need in patients with hyperthyroidism, anaesthetic requirements for halothane were found to be unchanged in hyperthyroid dogs (Babad & Eger, 1968). Increased cardiac output caused by hyperthyroidism will slow the induction of anaesthesia with inhalation agents and this is the most likely reason for the clinical impression of increased anaesthetic requirement.

While muscle relaxants are rarely required for thyroidectomy, they could be needed as part of emergency management of the hyperthyroid cat and selection is important if their use is considered (see chapter 8). Drugs, like vecuronium (50 µg/kg, i/v) or atracurium (0.25 mg/kg), which have minimal effects on the cardiovascular system (Stoelting, 1991) are to be considered as the agents of choice. Drugs such as pancuronium, which increase heart rate and activate the sympathetic nervous system (Stoelting, 1991), or d-tubocurarine and to a lesser extent metocurine, which cause histamine release (Stoelting, 1991), are undesirable. Reversal of neuromuscular blockade induced by non-depolarizing drugs using anticholinesterase drugs combined with anticholinergic drugs raises the question about drug-induced tachycardia. In this case, glycopyrrolate, which has less chronotropic effect than atropine, would be the more appropriate anticholinergic drug. Alternatively, edrophonium can be used for reversal and, if administered slowly, a significant decrease in heart rate rarely occurs.

Monitoring and Management of Problems arising under Anaesthesia

Monitoring should be directed towards the cardiovascular system as arrhythmias and cardiac arrest are the most common causes of mortality during surgery (Feldman & Nelson, 1987). Prior to induction, ECG limb leads and a doppler crystal and cuff are placed provided the cat does not become stressed. These allow the heart rate and rhythm to be assessed, the pulse rhythm to be heard and systolic blood pressure to be measured indirectly. A peripheral catheter is placed for administration of anaesthetic drugs, replacement fluids and emergency drugs. Hypoxaemia should be avoided by oxygenation via a face mask during induction if this can be accomplished without provoking resentment in the cat. Once anaesthesia has been induced and the trachea intubated, an oesophageal stethoscope should be introduced to monitor heart sounds, the ECG limb leads can be changed to an oesophageal ECG lead, an oesophageal thermistor probe can be placed to monitor body temperature and hypercarbia can be avoided by controlling ventilation with a respirator.

During the maintenance of anaesthesia, a balanced electrolyte replacement solution should be administered. The rate of fluid administration will depend on the cardiovascular status of the patient (conservative, 3–5 ml/kg/h, if heart failure is present) and the need of the patient (10–20 ml/kg bolus if significant blood loss occurs).

If heart failure is present, direct measurement of arterial blood pressure is considered helpful to determine the need for more aggressive management and the response to treatment. Measurement can be carried out from a percutaneously placed catheter in the dorsal pedal artery or from a catheter placed in the femoral artery via a cut-down (see Chapter 10). Another advantage of an arterial catheter is the ability to measure arterial blood-gas and pH status. This enables one to recognize and treat hypoxaemia and/or hypercarbia, two situations likely to increase the incidence of arrhythmias in hyperthyroid patients.

Since hyperthyroid cats are likely to have multisystemic disease, recognition and treatment of hypotension is important to prevent postanaesthetic organ dysfunction. Hyperthyroid patients may have exaggerated responsiveness to catecholamines and reduced doses of direct-acting vasopressors such as phenylephrine may be a more logical selection than ephedrine, which acts in part by provoking release of catecholamines (Stoelting *et al.*, 1988). Since some cats have a degree of renal insufficiency, preservation of renal blood flow during anaesthesia is important. In those cats with elevated serum concentrations of creatinine and BUN, infusion of a low dose of dopamine (2 μg/kg/min) can be administered to attempt to increase renal blood flow (Schwartz & Gewertz, 1988) and hypotension should be managed aggressively.

Since arrhythmias can precede cardiac arrest in the hyperthyroid patient, early recognition and treatment of them is imperative. In these cats, arrhythmias can usually be controlled by administration of β-adrenergic blocking agents, such as propranolol or esmolol. Propranolol (0.25 mg) is administered as an intravenous bolus to control tachyarrhythmias. Usually one dose is beneficial and effects will last 10–30 min. If arrhythmias recur, the dose of propranolol can be repeated. Esmolol, a newer agent, has the advantage of being a shorter acting agent and having very little β2 activity. It is administered as a loading dose (100–500 μg/kg, i/v) followed by an infusion (50–70 μg/kg/min) and its effects can be terminated rapidly if needed.

Cats, because of a large surface area relative to their small body size, rapidly lose body heat under anaesthesia (see Chapter 12). Hyperthyroid cats tend to be thin with little body fat and therefore, will lose body heat at a greater rate. The cat should be placed on a warming pad immediately after induction and maintained on this into the postanaesthetic period. During thyroidectomy, the surgical site is relatively small, and a second warming pad can be placed over the thorax and abdomen. Intravenous fluids and the inspired gases can also be warmed by placing fluid and gas lines under hot water containers. Oesophageal or rectal temperature should be continuously monitored during anaesthesia (Chapter 10).

Postoperative Management

Many potential complications are associated with thyroidectomy (Peterson, 1984) including hypoparathyroidism, Horner's syndrome, vocal cord paralysis, haematoma formation and airway obstruction.

The most serious complication is hypocalcaemia, which develops after the parathyroid glands are injured, devascularized or inadvertently removed in the course of bilateral thyroidectomy. After bilateral thyroidectomy, serum calcium concentration should be monitored on a daily basis for 4–7 days or until it has stabilized within the normal range (Feldman & Nelson, 1987). Thyrotoxicosis depletes bone calcium concentrations and following successful surgery, the serum calcium concentration may decline below normal for several days as skeletal reserves are restored (McDougall, 1981). This mild hypocalcaemia (serum calcium concentration 1.75–2.25 mmol/l) must be differentiated from severe, acute hypocalcaemia (serum calcium concentration < 1.75 mmol/l) associated with iatrogenic hypoparathyroidism. In the latter case, clinical signs associated with hypocalcaemia will develop within 1–3 days of surgery. If clinical signs of restlessness, abnormal behaviour, muscle cramping or muscle pain, muscle tremors, tetany or convulsions develop, in association with a serum calcium concentration of < 1.75 mmol/l, the cat should be treated (Feldman & Nelson, 1987). Severe tetany should be treated by administration of calcium gluconate intravenously to effect, with ECG monitoring for bradycardia. Tetany can then be controlled by the same dose of calcium gluconate diluted with an equal amount of normal saline and administered subcutaneously, three to four times daily (Feldman & Nelson, 1987). Cats with less severe signs should be treated with oral vitamin D and calcium supplementation (Feldman & Nelson, 1987). Plasma thyroid hormone concentrations decline, often to subnormal levels, within 24–72 h of a total thyroidectomy. This is not, however, an absolute indication to initiate thyroid hormone supplementation (Feldman & Nelson, 1987). Thyroid hormone levels should be checked 1 week after total thyroidectomy and if T_4 is < 12.87 nmol/l, supplementation with L-thyroxine should be started. If T_4 is > 12.87 nmol/l then the level should be checked again in 2 weeks (Nelson, 1993 pers. commum.).

Bilateral recurrent laryngeal nerve injury causes stridor and laryngeal obstruction due to unopposed adduction of the vocal cords and closure of the glottic aperture. Immediate endotracheal intubation is necessary to establish an airway, usually followed by tracheostomy (Roizen, 1990). Unilateral recurrent nerve injury usually goes unnoticed. If laryngeal nerve damage is suspected, function can be assessed at the end of surgery by placing the patient in sternal recumbency and viewing arytenoid cartilage movement during a light plane of anaesthesia.

Postoperative bleeding can lead to haematoma formation which can compromise the airway. If this occurs, the cat should be re-anaesthetized, the surgical area explored and all bleeding vessels ligated.

Urethral Obstruction

Disease of the lower urinary tract is a common health problem in cats. The reported incidence varies from 52 to 85 new cases per 10 000 cats each year (Fennell, 1975; Lawler *et al.*, 1985). The reported proportional morbidity rate in both male and female cats varies from 1 to 6% (Lees *et al.*, 1989). Males and females have similar risks of occurrence of non-obstructive forms of feline urologic syndrome (FUS), but urethral obstruction is almost exclusively an affliction of male cats. Occurrence is highly age-related; lower urinary tract disorders are diagnosed predominantly in cats aged 2–6 years. Urinary tract diseases can be categorized into one of several clinical syndromes based on how they are encountered in small animal practice (Lees *et*

al., 1989). Acute urethral obstruction can be life-threatening and can induce acute renal failure, while chronic partial obstruction can reduce renal function. Male cats presenting with acute urethral obstruction require some form of restraint, usually chemical in nature, to enable urine flow to be restored.

Clinical Signs and Laboratory Findings Relevant to Anaesthetic Management

Acute urethral obstruction induces bladder distension with increased bladder wall tension and intravesical pressure, and may cause haemorrhage and necrosis. The increased intravesical pressure is transmitted to the renal tubules where increased intratubular hydrostatic pressure reduces glomerular filtration rate. Altered regulation of renal blood flow also causes vasoconstriction of preglomerular vessels which reduces glomerular filtration rate. As complete obstruction continues, blood flow decreases and by 24 h only 50–60% is present (Bovee, 1982). After relief of acute obstruction, renal blood flow slowly returns and is approximately 60% of control levels after 24 h, but may take 2–3 days to return to normal (Bovee, 1982). Glomerular filtration rate is also affected, and after relief of a 24-h complete obstruction, is only approximately 40% of normal (Bovee, 1982). Even after 2–3 days, glomerular filtration rate remains decreased, due most probably to decreased resistance in the efferent glomerular arterioles (Bovee, 1982). The decrease in glomerular filtration rate that occurs with short periods of obstruction (24–36 h) is completely reversible (Klahr, 1983) however longer periods (72 to 96 hours) result in permanent loss of renal function (Klahr, 1983). With chronic partial obstruction, renal blood flow decreases progressively and after days to weeks glomerular filtration rate is variably reduced from 20 to 70% of normal. Thus, depending on the duration and degree of obstruction, renal function may be significantly reduced. An important anaesthetic consideration in these patients is to preserve existing renal function and prevent any further loss.

Hyperkalaemia is the most important abnormality associated with complete obstruction because this electrolyte abnormality may cause life-threatening cardiac arrhythmias. In experimental studies, the serum potassium concentration 48 h after obstruction was 7.6 ± 2.4 mmol/l, while at 72 h it was 10.9 ± 4.2 mmol/l (Finco & Cornelius, 1977). The first clinical signs of hyperkalaemia are usually weakness, absence of reflexes and other neuromuscular malfunctions which eventually lead to muscular and respiratory paralysis. At concentrations greater than 7 mmol/l, potassium causes progressive depression in excitability and conduction velocity (Schaer, 1977). The electrocardiographic abnormalities (Fig. 11.2) include peaking of the T wave, shortening and widening of the P wave, prolongation of the P–R interval, eventual disappearance of the P wave, widening of the QRS complex and irregular RR intervals, and sine wave type QRS complexes (Schaer, 1977). When the serum potassium concentration exceeds 8–9 mmol/l, sequential cardiac conduction abnormalities occur including delays at the atrioventricular junction, in the His–Purkinje system and in ventricular muscle. These conduction defects cause the heart block, idioventricular complexes and various escape beats and rhythms which appear on the electrocardiogram. Eventually, severe hyperkalaemia culminates in ventricular fibrillation or asystole (Schaer, 1977). The prompt recognition and treatment of arrhythmias frequently determine success or failure in the management of the critically ill patient (Schaer, 1975). Exposure of hyperkalaemic cats to anaesthetic agents may further aggravate cardiovascular depression and result in cardiac arrest (Raffe & Caywood,

1984). An essential part of the pre-anaesthetic preparation is to reduce the serum potassium concentration prior to administration of anaesthetic agents. Anaesthesia should be deferred until serum potassium concentrations are less than 6 mmol/l, especially in elective surgery (Schaer, 1975).

Other electrolyte abnormalities include hyperphosphataemia, hypermagnesaemia, hypocalcaemia and hyponatraemia (Schaer, 1977). Hypocalcaemia is usually mild and signs are rarely present because acidosis increases the ionized fraction (Lees *et al.*, 1989). Hyponatraemia is also mild and unlikely to pose a threat to the cat's life (Finco & Cornelius, 1977).

Cats with urethral obstruction have varying degrees of dehydration, evident clinically as well as by an increase in total protein concentration and a loss of body weight (Lees *et al.*, 1989). Correction of body fluid deficits prior to induction of anaesthesia is necessary because anaesthetic-induced peripheral vasodilation and myocardial depression accentuate pre-existing fluid deficits and may cause profound hypotension (Ilkiw, 1982).

Acidaemia occurs in obstructive uropathy and has important direct and indirect effects. Direct effects include decreased myocardial contractility, stroke volume and cardiac output; excitable membrane alterations leading to arrhythmias; central nervous system depression and dysfunction of metabolic pathways (Schaer, 1975). Indirect effects of acidaemia include alterations in transcellular potassium distribution; plasma protein binding; ionization of pharmacologic agents; activity of 2,3 DPG affecting oxygen

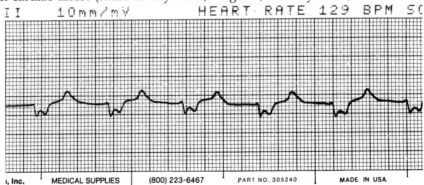

Fig. 11.2 Electrocardiogram from a cat with hyperkalaemia (plasma potassium concentration 9.1 mmol/l) showing absence of P waves, increased duration of QRS and increased voltage of T wave.

transport; tissue catabolism and parasympathetic activity (Schaer, 1975). Because of its far-reaching effects, acidaemia should be corrected prior to inducing anaesthesia (Schaer, 1975).

Elevation of blood urea nitrogen concentration occurs in obstructive uropathy. In one study, the blood urea nitrogen was 57 ± 39 mmol/l and 71 ± 37 mmol/l after obstructions of 48 and 72 h, respectively (Finco & Cornelius, 1977). Uraemic 'toxaemia' causes central nervous system and myocardial depression. In uraemia, the effects of general anaesthetic agents are potentiated and drug dosages should be decreased (Haskins, 1992).

Pre-anaesthetic Assessment and Preparation of the Patient

Fluid therapy and restoration of urine flow are the most important components of therapy for cats with urethral obstruction. In uraemic cats both are essential, as in one study 10 of 13 cats treated only by relief of obstruction died, whereas all cats treated by relief of obstruction and fluid therapy survived (Finco & Cornelius, 1977). Thus, fluid therapy should be started before unblocking the urethra, particularly in cats with severe signs (Lees *et al*, 1989). Knowledge of the duration of the obstruction and physical condition of the patient are essential. Generally, obstruction of less than 6 h does not affect homeostasis and patients can be anaesthetized in a routine manner (Raffe & Caywood, 1984). Cats with obstruction of 6–24 h need to be evaluated and stabilized on an individual basis, while cats with prolonged obstruction (greater than 24 h) should be stabilized prior to anaesthesia (Raffe & Caywood, 1984).

Before treatment is undertaken, blood should be collected for haematocrit, total protein, blood urea nitrogen, creatinine, serum electrolytes and, if possible, blood-gas and acid–base status. An electrocardiogram will allow the clinician to identify cats with cardiotoxic signs and serial electrocardiograms will allow assessment of therapy for hyperkalaemia. A catheter should be placed percutaneously into a peripheral vein for administration of fluids and drugs.

Hyperkalaemia can affect patient outcome when abnormal cardiac complexes and arrhythmias accompany serum potassium levels exceeding 8.0 mmol/l. Treatment regimes for hyperkalaemia include rapid volume replacement and/or administration of calcium gluconate, sodium bicarbonate, glucose or insulin and glucose. Rapid volume replacement will decrease serum potassium by dilution. Although potassium-free solutions have a greater dilutional effect on hyperkalaemia, lactated Ringer's solution is reported to combat hyperkalaemia by dilution (Lees *et al.*, 1989). One problem with administration of large quantities of fluid prior to removal of the obstruction is the risk of pulmonary oedema. Calcium is the physiological antagonist of the effects of hyperkalaemia on the heart and administration can be life-saving in severely hyperkalaemic cats. A dose of 0.5–1.0 ml/kg of 10% calcium gluconate should be titrated to effect slowly intravenously over 10 min with careful electrocardiographic monitoring to avoid bradycardia (Schaer, 1977). Although this treatment does not change serum potassium concentrations, it does gain time while other treatments are taking effect. Another treatment involves alleviating the metabolic acidaemia by intravenous administration of sodium bicarbonate. Treatment of acidaemia helps to decrease serum potassium concentration because part of the hyperkalaemia is induced by potassium ions moving extracellularly in exchange for hydrogen ions which are buffered intracellularly. If a laboratory measurement of base deficit is available, it can be used to calculate the amount of bicarbonate to be administered (see Chapter 13). The total calculated dose (mmol) of sodium bicarbonate is generally calculated using the formula: 0.3 × base deficit × cat's body weight (kg). Usually, one half of the calculated amount is administered over 20 min and the base deficit reassessed. Alternatively, the base deficit can be estimated on the basis of the relative magnitude of azotaemia and uraemia. A moderate base deficit (10 mmol/l) is expected with moderate azotaemia and uraemia, while a severe base deficit (15 mmol/l) is expected with severe azotaemia and uraemia (Lees *et al.*, 1989). Insulin-mediated transport of glucose into cells also moves potassium ions intracellularly, thereby lowering the serum potassium concentration. While some advocate administration of both dextrose and insulin (Schaer, 1975) others have found administration of dextrose alone to decrease serum potassium concentration due to endogenous insulin release (Lees *et al.*, 1989). With the first regime, a total dose of 0.5 units of regular insulin/kg is added to lactated Ringer's solution, together with 2 g of dextrose/unit of insulin. The fluids are administered so that 40% of the estimated deficit from dehydration is administered over the first few hours (Schaer, 1975). In the second regime, the initial fluid deficit is replaced using a solution which is made with half 0.45% saline and half dextrose 5% (Lees *et al.*, 1989).

If cats are not depressed, hyperkalaemic or uraemic, a balanced electrolyte solution, such as lactated Ringer's solution can be administered subcutaneously. Approximately 90 ml/kg, divided into three daily doses, has been recommended until the patient is no longer azotaemic and then tapered off over 1–3 days (Barsanti & Finco, 1984). In sicker cats, the amount of fluid to be administered depends on the severity of the dehydration, uraemic signs and hyperkalaemia. One recommendation is to deliver over 2–4 h a quantity of fluid equal to 5% of body weight if signs are mild, 8% if moderate and 12% if severe (Barsanti & Finco, 1984). However, these are guidelines only and actual volumes should be given according to individual requirements based on vital signs, hydration status and urine output.

Anaesthetic Management

Even in healthy animals, general anaesthesia depresses renal function by decreasing renal blood flow, glomerular filtration rate and electrolyte excretion and by increasing renal vascular resistance (Benson & Thurmon, 1987) (Chapter 2). This is due to both direct and indirect effects on renal function, with indirect effects thought to play a more important role. Indirect effects include changes in cardiovascular function as well as in sympathetic system and endocrine activity, while anaesthetic agents can directly affect tubular transport mechanisms. After short uncomplicated anaesthesia,

renal blood flow and glomerular filtration rate return to normal within a few hours. However, in the obstructed patient where renal blood flow and glomerular filtration are already decreased, the added depression induced by anaesthesia may have profound effects and every effort should be made to minimize these changes.

Generally, only a short period of restraint is needed to relieve the obstruction. Physical restraint alone or in combination with topical local anaesthetic may be sufficient in cats which are either severely weak from hyperkalaemia or very docile. Wrapping these cats in a towel or a cat restraining bag may help to protect the patient and veterinary staff (see Chapter 5).

A premedicant such as a μ-opioid agonist (for instance, oxymorphone, 0.05 mg/kg subcutaneously or methadone 0.1 mg/kg s/c or i/m), may be administered to smooth induction and recovery and to decrease the dose of anaesthetic agents. As uraemic people have been reported to succumb to vagally mediated cardiac arrest, an anticholinergic such as glycopyrrolate has been recommended for these cats (Haskins, 1992). Cats with minimal abnormalities can usually be restrained by intravenous administration of low dose ketamine (1–3 mg/kg) and diazepam (0.2–0.5 mg/kg) to effect. The administration of the dissociative agents, ketamine and tiletamine, to cats with renal failure is controversial. Pharmacokinetic studies following ketamine administration to cats found that the majority of the administered dose was eliminated unchanged by the kidneys (Baggot & Blake, 1976). This led to the initial recommendation that these agents should not be administered to cats with renal insufficiency. However, more recent pharmacokinetic studies after intramuscular (i/m) administration of ketamine reported recovery of cats prior to detection of ketamine or its metabolite in urine. The author of this study concluded that recovery from ketamine was due to redistribution of the drug, rather than metabolism (Waterman, 1983). Experience at Davis indicates that ketamine, in low doses, is a suitable agent for cats with urethral obstruction, provided they do not have significant renal failure and that they are given fluids as part of the management. Prolonged recoveries and mortality have occurred following induction of anaesthesia using ketamine or tiletamine in cats with advanced renal failure. Other induction agents, such as thiobarbiturates, have been recommended (Raffe & Caywood, 1984) but are best used only in cats which have normal homeostasis. Increased toxicity has been associated with administration of thiobarbiturates due to an increase in the non-ionized and unbound portion of the drug from metabolic acidosis, as well as increased permeability of the blood–brain barrier and disturbed cerebral metabolism in uraemia. Also, barbiturates are arrhythmogenic drugs and their use would be likely to exacerbate cardiac abnormalities.

Another suitable technique, provided excitement can be minimized, is mask or chamber induction and maintenance with the inhalant, isoflurane (Raffe & Caywood, 1984). Xylazine is not recommended for restraint because of adverse effects on cardiac rhythm, rate and output (Kolata, 1984).

Saffan, a mixture of the two steroids, alphaxalone and alphadolone (Chapters 8 and 12), has been used quite successfully for the induction of anaesthesia in uraemic cats and has the advantage of having minimal hypotensive effects provided the dose given does not exceed 2 mg/kg (total steroid). Reactions to Saffan, either to the steroids themselves or to the vehicle in which they are dissolved, have been described (Chapter 12) but, nevertheless, it has been shown to be a surprisingly safe anaesthetic for sick cats (Clarke & Hall, 1990). In critically ill cats propofol appears to be equally satisfactory when given slowly and in doses titrated to effect, but much more experience of the effects of this agent in cats is needed before its place can be firmly established (Editor, pers. comm.).

In critically ill, moribund cats which need chemical restraint, the preferred technique at Davis is to induce anaesthesia with a low dose of etomidate (0.5 mg/kg) and diazepam (0.5 mg/kg) titrated intravenously to effect. Although these drugs are injected into the intravenous delivery line during administration of fluid some haemolysis has been seen, especially in cats which are uraemic. This probably occurs because of the high osmolality of the etomidate solution.

Generally, because the surgical procedure is accomplished quickly, cats are not intubated and maintenance agents are not required. If the cat has systemic illness, it is best to intubate the trachea so that an oxygen-enriched gas can be delivered and the cat's lungs can be ventilated if necessary. Both hypoxaemia and hypercapnia should be avoided as they are likely to increase the incidence of arrhythmias. If a longer period of time is required, anaesthesia can be maintained with an inhalation agent. Isoflurane is preferable to halothane if arrhythmias are present. Methoxyflurane is not recommended because it has a nephrotoxic metabolite which may accentuate the tubular damage induced by prolonged urethral obstruction (Kolata, 1984).

Monitoring and Management of Problems arising under Anaesthesia

Monitoring should be directed towards recognition of arrhythmias and hypotension (see Chapter 10). Limb leads for ECG monitoring should be placed prior to administration of anaesthetic drugs. A doppler crystal and cuff can also be placed prior to induction and can be used to monitor systolic arterial blood pressure prior to and during maintenance of anaesthesia. Throughout the procedure, systolic arterial blood pressure should be maintained at 90 mmHg or greater to ensure adequate renal perfusion. If systolic arterial blood pressure falls below 90 mmHg, anaesthesia should be lightened, a fluid bolus should be administered and administration of an inotrope (dopamine, 5 μg/kg/min i/v) should be considered. The cat should be cocooned in a circulating warm water blanket to prevent hypothermia. Measurement of urine production, utilizing a closed technique following catheterization (Chapter 13), provides an index of renal function and should be > 1 ml/kg/h. If oliguria develops or persists despite adequate fluid therapy, other measures such as loop diuretics (frusemide, bolus 0.1 mg/kg followed by infusion 0.1 mg/kg/h, i/v) osmotic agents (mannitol, 0.25 mg/kg over 20 min i/v) or low-dose dopamine (2–3 μg/kg/min i/v) should be tried.

Postanaesthetic Management

Fluid therapy should be continued until azotaemia is resolved. Some cats will undergo a marked diuresis (postobstructive diuresis) following relief of the obstruction. This is believed to be due to both clearance of accumulated metabolites and transient inability of the proximal tubules to concentrate urine effectively. Substantial losses of water, sodium and potassium can occur during this diuresis and, since it may lead to volume depletion and reduced renal function, it is important that it be identified and adequate amounts of fluids administered. Measurement of urine volume every 2–4 h will help to identify diuresis and can be used to calculate fluid requirements.

Haematocrit, total protein, blood urea nitrogen, creatinine and serum electrolyte concentrations should be reassessed as needed to ensure adequate hydration and recovery of renal function. The time interval between measurements will depend on the degree of uraemia and the response to therapy.

Idiopathic Hepatic Lipidosis

Idiopathic hepatic lipidosis is the most commonly recognized hepatobiliary disorder in cats (fatty liver syndrome, see Chapter 4). No age, sex or breed predisposition has been found, but obesity appears to be a common underlying factor. Typically, the cat has been inappetant or eating very little for 5–7 weeks prior to presentation. Sometimes the onset of anorexia is preceded by a recognized stressful event. The syndrome can be defined as an acquired disorder of metabolism resulting in hepatocellular accumulation of triglycerides in quantities sufficient to be visible by light microscopy (Center, 1986). On post-mortem examination, the liver is yellow and greasy, has rounded edges and is often friable. Histology of abnormal hepatocytes reveals two forms of vacuolization: macrovesicular and microvesicular. Excessive accumulation of fat may induce cell necrosis; before that stage, liver damage appears to be reversible (Biourge *et al.*, 1990). The

pathogenesis of the disease is still not known but hepatic lipid may accumulate because fatty acid delivery to the liver is excessive, β-oxidation of fatty acids is impaired or transport of fat out of the liver is impaired (Jacobs *et al.*, 1990). Current theories include: chronic anorexia, protein-calorie malnutrition, amino acid deficiency and obesity (Zawie & Shaker, 1989).

Confirmation of hepatic lipidosis requires histopathologic examination of liver tissue and usually some form of chemical restraint is needed to obtain an ultrasound guided liver biopsy. Treatment of cats with idiopathic hepatic lipidosis involves proper fluid and nutritional therapy (see Chapter 13) and these cats also require anaesthesia for percutaneous tube gastrostomy to allow enteral feeding.

Clinical Signs and Laboratory Findings Relevant to Anaesthetic Management

Since these cats have not eaten for a period of time, they have significant weight loss, which may be extreme. Muscle wasting is evident and although appendicular and truncal fat stores may be depleted, abdominal and thoracic fat may be spared. They generally have an unkempt appearance and hair may be matted. These changes in body weight and composition will make the cats more susceptible to hypothermia under anaesthesia and in some cases change the pharmacokinetics of anaesthetic agents. Recovery from induction doses of thiobarbiturates in cachectic patients is liable to be prolonged (unpublished observations).

Many cats with hepatic lipidosis are chronically debilitated. Vomiting, diarrhoea, chronic anorexia and reluctance to drink all contribute to the dehydration in these animals (Center, 1991). Correction of body fluid deficits prior to induction of anaesthesia is necessary to prevent profound hypotension from anaesthetic-induced peripheral vasodilation and myocardial depression.

Most cats have varying degrees of anaemia which may be non-regenerative in nature. Both bone marrow depression and erythrocyte destruction have been reported (Barsanti *et al.*, 1977). Coagulation disorders, although unusual, may develop in severe disease as a result of hepatic insufficiency. In these cases, surface haemorrhages, haematuria and gastrointestinal blood loss may be found.

Cats with severe lipidosis may demonstrate obvious hepatic encephalopathy. In one study, 25% of cats had some neurological deficit at presentation, while signs of central nervous system dysfunction developed in the remaining cats as the disease progressed (Burrows *et al.*, 1981). Encephalopathic signs may include lethargy, behavioural changes, intermittent blindness, dementia, ptyalism, seizures, rage and coma. Changes in response to anaesthetic drugs can occur through changes in receptors such as gamma aminobutyric acid (GABA) and opioid, as well as changes in neurotransmitters.

Cats with hepatic lipidosis have varying degrees of hepatic dysfunction. Virtually all cats develop increased activity of serum alkaline phosphatase (ALP). Many cats also develop increased serum activities of alanine aminotransferase (ALT) and aspartate amino-transferase (AST). The increase in gamma-glutamyltransferase (GGT) is usually less than that of ALP. Cats with moderate to severe disease usually are hyperbilirubinaemic and appear jaundiced. These changes induce decreased hepatocyte function and drugs that are dependent on the liver for metabolism or excretion should be avoided. Serum albumin and globulin concentrations are usually within the normal range, although hyperglobulinaemia may develop with chronically impaired hepatic function.

Hyperglycaemia has been recognized in some cats with hepatic lipidosis. Overt diabetes mellitus is not commonly associated with severe hepatic lipidosis in cats and glucose intolerance may be the result of changed concentrations of endogenous catecholamines and glucocorticoids.

Pre-anaesthetic Assessment and Preparation of the Patient

Since cats may present in various stages of hepatic disease, it is important that the degree of hepatic impairment is defined during pre-operative preparation. Blood should be collected for full haematological and biochemical examination. Evaluation of liver function may detect severe lipidosis even before hyperbilirubinaemia has developed. Serum bile acid concentrations after a 12-h fast and 2 h after a meal may be used to detect functional impairment. Bile acid concentrations exceeding 20 μmol/l indicate impaired hepatic function and warrant biopsy for histologic diagnosis of the underlying liver disorder (Center, 1991).

Confirmation of hepatic lipidosis requires histopathologic examination of liver tissue. The coagulation status must be evaluated prior to liver biopsy, especially if the patient is jaundiced (Center, 1991). This should include prothrombin time, partial thromboplastin time, fibrinogen concentration and a platelet count. Prolonged clotting times, a fibrinogen concentration less than 0.5 g/l or a platelet count less than 50 × 10^9/l should be corrected prior to liver biopsy by administration of a transfusion of fresh whole blood or platelet-rich plasma depending on the haematocrit. A haematocrit of 0.25 l/l is generally recommended as the minimum acceptable level prior to anaesthesia and surgery (Dodman *et al.*, 1987) although, in this disease, it is generally unnecessary to transfuse prior to induction of anaesthesia provided the haematocrit is above 0.20 l/l. A blood cross-match, however, is carried out on these cats prior to liver biopsy or tube gastrostomy placement.

Cats that are dehydrated should be rehydrated prior to induction of anaesthesia by intravenous administration of a balanced electrolyte solution with appropriate potassium supplementation. Serum electrolyte concentrations should be monitored to guide fluid supplementation. Administration of glucose as a calorie supplement should be avoided until a well balanced nutritional ration is successfully ingested (Center, 1991).

Anaesthesia and Liver Disease

In patients with normal liver function, anaesthesia and surgery uniformly and consistently lower hepatic blood flow. In most instances, the decrease in hepatic blood flow induced by anaesthesia parallels and is proportional to the decrease in systemic arterial pressure or cardiac output. Maintenance of an adequate circulating blood volume tends to mitigate against decreases in hepatic blood flow. In conscious animals, there is a semireciprocal relationship between portal venous and hepatic arterial blood flows. Thus, hepatic arterial blood flow is regulated in response to changes in portal venous blood flow to prevent or reduce wide fluctuations in total hepatic blood flow. Animal studies imply that during anaesthesia this relationship is still extant, so that hepatic arterial resistance decreases as portal and hepatic arterial flows decrease (Brown, 1989b). However, this may not hold true for the inhalation agents cyclopropane, halothane and methoxyflurane where resistance in the hepatic artery increased as portal venous flow decreased (Brown, 1989b). Changes in P_aCO_2 also affect liver blood flow; hypocapnia has been reported to decrease hepatic blood flow significantly, while hypercapnia has the opposite effect. In animals with severe liver disease, the autoregulatory ability of hepatic arterial blood flow to increase is diminished or abolished (Gelman & Ernst, 1982). Therefore, hepatic arterial blood flow may not increase when portal blood flow and/or oxygen content in portal venous blood decrease. Conditions such as arterial hypotension or a decrease in cardiac output should be avoided in order to prevent hepatic oxygen deprivation.

Involvement of the liver in pharmacokinetics is reflected by elimination of drugs by biotransformation or by excretion of unchanged drugs into the bile. The hepatic elimination of drugs can be affected by either changes in hepatic blood flow or changes in the ability of the liver cells to biotransform and/or excrete a given drug. Other mechanisms of altered pharmacokinetics in liver disease include changes in the binding of drugs to albumin and globulin, as well as changes in volume of distribution.

Pharmacodynamic observations in cats with hepatic disease are limited. As mentioned earlier, changes in cerebral sensitivity to drugs, such as opioids, benzodiazepines and barbiturates, may be due to an increase in the number of opioid and GABA receptors (Jones et al., 1984).

Owing to pharmacokinetic and pharmacodynamic alterations, the response of the cat with hepatic disease to a drug is virtually unpredictable. Therefore, each drug must be carefully selected and, more importantly, carefully titrated to the desirable effect (Gelman, 1989).

Anaesthetic Management and Monitoring

Cats are generally premedicated with a low dose of a μ-agonist opioid (e.g. oxymorphone, 0.03 mg/kg or methadone 0.1 mg/kg subcutaneously). Opioids have little effect on the liver, appear to be safe if a low dose is administered and provide both sedation and analgesia. An anticholinergic, such as atropine, is also administered and although the pharmacological action may be prolonged in severe liver disease, this is of little consequence (Dodman et al., 1987). Phenothiazine tranquillizers, such as acepromazine, are best avoided as they may lower systemic vascular resistance and arterial blood pressure. Also, seizures have been reported after acepromazine administration in dogs with hepatic encephalopathy.

Prior to induction, a venous catheter is placed percutaneously for drug and fluid administration. At Davis the induction technique of choice for percutaneous tube gastrostomy placement is administration of isoflurane via a face mask or cat box. Isoflurane is the inhalant of choice, as liver blood flow is thought to be better preserved with isoflurane than with halothane or methoxyflurane. Although portal blood flow decreases during isoflurane anaesthesia, the decrease is not as dramatic as with halothane, and hepatic arterial flow has been found to increase (Gelman et al., 1984). Also, only a small percentage of isoflurane (7% not recovered) is metabolized compared with halothane (50% not recovered) and methoxyflurane (77% not recovered) (Berman & Holaday, 1989). Alternatively, if an injectable technique is preferred, etomidate would be a suitable induction drug. Etomidate has a high clearance in cats and is rapidly metabolized (Wertz et al., 1990). Although no studies have been carried out in cats with liver disease, in people with cirrhosis, clearance was not affected (Van Been et al., 1983). Induction of anaesthesia with thiamylal, thiopentone or Saffan is probably best avoided as these agents may cause prolonged recovery in cachectic patients. Depending on the condition of the cat, ketamine and diazepam may not be a suitable induction technique. In cats with hepatic encephalopathy, the central stimulant action of ketamine may precipitate seizures (Dodman *et al.*, 1987) while the central depressant effects of diazepam may be accentuated. Signs of hepatic encephalopathy have been observed during recovery from ketamine and diazepam in a dog with severe liver disease and prolonged sedation, as well as apnoea, in cats given a single dose of diazepam. Once anaesthesia is induced, the trachea is intubated and anaesthesia maintained with isoflurane and oxygen.

Administration of a balanced electrolyte solution at 5–10 ml/kg/h during maintenance of anaesthesia will help offset some of the drug-induced decrease in hepatic blood flow. Systolic arterial blood pressure should be monitored using the Doppler technique and maintained at 90 mmHg or above. If systolic arterial blood pressure decreases to 80 mmHg or less, the inhalant anaesthetic concentration should be decreased and/or a fluid bolus should be administered (5 ml/kg over 10 min). If systolic pressure remains low, drug administration should be considered. Ephedrine (0.1 mg/kg i/v) is perhaps a better choice than dopamine as ephedrine increases hepatic blood flow slightly by lowering hepatic arterial resistance (Brown, 1989b) whereas dopamine constricts hepatic arterioles (Brown, 1989a). Alternatively, if the haematocrit is less than 0.251/l, systolic arterial blood pressure often responds better to infusion of blood than administration of a vasoconstricting agent.

The technique for percutaneous tube gastrostomy placement (Allan, 1991; Bright *et al.*, 1991) involves passage of a gastroscope through the mouth to the level of the stomach. The stomach is inflated to push the abdominal contents away from the gastrostomy site and bring the stomach wall in contact with the abdominal wall. During inflation of the stomach it is important to monitor the patient closely for hypotension due to pressure on the vena cava and hypoventilation due to pressure on the diaphragm inhibiting respiration. Before the scope is removed from the stomach all air should be evacuated.

Administration of low doses of ketamine and diazepam, sufficient for chemical restraint, is the most commonly used technique to allow ultrasound-guided liver biopsy. However, the adverse affects of this drug combination in patients with hepatic encephalopathy should be borne in mind.

Postanaesthetic Management

Maintenance fluids should be administered in the postanaesthetic period. Cats recovering from liver biopsy should be watched closely for signs of haemorrhage. Signs of haemorrhage may include a delayed awakening from anaesthesia, pale mucous membranes, slow capillary refill time, rapid heart rate, decreasing haematocrit and total protein and abdominal paracentesis which is positive for blood. Haemorrhage should be treated initially by transfusion with fresh whole blood and, if bleeding continues, exploratory laparotomy.

The only known treatment for cats with hepatic lipidosis is dietary support, hence tube gastrostomy placement. Once the cat has recovered from anaesthesia, supplementation of food via the tube can be started. Recommendations for nutritional management are available (Biourge *et al.*, 1990; Riggs, 1991).

Hypertrophic Cardiomyopathy

Cardiomyopathies represent the majority of feline cardiovascular diseases (see Chapter 4). An incidence of 8.5% was found in cats autopsied at the Animal Medical Center between 1962 and 1976, compared with an incidence of 1.9% for congenital heart disease (Lui, 1977). In 1987, a direct link between decreased taurine concentration in the myocardium and dilated cardiomyopathy was proposed (Pion *et al.*, 1987) and the concentration of taurine in commercial cat food was increased. The incidence of dilated cardiomyopathy in one echocardiographic study has fallen from 28% in 1986 to 6% in 1989 (Skiles *et al.*, 1990). Hypertrophic cardiomyopathy is now the most prevalent feline cardiac disorder, its relative importance having increased with the decline in dilated cardiomyopathy (Atkins & Snyder, 1991). In one study, the age (mean ± SD) of cats diagnosed with hypertrophic cardiomyopathy was found to be 6.5 ± 4.0 years, with a significantly greater incidence in neutered male cats compared with neutered female cats (3.1 times) (Atkins et al., 1992).

Since it is common for cats with hypertrophic cardiomyopathy to live for more than 2 years after an initial bout of pulmonary oedema, these cats often require anaesthesia for elective procedures such as prophylactic dentistry. In fact, many cats with hypertrophic cardiomyopathy may be asymptomatic unless their condition is complicated by such things as aortic thrombosis, atrial fibrillation, anaemia, anaesthesia or fluid administration (Bonagura, 1989). In these cats, special anaesthetic considerations are required to prevent overt signs of cardiac failure.

Pathophysiology, Clinical Signs and Laboratory Findings Relevant to Anaesthetic Management

Hypertrophic cardiomyopathy is characterized by increased muscle mass due to a hypertrophied non-dilated left ventricle (Fox, 1988). Global left ventricular diastolic function is adversely affected causing elevated left ventricular end-diastolic pressure in the face of a normal or reduced end-diastolic volume (Fox, 1988). A decrease in early rapid diastolic filling results from reduced ventricular compliance and prolonged relaxation. Increased muscle stiffness may be caused by fibrosis or myocardial cell disorganization, while ventricular chamber stiffness results from increased muscle stiffness and hypertrophy. Mitral regurgitation develops from distortional changes in the mitral valve apparatus caused by hypertrophy, or from interference with normal mitral valve closure due to anterior wall motion of the mitral valve during mid-systole. The left atrium dilates and hypertrophies in response to increased end-diastolic pressures and pulmonary venous pressures eventually increase. Chronic elevation of left atrial and pulmonary venous

pressures makes cats prone to pulmonary oedema. Tachycardia, which reduces ventricular filling time, and arrhythmias, such as atrial fibrillation, which diminish effective left atrial contraction, can cause florid pulmonary oedema (Atkins et al., 1992). In hypertrophic cardiomyopathy, left ventricular function is hyperdynamic and ventricular ejection may be nearly completed during the first third of the systolic ejection period. Asymmetric hypertrophic cardiomyopathy has been reported in about 40% of affected cats. The importance of this pathology lies in the greater potential for left ventricular outflow tract obstruction during systole. The obstruction occurs when the anterior leaflet of the mitral valve moves to contact the septum during systole (Bonagura, 1989). Myocardial ischaemia contributes to the pathogenesis of hypertrophic cardiomyopathy in both people and cats (Bright & Gloden, 1991). Ischaemia is believed to result from inadequate capillary density per unit myocardial mass, narrowing of the intramural coronary arteries, microvascular spasm, decreased coronary perfusion pressure and elevated left ventricular diastolic pressure (Bright & Gloden, 1991).

Most symptomatic cats have an audible gallop rhythm or systolic cardiac murmur. The murmur may be related to either mitral regurgitation or left ventricular outflow obstruction and may vary with changes in heart rate, ventilation or body position. Audible crackles over the lung fields are suggestive of pulmonary oedema. A common presenting sign for cats with hypertrophic cardiomyopathy is acute dyspnoea from pulmonary oedema. Although these cats rarely require anaesthesia at presentation, they will often need anaesthesia at a future date and, at that time, it is important to ascertain whether pulmonary oedema has been a feature of the disease. Laboratory tests are usually normal unless there is increased serum potassium or skeletal muscle enzymes due to aortic obstruction secondary to aortic thromboembolism or unless renal infarction has occurred resulting in azotaemia. Radiographic examination reveals a valentine-shaped heart seen on the ventrodorsal view. This appearance is due to significant left atrial enlargement in conjunction with shifting of the cardiac apex towards the

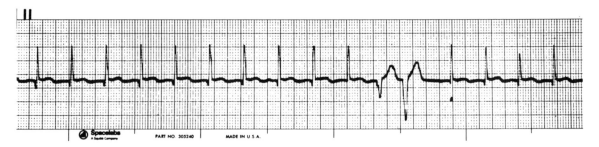

Fig. 11.3 Electrocardiogram from a cat with hypertrophic cardiomyopathy showing premature ventricular contractions.

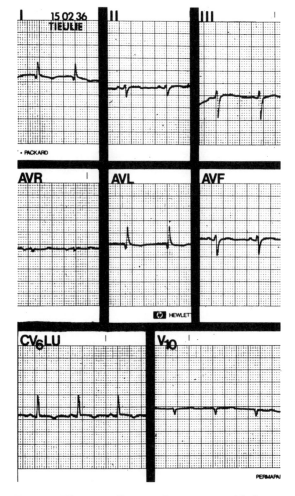

Fig. 11.4 Electrocardiogram from a cat with hypertrophic cardiomyopathy showing left axis deviation (which is sometimes referred to as left anterior fascicular block).

also develop, especially in chronic cases or when atrial fibrillation is present.

Electrocardiographic abnormalities have been reported in 35–70% of affected cats. The most commonly reported findings are conduction disturbances with left anterior fascicular block (Fig. 11.4) being the most consistent (Fox, 1988). Left ventricular enlargement patterns are present in some cases (Fig. 11.5) and arrhythmias occur in 25–59% of affected cats with ventricular premature complexes (Fig. 11.3) predominating (Fox, 1988).

Echocardiographic changes consist of hypertrophy of the ventricular septum and left ventricular free wall, decreased left ventricular internal dimensions, normal to elevated fractional shortening and, late in the disease, right ventricular dilation. Left atrial enlargement is often marked (Fox, 1988). Systolic anterior motion of the mitral valve, suggestive of hypertrophic obstructive cardiomyopathy, may be found.

Pre-anaesthetic Assessment and Preparation of the Patient

The safest approach to anaesthetic management of the patient with heart disease is to establish an accurate diagnosis of the disease and the extent of its progression, and to have a good understanding of the pathophysiology of the disease. With this knowledge, the anaesthetist is able to prepare the cat properly, to select an anaesthetic technique least likely to affect cardiovascular function and, should problems arise during the anaesthesia, to take remedial action on the basis of the pathophysiology that will improve the cat's status.

midline (Bonagura, 1989). Pulmonary oedema is typical of heart failure in cats with hypertrophic cardiomyopathy; however, pleural effusion may

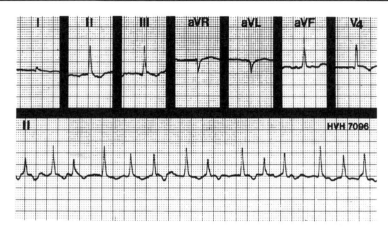

Fig. 11.5 Electrocardiogram from a cat with hypertrophic cardiomyopathy showing atrial fibrillation and increased QRS voltage and duration. The latter are indicative of left ventricular enlargement.

An important aspect of the history in cats with hypertrophic cardiomyopathy is to determine whether the cat has, at any time, been dyspnoeic, as these cats seem to be more likely to develop pulmonary oedema when anaesthetized. Physical examination should include auscultation of the heart and lung fields for evidence of arrhythmias or rales.

Pre-operative preparation for a cat with hypertrophic cardiomyopathy prior to anaesthesia should include full haematological and biochemical evaluation, a thoracic radiograph, an electrocardiogram and an ultrasound examination. Anaemia can be deleterious to a cat with hypertrophic cardiomyopathy since, under anaesthesia, heart rate is often increased to maintain tissue oxygenation. An increase in heart rate may lead to sudden decompensation as it decreases ventricular filling time. These cats may be very sensitive to fluid administration if left atrial and pulmonary venous pressures are elevated, and correction of the anaemia by packed red cell administration is best carried out slowly, with careful monitoring, prior to induction of anaesthesia.

If the cat has been treated with a diuretic such as frusemide, serum potassium concentration may be decreased and this may predispose the cat to arrhythmias during anaesthesia. Serum potassium concentration can be increased by intravenous administration of potassium chloride, 0.5 mmol/kg/h, and monitoring of serum potassium concentration every hour. An electrocardiogram can be used to determine the presence and type of arrhythmia. Premature ventricular contractions and/or atrial fibrillation are associated with hypertrophic cardiomyopathy and may induce pulmonary oedema by diminishing ventricular filling. Atrial fibrillation often precipitates clinical deterioration because of the dependence of the non-compliant left ventricle on atrial systole for its filling.

An echocardiogram is the most sensitive technique for evaluation of left ventricular hypertrophy, as well as allowing assessment of myocardial function. Hence, echocardiography is important not only in making the initial diagnosis, but also in assessment of the cat prior to anaesthesia.

If possible, arrhythmias and pulmonary oedema should be treated prior to anaesthesia. A stable rhythm maximizes cardiac output and minimizes the development of malignant arrhythmias during anaesthesia. Pulmonary oedema is treated by administration of diuretics (frusemide, 1 mg/kg i/v or i/m, twice or three times daily). After 24–36 h, the dose may be decreased to once or twice daily and changed from parenteral to oral administration. Pulmonary oedema is usually very responsive to potent diuretics and the dose should be reduced to the lowest effective dose. In cases of severe fulminating pulmonary oedema, the initial dose of frusemide may be increased to 2.0 mg/kg and supplemental oxygen therapy, administered via an oxygen cage, may be beneficial. Beta-adrenergic blocking drugs and calcium channel blocking drugs form the basis of medical treatment. Propranolol inhibits sympathetic cardiac stimulation and diminishes myocardial oxygen requirements by reducing heart rate, left ventricular contractility and systolic myocardial wall stress. Left ventricular diastolic compliance may improve indirectly through reduction of heart rate and myocardial ischaemia (Fox, 1988). Propranolol 2.5 mg is administered orally two to three times daily to cats weighing less than 6 kg and 5.0 mg to cats weighing more than 6 kg. Propranolol is usually administered 24–36 h after diuretic therapy has been initiated. If sinus tachycardia or ventricular arrhythmias are present, it may be administered with diuretics (Fox, 1988). Calcium channel blocking drugs have been found to be effective in both people and cats with hypertrophic cardiomyopathy, and are reported by some to be more effective in cats than β-blocking drugs (Bright & Gloden, 1991). Calcium channel blocking drugs have similar effects to β-blocking drugs in that they reduce heart rate, contractility, systolic pressure gradients and myocardial oxygen demand. However, they also enhance myocardial relaxation, directly dilate the coronary vasculature and relieve coronary vasospasm (Bright & Gloden, 1991). Diltiazem, a potent calcium channel blocking drug, has been evaluated in cats with hypertrophic cardiomyopathy (Bright *et al.*, 1991). Diltiazem, 1.75–2.5 mg/kg, administered orally every 8 h, was reported not to cause any adverse effects and all cats in the study became asymptomatic. Chronic β-blockade and/or calcium channel blockade should be continued up to and including the day of surgery.

Anaesthetic Management and Monitoring

Because of poor ventricular compliance, cats with hypertrophic cardiomyopathy are dependent on a large ventricular volume and maintenance of sinus rhythm for adequate diastolic filling. The atrial contribution to ventricular filling is important and may approach 75% of total stroke volume (Jackson & Thomas, 1993). If outflow obstruction is a component of the disease, factors such as increased contractility, decreased afterload and decreased preload increase outflow obstruction by reducing ventricular volume (Jackson & Thomas, 1993). Thus,

factors that usually impair contractile performance, such as myocardial depression, systemic vasoconstriction and ventricular over-distension characteristically improve systolic function (Jackson & Thomas, 1993). In this situation, the mitral regurgitation associated with hypertrophic cardiomyopathy with outflow obstruction, responds to pharmacologic intervention in a manner opposite to classic mitral regurgitation. Vasodilating agents augment the outflow obstruction with a resultant increase in mitral regurgitation, while vasoconstricting drugs attenuate obstruction and decrease mitral regurgitation (Jackson & Thomas, 1993).

Cats are generally premedicated with a μ-opioid agonist (such as oxymorphone, 0.03–0.05 mg/kg or methadone 0.1 mg/kg subcutaneously) and an anticholinergic such as glycopyrrolate (0.01 mg/kg subcutaneously). Opioid agonists have minimal effects on myocardial contractility, preload and afterload (Copland *et al.*, 1987). Glycopyrrolate is chosen in preference to atropine because it is less likely to induce sinus tachycardia or arrhythmias. If the cat will tolerate a facemask, oxygen is administered prior to, and during, induction of anaesthesia. An intravenous rather than mask or chamber induction is preferred to avoid excitement and increased circulating catecholamine. At Davis, the injectable drugs most commonly used to induce anaesthesia are etomidate and diazepam. One quarter (0.25 mg/kg) of the calculated dose of etomidate (1.0 mg/kg), followed by half (0.25 mg/kg) of the calculated dose (0.5 mg/kg) of diazepam are administered together with a replacement solution at a very slow rate. Depth of anaesthesia is assessed after 30 s and if the patient cannot be intubated another dose of etomidate and diazepam is administered. The dissociatives ketamine and tiletamine should be avoided, as drugs which stimulate the sympathetic nervous system increase heart rate, myocardial oxygen demand, shorten diastolic filling time (Mason & Atkins, 1991) and may increase outflow tract obstruction. Propofol, thiopentone and thiamylal should also be avoided. Propofol has been reported to impair regional myocardial function in ischaemic myocardium (Mayer *et al.*, 1993), while the increase in heart rate following thiobarbiturate administration is potentially deleterious because of the obligatory increase in myocardial oxygen consumption (Reves & Berkowitz, 1993). There are no reports of the use of Saffan in cats with cardiomyopathy. Once the cat has been intubated, anaesthesia is maintained with oxygen and isoflurane. Isoflurane is chosen over other inhalation anaesthetics because it induces less depression of the myocardium and is less arrhythmogenic. However, isoflurane does decrease systemic vascular resistance, a situation which may increase outflow tract obstruction (Gutgesell, 1988).

Balanced anaesthetic techniques, utilizing opioids and muscle relaxants, are often advocated for maintenance of anaesthesia in people and dogs with cardiovascular disease. These techniques generally allow lower inhalation agent concentrations to be administered and thus cardiovascular function is better preserved. Balanced techniques using muscle relaxants are well documented (Ilkiw, 1992) and are considered safe in these cats provided drugs with minimal effects on the cardiovascular system, such as vecuronium (50 µg/kg i/v) or atracurium (0.25 mg/kg i/v) (Stoelting, 1991) are used. Opioid techniques have not been described previously in cats, most probably because of the uncertainty of beneficial effects, as well as the worry of excitement in recovery (see Chapters 7 and 8). A recently completed study in cats (unpublished observations) demonstrated that opioids reduce the need for inhalant anaesthetics and in that study all recoveries were free of excitement (Pascoe et al., 1993). It is thus safe to utilize opioid/inhalant maintenance techniques in sick cats with cardiovascular disease. Fentanyl, at a loading dose of 5 µg/kg and an infusion of 0.4 µg/kg/min, is administered intravenously and the inhalant concentration decreased according to anaesthetic requirement. The fentanyl infusion is stopped 20 min before the end of surgery.

Monitoring and Management of Problems arising under Anaesthesia

A catheter is placed into the cephalic vein for administration of injectable anaesthetic drugs.

Limb leads are placed prior to induction and a lead II electrocardiogram is assessed prior to and during induction of anaesthesia. Once the cat is intubated and a stable plane of anaesthesia has been reached, an oesophageal ECG lead is usually introduced and the limb leads removed. A doppler crystal and cuff are also placed prior to induction of anaesthesia to allow the pulse to be monitored and indirect systolic arterial blood pressure to be measured prior to, during and after induction of anaesthesia. If pulmonary oedema is not present, extensive surgery is not planned, and the duration of anaesthesia short, blood pressure is monitored using an indirect technique and ventilation is not controlled unless hypoventilation occurs. Otherwise, an arterial catheter is placed percutaneously in the dorsal pedal artery or via a cut-down in the femoral artery. This catheter is used to monitor mean arterial pressure accurately and to collect arterial blood samples for measurement of blood gases and pH. For more extensive procedures, anaesthesia of long duration, or maintenance techniques which include opioids, ventilation is controlled using a ventilator. If pulmonary oedema is present, a small amount of positive end-expiratory pressure (5 cmH$_2$O) is added. Fluid administration and replacement of blood loss must be judicious to avoid hypotension or pulmonary oedema.

Intra-operative arrhythmias require aggressive therapy. Esmolol, a short-acting β-adrenergic antagonist, has the advantages of rapid onset and termination. It is administered as a loading dose of 100–500 µg/kg i/v, followed by an infusion of 50–70 µg/kg/min i/v. Diltiazem i/v has been rarely used in cats and dose rates have yet to be published.

Intra-operative hypotension should be managed by administration of vasoconstrictor agents such as phenylephrine, rather than inotropes or β-adrenergic agonists. Phenylephrine is administered intravenously at a loading dose of 5 µg/kg and an infusion of 0.1–3.0 µg/kg/min.

Postanaesthetic Management

If the cat has been on long-term treatment for hypertrophic cardiomyopathy with β-blocking drugs and/or calcium channel blocking drugs, these should be restarted immediately after surgery.

Postanaesthetic management should be directed towards early recognition of complications occurring as a result of anaesthesia. These include pulmonary oedema and arrhythmias and their management has been detailed above.

References

Allan, D.G. (1991) Special techniques. *In: Small Animal Medicine* (ed. D.G. Allen), p. 1035–1096. J.B. Lippincott, Philadelphia.

Atkins, C.E. & Snyder, P.S. (1991) Cardiomyopathy. *In: Small Animal Medicine* (ed. D.G. Allen) p. 269–297. J.B. Lippincott, Philadelphia.

Atkins, C.E., Gallo, A.M., Kurzman, I.D. & Cowen, P. (1992) Risk factors, clinical signs, and survival in cats with a clinical diagnosis of idiopathic hypertrophic cardiomyopathy: 74 cases (1985–1989). *J. Am. Vet. Med. Ass.* **201**, 613–618.

Babad, A.A. & Eger, E.I. (1968) The effects of hyperthyroidism and hypothyroidism on halothane and oxygen requirements in dogs. *Anesthesiology* **29**, 1087–1093.

Baggot, J.D. & Blake, J.W. (1976) Disposition kinetics of ketamine in the domestic cat. *Arch. Int. Pharmacodyn. Ther.* **220**, 115–124.

Barsanti, J.A. & Finco, D.R. (1984) Management of post-renal uremia. *Vet. Clin. N Am.: Small Anim. Pract.* **14**, 609–616.

Barsanti, J.A., Jones, B.D., Spano, J.S. & Taylor, H.W. (1977) Prolonged anorexia associated with hepatic lipidosis in three cats. *Feline Pract.* **7**, 52–57.

Bedford, P.G.C. (1991) *Small Animal Anaesthesia, The Increased Risk Patient.* Baillière Tindall, London.

Benson, G.J. & Thurmon, J.C. (1987) Anesthesia and the kidney: Special considerations. *In: Principles and Practice of Veterinary Anesthesia*, (ed. C.E. Short), p. 237–250. Williams & Wilkins, Baltimore.

Berman, M.L. & Holaday, D.A. (1989) Inhalation anesthetic metabolism and toxicity. *In: Clinical Anesthesia* (ed. P.G. Barash, B.F. Cullen & R.K. Stoelting), p. 323–338. J.B. Lippincott, Philadelphia.

Berman, M.L., Kuhnert, L., Phythyon, J.M. *et al.* (1983) Isoflurane and enflurane-induced hepatic necrosis in triiodothyronine-pretreated rats. *Anesthesiology* **58**, 1.

Bilezikian, J.P., Loeb, J.N. & Gammon, D.E. (1979) The influence of hyperthyroidism and hypothyroidism on the β-adrenergic responsiveness of the turkey erythrocyte. *J. Clin. Invest.* **63**, 184–192.

Biourge, V., MacDonald, M.J. & King, L. (1990) Feline hepatic lipidosis: Pathogenesis and nutritional management. *Compend. Cont. Ed. Pract. Vet.* **12**, 1244–1258.

Bonagura, J.D. (1989) Cardiovascular diseases. *In: The Cat. Diseases and Clinical Management* (ed. R.G. Sherding), p. 649–753. Churchill Livingstone, New York.

Bond, B.R. (1988) Hyperthyroidism and other high cardiac output states. In: *Canine and Feline Cardiology* (ed. P.R. Fox), p. 255–267. Churchill Livingstone, New York.

Bovee, K.C. (1982) Pathophysiology of urinary obstruction. *Post-Graduate Committee in Veterinary Science Refresher Course for Veterinarians* **61**, 179–192.

Bright, J.M. & Gloden, A.L. (1991) Evidence for or against the efficacy of calcium channel blockers for management of hypertrophic cardiomyopathy in cats. *Vet. Clin. Nth. Am.: Small Anim. Pract.* **21**, 1023–1033.

Bright, J.M., Golden, A.L., Gompf, R.E., Walker, M.A. & Toal, R.L. (1991) Evaluation of calcium channel blocking agents verapamil and diltiazem for treatment of hypertrophic cardiomyopathy. *J. Vet. Intern. Med.* **5**, 272–282.

Bright, R.M., Okrasinski, E.B., Pardo, A.D., Ellison, G.W. & Burrows, C.E.L. (1991) Percutaneous tube gastrostomy for enteral alimentation in small animals. *Compend. Cont. Ed. Pract. Vet.* **13**, 15–22.

Brown B.R. (1989a) Liver blood supply and regulation. *In: Anesthesia in Hepatic and Biliary Tract Disease* (ed. B.R. Brown), p. 17–32. F.A. Davis, Philadelphia.

Brown, B.R. (1989b) Effect of anesthetics on hepatic blood flow. *In: Anesthesia in Hepatic and Biliary Tract Disease* (ed. B.R. Brown), p. 49–60. F.A. Davis, Philadelphia.

Burrows, C.F., Chiapella, A.M. and Jezyk, P. (1981) Idiopathic feline hepatic lipidosis. The syndrome and speculations on its pathogenesis. *Florida Vet. J.* **10**, 18–20.

Cairoli, V.J. & Crout, J.R. (1967) Role of the autonomic nervous system in the resting tachycardia of experimental hyperthyroidism. *J. Pharmacol. Exp. Ther.* **158**, 55–65.

Center, S.A. (1986) Hepatic lipidosis in the cat. *Proc. 4th Ann. ACVIM Vet. Forum* **2**, 13.

Center, S.A. (1991) Hepatic lipidosis. *In: Consultations in Feline Internal Medicine* (ed. J.R. August), p. 451–462. W.B. Saunders, Philadelphia.

Clarke, K.W. & Hall, L.W. (1990) A survey of

anaesthesia in small animal practice: AVA/BSAVA report. *J. Ass. Vet. Anaesth.* **17**, 4–10.

Cohen, J. (1974) Role of endocrine factors in the pathogenesis of cardiac hypertrophy. *Circ. Res. (Suppl. II)* **35**, 49.

Copland, V.S., Haskins, S.C. & Patz, J.D. (1987) Oxymorphone: Cardiovascular, pulmonary, and behavioral effects in dogs. *Am. J. Vet. Res.* **48**, 1626–1630.

Dodman, N.H., Engelking, L.R. & Anwer, M.S. (1987) Pathophysiological changes of the hepatic system. *In: Principles and Practice of Veterinary Anesthesia*, (ed. C.E. Short), p. 221–237. Williams & Wilkins, Baltimore.

Feldman, E.C. & Nelson, R.W. (1987) Hyperthyroidism and thyroid tumors. *In: Canine and Feline Endocrinology and Reproduction* (ed. E.C. Feldman & R.W. Nelson), p. 91–135. W.B. Saunders, Philadelphia.

Fennell, C. (1975) Some demographic characteristics of the domestic cat population in Great Britain with particular reference to feeding habits and the incidence of feline urologic syndrome. *J. Small Anim. Pract.* **16**, 775–783.

Finco, D.R. & Cornelius, L.M. (1977) Characterization and treatment of water, electrolyte, and acid–base imbalances of induced urethral obstruction in the cat. *Am. J. Vet. Res.* **38**, 823–830.

Fox P.R. (1988) Feline myocardial disease. *In: Canine and Feline Cardiology* (ed. P.R. Fox), pp. 435–466 Churchill Livingstone, New York.

Gelman, S. (1989) Anesthesia and the liver. *In: Clinical Anesthesia* (eds. P.G. Barash, B.F. Cullen & R.K. Stoelting), p. 1133. J.B. Lippincott, Philadelphia.

Gelman, S. & Ernst, E.A. (1982) Hepatic circulation during sodium nitroprusside infusion in the carbon tetrachloride-treated dog. *Ala. J. Med. Sci.* **19**, 371.

Gelman, S., Fowler, K.C. & Smith, L.R. (1984) Liver circulation and function during isoflurane and halothane anesthesia. *Anesthesiology* **61**, 726–730.

Gompf, R.E. (1991) Cardiac and respiratory involvement in systemic diseases and problems. *In: Consultations in Feline Internal Medicine* (ed. J.R. August), p. 189–212. W.B. Saunders, Philadelphia.

Gutgesell, H.P. (1988) Myocardial and coronary anomalies. *In: Pediatric Cardiac Anesthesia* (ed. C.L. Lake), p. 351–361. Appleton & Lance, Norwalk.

Haskins, S.C. (1992) Anesthesia for urologic surgery. *In: Urologic Surgery of the Dog and Cat* (ed. E.A. Stone & J.A. Barsanti), p. 91–96. Lea & Febriger, Philadelphia.

Hayashi, Y., Sumikawa, K., Yamatodani, A. *et al.* (1989) Myocardial sensitization by thiopental to arrhythmogenic action of epinephrine in dogs. *Anesthesiology* **71**, 929–935.

Ilkiw, J.E. (1982) Anaesthesia and renal failure. *Post-Graduate Committee in Veterinary Science Refresher Course for Veterinarians* **61**, 145–149.

Ilkiw, J.E. (1992) Advantages of and guidelines for using neuromuscular blocking agents. *Vet. Clin. Nth. Am.: Small Anim. Pract.* **22**, 347–350.

Ingbar, S.H. & Woeber, K.A. (1981) The thyroid gland. *In: Textbook of Endocrinology* (ed. R.H. Williams), p. 117–247. W.B. Saunders, Philadelphia.

Jackson, J.M. & Thomas, S.J. (1993) Valvular heart disease. *In: Cardiac Anesthesia* (ed. J.A. Kaplan), p. 629–680. W.B. Saunders, Philadelphia.

Jacobs, G., Cornelias, L., Keene, B. *et al.* (1990) Comparison of plasma, liver, and skeletal muscle carnitine concentrations in cats with idiopathic hepatic lipidosis and in healthy cats. *Am. J. Vet. Res.* **15**, 1349–1351.

Jones, A.E., Schafter, D.F., Ferenci, P. *et al.* (1984) The neurobiology of hepatic encephalopathy. *Hepatology* **4**, 1235–1242.

Joyce, J.T., Roizen, M.F. & Eger, E.I. (1983) Effect of thiopental induction on sympathetic activity. *Anesthesiology* **59**, 19–22.

Klahr, S. (1983) Pathophysiology of obstructive nephropathy. *Kid. Intl.* **23**, 414–426.

Kobayashi, D.I., Peterson, M.E., Graves, T.K. *et al.* (1990) Hypertension in cats with chronic renal failure or hyperthyroidism. *J. Vet. Intern. Med.* **4**, 58–62.

Kolata, R.J. (1984) Emergency treatment of urethral obstruction in male cats. *Mod. Vet. Pract.* **65**, 517–521.

Kruse-Elliott, K.T., Swanson, C.R. & Aucoin, D.P. (1987) Effects of etomidate on adrenocortical function in canine surgical patients. *Am. J. Vet. Res.* **48**, 1098–1100.

Lawler, D.F., Sjolin, D.W. & Collins, J.E. (1985) Incidence rates of feline lower urinary tract disease in the United States. *Feline Pract.* **15**, 13–16.

Lees, G.E., Rogers, K.S. & Wolf, A.M. (1989) Diseases of the lower urinary tract. *In: The Cat Diseases and Clinical Management* (ed. R.G. Sherding), p. 1397–1454. Churchill Livingstone, New York.

Lui, S.K. (1977) Pathology of feline heart disease. *Vet. Clin. Nth. Amer.: Small Anim. Pract.* **7**, 323–339.

Marx, G.H., Matteo, C.V. & Orkin, L.R. (1973) Computer analysis of post anesthetic deaths. *Anesthesiology* **39**, 54–58.

Mason, D.E. & Atkins, C.E. (1991) Anesthesia for the Cardiac Patient. *In: Small Animal Medicine* (ed. D.G. Allen), p. 365–380. J.B. Lippincott, Philadelphia.

Massey, D.G., Becklake, M.R., McKenzie, J.M. *et al.*

(1967) Circulatory and ventilatory response to exercise in thyrotoxicosis. *New Engl. J. Med.* **276**, 1104–1112.

Mayer, N., Legat, K., Weinstable, C. *et al.* (1993) Effects of propofol on the function of normal, collateral-dependent, and ischemic myocardium. *Anesth. Analg.* **76**, 33.

McConnaughey, M.M., Jones, L.R., Watanabe, A.M. *et al.* (1979) Thyroxine and propylthiouracil effects on alpha- and beta-adrenergic receptor number, ATPase activities, and sialic acid content of rat cardiac membrane vesicles. *J. Cardiovasc. Pharmacol.* **1**, 609–623.

McDougall, I.R. (1981) Treatment of hyper- and hypothyroidism. *J. Clin. Pharmacol.* **21**, 365–384.

Muir, W.W., Werner, L.L. & Hamlin, R.L. (1975) Effects of xylazine and acetylpromazine upon induced ventricular fibrillation in dogs anesthetized with thiamylal and halothane. *Am. J. Vet. Res.* **36**, 1299–1303.

Nagel, M.L., Muir, W.W. & Nguyen, K. (1979) Comparison of the cardiopulmonary effects of etomidate and thiamylal in dogs. *Am. J. Vet. Res.* **40**, 193–196.

Pascoe, P.J. Ilkiw, J.E. & Fisher, L.D. (1993) The effect of two doses of morphine on the minimum alveolar concentration of isoflurane in cats. *Proc. Ann. Mtg. Am. Coll. Vet. Anes.* **18**, 25.

Peterson, M.E. (1981) Propylthiouracil in the treatment of feline hyperthyroidism. *J. Am. Vet. Med. Ass.* **179**, 485–487.

Peterson, M.E. (1984) Feline hyperthyroidism. *Vet. Clin. Nth. Am.: Small Anim. Pract.* **14**, 809–826.

Peterson, M.E. & Ferguson, D.C. (1989) Thyroid diseases. *In: Textbook of Veterinary Internal Medicine* (ed. S.J. Ettinger), p. 1632–1675. W.B. Saunders, Philadelphia.

Peterson, M.E. & Randolph, J.F. (1989) Endocrine diseases. *In: The Cat. Diseases and Clinical Management* (ed. R.G. Sherding), p. 1095. Churchill Livingstone, New York.

Peterson, M.E., Kintzer, P.P., Cavanagh, P.G. *et al.* (1983) Feline hyperthyroidism: Pretreatment clinical and laboratory evaluation of 131 cases. *J. Am. Vet. Med. Ass.* **183**, 103.

Peterson, M.E., Birchard, S.J. & Mehlhaff, C.J. (1984) Anesthetic and surgical management of endocrine disorders. *Vet. Clin. Nth. Am.: Small Anim. Pract.* **14**, 911–925.

Peterson, M.E., Kintzer, P.P. & Hurvitz, A.I. (1988) Methimazole treatment of 262 cats with hyperthyroidism. *J. Vet. Intern. Med.* **2**, 150–157.

Pion, P.D., Kittleson, M.D., Rogers, Q.R. *et al.* (1987) Myocardial failure in cats associated with low

plasma taurine: A reversible cardiomyopathy. *Science* **237**, 764–768.

Raffe, M.R. & Caywood, D.D. (1984) Use of anesthetic agents in cats with obstructive uropathy. *Vet. Clin. Nth. Am.: Small Anim. Pract.* **14**, 691–702.

Reves, J.G. & Berkowitz, D.E. (1993) Pharmacology of intravenous anesthetic induction drugs. *In: Cardiac Anesthesia* (ed. J.A. Kaplan), p. 512. W.B. Saunders, Philadelphia.

Riggs, C.M. (1991) Idiopathic feline hepatic lipidosis. *Feline Pract* **19**, 12–15.

Roizen, M.F. (1990) Anesthetic implications of concurrent diseases. *In: Anesthesia* (ed. R.D. Miller), p. 793–893. Churchill Livingstone, New York.

Schaer, M. (1975) The use of regular insulin in the treatment of hyperkalemia in cats with urethral obstruction. *J. Am. Anim. Hosp. Assoc.* **11**, 106–109.

Schaer, M. (1977) Hyperkalemia in cats with urethral obstruction. Electrocardiographic abnormalities and treatment. *Vet. Clin. Nth. Am.: Small Anim. Pract.* **7**, 407–414.

Schwartz, L.B. & Gewertz, B.L. (1988) The renal response to low dose dopamine. *J. Surg. Res.* **45**, 574–588.

Short, C.E. & Miller, R.L. (1978) Comparative evaluation of the anticholinergic glycopyrrolate as a preanesthetic agent. *Vet. Med. Small Anim. Clin.* **73**, 1269–1273.

Skeleton, C.L., Coleman, H.N., Wildenthal, K. *et al.* (1970) Augmentation of myocardial oxygen consumption in hyperthyroid cats. *Circ. Res.* **27**, 301–309.

Skiles, M.L., Pion, P.D., Hird, D.W. *et al.* (1990) Epidemiologic evaluation of taurine deficiency and dilated cardiomyopathy in cats. *J. Vet. Intern. Med.* **4**, 117 (Abstract 48).

Stehling, L.C. & Roizen, M.F. (1989) Pre-existing endocrine disorders. *In: General Anaesthesia* (eds. J.F. Nunn, J.E. Utting, & B.R. Brown), p. 392–401. Butterworths, London.

Stoelting, R.K. (1991) Neuromuscular blocking drugs. *In: Pharmacology and Physiology in Anesthetic Practice* (ed. R.K. Stoelting), p. 172. J.B. Lippincott, Philadelphia.

Stoelting, R.K., Dierdorf, S.F. & McCammon, R.L. (1988) Endocrine diseases. *In: Anesthesia and Co-Existing Disease* (eds. R.K. Stoelting, S.F. Dierdorf & R.L. McCammon), p. 473. Churchill Livingstone, New York.

Vaamonde, C.A. & Michael, U.F. (1981) The kidney in thyroid dysfunction. *In: The Kidney in Systemic Disease* (ed. W.N. Suki, & G. Eknoyan), p. 361–415. John Wiley, New York.

Van Been, H., Manger, F.W., Van Boxtel, C. *et al.* (1983)

Etomidate anaesthesia in patients with cirrhosis of the liver: Pharmacokinetic data. *Anaesthesia* **38**, 61–62.

Wase, A.W. & Foster, W.C. (1956) Thiopental and thyroid metabolism. *Proc. Soc. exp. Biol. Med.* **91**, 89.

Waterman, A.E. (1983) Influence of premedication with xylazine on the distribution and metabolism of intramuscularly administered ketamine in cats. *Res. Vet. Sci.* **35**, 285–290.

Weller, C.V., Wanstrom, R.C., Gordon, H. *et al.* (1932) Cardiac histopathology in thyroid disease. *Am. Heart J.* **8**, 8–18.

Wertz, E.M., Benson, G.J., Thurmon, J.C. *et al.* (1990) Pharmacokinetics of etomidate in cats. *Am. J. Vet. Res.* **51**, 281–285.

Wong, D.H.W. & Jenkins, L.C. (1974) An experimental study of the mechanism of action of ketamine on the central nervous system. *Can. Anaesth. Soc. J.* **21**, 57–67.

Zawie, D.A. & Shaker, E. (1989) Diseases of the liver. *In: The Cat, Diseases and Clinical Management* (ed. R.G. Sherding), p. 1015–1036. Churchill Livingstone, New York.

P.M. Taylor

12
Accidents and Emergencies

Introduction

There is no doubt that the safety of feline anaesthesia has increased during the last 10–20 years. This is largely due to better understanding of the physiology of anaesthesia and to the discovery of new, more specific drugs. However, the most important component of safe anaesthesia is the anaesthetist. As with any species, anaesthetic emergencies in the cat should, theoretically, be rare, as many can be prevented by forethought and good monitoring. In spite of this, certain problems may arise in the cat where particular knowledge about the species is lacking; it is, unfortunately, regarded as a small dog in an attempt to extrapolate information such as drug dosage. The cat is unique both physiologically and psychologically, and provision of consistently trouble-free anaesthesia in this species still presents a challenge.

In 1990, Clarke and Hall reported the results of the Association of Veterinary Anaesthetists and British Small Animal Veterinary Association (AVA/BSAVA) survey of anaesthesia in small animal practice which had been carried out in the United Kingdom. They reported an overall death rate of 1 per 552 general anaesthetics carried out in healthy cats. A significant number of these deaths occurred when the animals were not under close observation; death during unobserved recovery made a substantial contribution. The death rate in cats with pathological but not immediately life threatening conditions was very much higher: 1 per 30 anaesthetics. These death rates are very much higher than in man, where a survey conducted by the Association of Anaesthetists of Great Britain and Ireland (Lunn & Mushin, 1982) reported 1 in 10 000 solely attributed to the anaesthetic or 1 in 1667 where anaesthesia

contributed to death. In a number of other surveys carried out in medical anaesthesia, notably the Confidential Enquiry in Perioperative Deaths carried out in the United Kingdom, increased risk of death or serious anaesthetic accidents was associated with inexperienced anaesthetists (Campling et al., 1991/92).

Two main recommendations that should lead to safer anaesthesia in cats arise from these data: first that all anaesthetized cats should be monitored properly until they are fully conscious and second, that anaesthetists inexperienced in feline anaesthesia, even if familiar with other species, should be given the chance to learn the techniques of anaesthesia under adequate supervision.

In the AVA/BSAVA survey Clarke and Hall (1990) reported a number of non-fatal anaesthetic problems that occurred in dogs and cats. These include apnoea, cyanosis, prolonged recovery, cardiac arrest, swollen extremities, laryngeal spasm and blocked endotracheal tube. This survey, (Clarke & Hall, 1990), individual reports and anecdotal accounts suggest that such problems occur at least as commonly in cats as in other species.

Pre-operative Considerations

Temperament of the Cat

The cat's unique temperament and athleticism may lead to disasters at induction. If the cat becomes upset and is handled inappropriately (see Chapter 5) a violent struggle may ensue. A struggling cat will require a much higher dose of induction agent leading to hazards of overdose. It is also likely to have high circulating catecholamines which will cause cardiac arrhythmias. Hypoxia may develop from forceful restraint. A hazard unique to the cat is escape and they should be anaesthetized in a secure room; they easily escape from places that would be secure for other small domestic species, through windows or even up a chimney. The potential for injury to cat or handlers is best avoided by providing sympathetic handling, good sedation, and a quiet environment. Barking dogs and noisy activity are not conducive to smooth induction of anaesthesia in the cat.

The cat's temperament may result in unusual reactions to premedication. Morphine overdose may lead to manic behaviour although this is very rare if recommended doses (Chapter 7) are given. Variable responses to acepromazine have been reported (Hall & Clarke, 1991). A manic cat is not a good candidate for smooth induction of anaesthesia and is best allowed to recover completely before anaesthesia is attempted.

Size of the Cat

The cat's small size leads to a number of physical problems which may lead to accidents. Overdose of the anaesthetic agent is a significant hazard in the cat. This is largely a result of its size and overestimation of its weight. Even an adult cat is relatively very small as can be appreciated by comparison with the dog: 5 kg body weight indicates a large cat but a very small dog. It is easy to overdose a cat with, for instance, thiopentone where the therapeutic index is low. A 50-mg dose given to the supposedly 5 kg cat represents 20 mg/kg if the cat is a more common 2.5 kg; this may be sufficient to cause apnoea and serious cardiovascular depression.

Difficulty with intravenous injection and inadvertent perivascular injection may render superficial veins inaccessible. A quiet induction and use of catheters rather than needles should minimize this hazard.

The relatively high body surface area to volume ratio leads to significant heat loss and hypothermia (see below). Apparently small volumes of blood loss may in fact constitute a significant proportion of the circulating blood volume. It is essential to monitor such losses

carefully (Chapter 10) so that fluid or blood infusion is started before signs of hypovolaemia develop.

Access to a surgical site is often limited and the cat is likely to be completely covered by surgical drapes. Careful attachment of monitoring equipment and access to venous lines should be established before draping takes place. It is imperative that adequate means of monitoring the cat are established before surgery starts or it may be impossible either to detect or to remedy a problem until it is too late.

Prevention is Better Than Cure

Anaesthesia has been likened to flying and one of the most pertinent comparisons is the 'pre-flight check' where a routine check is carried out to ensure that all the equipment is functioning correctly. A full clinical examination (Chapter 6) of the cat either to ensure that it is healthy or to detect potential problems (Chapters 11 and 13) so they do not come as a surprise will go a long way to averting any accident. A full examination of the anaesthetic equipment (Chapter 9) and repair of any faults before anaesthesia is induced is of equal importance in preventing accidents.

Monitoring during anaesthesia is as important in preventing anaesthetic accidents as the pre-flight check (Chapter 10). It entails regular examination of clinical signs that convey information about the patient's physiological well-being. Examination is made regularly and frequently so that small changes can be detected and any necessary action taken before any abnormality becomes serious.

In spite of all precautions, accidents do happen and preparation for their eventuality may prevent a fatal result. Even if a breathing circuit and volatile anaesthesia are not to be used it is essential that means of resuscitation, including an oxygen supply and a means of supplying intermittent positive pressure ventilation (IPPV) is immediately available, should any problem occur. Many anaesthetic accidents could have a satisfactory outcome if resuscitation were to be applied immediately they occurred.

Accidents During Anaesthesia

The main requirement for the well-being of the cat during anaesthesia is that tissue perfusion is adequate to supply oxygen and to remove waste products. Most serious or fatal anaesthetic accidents lead to tissue hypoxia and cell damage or death. The brain is the most easily damaged and hypoxic episodes during anaesthesia, whatever the cause, result in brain damage ranging from death to a degree of neurological deficit.

Adequate tissue perfusion with oxygenated blood is best assured by maintenance of the 'ABC' of resuscitation: Airway, Breathing and Circulation. Accidents occurring during anaesthesia will be considered under those headings.

Obstruction of the Airway

The cat has a small, delicate trachea and larynx which are easily damaged and blocked. If obstruction is complete and undetected death through hypoxia is rapid. Partial obstruction is more common and causes insidious respiratory insufficiency leading to hypercapnia and hypoxia. Initially, a partially obstructed airway in an anaesthetized cat leads to laboured attempts to breathe so that it may appear as though anaesthesia is too light. This may progress to shallow breathing and even apnoea, particularly during deep anaesthesia. The airway should be cleared as soon as any problem is detected.

Obstruction by fluid or debris
Obstruction is commonly caused by blood, saliva or other secretions. Although it is now generally considered unnecessary to use an anticholinergic drying agent as a routine premedication before general anaesthesia (see Chapter 7) atropine or glycopyrrolate given early in the course of anaesthesia probably help to prevent the partial airway obstruction which is not uncommon in the cat. Its very small trachea is easily blocked with one bubble of saliva when the swallowing and cough reflexes are absent during general anaesthesia.

Obstruction of the airway by fluid or other debris is more likely to be a problem if an endotracheal tube is not used, although intubation does not guarantee a clear airway (see below). It is essential that an endotracheal tube is used for any surgery of the head and neck, as it is impossible to ensure a clear airway without. Whenever intra-oral surgery is undertaken the pharynx should be packed with moist gauze bandage to prevent leakage of fluid into the trachea (Fig. 12.1). The throat pack should be secured outside the mouth to prevent its aspiration. On occasions, such as hard palate surgery, the endotracheal tube will obscure the surgical site and is in danger of being displaced or kinked throughout surgery. In this case it is safer to bring the proximal end of the endotracheal tube out through a pharyngotomy incision (Fig. 12.2). The cat is anaesthetized and intubated in the usual manner, a stab incision is made through the pharyngeal wall and the end of the endotracheal tube is grasped with forceps and pulled through the incision and then attached to the breathing circuit. The throat can still be packed in the usual manner. The process is reversed at the end of anaesthesia and the incision sutured. Such incisions usually heal well.

Problems associated with intubation
Intubation should always be performed if there is any doubt about maintenance of a clear airway. There are many instances where intubation is essential, including surgery of the head and neck as above, whenever IPPV is required and whenever regurgitation is likely to occur, as in any gastrointestinal surgery. It is usually safer to intubate the trachea for major surgery or prolonged anaesthesia as this gives better control of the airway should any problem arise. However, the cat has a small and delicate larynx easily damaged by rough treatment. It also has well-developed protective reflexes making laryngeal spasm a common hazard of intubation. Consequently, intubation should be performed with particular care in this species. Fortunately the cat has no excess pharyngeal tissue and generally maintains a good airway without an endotracheal tube, so intubation is often unnecessary

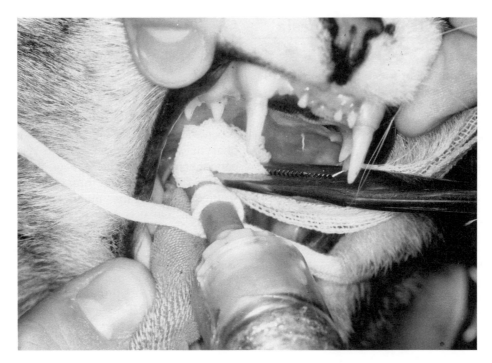

Fig. 12.1 The pharynx is packed with moist, non-fraying, gauze bandage to prevent fluid from leaking around the endotracheal tube into the trachea. The proximal end of the bandage is secured at the mouth.

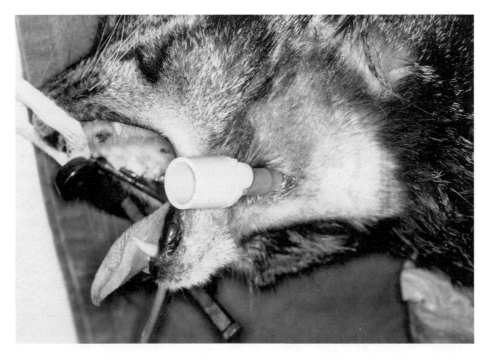

Fig. 12.2 Better access to the mouth and a safer airway is ensured if the endotracheal tube is brought out through a pharyngotomy during oral surgery.

for short periods of anaesthesia when a mask can be used to administer oxygen and the anaesthetic.

Intubation is performed after the laryngeal reflexes have been suppressed by local anaesthesia, neuromuscular blockade or deep anaesthesia. Local anaesthetic techniques are the most commonly used, often with lignocaine sprays developed for human use. Pure lignocaine spray is best, as some of the additives in the medical products have caused chemical irritation of the larynx (Watson, 1992; Taylor 1992, 1993). Even plain lignocaine has been reported to increase tracheal mucus secretion *in vivo* in cats (Somerville *et al.*, 1990) but this is probably insufficient to cause a clinical problem. Application of the spray itself usually causes some reaction such as closing of the glottis and sometimes coughing. No attempt should be made to intubate until the glottis has opened again and the analgesic solution has had time to take effect, or laryngeal spasm may develop.

Neuromuscular blockade with suxamethonium (0.2 mg/kg i/v) (Chapter 8), given immediately after induction of anaesthesia is used to ensure complete laryngeal relaxation which allows atraumatic passage of the endotracheal tube (Hall & Clarke, 1991). Although this method ensures smooth passage of the tube it is not commonly employed as, with care, intubation is relatively straightforward after local desensitization. If neuromuscular blockade is used it is essential that the cat can be ventilated with oxygen using a face mask to ensure that it is well oxygenated during intubation and in case there is any problem with intubation.

Use of very deep anaesthesia for intubation is not recommended as the depth necessary to produce laryngeal relaxation is only achieved after considerable overdose.

There is often a temptation to use a tube that is too small because this is easier to place, but this constitutes partial airway obstruction. It is better to use an uncuffed tube to allow a reasonable size to be used (4.0–5.0 mm in the adult cat) without the additional laryngeal trauma that the cuff itself may cause. Damage may also be inflicted with the laryngoscope. It is possible to intubate the cat by direct vision but

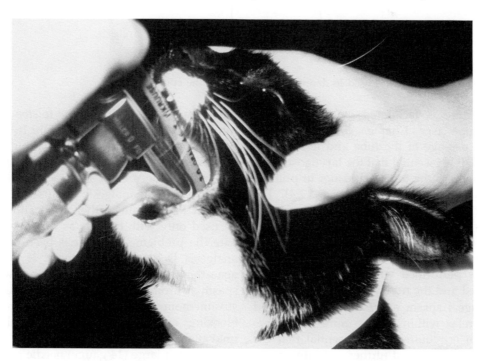

Fig. 12.3 Intubation is facilitated with use of a laryngoscope and small Mackintosh blade. Careful positioning by the assistant to extend the head and neck ensures a straight route for the tube.

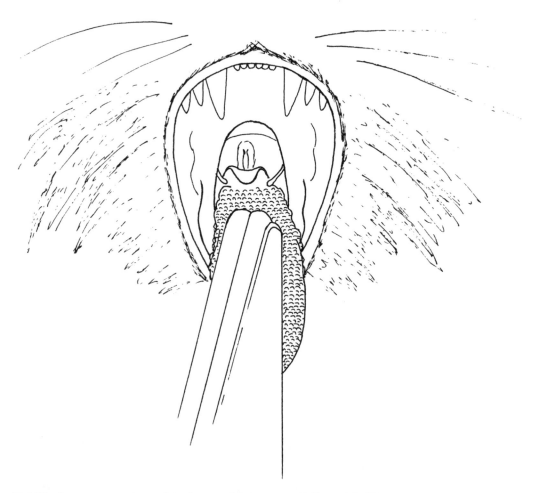

Fig. 12.4 The laryngoscope is used to depress the tongue, not the epiglottis.

the procedure is facilitated by the use of a laryngoscope (see Chapter 5), resulting in smoother passage of the tube and less trauma (Fig. 12.3). It is essential that the laryngoscope is used to depress the tongue and not to pull the epiglottis forward and down (Fig. 12.4). The laryngoscope blade should not touch the epiglottis as this will cause considerable trauma and oedema. The laryngoscope can be used with the cat in any position, but intubation is most commonly performed with the cat prone, the head raised and the neck extended (Fig. 12.3).

If laryngeal spasm occurs at intubation and does not relax within 10–20 s immediate remedial action is required. It is essential that the larynx is not stimulated further and attempts to intubate should cease immediately. Serious accidents at intubation in medical anaesthesia may be associated with failure to *stop* trying to intubate (Feldman *et al.*, 1989). It may be necessary to deepen anaesthesia but in any case oxygen should be supplied by mask so that any air that does enter the trachea is oxygen-enriched. If local analgesic was used at the first attempt to intubate further application should be used only with caution as this may exacerbate the problem. If none has been used local analgesia is a logical treatment. If deepening anaesthesia and extra time do not resolve the spasm neuromuscular blockade is indicated if suxamethonium or another neuromuscular blocking agent is immediately available. If unavailable, a temporary airway can be provided with a large (14 gauge) needle or catheter placed in the trachea percutaneously. If all else fails a tracheotomy can be performed but this is extremely difficult to manage in the cat (Chapter 13) and best avoided if possible.

Laryngeal spasm may occur at extubation. The tube should be removed gently and preferably when the cat is still quite deeply anaesthetized. It should not be left in until the cat is coughing or gagging on the tube. If any difficulty was experienced at intubation extubation should be performed when the cat is still anaesthetized deeply enough to re-intubate or otherwise manipulate the cat if further problems occur. A struggling, half-conscious cat with laryngeal spasm is highly likely to become hypoxic and is extremely difficult to manage. Another hazard of delaying extubation is that the tube may be chewed in half by cats emerging from anaesthesia with aspiration of the distal portion of the tube. Such an event usually requires prompt action that includes re-anaesthetizing the patient to retrieve the aspirated tube end.

If the larynx is damaged during intubation the ensuing swelling may cause airway obstruction after the tube has been removed. Trauma due to difficulty at intubation was considered likely to have caused death due to obstruction in a number of cats in the AVA/BSAVA survey (Clarke & Hall, 1990). If intubation was difficult the cat must be very closely observed for some hours after recovery as oedema may take time to develop. Treatment with steroids and diuretics may be indicated.

Although the use of an endotracheal tube makes it a great deal easier to ensure that the airway is clear it does not guarantee it; monitoring is still necessary. The tube itself may become blocked with fluid or other debris and may be kinked or compressed by surgical equipment or when the cat's position is changed. This is a particular hazard during head and neck surgery or when positioning the cat for radiography.

Respiratory Insufficiency

Inadequate respiration is often difficult to detect unless specific monitors are used (Chapter 10). Hypercapnia is notoriously difficult to detect clinically but results in acidosis, myocardial sensitization leading to cardiac arrhythmias and, if severe, increased CNS depression. Hypoxaemia is also difficult to detect clinically as cyanosis is notoriously unreliable unless hypoxaemia is severe.

Apnoea requires immediate action. It is not uncommon immediately after intravenous induction, regardless of the agent used. If this happens the pulse should be palpated immediately to ensure that cardiac arrest has not occurred. If apnoea persists for longer than 15–30 s the cat should be ventilated with the breathing circuit via endotracheal tube or a mask, or by using an Ambu bag resuscitator. Once ventilated the cat is safe while investigation of the cause and decision about the next course of action can be undertaken. Apnoea during anaesthesia is treated in much the same way. If the cardiovascular system is stable ventilation ensures that the animal is safe while the cause and treatment of the respiratory arrest are considered.

If the cat is breathing, even with a low minute volume, it is unlikely to be hypoxaemic if the inspired gas is oxygen-enriched. However, respiration that appears, on clinical grounds alone, to be inadequate can generally be expected to cause hypercapnia.

A hazard of the use of pulse oximeters (see Chapter 10) has received attention recently in the medical literature and the principle is equally applicable to the cat (Davidson & Hosie, 1993; Hutton & Clutton-Brock, 1993; Lear & Morgan 1993; Mak, 1993). Pulse oximeters measure oxygen saturation but supply no information about carbon dioxide. A number of cases have been reported where severe respiratory depression was missed because the patients were adequately oxygenated and therefore appeared normal on pulse oximetry (Davidson & Hosie, 1993; Lear & Morgan, 1993). These patients were breathing oxygen-enriched air and thus remained adequately oxygenated in spite of a low minute volume. Very marked hypercapnia developed because of the hypoventilation. This is not the fault of the pulse oximeter but of interpretation of the information it provides. It is important to remember that adequate oxygenation does not imply adequate respiration if oxygen-rich gas is inspired. However, it is probably safe to assume that adequate oxygenation does imply adequate respiration if the cat is breathing air.

Respiratory depression is commonly caused by overdose of anaesthetic, partial airway obstruction and pulmonary disease. If respiratory depression is suspected the inspired concentration of anaesthetic should be reduced if possible. The most important treatment for respiratory depression is IPPV. This can be started manually or with a ventilator and allows time to consider why depression developed and what longer term remedial action is required. Its effect is immediate, however, and other than some depression of cardiac output is less harmful than respiratory depression and apnoea.

Excessive dead space in the breathing circuit will lead, insidiously, to hypercapnia as the cat rebreathes too much of its expired gases. This is a particular hazard in the cat where a few extra millilitres in connecting tubing may constitute a significant proportion of its tidal volume. Endotracheal tubes should be kept as short as possible. Commercially available tubes are always too long and should be cut to size before insertion. A suitable length is from the mouth to the point of shoulder. Many breathing circuits are unsuitable for cats for the same reason as, designed for larger animals, they have a large Y-piece at the patient end which leads to rebreathing and carbon dioxide retention in animals the size of a cat (see Chapter 9).

Increased work of breathing will also lead to respiratory depression. This may be caused by pressure on the chest wall from the weight of surgical equipment or by surgical assistants leaning on the thorax. Increased respiratory effort is also required to work the heavier types of one-way valve in circle systems and many circle systems are unsuitable for use in cats for this reason as well as the large dead space discussed above. These considerations are particularly important in the cat because of its small size.

Aspiration of stomach contents
Aspiration of stomach contents may lead to immediate tracheal obstruction or development of fatal pneumonia and thus prevention is essential. The cat has a well developed vomit-

ing reflex and whenever possible anaesthesia should not be induced when the stomach is full. Vomiting is most likely to occur during induction or in recovery when the cat is not fully conscious, and may lead to inhalation of stomach contents. Starvation for 6 h should ensure an empty stomach and decrease the chances of such an eventuality. Parturient queens and cats with intestinal obstruction have slower gastric emptying than normal cats. Particular care should be taken to prevent inhalation in these cases since it may not be possible to prevent vomiting or regurgitation of stomach content.

Where vomiting is likely anaesthesia should be induced by a rapid intravenous technique, the cat should be held with the head up and intubated immediately. If a cuffed tube is used the cuff should be inflated before the cat is placed in a horizontal position. Ideally suction should be available at induction in high risk cases.

If vomiting occurs at induction the cat's mouth should be held open and the head lowered over the edge of the table so that vomit is not aspirated. The mouth, pharynx and if necessary the trachea must be cleared immediately if any obstruction remains. If any material is aspirated the cat should at least be give prophylactic antibiotic cover and be kept under careful observation postoperatively (Chapter 13).

A more insidious problem is where aspiration occurs during anaesthesia through leakage of regurgitated material into the trachea and lungs. The first signs may be slow onset of respiratory distress and hypoxia during anaesthesia or in the recovery period. As much material as possible should be aspirated, the cat should be given oxygen-enriched gas to breathe and antibiotic cover. The prognosis after aspiration of stomach content is relatively poor and major effort to prevent aspiration is justified.

Accidents relating to specific anaesthetic agents
Thiopentone is irritant, and perivascular injection may cause inflammation and skin sloughing. However in the cat there is no need for solutions more concentrated than 2.5% or, even

better, 1.25%, and problems with perivascular injection with this drug are easily prevented.

Saffan has been used in the cat for many years with good results. Indeed, in the AVA/BSAVA survey reported by Clarke and Hall (1990) it was associated with fewer deaths than any other anaesthetic agent used in cats. However, Saffan does appear to be responsible for a number of aberrant reactions. Swollen paws and ears are commonly reported but rarely cause any serious problem. However, oedema in the larynx and pulmonary oedema may be far more serious (Stogdale, 1978; Hale, 1989). Bronchial spasm may also occur (Dodman, 1980). The drug has now been withdrawn from the human market because of these reactions, thought to be due to the solvent cremaphor EL. The cat is more tolerant of the product and Saffan remains available for use in the cat. There is no doubt that it is useful in the cat but the potential hazards of anaphylactoid reaction must be borne in mind.

There are no reports of successful treatment of the more serious reactions to Saffan, particularly bronchial spasm but adrenaline (1 ml of 1 : 10 000) injected down the endotracheal tube (Clarke, pers. comm.) appears the most promising approach.

Propofol has been widely used in the cat and is often recommended for use in high risk cats (see Chapters 8 and 11). It causes at least as much cardiorespiratory depression as thiopentone and may cause apnoea at induction. It is essential to be prepared to ventilate for a short period immediately after induction as the apnoea may last several minutes. It appears that apnoea is less likely after slow injection. Propofol has also been reported to cause twitching and muscle spasm in dogs (Davies, 1991) which may interfere with a surgical procedure although is rarely life threatening. CNS excitement has also been associated with the use of propofol in man (Shearer, 1990) and must be regarded as a potential hazard in the cat although it has not so far been reported in this species.

Circulatory Abnormalities

Adequate circulation is dependent on many factors and failure of any of these may lead to cardiovascular collapse during anaesthesia. The main requirement of the circulation is that sufficient oxygen is supplied to the tissues; thus tissue perfusion is at least as important as the oxygen content of the blood. The most common causes of circulatory failure during anaesthesia are hypovolaemia or inadequate cardiac output. Cardiac output is most likely to fall as a result of anaesthetic-induced myocardial depression but endotoxaemia also causes myocardial depression and cardiac arrhythmias, if severe, also reduce output.

Hypovolaemia
Untreated hypovolaemia may lead to serious mishaps during anaesthesia, particularly when drugs that prevent the normal physiological response to blood loss and hypotension are used. In particular, acepromazine may cause severe cardiovascular collapse in an otherwise a well compensated, hypovolaemic cat. At least the circulating blood volume should be restored before induction of anaesthesia (see Chapter 13). Potential problems should be anticipated from the history (see Chapter 6) and treated accordingly before anaesthesia (Chapter 13).

Hypovolaemia may also develop during surgery as a result of blood loss. In the cat an apparently small volume constitutes a significant proportion of the circulating blood volume and can be lost remarkably quickly during surgery that does not appear to cause particularly marked bleeding. For instance, in a 3-kg cat the circulating blood volume is in the order of 170 ml, thus 17 ml is 10% of the circulating blood volume. This represents only a few blood soaked swabs which may not draw attention to their significance unless the problem is anticipated and a careful watch made. It is far better to start to replace blood loss before hypovolaemia develops and thus prevent an emergency. This is easily done if blood loss is estimated (see Chapter 10) by such methods as counting swabs.

Signs of hypovolaemia during anaesthesia may be insidious, but it should be suspected when tachycardia develops without obvious surgical stimulation, when anaesthesia deepens unexpectedly and when the cat fails to regain consciousness normally. A weak thready pulse and pale mucous membranes are also seen, but may be difficult to assess objectively during anaesthesia. Unfortunately the tachycardic response to hypovolaemia may be blunted by anaesthetic drugs and severe hypovolaemia can develop before marked clinical changes are noticed in the anaesthetized cat. It is thus extremely important in this small species to estimate and replace losses before they become severe.

Treatment should be aimed at restoring the circulation first, with warmed isotonic crystalloids, and colloids or blood in severe cases. Any extracellular fluid (ECF) or intracellular fluid (ICF) deficit can be replenished later after the circulation has been restored (see Chapter 13). The cat's small size is now an advantage as it is easy to replace the small volumes involved.

Myocardial depression

Myocardial depression is difficult to detect specifically but will result in hypotension, a weak thready pulse and, if caused by anaesthetic overdose, will be accompanied by other signs of deep anaesthesia. If suspected, the inspired anaesthetic concentration or the infusion rate of intravenous agents should be reduced. If these measures are insufficient to improve the circulation a more serious underlying cause is likely, such as endotoxaemia or myocardial hypoxia, and cardiac support should be considered (Chapter 13).

Cardiac arrhythmias

Cardiac arrhythmias are not uncommon during anaesthesia although they are only a serious hazard if severe enough to affect cardiac output. Many volatile agents sensitize the heart to arrhythmogenic stimuli, and in cats arrhythmias are more common during volatile anaesthesia, particularly halothane (Purchase, 1966), than during intravenous anaesthesia. Arrhythmias are caused by intubation, hypercapnia, hypoxaemia, electrolyte and acid–base imbalance and hypovolaemia.

Cats that have some pathological condition predisposing towards arrhythmias should have this treated or controlled as far as possible before surgery (see Chapter 11). Arrhythmias which develop during the course of anaesthesia

in the healthy cat are rarely a significant problem although the underlying cause, such as hypovolaemia, may be life threatening.

Premature ventricular contractions are the most frequent arrhythmia seen in cats other than bradycardia (Cohen & Tilley, 1979; Trim, 1987). These may be seen at induction and also occur during intubation under light anaesthesia. They are abolished if the larynx is desensitized with local anaesthetic solution. Such arrhythmias are usually self limiting, disappear with the onset of stable anaesthesia and do not need treatment.

Premature ventricular contractions that occur during anaesthesia are generally related to hypercapnia and increased myocardial sensitivity or with deep anaesthesia and myocardial hypoxia. Occasionally they may occur in response to stimulation in a cat that is too lightly anaesthetized. During halothane anaesthesia irregular electrocardiograms are not uncommon (Muir *et al.*, 1959) and have the appearance of multifocal extrasystoles but do not affect the arterial blood pressure.

The common non-life-threatening premature ventricular contractions can usually only be identified with an ECG as they do not affect blood pressure, suggesting that cardiac output is probably also little affected. If they occur during anaesthesia they generally respond to increased ventilation with IPPV suggesting that hypercapnia is the most likely cause. The inspired oxygen concentration should also be increased and anaesthetic administration reduced (Cohen & Tilley, 1979). A change from halothane to isoflurane or enflurane is usually also effective (Hubbell *et al.*, 1984). Volume expansion with isotonic fluid is also indicated, as is bicarbonate administration if metabolic acidosis is present (Trim, 1987). It is important to decide whether the arrhythmia is affecting the circulation in deciding how aggressive treatment should be. If there are no signs of circulatory failure, such as a fall in blood pressure, weakening or irregularity of the pulse or an unexpected increase in anaesthetic depth, it is probably unnecessary to take any further action unless the arrhythmia becomes more persistent.

If arrhythmias are frequent (two or more premature ventricular contractions in succession or more than five or six per minute) or worsening in spite of the remedial action described above, treatment with lignocaine (1–2 mg/kg) is indicated. This should be injected intravenously over approximately 1 min. This is most easily accomplished by diluting the lignocaine in saline to ensure accurate dosing. A 1 mg/kg dose in a 3-kg cat is only 0.15 ml of the standard 2% solution. The anti-arrhythmic effect lasts about 10 min and may need repeating if the cause has not been eliminated. This is an extremely uncommon requirement during anaesthesia in cats that do not have any underlying cardiac or metabolic disease. In 1979, Cohen and Tilley considered that the use of lignocaine as an antiarrhythmic agent in the cat was extremely dangerous. However, there have been several recommendations for its use subsequently (Trim, 1987) but it is extremely important not to overdose.

Vagal reflexes leading to bradyarrhythmias and sinus arrest are not uncommon in cats undergoing enucleation of the eye. This was reported as a probable cause of death in two cats in the AVA/BSAVA survey (Clarke & Hall, 1990). Anticholinergic premedication may not protect against this, particularly if over 1–2 h has elapsed since premedication. It is essential that venous access is secured and anticholinergics are easily accessible for any surgery about the eye and neck that may stimulate the vagus. Bradyarrhythmias are a recognized response to some surgical manipulations in man and are generally thought to be a vagal reflex that can be prevented or treated with anticholinergic drugs (Doyle & Mark, 1990).

Cardiac abnormalities relating to specific anaesthetic agents
In the dog, atropine premedication increases the incidence of arrhythmias, in particular second degree atrioventricular (AV) block and premature ventricular contractions and is thus probably contraindicated for use on a regular basis (Muir, 1978). Similar information is not available in the cat and atropine is probably more widely used in this species for its effect as a drying agent. It is also notable, if somewhat paradoxical, that the cardiac irregularities as reported by Muir *et al.* (1959), appearing as

multifocal premature ventricular contractions, are less common in cats premedicated with atropine. Atropine may even sometimes be used effectively to treat such irregularities during anaesthesia.

The α_2-adrenoceptor agonist agents xylazine and medetomidine cause marked bradyarrhythmias and a decrease in cardiac output (see Chapter 7). They can be expected to enhance the general cardiodepressant effect of general anaesthetics and are likely to exacerbate myocardial hypoxia. If severe cardiovascular depression develops in a cat which has been given either xylazine or medetomidine it would be logical to antagonize their effect with atipamezole (see Chapter 7) as part of the resuscitation routine. Xylazine also potentiates myocardial sensitivity to catecholamines under halothane anaesthesia in dogs (Muir *et al.*, 1975). Thus, if α_2-adrenoceptor agonist drugs are used prior to halothane anaesthesia, without protective drugs such as the phenothiazines (see below), considerable care must be taken not to allow hypercapnia or other arrhythmogenic stimuli to develop.

Ventricular arrhythmias, particularly bigeminy, are not uncommon after thiamylal and thiopentone induction. These are rarely life threatening and are less common in the cat than in the dog. This may be because they are related to the concentration of the injected solution (Cohen & Tilley, 1979) as lower concentrations (2.5% or less) can easily be used in the cat. There is some suggestion that ketamine may enhance halothane-induced sensitivity of the heart to catecholamine-induced arrhythmias in the cat (Bednarski *et al.*, 1988) but this is not always consistent (Bednarski & Majors, 1986).

Acepromazine is widely used for premedication and causes some hypotension through its α_1-blocking action. This may cause cardiovascular collapse in the hypovolaemic cat and has undoubtedly caused a number of accidents when used before volume restoration in such animals. It does, however, have a marked cardioprotective effect against catecholamine induced ventricular arrhythmias, at least in the dog, (Muir *et al.*, 1975) which may be of considerable benefit in the hypercapnic, acidotic and hypoxaemic cat.

The volatile anaesthetic agents all cause marked cardiovascular depression (see Chapter 9) as well as myocardial sensitization to catecholamines. As in other species, halothane sensitizes the feline heart much more than isoflurane (Bednarski & Majors, 1986). However, it is the cardiorespiratory effects that are most significant in causing anaesthetic accidents, and it is extremely easy to overdose the cat with these agents and cause cardiovascular collapse as well as respiratory depression. Careful monitoring of the depth of anaesthesia and the state of the cardiovascular and respiratory systems are essential when these potent agents are used. Theoretically, apnoea occurs before cardiac arrest with overdose of most volatile agents. In practice they may occur very close together and such a catastrophe is much better avoided by careful monitoring (see Chapter 10).

Other Complications of Anaesthesia

Temperature abnormalities

Hypothermia. There may be a very marked fall in body temperature during anaesthesia, particularly when the room is cold or when a large area of the body is prepared for surgery using cold fluids or alcohol. Kittens and geriatric cats are less well able to thermoregulate and are at particular risk of developing hypothermia. Serious effects of hypothermia (30–35°C) include a progressive decrease in anaesthetic requirement, decreased cardiac and ventilatory function, and a very prolonged recovery from anaesthesia. Core temperatures less than 32°C may be life-threatening. Reports of anaesthetized human patients indicate that there is increased morbidity and mortality in the days following anaesthesia in patients that were hypothermic during surgery compared with those that remained normothermic.

Haskins (1981) found no correlation between the degree of hypothermia and the anaesthetic drug combinations used in anaesthetized cats. In this study the greatest decrease in body

temperature occurred during preparation of the surgical site before the beginning of surgery. Once a cat's body temperature has decreased it may be difficult to return it to normal until the animal begins to recover from anaesthesia. Therefore, it is advisable to make every effort to prevent any decrease in body temperature and to monitor temperature throughout surgery and during recovery (see Chapter 10) so that further action can be taken as soon as possible if the temperature begins to fall.

Heat loss can be minimized if the cat is anaesthetized in a warm environment and insulated from the outset. A plastic covered foam pad between the cat and surgery table help to minimize heat loss. Placing the cat on a circulating warm water heating pad is generally inefficient in slowing heat loss (Hubbell *et al.*, 1985) but the pad is more effective when placed over the cat to warm the surrounding air (Haskins, 1981) although care must be taken not to burn the skin. Parts of the cat distant from the surgical site may be wrapped in plastic bubble packing sheets, plastic kitchen wrap (Saran Wrap®), or aluminium fabric used in camping. Warmed gel packs usually used as cold packs, examination gloves filled with warm water, or 'Safe and Warm'® heat packs can be placed around the cat. Heat exchangers (Thermovent®; Portex), which retain water lost from the respiratory tract, can be used in the breathing circuit. Small models are available which add little to respiratory dead space even in the cat. Intravenous fluids should be warmed either by coiling the infusion line on the circulating warm water pad and covering the tubing with a warm gel or water bag, passing the coil through a warm water bath kept at 37°C, passing the tubing through a bottle of warm water (which will need to be changed frequently), or attaching an electrical fluid warmer to the infusion set.

Some cats increase their body temperature during recovery from anaesthesia by increasing muscular activity, shivering, and increasing metabolism. Other cats may become colder during recovery after the heating pad, drapes and lights are removed. It is important to continue to monitor rectal temperature during recovery until an upward trend in body temperature occurs. Heated cage floors are an inadequate heat source for active rewarming of some patients. It may be necessary to surround the cat with warm air by wrapping it in the circulating warm water pad or blowing in hot air with a hair dryer or fan heater.

Hyperthermia. Hyperthermia may occasionally occur in cats during anaesthesia. The clinical signs are insidious in the unconscious animal and temperature monitoring is the only way to detect it in the early stages. An increase in temperature during anaesthesia may be due to excessive application of heat, pyrexia of bacterial or viral origin, malignant hyperthermia syndrome, or may occur for no apparent reason. Overheating may develop when the cat has a heavy hair coat and is anaesthetized lying on a warm water pad and covered with drapes in a warm room. Malignant hyperthermia syndrome (MH) is extremely rare in cats but has been reported (de Jong *et al.*, 1974; Bellah *et al.*, 1989). Features of this syndrome are increased rectal temperature, hypotension, premature ventricular contractions, and severe hyperkalaemia developing during halothane anaesthesia, progressing to cardiac arrest and early onset (within 10 min) of rigor mortis. Investigations of the MH syndrome in human beings and in pigs have identified an inherited abnormality of calcium control in the sarcoplasmic reticulum in skeletal muscle. When triggered by administration of halothane or isoflurane anaesthesia, or by injection of suxamethonium, this abnormality allows a massive increase in muscle metabolism and sympathetic stimulation (Gronert *et al.*, 1988). The significant increase in CO_2 production is detected by capnometry or by observation of a dramatic increase in respiratory effort with rapidly changing sodalime colour and heating of the sodalime canister, and measurement of respiratory acidosis (increased P_aCO_2). Rectal temperature increases and abnormal cardiac rhythm develops (Nelson, 1991). Treatment of MH involves discontinuing halothane or isoflurane administration, changing sodalime (if used) and tubing, and surface cooling of the patient with ice packs and cold water, as well as making use of evaporation. Respiratory and metabolic acidoses are treated by artificial ventilation with large tidal volumes and intravenous injection of sodium bicarbonate, 1–2 mEq/kg, respectively. Specific treatment for MH is intravenous injection of dantrolene (Dantrium®), a muscle relaxant with an intracellular action. A recommended intravenous dose for treatment of MH in dogs is 3 mg/kg. A repeat prophylactic dose 10–12 h later has been recommended. Prophylactic use of dantrolene is recommended for patients with litter mates or relatives known to be MH-susceptible, although anaesthesia has been administered successfully without dantrolene to known MH-susceptible human patients using non-triggering anaesthetic agents, primarily benzodiazepines, opioids, thiopentone, nitrous oxide, and non-depolarizing neuromuscular blocking agents (Hackl *et al.*, 1990).

An increase in rectal temperature occurring after an otherwise uncomplicated anaesthesia may have other origins. Not uncommonly, cats exhibiting excessive muscular activity during recovery from ketamine or tiletamine–zolazepam anaesthesia develop a temperature of 40°C or higher. Administration of an opioid such as butorphanol and/or acepromazine to provide sedation and analgesia is followed by a gradual decrease in temperature.

Trauma

As in other species the cat may be damaged through physical injury when it is unconscious and unable to protect itself or move away from the source of injury. Diathermy injuries and burns from over-hot heating pads are an obvious example. They may be particularly serious in the cat as a result of its size; an area that would be trivial in a large dog may constitute a significant proportion of a cat's body surface. Similarly, care should be taken where alcohol has been used to clean the skin before cautery is used immediately as this may set fire to the cat and affect a large proportion of its body surface. Delicate areas of the cat, particularly the ears, are easily damaged inadvertently when ancillary surgical equipment is used close to the cat's body.

The dangers of inflammable anaesthetics are the same in cats as in other species. However, a minor fire may cause more damage to a cat as a

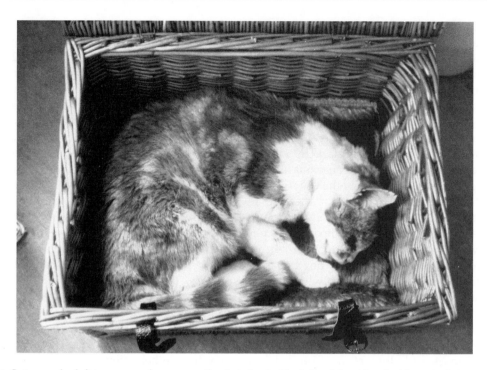

Fig. 12.5 Cats may be left to recover from anaesthesia in basket but should not be shut in out of view until able to maintain a sternal position. While in lateral recumbency the head and neck should be straightened to allow a clear airway.

result of its small size. If inflammable anaesthetics are used it is essential that all sources of ignition are excluded. Oil and grease should not be used on oxygen and nitrous oxide supplies as these may ignite, burn and explode. Compressed gas cylinders should be stored where they cannot fall and break open the valve as the explosion or consequent jet propelled cylinder is lethal.

Accidents in Recovery

The consequences of unnoticed or non-fatal problems occurring during anaesthesia often become apparent in the recovery period. In this respect the cat is no different from other species but a number of points are particularly pertinent. In the AVA/BSAVA survey carried out by Clarke and Hall (1990) a significant number of cats died, unobserved, in the recovery period suggesting that this is a particularly hazardous period in this species. Any of the problems seen during anaesthesia may occur in the recovery period. If recovery is prolonged there is a greater chance of these developing. There is a temptation to reduce monitoring as the anaesthetic has ended; however, until the cat is fully conscious and able to retain a sternal position most of the hazards of anaesthesia remain. When anaesthetized or semi-conscious it must remain under direct observation until it can maintain normal homeostasis on its own.

Obstruction of the Airway

While unconscious, or in the early stages of regaining consciousness, normal protective airway reflexes are absent or depressed. The cat is unable to clear the airway by coughing or swallowing and is as vulnerable to airway obstruction as during anaesthesia. It is essential to ensure a clear airway in this period; any saliva or other debris should be cleared from the mouth when the endotracheal tube is removed and the cat is placed in a recovery area. A few moments should be spent watching the respiratory pattern before the cat is left. It should recover in a cage or other position where it can easily be observed and the room should be attended until the cat is in sternal recumbency. If recovering in a cage there should be enough room to extend the head and neck in a normal position (Fig. 12.5).

Laryngeal spasm (see above) may occur in recovery, particularly as the endotracheal tube is removed or if fluids and other debris collect in the larynx. Treatment is as already described. In recovery it usually resolves but on occasions it may be necessary to reintubate to ensure an airway while alternative treatment is contemplated.

Vomiting may occur as the cat regains consciousness. This may be particularly hazardous as it occurs at a stage when the cat has weak laryngeal reflexes and may inhale solid material which blocks the trachea. If it occurs, the cat's mouth should be held open with its head lowered and all foreign material removed.

Respiratory and Cardiovascular Depression

Cardiorespiratory depression from residual effects of the anaesthetic agents or any problem such as blood loss or hypoxaemia that occurred during anaesthesia will not suddenly cease when the anaesthetic is switched off. These systems must be monitored and physiological support supplied as necessary during recovery in the same way as during anaesthesia. Probably the most common cause of respiratory inadequacy in the recovery period is an obstructed airway as discussed above. If the cat is still too weak or centrally depressed to make the necessary effort to breathe against the obstruction respiration will be inadequate or may even cease and the cat will die of hypoxia. Cats with diseased lungs or those undergoing thoracic surgery where the lungs have been compressed are at greater risk and oxygen should be supplied for the first few hours of the recovery period.

Unless replaced significant blood loss that continues in the recovery period is likely to cause cardiovascular collapse. If the cat is still unconscious some of the clinical signs may be

missed if not specifically investigated. Fluid replacement should continue in the recovery period to replace abnormal losses and provide daily requirements in the same way as during anaesthesia.

The full effects of any drugs such as opioid analgesics or tranquillizers given at the end of anaesthesia will not reach their full effect immediately and may increase cardiorespiratory depression during recovery. Good monitoring is essential to detect this and show when provided supportive measures, such as intravenous fluids, oxygen or even IPPV, may be necessary.

Hypothermia

The small size of the cat and the ease with which it loses heat make hypothermia a particular problem during recovery from anaesthesia in cats. If temperature is not measured during anaesthesia intraoperative hypothermia may not be noticed and its effects may only become apparent when the cat fails to regain consciousness after anaesthesia. Hypothermia delays recovery and if no attempt is made to rewarm the cat the problem is self perpetuating. It is far better to prevent heat loss during anaesthesia (see above) than to rewarm the cat during recovery. The cat will be unable to regulate its temperature until it has regained consciousness thus heat conservation must continue into the recovery period (Fig. 12.6). If the cat has become hypothermic it is essential to ensure adequate cardiovascular and respiratory function during rewarming.

Prolonged Recovery

Hypothermia, deep or prolonged anaesthesia, heavy premedication, hypovolaemia, electrolyte abnormalities or failure to detoxify anaesthetics due to liver or kidney failure may prolong recovery. Liver or kidney failure may be caused by poor hepatic and renal perfusion resulting from anaesthetic-induced cardiovascular depression or to hypovolaemia.

Anaesthetic agents with long duration of action are particularly likely to prolong recovery, and if they also cause hypothermia the two

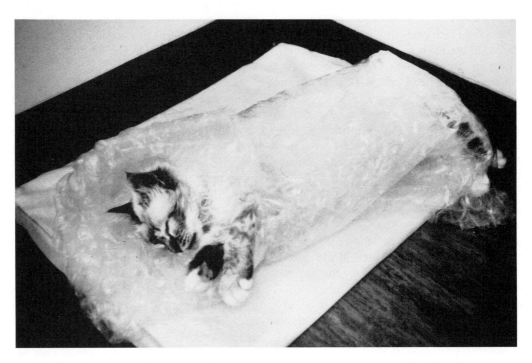

Fig. 12.6 Plastic bubble wrap is light and well tolerated and can be used to prevent heat loss during recovery as well as during anaesthesia.

effects perpetuate each other. Whatever agents are used recovery will tend to be longer after long procedures.

If recovery is prolonged, physiological support is essential. Cardiovascular support with intravenous fluids is particularly important. The cat should be warmed slowly at the same time and oxygen supplied by nasal tube, mask or an incubator (see Chapter 13). Prolonged recovery increases the period of time in which normal homeostasis and protective reflexes are depressed and, if the cat is unconscious, monitoring should be as thorough as during anaesthesia. Clarke and Hall (1990) commented that although the cause of death of some cats during recovery was not precisely known it occurred when they were not under observation. They point out the lesson to be learned is that, to prevent accidents, monitoring is essential from the time the anaesthetic drugs are given until recovery to full consciousness. If recovery is prolonged so must monitoring be.

Excitement

Excitement during emergence from anaesthesia is not uncommon in the cat. It should be prevented as it increases oxygen requirements, may damage the surgical site or cause other self inflicted injury and is presumably extremely unpleasant for the cat.

Excitement is most common after anaesthesia with Saffan (Dodman, 1980), methohexitone or ketamine and is best prevented with suitable premedication. The cat also responds extremely well to a quiet environment and excitable recoveries can often be prevented entirely if the cat is allowed to recover undisturbed.

Pain may cause excitable behaviour during recovery and bulky bandages, particularly on the hind limbs, may distress the cat and cause abnormal behaviour. Pain-free recovery undoubtedly contributes to a smooth emergence from anaesthesia and analgesics should be given in any case that can be expected to experience pain postoperatively (see Chapter 7).

Hypoxia causes restlessness which may appear like seizures. Such activity is extremely harmful in a hypoxic cat as it increases oxygen demand. Oxygen should be supplied by mask, nasal tube or oxygen cage (Chapter 13) in any case where postoperative hypoxaemia may develop, such as after any surgery that may have compressed or otherwise damaged the lung.

Renal Failure

Renal failure following anaesthesia is an insidious accident as it may take a few days to become apparent and may not be attributed to the anaesthetic. It is a sure sign, however, that some mishap occurred during anaesthesia. The kidney autoregulates renal blood flow so that, if hypotension develops, renal blood flow is maintained. However, if hypotension is severe, blood flow will be compromised and prerenal failure may develop (see Chapter 2). The precise mean arterial pressure at which renal blood flow begins to fall depends on a number of factors such as the anaesthetic drugs used and is not reported specifically in the cat. However, in man, renal blood flow begins to decrease when the mean arterial pressure decreases below 80 mmHg. During anaesthesia mean arterial pressures below 60 mmHg are likely to compromise renal blood flow. In addition, certain drugs used in anaesthesia may affect renal autoregulation so that renal blood flow is much more dependent on the systemic blood pressure. Hypovolaemia from untreated blood loss or pre-existing fluid deficit exacerbates the problem.

Autoregulation is largely under the control of renal prostaglandins, thus nonsteroidal anti-inflammatory drugs (NSAIDs) destroy the normal protection of renal blood flow. Renal failure following anaesthesia when NSAIDs were given pre-operatively has been reported in the dog (Smitherman, 1992; Dobromylskyj, 1992; Elwood *et al.*, 1992; McNeil, 1992). Although the problem has not been demonstrated with clinical use of NSAIDs in the cat, a similar effect may be expected. If NSAIDs are to be used conditions likely to cause prerenal failure should be avoided by preventing hypotension

from developing; adequate fluid replacement and avoiding overdose of hypotensive agents such as halothane are the best way to prevent the problem. NSAIDs should not be given when cardiovascular or renal disease already exists.

Renal failure may also become apparent in cats that are living a normal life in compensated chronic renal failure. This is generally seen in the older cat who maintains adequate renal function with high water intake and urine output. If such a cat is deprived of water for too long its kidney function will decompensate and uraemia will develop. This problem is best prevented by ensuring the cat has access to water up until the time of premedication and that at least its daily water requirements (see Chapter 13) are infused during and after anaesthesia until it is able to feed and drink again itself. The problem is likely to occur if owners mistakenly deprive these cats of water as well as food overnight in preparation for anaesthesia and surgery.

Problems in recovery relating to specific anaesthetic agents

The short-acting barbiturates are cumulative and, if used in incremental doses to maintain anaesthesia, will result in seriously prolonged recovery with the particular problem of hypothermia. There are now sufficient non-cumulative intravenous anaesthetics available, for instance propofol, Saffan and etomidate to make use of incremental thiopentone unnecessary. Pentobarbitone has a long duration of action after a single dose resulting in long potentially hypothermic recoveries. It now has little place in clinical feline anaesthesia.

Xylazine/ketamine or medetomidine/ketamine combinations are widely used in the cat. The higher doses are long acting and may lead to prolonged, hypothermic recoveries. The cardiovascular depression caused by the α_2-agonist component may also contribute to prolonged recovery. In the AVA/BSAVA survey (Clarke & Hall, 1990) a number of cats died in recovery after receiving xylazine and ketamine. However, Arnbjerg (1979) reported a death rate of 1 in 2333 after xylazine/ketamine where a low xylazine dose (0.5 mg/kg) was used. The AVA/BSAVA survey deaths were not observed and may have been due to airway obstruction unrelated to any particular drug combination. However, a prolonged recovery increases the chances of unobserved accident. Use of lower doses of the α_2-agent appears to be the safest way to use the combination.

In the AVA/BSAVA survey (Clarke & Hall, 1990) Saffan appeared to be particularly safe with the death rate at 1 in 986. However, there were a number of deaths in recovery from Saffan due to obstruction of the airway. Trauma to the larynx cannot be ruled out but drug-induced laryngeal oedema may have contributed. Laryngeal or pulmonary oedema and bronchial spasm remain a potential hazard of Saffan and may be difficult to treat. Airway obstruction may not develop until the recovery period when the endotracheal tube is removed. Swelling of ears and paws is a well-recognized hazard of Saffan (Hall & Clarke, 1991) but resolves during recovery and does not appear to cause any problem.

Problems Associated With Specific Surgical Procedures

Trauma

Management of the injured cat follows the same general principles as in other species. Unless it has an immediately life-threatening condition needing repair, such as an open pneumothorax, the injured cat is best not anaesthetized for 24 h. Ideally, the cat should be managed with fluid therapy and analgesics before surgery is undertaken. This will allow time for the cardiovascular and endocrine systems to stabilize following the injury, for the circulating blood volume to be restored and allows time for full assessment of the injuries. Myocardial bruising leading to cardiac arrhythmias may not become apparent for 24 h; if present, surgery should be delayed until normal cardiac function is restored. Damage to the urinary system is most easily detected by assessing urine output and may be missed in the first hours after injury.

The precise anaesthetic technique will depend on the nature of the injuries. Chest injury alone or accompanying other injuries has the most bearing on the anaesthetic technique. Any chest injury is likely to include lung contusion which impairs oxygenation, so 100% oxygen should be administered before, during and in recovery from anaesthesia. It is best to use a rapid intravenous induction technique without heavy sedation if the cat will tolerate this without a struggle. This allows complete care of the airway and respiratory system in contrast with heavy sedation which may simply depress ventilation. When any painful chest injury has occurred analgesic premedication with an opioid will often improve respiration and calm the cat sufficient to allow a smooth induction. Over infusion of fluid must be avoided to prevent pulmonary oedema. Trim (1987) suggests giving half the amount normally infused in a healthy cat.

A cat with fractured limbs, pelvis or ribs should always be examined for chest injuries, particularly a pneumothorax. Pneumothorax causing obvious respiratory embarrassment should be drained but if mild can be left to resolve as long as it is improving. The pleural cavity should be drained if possible using local anaesthesia as described in Chapter 13. If the cat is difficult to handle it is better to anaesthetize it and keep it well oxygenated. An already hypoxic cat which starts to struggle is at greater risk. If anaesthesia is required the cat should, if possible, be pre-oxygenated for a few minutes before induction to ensure adequate oxygenation during intubation. This is only beneficial if the cat remains calm as struggling will increase its oxygen demand. Induction should be by rapid intravenous injection without heavy premedication which may depress ventilation. The trachea should be intubated immediately and the cat given 100% oxygen to breathe. IPPV may be required but if the cat is able to breathe spontaneously there is less danger of worsening the original lung damage.

It is essential to ventilate immediately after induction if an open pneumothorax with paradoxical respiration is present. Positive inspiratory pressure immediately resolves lung collapse in such conditions and management of the respiratory system is straightforward thereafter. In cases where the chest is open or will be opened during surgery it is better to use a neuromuscular blocking agent and initiate IPPV from the start. Use of a neuromuscular blocking agent prevents any fighting against IPPV and allows a smooth transition to maintenance of anaesthesia.

Ruptured diaphragm

Anaesthesia for repair of a ruptured diaphragm requires special consideration. It is a relatively common injury in the cat and contributes to significant mortality in the species (Clarke & Hall, 1990). There are two critical periods: induction and the point at which abdominal viscera are removed from the chest.

The problems are proportional to the degree of lung collapse. At induction the change in respiratory mechanics and control may precipitate complete lung collapse and it is important that as much preparation as possible is carried out before induction of anaesthesia so that surgery to correct the problem is not delayed. The cat should be handled calmly but firmly and as long as it is kept in an upright position will tolerate pre-operative preparation. It should be held standing supported on its hind legs for clipping and scrubbing of the surgical site. Opioid analgesic premedication may help this procedure. Acepromazine is contraindicated if the cat is hypovolaemic but it may be beneficial if the cat is not severely depressed as it will decrease struggling. Alpha$_2$-agonist agents are best avoided in these circumstances as they are potent depressants.

As described above, the cat should be oxygenated by breathing 100% oxygen for a few minutes before induction if possible. Venous access must be secured before induction. Anaesthesia should be induced by rapid intravenous injection. All short-acting agents have been used for this operation and none is particularly recommended. The cat should be held in an upright position and intubated rapidly. The short-acting agent suxamethonium may be used to facilitate this and ensure laryngeal spasm does not occur. In practised hands desensitization of the larynx is adequate. Suction should be available at induction in case vomiting or regurgitation occur. IPPV should be started as soon as the cat is intubated and surgery begun as soon as possible. The cat should not be placed on its back until full control of the airway and ventilation is achieved. The ventral parts of the lungs will have been compressed by abdominal viscera and placing the cat on its back may compress the last remaining normal lung in the dorsal regions.

Cardiovascular collapse may occur as the abdominal viscera are removed from the chest. This is presumably due to sudden mechanical changes in the circulation. The lungs expand, increasing the size of the vascular bed, and blood may pool in the abdominal organs involved. Vagal stimulation from the surgical manipulation may contribute. The vena cava may be compressed or twisted as the abdominal viscera are extracted from the thorax further contributing to the cardiovascular upset by impeding venous return to the heart. Release of endotoxin and reperfusion injury may cause further cardiovascular depression. The vagal effects are best prevented by the use of anticholinergics given around the time of induction. The effects on the cardiovascular system are best managed by reducing the anaesthetic depth and increasing the rate of fluid infusion until the cat's condition is stable again.

Postoperatively, it is essential that the pleural cavity is drained of air and fluid and this is facilitated if a chest drain is placed before the diaphragmatic rupture is repaired. Suction is then applied as the chest is closed and is repeated during recovery when the cat can be moved around to clear all pockets of gas and fluid. The chest drain is usually removed a few hours after surgery if no further air or fluid can be aspirated. Oxygen, ideally in an oxygen cage or incubator, should be supplied in the first few hours after repair of a ruptured diaphragm until respiration has stabilized. Good postoperative analgesia will improve the quality of respiration and prevent agitation.

Head trauma

Any animal that has sustained a head injury and requires anaesthesia for this or other injury has a number of special needs that require attention so that the condition is not exacerbated. Little has been reported that applies specifically to the cat, but treatment is based on the same general principles in all mammals. Muir (1989) reviewed the effects of brain injury and described the physiology and treatment of the ischaemic and postischaemic brain.

One major aim during anaesthesia is to prevent a rise in intracranial pressure (ICP). It is important to ensure adequate respiration and gas exchange. Hypoxia, hypercapnia and acidosis increase cerebral blood flow and thus increase ICP. A P_aCO_2 between 3.3 and 4.7 kPa (25–35 mmHg) and P_aO_2 above 8 kPa (60 mmHg) is generally recommended (Muir, 1989) and most easily ensured during anaesthesia by using IPPV throughout. Head elevation and extending the neck may help to decrease ICP. Adequate cerebral perfusion is essential and it is important to ensure that the systemic circulation is maintained. It is equally important not to overtransfuse as this may exacerbate cerebral oedema and raise ICP. There is some controversy as to the best fluid therapy to give following brain ischaemia (Muir, 1989), but the most important aspect for emergency anaesthesia is to restore any systemic fluid deficit, according to the cat's needs, as described in Chapter 13.

A number of anaesthetic and sedative drugs are usually not recommended for anaesthesia of the cat with a head injury, most notably ketamine, as it increases ICP. Opioids may increase ICP as a result of respiratory depression and consequent hypercapnia but do not cause any problem if IPPV is used. Barbiturates are suitable agents to use as they decrease cerebral metabolic rate, increase the threshold for seizures and may protect against further deterioration of the cerebral injury. Benzodiazepines also help to prevent seizures. Isoflurane is the inhalation anaesthetic of choice as it has less effect on cerebral blood flow than halothane, which increases it.

The choice of which anaesthetic to use is probably less important than careful physiological support of the circulation and gas exchange. Equally, a smooth induction and recovery and prevention of seizures or excitement is of vital importance.

Thoracic Surgery

Thoracic surgery, whether for repair of injury or as an elective procedure, is managed in the cat according to the same general principles as in other species. IPPV is obviously required but it is quite common to initiate ventilation without neuromuscular blocking agents in the cat. However, ideally, neuromuscular blocking agents should be used during thoracotomy in the cat as in other species because relaxation of the chest wall may lead to better oxygenation in the period before and after the chest is open and will allow easier initiation of IPPV, thus ensuring as little disruption to the cardiovascular system as possible. Better surgical access and easier co-ordination of IPPV with the needs of the surgeon are also achieved. Postoperative care is similar to that described for repair of a ruptured diaphragm in that the pleural cavity should be drained using a chest drain placed during the surgery, oxygen should be supplied immediately after surgery and good analgesia should be provided.

Eye Surgery

Eye surgery in the cat has similar requirements as in other species. In particular, in intraocular surgery, whether elective or for repair of corneal injuries, intraocular pressure should be kept low and sudden increases avoided. Smooth intubation and extubation and a steady plane of anaesthesia are essential to prevent coughing or gagging on the tube as this increases intraocular pressure and may cause eye contents to be extruded through an incision or tear in the cornea. Vomiting also increases intraocular pressure and must be prevented as far as possible. Anaesthetic agents known to cause nausea and vomiting (such as ether) should be avoided. Opioids are routinely used in cats undergoing intraocular surgery and do not appear to increase the incidence of vomiting (Personal data).

Neuromuscular blockade considerably improves the surgical field for any surgery of the globe and this beneficial effect has been well demonstrated in dogs (Young et al., 1991). Relaxation of the ocular muscles produces a central, still eye that is slightly prolapsed, making access easier and reducing the need for potentially traumatizing clamps. There are few reports of the clinical use of neuromuscular blockade in the cat but personal experience has shown that muscular relaxation with vecuronium (0.1 mg/kg) has similar benefit for ocular surgery in cats as in dogs and has not been associated with any intraoperative or post-operative problem.

Caesarean Section

There are numerous reports of anaesthetic techniques for use in the dog but very little is published that refers specifically to the cat (Dodman, 1979; Benson & Thurmon, 1984; Gilroy & DeYoung, 1986). Trim (1987) has extrapolated relevant information from other species and applied them to the cat.

Caesarean section in the cat is usually an emergency procedure carried out due to dystocia or uterine inertia. As a consequence, there is often little time for pre-operative preparation and a basic understanding of the potential problems and their causes is essential. Pregnancy induces a number of physiological changes in the dam, most notably an increase in blood volume and cardiac output and a fall in blood pressure. In all domestic species the enlarged uterus takes up much of the abdomen and when the dam is placed on her back the heavily gravid uterus compresses the vena cava, thus reducing venous return and cardiac output. In addition, the lungs are also compressed through weight on the diaphragm so marked hypoxaemia and hypotension result. To mini-mize these effects, the cat should be tilted at an angle of 30° to one side until the kittens have been delivered.

Most parturient animals require less anaes-thetic than when non-pregnant and the cat appears to be no exception. One half to two-thirds of a normal induction dose of any intravenous agent should be given initially and this will often prove sufficient. During main-tenance of anaesthesia lower vaporizer settings for volatile agents or infusion rates of intrave-nous agents should be used.

Intestinal motility is decreased and gastric

emptying time is increased in late pregnancy and this may often lead to a cat presenting for caesarean section with a full stomach, even if it has not eaten for several hours. A rapid intravenous induction or smooth inhalation induction, each followed by intubation, nor-mally avoids any problem at induction but vomiting during recovery is a significant hazard and may lead to inhalation of vomit if it occurs when the cat is still semi-conscious. Cats recovering from caesarean section should be observed continuously until they are easily able to maintain sternal recumbency and are close to being able to stand.

Although few data are available that relate specifically to placental transfer in the cat it can generally be assumed that any drug that crosses the blood–brain barrier, such as an anaesthetic, will cross the placenta. Thus the agents used to anaesthetize the dam will affect the fetuses as well. There are no hard and fast rules about which drugs should be used for caesarean section in the cat; it is largely a matter of personal preference. There is no doubt that all intravenous agents result in less active kittens than when inhalation agents are used alone and it is quite common practice to use halothane for induction as well as for maintenance (Trim, 1987). The parturient queen is often easy to handle and induction by this method is usually smooth and intubation straightforward. The kittens eliminate halothane rapidly and suffer little depression. Theoretically, halothane results in slow uterine involution and uterine bleeding but this is rarely a problem in the cat. Oxytocin (0.5–3.0 iu, by slow i/v injection) can be given if necessary. Isoflurane should be an even better choice than halothane as it is more rapidly eliminated.

If intravenous agents are used, it should be appreciated that the longer the period that elapses between injection of the anaesthetic and removal of the kittens the more redistribu-tion that will occur and the more anaesthetic the fetuses will receive. Pre-operative clipping and scrubbing will reduce this period. A single induction dose of thiopentone does not appear to affect healthy kittens adversely but α_2/ketamine induction may cause marked depres-sion. Saffan has been widely used, but even after a small induction dose the kittens appear quite 'sleepy' although the cardiopulmonary depression is minimal. Use of propofol has not been reported for caesarean section in the cat but is probably one of the better intravenous agents to use for this purpose.

The most important consideration for the fetuses is that they are well oxygenated. This is best ensured by pre-oxygenation of the dam before induction if she will tolerate it and by supplying oxygen-enriched inspired gas during anaesthesia even if no inhalation agent is used. If caesarean section has been delayed and fetal hypoxia has already developed as is often, unfortunately, the case in the cat, it is essential that the condition is not made worse by the anaesthetic management. In such cases intravenous fluids should also be given to prevent hypotension, particularly if the dam has been anorexic for some time.

GI Tract Emergencies

Anaesthesia of cats with gastrointestinal emergencies is similar to that in other carnivores. The circulating blood volume should be restored before induction of anaesthesia, if necessary with a plasma substitute (see Chapter 13). Some restoration of the rest of the ECF with isotonic solution is preferable but preparation should not take more than a few hours as ECF will continue to be lost until surgical correction of the problem has been made. It is relatively easy to restore circulating blood volume and the ECF deficit in a cat because the actual volumes are small. Anaesthetic and sedative agents which cause marked cardiovascular depression should not be used as a degree of hypovolaemia is likely to remain or redevelop before surgical correction is made. Acepromazine may cause a cat that has compensated for hypovolaemia by vasoconstriction to collapse through vasodilatation. Alpha$_2$-agonist agents are also best avoided as they are potent cardiovascular depressants.

Care at induction is required to prevent aspiration of stomach contents as vomiting or regurgitation is likely to occur. Means of suction should be available to clear the pharynx of any regurgitated material. Induction of anaesthesia

should be by rapid intravenous anaesthesia so that the airway can be controlled as soon as possible. Induction and intubation is best carried out with the cat sitting up and kept in this position until intubated. It is preferable to use a cuffed tube in these circumstances and the cat's head is not lowered until the cuff is inflated.

Vomiting may also occur in recovery and good monitoring is essential until the cat has good control of its airway. Suction should remain available in this period. Control of fluid and electrolyte balance (Chapter 13) should continue in the postoperative period.

Emergency Resuscitation

The fundamental principles of anaesthesia are that the airway, breathing and circulation – the A,B,C – are maintained. This applies in the cat just as in any other species (Robello & Crowe, 1989). Henick *et al.* (1987) demonstrated that an effective circulation of oxygenated blood can be achieved in the cat through external cardiac massage and IPPV via an endotracheal tube. Emergency resuscitation is required when the heart fails in either asystole, ventricular fibrillation or electromechanical dissociation. If apnoea occurs without cardiac failure, support is relatively straightforward as described above under respiratory emergencies. Full cardiopulmonary resuscitation (CPR) is only required when the circulation fails as well and is based on the A,B,C. The resuscitative procedure should incorporate the following:

AIRWAY	– ensure clear airway, intubate if necessary
BREATHING	– ventilate with oxygen – turn off the anaesthetic
CIRCULATION	– cardiac massage

To be successful, cardiopulmonary resuscitation must start within a few minutes of cardiac arrest. Some CNS damage is evident after 3–5 min and long-term success is highly unlikely if more than 15 min have elapsed (Muir, 1989).

Ventilation is provided manually using a breathing circuit or Ambu bag. Cardiac massage is performed by external compression of the chest wall with the cat in lateral recumbency with a small flat sandbag under the chest. Cardiac compression should be performed at 80 per minute and co-ordinated with ventilation. It is now considered best to ventilate simultaneously with every second to third cardiac compression (Robello & Crowe, 1989) as this increases pressure within the chest and forces more blood into the systemic circulation. It is relatively easy to provide effective cardiac output by external massage in the cat. Muir (1993) considers that it is not improved in this species by using internal massage.

Once cardiac massage and ventilation are under way some sort of circulation of oxygenated blood should be established allowing a little time to decide on further treatment. The precise treatment for each individual will depend on the cause. If cardiopulmonary arrest followed anaesthetic overdose ventilation with oxygen, cardiac massage and intravenous fluids are required. If it followed release of vasoactive substances from freeing ischaemic, torsed viscera sodium bicarbonate and inotropic support from, for instance, dopamine or dobutamine infusion is required (see Chapter 13). If arrest results from a tension pneumothorax pressure in the thorax must be released by an intrapleural catheter before resuscitation can have any effect.

High vagal tone may result from manipulation and can be blocked with 0.02 mg/kg atropine. Intravenous fluids are required to maintain blood volume and provide venous return. Sodium bicarbonate is usually recommended to combat acidosis but should not be overdosed. One mEq for every 10 min inadequate circulation is often recommended (Trim, 1987) unless pH and P_aCO_2 measurements can be made. This stage is often represented as:

Drugs — establish intravenous access
— give intravenous fluids, sodium bicarbonate
— support the heart with inotropes (e.g. dobutamine)
— block vagal tone

If intravenous access cannot be established, atropine, adrenaline and lignocaine can be given

via the endotracheal tube and forced into the large absorptive area of the lungs by ventilation. The intra-osseous route can be used for fluid infusion (see Chapter 13) and has proved effective in dogs (Hodge *et al.*, 1987) .

Many of these procedures will restart co-ordinated cardiac activity, but if unsuccessful it is necessary to diagnose the electrical status of the heart which can only be done from an ECG. If the heart is in asystole cardiac massage and ventilation should continue and intracardiac adrenaline is given (0.25–0.5 ml of 1 : 10 000 solution) at 5-min intervals. This may cause fibrillation in a cat anaesthetized with halothane but the risk is reduced if acepromazine was used as premedication. Lignocaine 1 mg/kg may be given before adrenaline injection.

Ventricular fibrillation is extremely difficult to treat without a defibrillator if cardiac massage has not already been effective. If a defibrillator is available it should be used as soon as possible as early defibrillation is usually the most successful; 25–50 W/s is used with the paddles placed either side of the chest over the 6th left intercostal space near the sternum and over the right intercostal space more dorsally (Trim, 1987). Ventilation and cardiac massage should be continued between attempts at defibrillation. Lignocaine (1–2 mg/kg) may be required to preserve sinus rhythm.

Electromechanical dissociation occurs when, in spite of sinus rhythm, little cardiac output occurs. Calcium gluconate (10 mg/kg) enhances myocardial contractility and inotropic support with dobutamine or dopamine is essential. Sodium bicarbonate should be given if acidosis has developed but should not be given in excess or this may itself cause arrhythmias. A pH between 7.3 and 7.4 is sufficient.

Use of the ECG is represented by:

ECG — *if asystole* – adrenaline i/v, intratracheal
— calcium chloride
— *if ventricular fibrillation* – defibrillate
— lignocaine i/v,
— *if electromechanical dissociation* – calcium chloride
— inotrope infusion

After resuscitation it is essential to provide physiological support until the cat is able to sustain normal homeostasis. This includes

Table 12.1 Emergency kit for cardiopulmonary resuscitation in cats. (Suggested requirements. Precise volume and concentrations of drugs is dependent on commercial formulations available)

Adrenaline	1:1000	5 × 1-ml ampoules
Atropine	0.5–0.6 mg/ml	3 × 1-ml ampoules
Calcium gluconate	100 mg/ml	2 × 10-ml ampoules
Lignocaine	20 mg/ml	2 × 5-ml ampoules
Sodium bicarbonate	1–2 mEq/ml	2 × 20-ml ampoules
Dexamethazone	2–4 mg/ml	2 × 10-ml ampoules
Dobutamine/dopamine	As available – dilute to 250 μg/ml for infusion	
Saline or water	For dilution 100-ml ampoules	
Endotracheal tubes	2.5 and 4.5 mm plain with connectors attached to fit available breathing circuit or resuscitator with oxygen	
Syringes	1, 2, 5 and 10 ml	
Hypodermic needles	25, 21, 18 gauge, 1-5 cm	
ECG electrodes		
File for glass ampoules		
Infusion set	e.g. 500 ml lactated Ringers and giving set. Small flat sandbag	

continuation of IPPV as necessary, continued fluid and electrolyte administration to counteract acidosis and hypovolaemia, prevention of cerebral oedema with corticosteroids and diuretics, and circulatory support as required with inotropes such as dobutamine. This is described in Chapter 13.

There are many reports of cardiopulmonary resuscitation and most national medical health authorities or organizations such as the American Heart Association and the Resuscitation Council of the UK publish a regular update on the latest recommendations (Baskett, 1992). The techniques apply as well to the cat as to man. It is also important that a cardiac resuscitation routine should be agreed within any veterinary clinic in order to ensure that all clinicians and nurses know what to do in the event of an emergency.

A box of drugs and equipment should be maintained and checked regularly in an easily accessible place where it is most likely to be needed. It should include easy to follow instructions which give doses of drugs. Recommended contents are shown in Table 12.1.

References

Arnbjerg, J. (1979) Clinical use of ketamine–xylazine in the cat. *Nord. Vet. Med.* **31**, 145–154.

Baskett, P.J.F. (1992) Advances in cardiopulmonary resuscitation. *Brit. J. Anaesth.* **69**, 182–193.

Bednarski, R.M. & Majors, L.S. (1986) Ketamine and the arrhythmogenic dose of epinephrine in cats anesthetized with halothane and isoflurane. *Am. J. Vet. Res.* **47**, 2122–2125.

Bednarski, R.M., Sams, R.A., Majors, L.S. & Ashcraft, S. (1988) Reduction of the ventricular arrhythmogenic dose of epinephrine by ketamine administration in halothane-anesthetized cats *Am. J. Vet. Res.* **49**, 350–354.

Bellah, J.R., Robertson, S.A., Buergelt, C.D. & McGavin, A.D. (1989) Suspected malignant hyperthermia after halothane anesthesia in a cat. *Vet. Surg.* **18**, 483–488.

Benson, G.J. & Thurmon, J.C. (1984) Anesthesia for cesarean section in the dog and cat. *Mod. Vet. Pract.* **65**, 29–32.

Campling, E.A., Devlin, H.B. Hoile, R.W. & Lunn, J.N. (1991/1992). The report of the national confidential enquiry into perioperative deaths. The National Confidential Enquiry into Perioperative Deaths, London.

Clarke, K.W. & Hall, L.W. (1990) A survey of anaesthesia in small animal practice: AVA/BSAVA report. *J. Ass. Vet. Anaesth.* **17**, 4–10.

Cohen, R.B. & Tilley, L.P. (1979) Cardiac arrhythmias in the anesthetized patient. *Vet. Clin. N. Am.: SAP* **9** (1), 155–167.

Davidson, J.A.H. & Hosie, H.E. (1993) Limitations of pulse oximetry: respiratory insufficiency – a failure of detection. *Brit. Med. J.* **307**, 372–373.

Davies, C. (1991) Excitatory phenomena following the use propofol in dogs. *J. Vet. Anaesth.* **18**, 48–51.

de Jong, R.H., Heavner, J.E. & Amory, D.W. (1974) Malignant hyperpyrexia in the cat. *Anesthesiology* **41**, 608–609.

Dobromylskyj, P. (1992) Intraoperative use of flunixin meglumine. *Vet. Rec.* **131**, 520.

Dodman, N.H. (1979) Anaesthesia for caesarean section in the dog and cat: a review. *J. Small Anim. Pract.* **20**, 449–460.

Dodman, N.H. (1980) Complications of Saffan anaesthesia in cats. *Vet. Rec.* **107**, 481–483.

Doyle, D.J. & Mark, P.M.S. (1990) Reflex bradycardia during surgery. *Can. J. Anaesth.* **37**, 219–222.

Elwood, C., Boswood, A., Simpson, K. & Carmichael,

S. (1992) Renal failure after flunixin meglumine administration. *Vet. Rec.* **130**, 582–583.

Feldman, S., Harrop-Griffiths, W. & Hirsch, N. (1989) *Problems in Anaesthesia: Analysis and Management.* Heinemann, Oxford.

Gilroy, B.A. & DeYoung, D.J. (1986) Cesarean section. Anesthetic management and surgical technique. *Vet. Clin. North. Am. (SAC)* **16**, 483–494.

Gronert, G.A., Mott, J. & Lee, J. (1988) Aetiology of malignant hyperthermia. *Brit. J. Anaesth.* **60**, 253–267.

Hackl, W., Mauritz, Winkler M., Sporn, P. & Steinbereithner, K. (1990) Anaesthesia in malignant hyperthermia susceptible patients without dantrolene prophylaxis: a report of 30 cases. *Acta Anaesthesiol. Scand.* **34**, 534–537.

Hale, G.J. (1989) Respiratory obstruction after anaesthesia. *Vet. Rec.* **125**, 211.

Hall, L.W. & Clarke, K.W. (1991) *Veterinary Anaesthesia.* Baillière Tindall, London.

Haskins, S.C. (1981) Hypothermia and its prevention during general anesthesia in cats. *Am. J. Vet. Res.* **42**, 856–861.

Henik, R.A., Wingfield, W.E., Angleton, G.M. & Porter, R.E. (1987) Effects of body position and ventilation/compression ratios during cardiopulmonary resuscitation in cats. *Am. J. Vet. Res.* **48**, 1603–1606.

Hodge, D., Delgado-Predes, C. & Fleisher, G. (1987) Intraosseous infusion flow rates in hypovolaemic 'pediatric' dogs. *Ann. Emerg. Med.* **16**, 304–307.

Hubbell, J.A.E., Muir, W.W., Bednarski, R.M. & Bednarski, L.S. (1984) Change of inhalation anesthetic agents for management of ventricular premature depolarisations in anesthetized cats and dogs. *J. Am. Vet. Med. Ass.* **185**, 643–646.

Hubbell, J.A.E., Muir, W.W. & Harrison, E.E. (1985) Effect of warm water heating blankets on anesthetic heat loss in dogs and cats (abstract). *Vet. Surg.* **14**, 338.

Hutton, P. and Clutton-Brock, T. (1993) The benefits and pitfalls of pulse oximetry. *Brit. Med. J.* **307**, 457–458.

Lear and Morgan (1993) False reassurance of pulse oximetry – misunderstanding leads to dangerous practice. *Brit. Med. J.* **307**, 733.

Lunn, J.N. & Mushin, W.W. (1982) Mortality associated with anaesthesia. *Anaesthesia* **37**, 856.

Mak, V. (1993) False reassurance of pulse oximetry – take note of inspired oxygen concentration. *Brit. Med. J.* **307**, 732–733.

McNeil, P.E. (1992) Acute tubulo-interstitial nephritis in a dog after halothane anaesthesia and administration of flunixin meglumine and trimethoprim-sulphadiazine. *Vet. Rec.* **131**, 148–151.

Muir, W.W. (1978) Effects of atropine on cardiac rate and rhythm in dogs. *J. Am. Vet. Med. Ass.* **172**, 917–921.

Muir, W.W. (1989) Brain hypoperfusion post resuscitation. *Vet. Clin. North. Am. (SAC)* **19**, 1151–1166.

Muir, W.W. (1993) Cardiopulmonary cerebral resuscitation. *Proc. Am. Coll. Vet. Internal Med. Forum* **11**, 18–22.

Muir, B.J., Hall, L.W.H. & Littlewort, M.C.G. (1959) Cardiac irregularities under halothane anaesthesia, *Brit. J. Anaesth.* **31**, 488–489.

Muir, W.W., Werner, L.L. & Hamlin, R.L. (1975) Effects of xylazine and acetylpromazine upon induced ventricular fibrillation in dogs anesthetized with thiamylal and halothane. *Am. J. Vet. Res.* **36**, 1299–1303.

Nelson. T.E. (1991) Malignant hyperthermia in dogs. *J. Am. Vet. Med. Assoc.* **198**, 989–994.

Purchase, I.F. (1966) Cardiac arrhythmias occurring during halothane anaesthesia in cats. *Brit. J. Anaesth.* **38**, 13–22.

Robello, C.D. & Crowe, D.T. (1989) Cardiopulmonary resuscitation: current recommendations. *Vet. Clin. North. Am. (SAC)* **19**, 1127–1149.

Shearer, E.S. (1990) Convulsions and propofol. *Anaesthesia* **45**, 2255–2256.

Smitherman, P. (1992) Intraoperative use of flunixin meglumine. *Vet. Rec.* **131**, 471.

Somerville, M., Karlsson, J.A. & Richardson, P.S. (1990) The effects of local anaesthetic agents upon mucus secretion in the feline trachea *in vivo. Pulm. Pharmacol.* **3**, 93–101.

Stogdale, L. (1978) Laryngeal oedema due to Saffan in a cat. *Vet. Rec.* **102**, 283–284.

Taylor, P.M. (1992) Use of Xylocaine pump spray for intubation in cats. *Vet. Rec.* **130**, 583.

Taylor, P.M. (1993) Veterinary use of Xylocaine spray. *Brit. J. Anaesth.* **70**, 113.

Trim. C.M. (1987) Sedation and anaesthesia. *In: Diseases of the Cat.* (ed. J. Holzworth), pp. 43–67. W.B. Saunders, Philadelphia.

Watson, A.K. (1992) Use of Xylocaine pump spray for intubation in cats. *Vet. Rec.* **130**, 455.

Young, S.S., Taylor, P.M. & Barnett, K.C. (1991) Anaesthetic regimes for cataract removal in the dog. *J. Small Anim. Pract.* **32**, 236–240.

13
Perioperative Supportive Care

S.C. Haskins and J. Aldrich

Introduction

Effective intensive care of the critically ill cat requires a comprehensive and co-ordinated team effort. Such an effort usually requires some prior preparation in terms of knowledge, technical expertise, and equipment and supplies; it usually evolves over time as each new bit of expertise accumulates and complements existing protocols.

The core of a comprehensive care effort is the patient care checklist (Table 13.1). Most treatment gaps are generated by the omission of simple but important aspects of the total effort.

Insertion and Care of Indwelling Catheters

Perioperative supportive care of sick cats may require relatively long-term use of vascular and urinary catheters. A few specific points are relevant to their use in this way in contrast to that during anaesthesia alone.

Vascular Catheters

Insertion of intravenous catheters for drug and fluid administration during anaesthesia has been described in Chapter 8. A number of points pertinent to their use for longer term perioperative care are emphasized here. Percutaneous insertions are generally associated with a lower infection rate compared to cutdown insertions. A cutdown should be implemented when the vessel is small and/or difficult to catheterize percutaneously or if multiple percutaneous attempts have failed.

Table 13.1 Daily patient care checklist

I.   Cardiopulmonary function?
   A. Cardiovascular
     1. Electrical activity of the heart
      a. Rate, rhythm
     2. Mechanical activity
      a. Pulse quality
      b. Arterial blood pressure
      c. Cardiac output
     3. Tissue perfusion
      a. Capillary refill time
      b. Urine output
      c. Toe-web temperature
   B. Pulmonary
     1. Central control
      a. Rate, rhythm
     2. Ventilation
      a. Tidal volume
      b. Carbon dioxide
     3. Oxygenation
      a. Colour
      b. Blood oxygenation
II. Hydration?
   A. Physical evidence of dehydration
     1. Skin pliability, dry mucous membranes, blood/urine concentration
   B. Historical evidence
   C. Input/output balance
III Nutrition?
   A. 3 days without nutrition
   B. Doing poorly for no other reason
   C. Weight or fat/protein loss
   D. Hypoproteinaemia or lymphopaenia
IV. Infection control?
   a. Aseptic diagnostic/therapeutic procedures and fluid administration
   b. Indwelling catheter care
V.   Patient comfort?
   a. Well padded?
VI. Mentation, activity, behaviour?
VII. Status of other organ systems?
VIII. Body temperature?
IX. Record keeping?

Indwelling vascular catheters expose the patient to the risk of local and systemic infections. Appropriate aseptic safeguards during the insertion and maintenance of an indwelling catheter decrease the risk of untoward mechanical or infectious complications.

A wide area of hair should be clipped over the vessel to be catheterized. The area should be sufficiently large so that the catheter will not be accidentally contaminated during insertion. The skin is prepared as for surgery. A 1–2% tincture of iodine is the antiseptic solution of choice, but chorhexidine, iodophors and 70% alcohol could be used. Benzalkonium-like compounds and hexachloraphene are not recommended. Sterile drapes should be used if it is necessary or helpful to extend the aseptic field beyond the margins of the prepared area. Hands should be well washed and sterile gloves should be worn, if necessary, to prevent contamination of either the catheter or the skin puncture site during insertion.

Proper positioning and immobilization of the vessel greatly facilitates catheter insertion. Vessels are most effectively immobilized by stretching them between two points of traction. Insufficient traction allows the vessel to roll laterally or wrinkle longitudinally. Excessive traction may collapse the vessel. It is often helpful with tough skin to make a small skin incision to minimize resistance to catheter insertion and help prevent tearing the end of the catheter. This is easily accomplished by puncturing the skin with a hypodermic needle and enlarging the hole with the cutting edge of the bevel.

When the catheter is inserted there should be minimal skin–catheter interaction and the catheter should be directed as close as possible to the longitudinal axis of the vein to avoid penetrating the deep wall of the vessel. With the commonly used 'catheter over the needle' type, once catheter and needle are within the lumen of the vessel, the catheter is first advanced fully into the vein, and then the needle is removed to avoid penetrating or damaging the deep wall of the vein. It is important that the needle and catheter tip are fully through the superficial wall of the vessel or the catheter will not advance. A damaged catheter also will not advance and may damage the vein.

Once the catheter is in place it should be capped with an infusion plug and flushed with heparin saline (1000 units of heparin per 250–500 ml saline). The catheter should be sutured close to the skin puncture site to prevent it from sliding in and out which would predispose to the introduction of infectious agents and enhance mechanical trauma to the vessel. On a limb the catheter may be fixed by tape (Chapter 8) but is best sutured on flat body sufaces.

An antibiotic–antifungal ointment should be placed at the skin puncture and the site wrapped occlusively. The catheter should be sufficiently bound by the wrap so that accidental extraction of the catheter is prevented.

Maintenance of Indwelling Catheters and Infusion Apparatus

Indwelling catheters should be redressed and inspected every 24–48 h. All soiled bandage material should be discarded. The puncture site should be cleaned with antiseptic solutions and fresh antibiotic–antifungal ointment and the occlusive wrap reapplied.

The skin puncture site and the vessel should be inspected at each redressing. There is normally a very small ring of inflammation at the puncture site. Signs of untoward effects of the indwelling catheter may dictate removal. Cellulitis is characterized by warm, erythematous and tender skin around the insertion site. Phlebitis may be caused by mechanical, chemical or infectious irritation of the vein, and is recognized as warm, erythematous skin overlying a tender, indurated vessel. Purulent thrombophlebitis is heralded by all of the signs of simple phlebitis plus free exudate which may drain exteriorly with or without palpation or may drain internally resulting in a severe septicaemia. Thrombotic occlusion of the vessel is recognized by hardening or ropiness of the vessel. It may be associated with an impaired ability to infuse fluids or withdraw blood samples. An occult i/v-site infection may occur in the absence of local inflammatory, thrombotic or exudative signs. Unexplained fever and leucocytosis may be the only early signs. The diagnosis may be confirmed by culturing the catheter tip.

The catheter should be removed if there is evidence of cellulitis, phlebitis, thrombosis, purulent thrombophlebitis or catheter-associated bacteraemia or septicaemia; if the catheter ceases to function properly due to thrombosis or catheter occlusion by clot or kink; after about 3 days assuming there is another location to move it to; if the patient begins to lick or chew at the bandages; and when it is no longer required.

Infusion fluids and administration tubing must be sterile. Connections should not be disconnected unless absolutely necessary and then must be done aseptically. All injection caps should be cleaned well with an antiseptic solution prior to needle insertion. The fluid bottles and all administration tubing should be changed every 24–48 h. Tubing should be changed after blood or colloid infusion. The primary catheter or infusion line should not be used for the collection of blood samples except in emergencies. The fluid bottle should be clearly marked if any drug or concentrate has been added to the bottle. The name of the responsible person, time and date that the bottle is started should be indicated on the bottle. In-line filters are not necessary for infection control for routine fluid administration. They may be necessary for amino acid solutions.

Insertion and Maintenance of a Urinary Catheter

A number of conditions, such as those affecting the cardiovascular system, as well as primary urinary tract disease may lead to oliguria or even anuria, as descibed below under sepsis and will necessecitate monitoring the urinary output. In cats this is rarely performed during anaesthesia and it is more common to empty the bladder by gentle manual compression before and after surgery. When it is required during surgery it is most satisfactory to use a catheter and this can then be used to continue monitoring postoperatively. Postoperative monitoring with a catheter is often required following relief of urethral obstruction (see Chapter 11).

Intermittent or indwelling urinary catheters predispose to mechanical and septic cystitis and urethritis. Sterile introduction of a urinary catheter often requires a second person to help position the patient. The hair around the prepuce or vulva should be clipped and the area washed with a povidone–iodine soap solution. The prepuce or vestibule should be flushed with povidone iodine solution. The prepuce should be retracted and the penis gently washed with the povidone–iodine solution. The female urethra can be visualized with an otoscope although it is usually possible to pass a catheter blindly by sliding it along the floor of the vestibule.

A long, soft sterile catheter should be used. Depending upon the size of the cat a 3.5 Fr or 5 Fr catheter should be used. The catheter should be generously lubricated and inserted into the urethra and advanced until urine can be obtained. Introducing excessive lengths of catheter should be avoided because it enhances the mechanical trauma to the bladder. The catheter should be sutured in place (to the prepuce or labia) to minimize its sliding in and out which predisposes to infection and mechanical trauma. In the UK 'Jackson' urinary catheters are available for male cats but are too long for females. These catheters are designed with a flange around a Luer fitting at the proximal end so they can be sutured to the prepuce and a urine collection system fitted. They are sufficiently long to enter the bladder but not so long that they curl around in the bladder and damage the bladder wall.

The catheter must be attached to a closed drainage system; all joints should be firmly attached or taped to prevent accidental disconnection. The collection system should be positioned so that it drains downhill; urine should not be allowed to drain back into the bladder. Draining the collection reservoir or needle puncture of the collection tube to obtain a urine sample must be accomplished aseptically. Three to five millilitres of 3% hydrogen peroxide or 0.25% acetic acid in the collection reservoir will help prevent bacterial growth. The collection tubing should be taped to the hind leg or abdomen to prevent accidental traction on the catheter and suture sites. Enough slack should be provided in the tubing to allow the patient a full range of motion of the hind leg. Irrigation of the catheter with antiseptic or antibiotic solutions is discouraged. Antibiotic flushes have not been shown to prevent urinary infections, only to delay them and to select for resistant infections. The bag should be drained only every 8–12 h unless hourly output measurements are desired.

The prepuce or vestibule should be flushed with a dilute iodine solution three times daily to prevent migration of infectious agents into the bladder along the outside of the catheter.

Long-term catheterization of the urinary bladder carries significant risk of infection and requires meticulous care. This is feasible in the comatose or paralysed cat but is more difficult in a more mobile animal. Alternatives are to nurse the cat in/on disposable nappies which are regularly weighed to estimate urine production. Urine production can be measured in more mobile cats by providing a litter tray with non-absorbing granules that drains into a receptacle below. Urine can be collected from the lower section and its volume measured quite accurately.

Maintaining an Effective Circulating Volume

Most of the signs of an ineffective circulating volume are due to compensatory efforts to restore an effective circulating volume. The first priority in fluid therapy is therefore the restoration of an effective circulating volume. Vasoconstriction, in an effort to maintain an adequate arterial blood pressure for cerebral and coronary circulation, causes pale mucous membrane colour, prolonged capillary refill time, and cold appendages. Tachycardia is an effort to increase cardiac output. A weak, thready pulse quality is due to small stroke volumes secondary to the tachycardia and, in hypovolaemia, to poor venous return; in heart failure to poor contractility. Oliguria or anuria is attributed to vasoconstriction and, perhaps, low arterial blood pressure. Decreased skin pliability (the decreased tendency for skin to return to its normal resting position after it has been lifted

into a fold) suggests an interstitial fluid deficit. Low measured central venous pressure is an indication of a low circulating blood volume and a low arterial blood pressure indicates suboptimal compensation.

Diagnosing an ineffective circulating volume is not always a clear-cut decision. A cat can be mildly hypovolaemic, exhibiting some mild compensatory changes, and still have an effective circulating volume; compensation is adequate. As the compensatory mechanisms become overwhelmed by the disease process, tissue perfusion and eventually blood pressure begin to suffer; circulation becomes ineffective, and tissue hypoxia and lactic acidosis result. In evaluating a cat's condition, when the signs are not clear, it is generally best to assume an inadequate circulating volume and to treat accordingly with aggressive fluid therapy.

Crystalloids

It is usual to start with an ECF replacement crystalloid fluid (a polyionic, isotonic fluid with bicarbonate, lactate, acetate, or gluconate). It may require a volume of fluids equivalent to one blood volume (50–55 ml/kg in the cat), or more, to restore an effective circulation in severe hypovolaemia.

The condition of cats with pre-existing pulmonary oedema, cerebral oedema, or heart failure may deteriorate with aggressive fluid therapy. Fluid administration should be conservative but sufficient to restore adequate blood volume in these patients. Measurements of central venous pressure and arterial blood pressure can be helpful in fine-tuning fluid therapy.

In some circumstances it is desirable to achieve the greatest cardiovascular benefit with the least volume of infused fluids. Hypertonic saline, compared to isotonic saline, in a similar sodium load, but in a much smaller volume, has been reported to generate better volume expansion, and higher cardiac output, blood pressure, and tissue perfusion. The deleterious effects of hypertonic saline include: (1) cardiovascular depression if too hypertonic or administered too fast; (2) an increase in sodium and chloride concentration and osmolality, and a decrease in potassium and bicarbonate concentrations; (3) arrhythmias; and (4) haemolysis and haemoglobinuria if administered into small peripheral veins.

Colloids (see Tables 13.2 & 13.3)

Albumin
One important function of plasma albumin is to provide osmotic (oncotic) pressure at the capillary membrane to help prevent plasma fluid from leaking into the interstitium (Guyton, 1986; Kohn & Dibartola, 1992). Albumin provides approximately 80% of the colloid osmotic pressure (COP) of normal plasma (Falk *et al.*, 1989). About 40% of the total albumin pool is in the intravascular space, 60% in the extravascular space. In response to reduction of plasma COP, albumin is mobilized from extravascular stores (skin, muscle, viscera). Albumin synthesis is also increased. Exogenously administered albumin equilibrates between intravascular and extravascular spaces over 7–10 days. Less than 10% of the administered albumin leaves the intravascular space within the first 2 h (Falk *et al.*, 1989).

Excessive haemodilution is a common limitation to crystalloid fluid administration. Excessive anaemia is often defined as a packed cell volume below 20%, but higher red cell concentrations may be required in patients with cardiovascular disease. Excessively low colloid concentrations are often defined as a total plasma protein concentration below 35 mg/l or an albumin concentration below 15 mg/l. If the colloid concentration is likely to be reduced below this with crystalloid therapy, plasma or a plasma substitute, such as dextran or hetastarch should be administered. Colloids, compared to crystalloids, are more effective blood volume expanders (Dawidson *et al.*, 1980; Falk *et al.*, 1989) and could be considered when the patient does not appear to be responding appropriately to crystalloid fluid therapy.

Commercial colloidal solutions are generally iso-osmotic and hyperoncotic. Colloids of less than m.w. 50 000 are rapidly excreted in the urine and exhibit a short duration of action (2–4 h): dextran 40 (m.w. 40 000); gelatins (m.w. 35 000); mannitol (m.w. 182); glucose (m.w. 180).

Plasma infusion will result in an increase in plasma volume of about 50% of the infused volume. Albumin comprises approximately 50% of the plasma proteins and 80% of the plasma colloid oncotic pressure. There are approximately 5 g albumin per kilogram of body weight in the ECF; 40% of the total is in the intravascular space; 60% in the interstitial space.

Hetastarch
Hetastarch (HES) is a modified amylopectin; a branched glucose polymer. Hydroxylation

Table 13.2 Characteristics of common colloid solutions (Huse & Yacobi, 1983; Klotz, 1987; Falk *et al.*, 1989; Griffel & Kaufman, 1992)

| Colloid | Molecular weight | | | Intravascular half-life (h) | Duration (h) | COP (mmHg) | Osmolality (mOsm/l) | Water binding capacity (ml/g) | |
	Range (in 1000s)	Mw=	(Da) Mn=					Max	Sustained
5% Albumin	66–69	69	69	18	>24	20	–	28–35	25
Plasma	–	119	88	–	–	–	290	20	13–18
6% Hetastarch	10–1000	450/0.7*	69	2–67	24–36	30	310	–	20
10% Pentastarch	150–350	264/0.5*	–	35	–	40	–	–	30
6% Dextran	70	15–160	70	41	23–26	12–24	300	24–29	20–25
10% Dextran	40	0–80	40	26	3	2–4	–	29–37	20
Gelatins	5–100	35	6	2–4	–	–	–	–	–

* 0.7 and 0.5 = % hydroxylation of the starch molecules (the greater the hydroxylation, the slower the metabolism).
= Mw = weighted average of distribution of the molecular weights =
<u>Sum (weight of all molecules of each size x molecular weight).</u>
        Total weight of all molecules
= Mn = simple numerical average of all of the molecular weights = Total weight of all molecules/Total number of molecules.

makes the molecule more resistant to degradation by serum amylase (Griffel & Kaufman, 1992). Six per cent HES solution has an average molecular weight of 450 000 (Table 13.2). Half-life ($t\frac{1}{2}$) is dependent upon the degree of hydroxylation and molecular size. Elimination kinetics are complex because of the heterogeneity of hetastarch solutions: 18% has a $t\frac{1}{2}$ of 2 h; 17% of 8.5 h; and 30% of 67 h (Klotz, 1987). Starches are metabolized by plasma and interstitial α-amylase. Ten per cent pentastarch has smaller, more homogeneous particle sizes with less hydroxyethyl substitution (Table 13.2).

Dextrans

Dextrans are mixtures of polysaccharides produced by the bacteria *Leuconostoc mesenteroides* grown on sucrose media. Different molecular weights can be produced by acid hydrolysis of macromolecules. Molecular weights above 50 000 are widely distributed in the body and are metabolized by dextrinases at the rate of

70 mg/kg of body weight/day (Griffel & Kaufman, 1992). Elimination half-lives of various sized dextran molecules are variable: m.w. 18 000–23 000 = 20 min; m.w. 28 000–36 000 = 30 min; 44 000–55 000 = 7.5 h; 55 000–69 000 = >12 h (see Table 13.2) (Falk *et al.*, 1989). Dextran 40 lowers blood viscosity to a greater extent than does dextran 70. Dextran 40 has been associated with renal failure. Dextran 70 is most commonly used for blood volume expansion because of its longer duration of action. The solution has a refractometric index of 4.4 g/dl.

Dextrans produce a dose-related defect of primary haemostasis which is somewhat greater than that due to simple dilution (Concannon *et al.*, 1992). When administered in large volumes, dextrans can induce a von Willebrand's-like syndrome. Prolongation of APTT is attributed to a reduction of VIII:C activity. Prolonged bleeding time and decreased platelet adhesiveness is attributed to inhibition of the vWf:ag activity.

Table 13.3 Comparative advantages and disadvantages of colloid solutions*

Colloid	Advantages	Disadvantages
Whole blood	Red cells and plasma	Transfusion reactions Transmissible disease
Packed red cells	Red cell concentrate	Transfusion reactions
Plasma	Sustained COP Drug transport Toxin adsorption	Transmissible disease Cost Allergic reactions
Starches	No interference with RBC antigen testing	Coagulopathies (rarely) Anaphylaxis (rarely) Elevated serum amylase
6% Hetastarch		Cost
10% Pentastarch		
Dextran		Anaphylaxis Coagulopathies
D40	Improves viscosity	Acute renal failure Duration < 3 h
D70	Duration >D40;<Hetastarch	

* Inherent in all colloid solutions is the advantage that they support vascular compartment colloid oncotic pressure and that they are effective blood volume expanders compared to crystalloids. Also inherent is the risk of vascular overload.

While it is not expected that even large doses would induce bleeding in normal patients, dextrans should be used conservatively in patients with bleeding tendencies (Table 13.3).

Blood Transfusion

The practice of transferring blood, plasma or other constituents of blood from one animal to another makes a valuable contribution to the whole treatment (Pichler & Turnwald, 1985; Turnwald & Pichler, 1985; Auer & Bill, 1986; Authement, 1992; Brooks, 1992; Giger, 1992; Stone & Cotter, 1992). The specific storage characteristics of feline blood have not been extensively studied and the protocol for transfusion therapy in the cat that is usually used at Davis is reported below. Inevitably, much is extrapolated from information in other species.

Blood Products

The characteristics of the blood constituents must be considered when collecting and storing blood and blood products. Red blood cells gradually lose their viability during storage due to loss of ATP. Red cell metabolism causes a decrease in pH, 2,3 diphosphoglycerate (2,3-DPG), and calcium concentrations and an increase in ammonia. Citrate-phosphate-dextrose-adenine (CPDA-1) is an anticoagulant which maintains acceptable red cell viability for 35 days when red cells are stored between 1 and 6°C.

Platelets are viable for only a short time and it is preferable to administer them within 6 h of collection if in whole blood. Platelet-containing products are stored at room temperature with frequent, gentle agitation until administered.

Coagulation factors V, VIII and von-Willebrand's factor are labile and plasma containing these factors must be frozen within 6 h of collection to maintain reasonable concentrations. The vitamin-K dependent coagulation factors are II, VII, IX and X and these are stable for up to 5 years when properly stored. Plasma is a source of albumin which is stable for up to 5 years when properly stored.

Fresh whole blood
Fresh whole blood contains red blood cells, platelets, coagulation factors and albumin. It is desirable to administer fresh, whole blood within 4–6 h of the time of collection in order to preserve the viability of platelets and the labile coagulation factors.

Stored whole blood
Fresh whole blood which has not been administered within 4–6 h can be refrigerated between 1 and 6°C for 35 days after collection into CPDA-1. Platelets will not be viable and the blood will be deficient in the labile coagulation factors (V, VIII, and von Willebrand's factor) but will contain vitamin-K dependent coagulation factors (II, VII, IX, X) and albumin.

Red blood cells
Recent trends in transfusion medicine reflect an emphasis on administering only the blood constituents required. The exclusive use of whole blood can be beneficial even when only some of its components are needed; however, the use of component portions of whole blood, which contain the desired elements, has benefits: (1) extended use of a limited resource (blood and blood donors); (2) decreased exposure to antigenic sites on red blood cells, platelets, white blood cells and soluble antigens in plasma; (3) limiting the quantity of fluid administered in cases where there is potential for fluid overload; (4) extended shelf-life and immediate availability of some components (red blood cells); and (5) convenience of blood collection when time allows rather than in an emergency. Separation of whole blood into its component parts requires trained personnel and appropriate equipment. It has been reported that when a blood component programme was implemented, the overall use of transfusion therapy increased while the proportion of patients given whole blood decreased (Stone *et al.*, 1992).

One unit of packed red blood cells is obtained by centrifugation and separation of one unit of whole blood into the red cell and plasma components. When collected into CPDA-1 and refrigerated between 1 and 6°C the red blood cells retain acceptable viability for 35 days. This product has the same amount of red blood cells as in the original unit of whole blood but about 80% of the plasma and anti-coagulant has been removed. It is not a source of platelets.

Plasma

Fresh whole blood is separated by centrifugation to obtain various plasma products. The stability of the various constituents depends on proper handling and storage, as discussed above.

Fresh-frozen plasma has been separated from cells within 6 h of blood collection, frozen at −20°C or lower, and thawed just before use. It supplies all coagulation factors and plasma proteins, but no platelets. It has a shelf-life of 1 year after collection if properly stored.

Frozen plasma obtained from fresh whole blood more than 6 h after collection is frozen plasma but not fresh-frozen plasma, in that it is depleted of labile coagulation factors. Fresh frozen plasma which has been properly stored for 1 year can be relabelled as frozen plasma and stored for an additional 4 years as a source of the vitamin-K dependent coagulation factors, II, VII, IX, X and albumin.

Platelet-rich plasma is obtained immediately after blood collection by centrifugation at room temperature. It contains about 75% of the platelets in the original unit of whole blood. It should be administered within 6 h of collection. This product is maintained at room temperature throughout and is a source of platelets, coagulation factors and albumin.

Other blood products include cryoprecipitate and the supernatant plasma left after cryoprecipitation. Cryoprecipitate is the cold precipitated material obtained from thawing fresh frozen plasma. It is a concentrated source of Factor VIII, vonWillebrand's factor and fibrinogen. The supernatant plasma contains the vitamin-K dependent factors (II, VII, IX, X), antithrombin III and albumin. Deficiencies of Factor VIII (haemophilia A) and von Willebrand factor are indications for the use of cryoprecipitates but although these diseases have been described in cats there is little clinical experience with the use of these products in this species.

Blood Donors

At Davis, blood donor cats weighing more than 4 kg are preferred. Cats of this size can usually donate 50 ml of blood every 3 weeks without exhibiting signs of hypovolaemia. Evaluation as a donor begins with a physical examination, including an evaluation of temperament, and routine health screening with a full haematological examination including examination of a blood smear for *Haemobartonella*, serum biochemical examination, urinalysis, as well as FeLV and FIV testing. These health screens are repeated yearly. Blood typing should be performed and donors selected according to the expected distribution of blood types in the cat population in each clinic area. The predominant blood type is A. Precollection minimum packed cell volume is 30%, minimum total protein is 70 g/l.

Collection and Storage of Blood

Sedation is required to collect blood from most donor cats. At Davis, ketamine (approximately 2.5 mg/kg) and diazepam (approximately 0.4 mg/kg) are administered intravenously. Fresh whole blood is collected into CPDA-1 which prevents coagulation by inhibiting the calcium-dependent steps of coagulation and also provides a glucose substrate for ATP synthesis. Heparin is an anticoagulant but it has no preservative properties; it causes platelet activation and is not recommended for blood collection.

Twenty-five millilitres of blood is collected aseptically into a 35-ml syringe containing 10 ml of CPDA-1 (Fig. 13.1). Venepuncture is performed with a 21 SWG 'butterfly' catheter since two syringes are usually filled in sequence making a total of 50 ml of blood per collection. Suction is applied gently in order to avoid damage to red cells. Frequent gentle mixing of the collected blood is performed during the collection. For component product preparation, the blood is then transferred into commercially available blood transfer packs and stored as discussed above. Alternatively, blood may be collected directly into plastic bags or glass

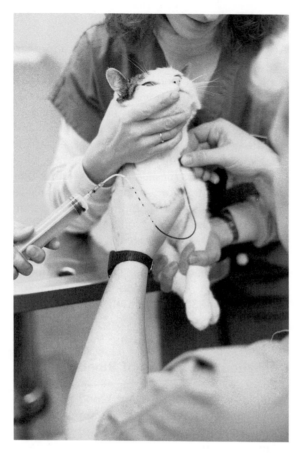

Fig. 13.1 Twenty-five millilitres of blood is collected from the jugular vein of an anesthetized cat into a 35-ml syringe containing 10 ml of CPDA-1.

collection systems specifically designed for this purpose.

Refrigerator temperatures are maintained between 1 and 6°C and freezer temperatures at −20°C or lower. Refrigerators and freezers used for blood and blood product storage should not be opened frequently in order to avoid fluctuations in temperature. The internal temperatures of the refrigerator and freezer should be monitored twice daily, preferably with a system that has a sensor inside the freezer and a gauge outside so that monitoring can be done without opening the freezer. Frozen blood products must be protected against temperature rises due to defrosting cycles. The blood product may be surrounded by prefrozen artificial ice packs which have been previously frozen at −20°C or lower.

Blood products are sterile preparations and must be handled as such. Before administration each product should be inspected. Excessive haemolysis, brown discoloration of the plasma portion or a leaking container all indicate that the product should be discarded. Products should not be left at room temperature for extended periods since this promotes bacterial growth.

Blood samples for future cross matching are obtained by drawing 5 ml of blood into a 6-ml syringe containing 1 ml of CPDA-1. The mixture is then placed in a sterile plain tube and can be stored between 1 and 6°C for up to 5 weeks.

Techniques of Administration of Blood

Blood is usually administered intravenously. When venous access cannot be obtained an alternative route is intraosseous. Sites for placement of an intraosseous catheter include proximal humerus, proximal femur, proximal tibia, and iliac crest. At Davis, the preferred sites are the proximal humerus or proximal femur. Intraosseous needles used to aspirate bone marrow are suitable. The rate of absorption of substances injected into the intraosseous space is almost the same as if injected into a peripheral vein. The technique has been described and the indications and contraindications reviewed (Otto *et al.*, 1989).

Citrate anticoagulated blood and blood products should not be contaminated with calcium-containing fluids which would reactivate coagulation pathways. Blood products may be diluted with 0.9% NaCl, or any calcium-free isotonic crystalloid, to improve flow characteristics, and these solutions may also be used to flush the intravenous line at the end of the transfusion.

Catheter and needle size should be as large as is practical and infusion rates should be moderately slow to reduce red cell damage and platelet activation caused by turbulent flow. A blood filter should be used when delivering blood products.

The volume and rate of transfusion depends on the patient's needs. Slow administration is preferred, especially with products containing red blood cells. For the average-sized adult cat requiring one unit of blood (total volume 60 ml) not in emergency, the administration time is usually 2–3 h.

Refrigerated products are usually warmed to body temperature before administration by immersion in a water bath or passing the administration tubing through a warming device such as a bowl of water. The infusion must not exceed 37°C. Frozen products are allowed to thaw at room temperature for 15 min, after which they may be immersed in a warm water bath or thawed in a microwave (high setting for 10-s intervals, gently agitating the plasma in between each interval until the product is thawed). Red blood cells may need to be diluted to improve flow characteristics, for instance 0.5–1.0 ml of 0.9% NaCl per millilitre of packed red blood cells.

During transfusion the patient is monitored for patency of the delivery system and for signs of vascular overload or immune-mediated reactions. The transfusion is given slowly for the first 15 min, then the rate is increased so as to deliver the total unit over the desired time, usually 2–3 h. Temperature, pulse and respiration are monitored at 30 min and hourly thereafter. Signs of vascular overload include increased respiratory rate and vomiting. Signs of immune-mediated reactions include restlessness, nausea, vomiting, tachypnoea, tachycardia, hypotension, increased temperature, urticaria and muscle tremors. In one report the first sign of an immune mediated reaction in Type B cats who were administered Type A blood was apnoea (Auer & Bell, 1983).

If an adverse reaction is observed the transfusion is stopped. If the signs are mild, they may resolve promptly when the transfusion is stopped. Severe effects should be treated with dexamethasone sodium phosphate (2 mg/kg i/v) or prednisolone sodium phosphate (10 mg/kg i/v). At Davis, if an antihistamine is indicated, benadryl 0.5 mg/kg is administered slowly intravenously. During the transfusion food and water are not allowed as this seems to be associated with occasional vomiting.

Whenever red blood cells are administered, the expected rise in packed cell volume (PCV) should be calculated. Administration of 2 ml/kg of whole blood in anticoagulant will raise the

PCV by approximately one percentage point. For a 4-kg cat, 60 ml of whole blood in CPDA-1 should raise the PCV by approximately 7 percentage points. If the expected rise is not achieved then causes of continued red blood cell loss should be sought.

The Feline Blood Group System

Erythrocytes contain cell membrane surface antigens which are species specific. Platelets, leukocytes and other tissues also contain such antigens. Some blood group antigens are in soluble form in plasma, saliva, milk and other body fluids. These antigens vary in their antigenicity and therefore some are of greater clinical significance than others.

Antigens produced by closely linked (allelic) genes are classified together in a blood group system. The feline blood group system is AB. There are three types: A, B, and AB. Types A and B are due to the action of two different alleles at the same gene locus and A is completely dominant over B. It has been suggested that the rare type AB is due to a third allele which allows codominant expression of A and B (Giger, 1992).

The frequency of blood types in various populations of cats has been reviewed (Auer & Bell, 1986; Giger et al., 1989; Giger, 1992). Blood types were found to vary geographically and between breeds of cats. Type A was the most common comprising over 98% of approximately 3000 DSH/DLH cats surveyed in the United States. The frequency of type B ranged from 3% in Manchester, UK to 26% in Brisbane, Australia. In British Shorthair, Cornish and Devon Rex breeds the percentage of type B cats was about 50%. Type AB is extremely rare but has been reported in Birman, British Shorthairs and Scottish Fold cats.

Some kittens which result from a mating between a type B queen and a type A male will have blood type A. When the nursing kitten absorbs colostral maternal antibodies these alloantibodies will lyse the kitten's red blood cells causing neonatal isoerythrolysis (Hubler et al., 1987; Gandolfi, 1988; Johnson, 1990; Giger, 1991).

Blood Cross Matching and Blood Typing

All recipient cats should be either blood typed or cross matched. Blood typing will identify incompatibilities within the AB blood group system while cross-matching identifies incompatibilities both within and without the blood group system.

The major cross match is performed by combining the recipient's plasma with the donor's red cells and determines if the recipient has antibodies against donor red cells sufficient to cause visible agglutination or haemolysis. The minor cross match combines the donor's plasma with the recipient's red cells. A reaction in this test may not indicate a clinically significant transfusion reaction because the donor antibodies are rapidly diluted within the recipient but it is none the less desirable to avoid such a transfusion. Agglutination is checked both grossly and microscopically in the major and minor tests. Significant agglutination (or haemolysis if observed) indicates incompatibility.

Blood typing for cats has been described (Auer & Bell, 1981; Giger, 1992). In this test the naturally occurring alloantibodies in the serum of any type B cat and in type A cats with sufficiently high titres are used to determine the blood type of the unknown cat. The unknown's red cells are added to either the anti-A or the anti-B serum. The anti-A serum will cause the agglutination of type A red cells and the anti-B serum will cause the agglutination of type B red cells. Type AB red cells will agglutinate with both sera.

All feline blood donors should be typed. This service, or a supply of the necessary antibody, is available through a few North American veterinary teaching hospitals and commercial laboratories.

Transfusion Reactions

Cats have naturally occurring (alloantibodies) against the other blood types and these can be haemagglutinins and haemolysins. Because type B cats normally possess strong hemagglutinins and haemolysins against type A there is a risk of severe transfusion reaction if a type B cat is transfused with type A red cells. Type A cats possess lower levels of alloantibodies. In one report over 50% of type B cats experienced a severe reaction to as little as 1 ml of a suspension of type A red cells (Auer, 1982, 1983).

In addition to naturally occurring blood group associated antibodies, incompatibility may also occur due to antibodies acquired as a result of previous transfusion(s) or to antibodies which fall outside the AB system. Transfusion reactions can be severe.

Indications for Blood and Blood Product Transfusion

Transfusion therapy is a valuable tool in the management of patients requiring red blood cells, platelets, proteins and/or coagulation factors. The decision to transfuse is based on laboratory data and clinical assessment of the patient. Deciding factors include haemoglobin concentration, albumin concentration, circulating blood volume, interstitial fluid volume, platelet count and coagulation status. Each individual has a minimum haemoglobin concentration below which oxygen delivery to the cells will be significantly decreased and each individual is different. The decision to transfuse red blood cells depends on the clinical assessment of the individual patient rather than on a pre-established minimum haemoglobin level. (Consensus Conference, 1988). A combination of anaemia, hypovolaemia, and circulatory impairment can severely compromise oxygen delivery even though each individual deficit may not be severe. The constituents of blood products are listed in Table 13.4. The product which represents the lowest common denominator, and thus will meet all of the specific needs of the patient, is the fluid of choice. For instance, a patient that is anaemic, hypovolaemic and dehydrated, but is not hypoproteinaemic and does not have a bleeding tendency should receive a combination of red blood cells and crystalloids. Transfusions of unneeded and potentially antigenic constituents should be avoided.

Indications for colloid transfusion have been discussed (see colloids above). An albumin deficit can be corrected by administration of plasma or plasma substitute

Table 13.4 Constituents of blood products

Product	RBC	Platelets	Labile coagulation factors (V, VIII, vW)	Vit-K dependent coagulation factors (II, VII, IX, X)	Albumin
Fresh whole blood (<6 h of collection, not refrigerated)	+	+	+	+	+
Stored whole blood (up to 35 days)	+	−	−	+	+
Red blood cells	+	−	−	−	−
Fresh frozen plasma (separated < 6 h of collection; after 1 year, relabel as 'frozen plasma')	−	−	+	+	+
Frozen plasma (separated > 6 h of collection; 5 years storage time)	−	−	−	+	+
Platelet-rich plasma (separated immediately; not refrigerated; administered within 6 h)	−	+	+	+	+

(dextran, hetastarch). Plasma substitute is usually much cheaper.

Ten per cent of an average human adult's total clotting factors is contained in 225 ml of fresh frozen plasma. For human patients with coagulopathies, fresh frozen plasma is dosed at 10 ml/kg with subsequent doses dependent on re-evaluation of the coagulopathy (Bontempo, 1993). At Davis, the starting dose of fresh frozen plasma for a 4-kg cat with a coagulopathy is approximated to be 10 ml/kg, which is roughly the amount of plasma obtained from 50 ml of blood.

Bleeding does not usually occur with platelet counts greater than 30 000, but platelet transfusion may be required if counts are less than this. However, there is often little evidence of clinical bleeding with counts much lower than 30 000.

Abnormalities of Electrolyte Balance

Normal values for the various fluid compartments and electrolyte concentrations are listed in Table 13.5. Note that red cell, plasma, and blood volume, haematocrit, and bicarbonate are slightly lower, and sodium and chloride are slightly higher than published values for dogs and people.

Sodium

The causes of hyponatraemia are listed in Table 13.6 (Maxwell & Kleeman, 1987; Rose, 1989). Hyponatraemia is the main cause of hypo-osmolality. Aldosterone augments sodium reabsorption and antidiuretic hormone (ADH) augments free water reabsorption; a lack of aldosterone or an excess of ADH promotes

Table 13.5 Normal values for cats

Red blood cell volume (ml/kg)	12–20	Sodium (mEq/l)	148–158
Plasma volume (ml/kg)	37–49	Potassium (mEq/l)	3.5–5.0
Blood volume (ml/kg)	54–66	Chloride (mEq/l)	113–120
Interstitial volume (ml/kg)	140–240	Bicarbonate (mEq/l)	17–22
ECF volume (ml/kg)	200–300		
Intracellular volume (ml/kg)	300–400		
Total body water (ml/kg)	580–620		
Packed cell colume (%)	25–45	Arterial pH	7.34–7.43
Haemoglobin (g/dl)	8–15	Arterial PCO_2 (mmHg)	28–35
Red cell diameter (μm)	5.5–6.3	Arterial PO_2 (mmHg)	100–115
Total plasma protein (g/dl)	6–7.5	Haemoglobin P_{50} (mmHg)	36–38
		Base deficit (mEq/l)	−1 to −8
Heart rate (/min)	110–170		
Mean arterial pressure (mmHg)	80–120		
Cardiac output (ml/kg/min)	120		
Breathing rate (/min)	24–42		
Minute ventilation (ml/kg/min)	200–350		
Oxygen consumption (ml/kg/min)	3.8		

Table 13.6 Causes of hyponatraemia (Maxwell & Kleeman, 1987; Rose, 1989)

Hypoadrenocorticism (hypoaldosteronism)
Appropriate ADH secretion
  Ineffective circulating volume
Inappropriate ADH secretion
  Hypothalamic disease
  Pulmonary disease
  Following major surgery
  Vasopressin therapy
Iatrogenic
Diuresis
  Compensated end-stage renal disease
  All diuretics except osmotic diuretics
Primary polydipsia
False hyponatraemia
  Hyperglycaemia
  Hyperlipaemia
  Hyperproteinaemia
Reset osmostat

hyponatraemia. Diuretics inhibit sodium reabsorption, increase urine sodium concentration, and diminish urinary free water loss; the retained free water induces hyponatraemia. Hyperglycaemia (or hypermannitolaemia) osmotically attracts water to the ECF and dilutes the electrolytes therein. Each g/l (5.3 mmol/l) of glucose decreases the measured sodium concentration by about 2 mEq/l and hyperproteinaemia decreases the measured sodium concentration when measured by flame photometry but not when measured by ion-specific potentiometry. The causes of hypernatraemia and hyperosmolality are listed in Tables 13.7 and 13.8.

In most clinical circumstances, sodium concentration abnormalities are secondary to specific losses or to normal compensatory processes for extracellular volume depletion. Volume restoration and correction of the underlying disease process will, therefore, allow the cat to restore its own sodium balance in almost all circumstances. It is relatively important not to alter the sodium concentration of the deficit repair fluids on the first day to 'help' the patient. A rapid change in the extracellular sodium concentration or osmolality may cause deleterious transcellular fluid shifts. If sodium imbalance persists after repair of the dehydration, it may be primary and it may be prudent then to alter the sodium concentration of subsequent fluids.

Table 13.7 Causes of hypernatraemia (Maxwell & Kleeman, 1987; Rose, 1987)

Water loss in excess of sodium
  Vomiting, diarrhoea, diuresis
  Enhanced insensible losses – fever
Diabetes insipidus
Insufficient free water intake
  Inaccessibility
  Primary hypodipsia
  Iatrogenic
Excessive sodium intake
  Hypertonic sodium chloride or sodium bicarbonate
  Cation exchange resins
  Sodium ingestion
Reset osmostat

Table 13.8 Causes of hyperosmolality (Maxwell & Kleeman, 1987; Rose, 1989)

Hypernatraemia
Hyperglycaemia
Elevated blood urea nitrogen (ineffective transcellular osmole)
Hypermannitolaemia
Ketoacidosis
Lactic acidosis
Phosphate and sulphate acidosis (oliguric renal failure)
Ethylene glycol intoxication
Ethanol (or methanol) intoxication (ineffective osmoles)
Salicylate intoxication (minor effect)

Potassium

The potassium balance is most easily identified by measuring the plasma or serum potassium concentration (plasma concentrations tend to be slightly lower). Hypokalaemia is very common (Table 13.9) (Maxwell & Kleeman, 1987; Rose, 1989). Many fluid losses contain potassium in concentrations in excess of normal extracellular fluid and if the losses are severe or prolonged, they will result in total body potassium depletion. The kidney, in its attempts to conserve sodium in a dehydrated patient, generates a very high urine potassium concentration, which then can be a source of considerable potassium loss. Many critically ill cats are anorexic and thus have no dietary replacement of the lost

Table 13.9 Causes of hypokalaemia (Maxwell & Kleeman, 1987; Rose, 1989)

Insufficient intake
  Anorexia
  Maintenance fluids with low potassium concentrations
Excessive losses
  Vomiting, diarrhoea, diuresis
  Dialysis with potassium-free fluids
Hypermineralocorticism
  Appropriate – dehydration
  Inappropriate – Addison's disease
Hypochloraemia
Diuretic therapy
Carbonic anhydrase inhibitors
Renal tubular acidosis (proximal and distal)
Carbenicillin and some other penicillin derivatives (due to renal tubular sodium reabsorption with a non-reabsorbable anion)
Intracellular redistribution
  Insulin and glucose
  Bicarbonate
  β_2-agonists
  Inorganic metabolic alkalosis (hydrogen loss or bicarbonate retention)
  Familial periodic hypokalaemic paralysis
Diabetic ketoacidosis

Table 13.10 Consequences of hypokalemia (Maxwell & Kleeman, 1987; Rose, 1989)

Skeletal muscle weakness, fatigue, myalgia, paresis
Gastrointestinal and urinary bladder hypomotility
Increased vascular resistance – acute hypokalaemia
Decreased vascular resistance – chronic hypokalaemia
Electrocardiographic abnormalities – flattened T-waves, U-waves, prolonged Q–U interval, diminished R-wave amplitude, heart block, asystole, fibrillation
Decreased myocardial contractility
Decreased renal blood flow and glomerular filtration; impaired concentrating ability, sodium retention, increased renin release
Decreased aldosterone release
Carbohydrate intolerance
Metabolic alkalosis
Digitalis toxicity

Table 13.11 Guidelines for potassium supplementation of deficit replacement solutions

Plasma potassium measured (mEq/l)	Concentration estimated	Suggested potassium concentration of the solution used to treat the deficit (mEq/l)
Above 5.5	High	0–5
3.5–5.5	Normal	5
	Low	
3.0–3.5	Mild	20
2.5–3.0	Moderate	30
2.0–2.5	Severe	40
Less than 2.0	SEVERE	50

potassium. The complications of hypokalaemia are listed in Table 13.10. If the animal is known or suspected of being hypokalaemic, the fluids should be supplemented with extra potassium in concentrations of 20–50 mEq/l (Table 13.11). In some cases, depending upon the rate of fluid administration, it may be necessary to supplement to even higher concentrations.

A cat might be hyperkalaemic if it has oliguric or anuric prerenal, renal, or postrenal disease, or if it has hypoadrenocorticism (Table 13.12). Obviously, the potassium concentration of administered fluids should not be increased in hyperkalaemic patients, but it is probably not necessary to administer potassium-free solutions (such as saline); regular ECF replacement solutions contain very low potassium concentrations (4–5 mEq/l) and should be quite safe since the potassium concentration will be lowered by the treatment of the underlying disease process. Life-threatening hyperkalaemia is defined by severe electrocardiographic disturbances (Table 13.13). Calcium (0.2 ml/kg 10% $CaCl_2$ i/v), by virtue of its effect on membrane threshold potential, antagonizes the effect of hyperkalaemia and returns the electrical performance of the heart toward normal. However, its effects are short-lived, lasting only until the calcium is redistributed. Insulin and glucose (0.1–0.25 units of regular insulin/kg by i/v bolus and 0.5–1.5 g of glucose/kg, administered i/v as an infusion over 2 h) is one treatment for hyperkalaemia. Cats should be monitored to

Table 13.12 Causes of hyperkalaemia (Maxwell & Kleeman, 1987; Rose, 1989)

Excessive intake
Oliguric or anuric renal disease
  Prerenal
  Renal failure
  Urethral obstruction
  Ruptured bladder
Hypomineralocorticism
Hyporeninism/hypoangiotensinism
Extracellular redistribution
  Inorganic metabolic acidosis
  Hypoinsulinaemia
  β_2-adrenergic blockade
  Familial periodic hyperkalaemic paralysis
Tissue damage or catabolism
  Trauma, burns
  Rewarming and washout of ischaemic tissues
  Severe exercise
  Succinylcholine
  Acute tumour lysis syndrome
Pseudohyperkalaemia
  Haemolysis (Akita)
  Thrombocytosis (serum)
  Leukocytosis
Angiotensin converting enzyme inhibitors
Potassium-sparing diuretics

Table 13.13 Consequences of hyperkalaemia (Maxwell & Kleeman, 1987; Rose, 1989)

Muscle weakness, paralysis
Cardiac arrhythmias
  Ectopic pacemaker activity, fibrillation
  Asystole
  Enhanced repolarization – tall, tented T-waves
  Depressed depolarization – small P-waves, prolonged PR interval, widened QRS complexes, bradycardia, sine-wave pattern

make sure that they do not get excessively hypoglycaemic. Bicarbonate will also cause the intracellular redistribution of potassium if it is administered to treat acidosis. Sympathomimetic drugs with β_2-agonist activity will also cause intracellular redistribution of potassium but their therapeutic margin is too narrow for routine use.

Table 13.14 Causes of metabolic acidosis (Maxwell & Kleeman, 1987; Rose, 1989)

With a normal anion gap
Gastrointestinal loss of bicarbonate
  Diarrhoea
  Vomiting with reflux from the duodenum
Renal loss of bicarbonate
  Proximal tubular acidosis
  Carbonic anhydrase inhibitors
Renal hydrogen retention
  Distal tubular acidosis
  Hypomineralocorticism
Intravenous nutrition
Ammonium chloride
Compensation for respiratory alkalosis
Dilutional acidosis (large-volume saline
  administration)
Hyponatraemia
Hyperchloraemia
Hyperproteinaemia

With an elevated anion gap
Lactic and pyruvic acidosis
Ketoacidosis
Phosphate and sulphate acidosis (oliguric renal
  failure)
Ethylene glycol intoxication
Ethanol or methanol intoxication
Salicylate poisoning
Extensive rhabdomyolysis

Metabolic Acidosis

Metabolic acidosis is common in critically ill patients (Table 13.14). The metabolic contribution to the acid–base balance is easily identified by measuring the bicarbonate concentration or total carbon dioxide content, or by calculating the bicarbonate concentration or base deficit from pH and PCO_2 measurements. If these measurements are not available, then the acid–base disturbance should be estimated, based upon the magnitude of the underlying disturbance. A cat could be expected to be mildly, moderately, or severely acidaemic if it is mildly, moderately, or severely, respectively, affected by a disease process that is known to be associated with acidaemia: hypovolaemic or traumatic shock, septic shock, ketoacidotic diabetes mellitus, oliguric or anuric renal failure. Treatment should focus on the underlying disease process.

Alkalinizing therapy may be indicated if the metabolic acidosis is severe: base deficit > 10 mEq/l, bicarbonate concentration < 14 mEq/l or if the pH decreases below 7.2.

The quantity (mEq) of bicarbonate to administer can be calculated by multiplying the base or bicarbonate deficit to be corrected (usually less than the entire deficit) $\times$ 0.3 $\times$ body weight in kilograms, where $0.3 \times BW_{kg}$ is an estimate of the extracellular fluid volume and the early redistributive fluid space of the administered bicarbonate. Bicarbonate therapy should be conservative, both in terms of total dose (usually only a portion of the deficit is corrected, such as a half or two thirds) and rate of administration (the total dose should not be administered faster than over 30 min). The deleterious effects of bicarbonate administration include: (1) cardiovascular collapse (hypotension, restlessness, vomiting and death) if administered too rapidly; (2) an exaggeration of pre-existing hypokalaemia; (3) a transient increase in carbon dioxide tension (P_aCO_2) and hypercapnia in a patient with ventilatory compromise; and (4) a paradoxical intracellular acidosis secondary to the intracellular distribution of carbon dioxide.

Metabolic alkalosis is much less common (Table 13.15) and usually reponds to restoration of the fluid deficit. Normal saline may be the replacement solution of choice in such cases.

Table 13.15 Causes of metabolic alkalosis (Maxwell & Kleeman, 1987; Rose, 1989)

Gastric losses
  Vomiting due to a pyloric obstruction
  Gastric suctioning
Diuretics
Hypermineralocorticism
Hypochloraemia
Hypokalaemia
Compensation for respiratory acidosis
Excessive alkalinization therapy
Contraction alkalosis
Carbenicillin and other penicillin derivatives
Citrate and ketone metabolism
Hypernatraemia
Hypoproteinaemia

Total Body Water and Electrolyte Restoration Therapy

Deficit

It is not always straight-forward to assess whether or not a cat is dehydrated, and, if so, the magnitude of the dehydration, because the signs of dehydration can be obscure. The judgement must, however, be made to the best of the clinician's ability. A cat may be determined to be dehydrated qualitatively by the signs of dry skin and mucous membranes, oliguria, blood and urine concentration, and signs of compensatory peripheral vasoconstriction. However, these signs do not provide a quantitative estimate of the volume of fluid which should be administered. An acute change in body weight could be used as a quantitative guide to the volume of the deficit; lean body mass is neither lost nor gained sufficiently rapidly to affect day-to-day changes in body weight. Large volumes of fluid can, however, accumulate in the intestinal lumen, the peritoneal or pleural cavities, or in tissues around fracture or trauma sites, resulting in a diminution of the effective extracellular fluid volume without a change in body weight. Skin pliability is often used to evaluate the magnitude of the existing deficit, but there are large individual variations. The cat is credited with being dehydrated by 5% of the total body weight when the skin, after being lifted into a fold, returns perceptibly slowly to its resting position; the estimated deficit increases to 12% if the skin remains standing in the fold.

Any ECF replacement solution (a solution with electrolyte concentrations which are equivalent to normal extracellular concentrations) can be used to restore the deficit. These replacement fluids should be administered without alteration when the dehydration is known to be due to an accumulation of fluids within the intestinal lumen, or peritoneal and pleural cavities. The potassium concentration of this deficit repair solution may need to be supplemented if potassium is depleted (Table 13.11). Hypokalaemia should be expected if the history includes abnormal gastrointestinal losses, dehydration, or anorexia. Administration of higher potassium concentrations should be monitored by regular or continuous electrocardiographic assessment to look for the electrical changes associated with iatrogenic hyperkalaemia (Table 13.13). Potassium should not be administered faster than 0.5 mEq/kg/h. Volume restoration alone will enable many patients to self-correct mild to moderate metabolic acidosis but those with moderate to severe metabolic acidosis may benefit from bicarbonate therapy.

Maintenance (Normal Ongoing Losses)

The volume of fluids required to replace the normal daily ongoing losses is determined from Table 13.16. Fluids used for maintenance are distinctly different from those used to replace deficits in that the sodium concentration should be 40–50 mEq/l and the potassium concentration should be 15–20 mEq/l.

Ongoing Abnormal Losses

Initially it is usually not known how much fluid the cat will lose over the upcoming day and therefore it seems most practical to replace the losses after they occur and can be quantitated. If the loss occurs via transudation into one of the

Table 13.16 Daily water requirements for cats*

Body weight (kg)	ml/day	ml/kg/day	ml/h
1.0	80.0	80	3
1.5	108.4	72	5
2.0	134.5	67	6
2.5	159.1	64	7
3.0	182.4	61	8
3.5	204.7	58	9
4.0	226.3	57	9
4.5	247.2	55	10
5.0	267.5	53	11

* 80 kcal kg$^{0.75}$; *Nutritional Requirements of the Cat*, (1987) National Research Council, Bethesda, MD.

major body cavities, into the tissues, or via burn wounds, they should be replaced with an unaltered ECF replacement solution. If the loss occurs via vomiting, diarrhoea, or diuresis, the replacement solution should be supplemented with potassium (10 mEq/l).

Administration of Fluids

There are many acceptable ways to administer the prescribed fluids. The intravenous route is by far the most immediate and reliable. Fluids can also be administered via an intramedullary needle, or even subcutaneously and orally in several divided daily doses. Fluids can be administered intraperitoneally; in general fluids are well absorbed but infection and visceral damage are a risk.

Intravenously administered fluids can be mixed into one large mixing container, or successively 'piggy-backed' into one administration line, or administered in series. Fluids should be administered over as many hours of the day as possible so that the patient may have as much time as possible to redistribute and fully utilize the administered fluids and electrolytes. The faster the fluids are administered, the more that will be excreted as urine and be unavailable to the cat. Fluids should not be administered continuously by the intravenous route when the patient cannot be frequently and regularly observed. Burettes should be used with intravenous fluid administration in animals as small as cats to (1) provide some safeguard against accidental excessive fluid administration and (2) to monitor accurately the amount of fluids that have been administered (Fig. 13.2) (Chapter 10). Fluid pumps greatly facilitate continuous administration of accurate volumes of fluids.

Enteral and Parenteral Nutrition

Acute protein-energy malnutrition predisposes to impaired immune competence, poor wound healing and an increased incidence of wound dehiscence, as well as wound and systemic sepsis. It also leads to cardiac, skeletal and

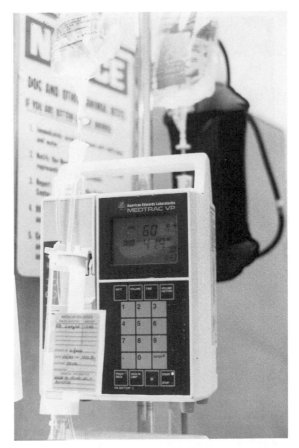

Fig. 13.2 A burette is recommended for fluid administration in cats so as to limit the amount of fluids which can accidentally be administered. Fluid pumps facilitate the accurate administration of fluids over time.

smooth muscle weakness, and major organ failure and death. It should be assumed that nutritional supplementation is necessary whenever a critically ill, stressed cat has been without nutrition for 3 days. An acute body weight loss of more than 5–10% which is not due to fluid loss, persistent hypoalbuminaemia, persistent lymphopaenia, or the clinical impression that the cat is 'doing poorly' in the absence of other, more likely causes, are indications for nutritional support.

Enteral

Enteral feeding should be used whenever the intestinal tract (motility, digestion, and

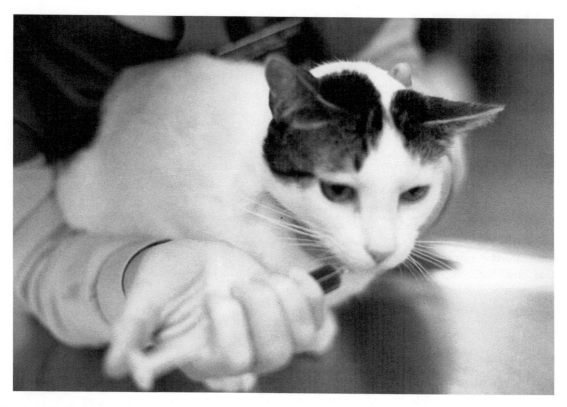

Fig. 13.3 Small amounts of a liquid gruel or a commercial liquid meal can be syringed into the corner of a cat's mouth if it will not eat voluntarily. Do not place the liquid in the pharynx as this might predispose to aspiration but rather allow the cat to swallow voluntarily.

absorption) is functional. Enteral feeding preserves normal gut epithelial structure and function. Small quantities of commercial foods (moist, semimoist, and dry; cooked or raw) can be offered. It may help to warm the food or to provide a topping of gravy or chicken/beef broth to make it more appetizing. Sometimes cats will eat foods like peanut butter with or without honey, commercial nutrient pastes, or one of the commercial liquid meal replacement diets when other foods have been refused. If the cat will not eat the food voluntarily, perhaps it will eat with coaxing or if the food is placed into the mouth (Fig. 13.3). The food should not be forced into the back of the mouth since the food may cause airway obstruction or may be aspirated into the trachea. For cats that feel well enough to clean themselves, the food material can be applied to the lips or feet and be consumed during cleaning. Diazepam (0.1 mg/kg i/v) or oxazepam have

been reported to stimulate appetite in some patients.

A 5-Fr nasogastric tube can be inserted without general anaesthesia and is normally well tolerated (Fig. 13.4). An oesophagostomy or gastrostomy tube is also effective (Fulton & Dennis, 1992). Once an indwelling tube is placed, the required kcal/day is determined (Table 13.17) and feeding can be instituted. Initial volumes should be conservative: 0.5–1 ml/kg/h, to make sure that the cat will be able to mobilize and utilize the material without problems. If abdominal discomfort or restlessness develop, or if the cat salivates, retches, or vomits, the volume of the nutrient solution or its concentration may be too high. If an indwelling stomach tube is in place, it should be periodically aspirated through to make sure that the nutrient solutions are not accumulating in the stomach. Persistent residual material in excess of 50% of what was instilled suggests that the

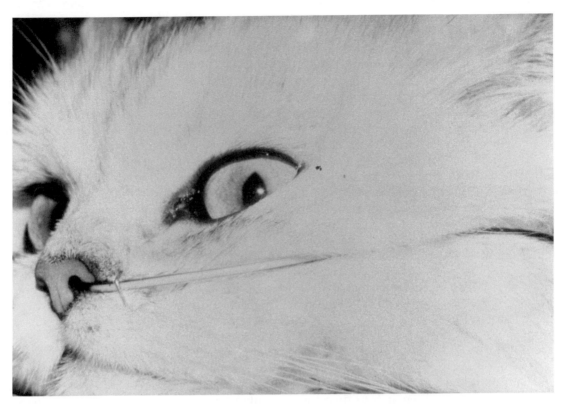

Fig. 13.4 A nasogastric tube can be placed for enteral feeding of liquid diets.

Table 13.17 Energy requirements for cats

Average body weight (kg)	Estimated basal energy expenditure* (kcal/day)	Estimated energy expenditure= (kcal/day)	(kcal/h)
1	70	105	4.4
1.5	95	142	5.9
2	118	177	7.4
2.5	139	209	8.7
3	160	239	10.0
3.5	179	269	11.2
4	198	297	12.4
4.5	216	324	13.5
5	234	351	14.6

* $70 \times BW \, kg^{0.75}$

= Average energy requirements for the critically ill patient; calculated as $1.5 \times$ basal energy expenditure (BEE). Caged animals with minimal activity and minor disease stress perhaps might be more closely approximated by $1.25 \times$ BEE. Normal canine activity or very severe disease stress in either the dog or cat perhaps would be more accurately approximated by 1.75 or $2.0 \times$ BEE. Lactation, late-stage pregnancy, and heavy exercise may increase energy requirements 4–$6 \times$ BEE.

gut is not working properly. If the gastrointestinal tract is moving the nutrient solutions forward, subsequent feeding can be increased. The abdomen should be auscultated at regular intervals; the presence of gut sounds suggests that the gastrointestinal tract is functional. If diarrhoea develops one or more of the following should be considered: (1) reduce the volume and feed more frequently; (2) decrease the concentration (osmolality) of the solution; (3) treat hypoproteinaemia (which impairs absorption of enteric nutrients); (4) change to a different carbohydrate (lactose-free) or protein source; or (5) change to an entirely different foodstuff.

Cats have somewhat different nutritional requirements from dogs or people (Rogers *et al.*, 1986) in that they have higher total protein, arginine and taurine requirements, and require all essential fatty acids. Cats, except for short-term (1-week) feeding, require an animal protein and fat source (as opposed to a milk or vegetable-based food stuff).

Parenteral

Parenteral nutrition is indicated whenever the gut is not working well enough to digest and absorb sufficient quantities of nutrients (Lippert *et al.*, 1989). Parenteral nutrition solutions are very hypertonic (1500–2000 mOsm/l) and must be administered via a large central vein so that they may be rapidly diluted to minimize the incidence of phlebitis and thrombosis. Catheters must be inserted and maintained aseptically (see above). An intravenous nutrition catheter is a dedicated catheter; it is not used for any other purpose such as blood sampling or drug administration.

The nutrition solution should be mixed under aseptic conditions. The following formula is appropriate for the most sick cats:

    250 ml 50% dextrose
    500 ml 8.5% crystalline amino acid solution
       with electrolytes
    250 ml 20% intralipid
    1 ml of a multi-vitamin B solution
    10 mEq potassium phosphate

This formulation provides 1.08 kcal/ml, 12.4% glucose, and 40 mEq K+/l. There are 3.9 g protein/100 kcal. Kcal are supplied as 39% glucose, 46% fat, and 15% protein. The daily requirement (kcal/day) is determined (Table 13.17) and the hourly infusion rate set by dividing the total volume to be administered by 24 h. The infusion is started at 50% of this value. The blood glucose is checked after 4 h. If the blood glucose is less than 13.3 mmol/l (250 mg/dl), increase the infusion rate to 75% of the calculated infusion rate and remeasure the blood glucose in 4 h. If the blood glucose is less than 13.3 mmol/l (250 mg/dl), the infusion rate is increased to 100%. If the blood glucose exceeds 16 mmol/l (300 mg/dl) at any measurement, the glucose infusion rate should be decreased.

If the cat is glucose intolerant (the calculated 100% infusion rate cannot be achieved without unacceptable hyperglycaemia) the following course of action should be taken: (1) accept the highest infusion rate that the animal will tolerate as partial nutrition is better than no nutrition at all; (2) decrease the glucose concentration in the solution and replace its energy-equivalents with lipid; or (3) add exogenous insulin to the nutrient solution (start with 1–4 unit/10 g dextrose) to supplement the cat's endogenous insulin output. Sepsis, and other stressors, are common causes of glucose intolerance.

Cats should be weaned off high glucose infusions to avoid a rebound hypoglycaemia. The infusion rate is decreased by 50%, and the blood glucose is measured 2 h later. If the blood glucose is normal or still high, stop the glucose infusion and recheck the blood glucose again 2 h later.

Respiratory Complications

Respiratory inadequacy/failure is heralded by (Table 13.18): markedly increased or decreased ventilatory rate and effort; an anxious expression, restlessness, anxiety; open mouth breathing; abducted elbows; minimal concern for the events occurring around them; abnormal breathing sounds; an extended head and neck; cyanotic discoloration of the mucous

Table 13.18 Categorization of respiratory distress

Major presenting sign	Anatomical location of problem	Additional presenting signs	Pathophysiology of problem	P_aCO_2	P_aO_2
Decreased ventilatory efforts	Neuromuscular Medulla Cervical spine N–M Junction		Hypoventilation	Increases	Decreases
Increased ventilatory efforts			Decreased inspired O_2	Variable	Decreases
			Increased inspired CO_2	Increases	Variable
	Big airway obstruction	'Snoring' 'Squeaking'	Hypoventilation	Increases	Decreases
	Little airway obstruction	'Wheezing'	Hypoventilation	Increases	Decreases
	Chest wall problem Open pneumothorax 'Flail chest' Abdominal enlargements		Hypoventilation	Increases	Decreases
	Pleural space filling problem Fluid Air Intestines	Decreased auscultability	Hypoventilation	Increases	Decreases
	Pulmonary Parenchymal	'Crepitation' Rales	Venous admixture Anatomical shunt Physiological shunt V/Q mismatch Diffusion impairment	Decreases [variable]	Decreases
	'Look-alikes' Hyperthermia Ketoacidosis Hypotension Hypovolaemia Heart failure Tamponade		Medullary stimulation	Decreases	Increases
	Thromboembolism		Venous admixture	Decreases [variable]	Decreases

membranes; abnormal radiographic findings; and abnormal blood gas measurements: P_aO_2 below 50–60 mmHg (Table 13.19) or P_aCO_2 above 60–70 mmHg.

Cats with respiratory failure associated with decreased ventilatory efforts (Table 13.20) should be intubated and ventilated until the underlying disease can be determined and treated.

Large Airway Obstruction

Complete large airway obstruction is characterized by complete absence of sounds or air

Table 13.19 Hypoxaemia

Low inspired oxygen concentration
Hypoventilation
Venous admixture
   Low ventilation/perfusion regions
   No ventilation/perfusion regions (atelectasis; small
     airway and alveolar collapse)
   Anatomical shunts
   Diffusion impairment

movement and vigorous attempts to breath associated with retraction of the chest wall. Incomplete large airway obstruction is heralded by stertorous snoring or high-pitched 'squeaking' sounds. The oropharynx should be examined first and the cat anaesthetized if necessary. Sedatives are not recommended under life-threatening conditions because they may cause excessive respiratory depression without causing sufficient CNS depression to allow a thorough pharyngeal examination.

If the cause of the obstruction cannot be removed easily or if the larynx is malfunctioning, the obstruction should be bypassed by endotracheal intubation. A stiff urinary catheter can be placed (Fig. 13.5) and used as a stylet for oxygen insufflation or for high-frequency jet ventilation. Tracheostomy should only be performed as a last resort life-saving procedure in emergency.

Small Airway Obstruction

Small airway (bronchiolar) obstruction is heralded by mid-pitched, sometimes musical,

Table 13.20 Causes of respiratory failure

Decreased ventilatory efforts
Medullary dysfunction
   Intracranial (trauma; contusion; haemorrhage; oedema; neoplasia; cingulate, tentoral, cerebellar herniation;
     thromboemboli)
   Extracranial (anaesthetic and sedative drugs; visceral organ failure; severe hypoxia; hypoglycaemia; severe
     hypo- or hyperosmolality)
Spinal cord efferent motor nerve dysfunction (trauma; disc disease; myelography; laminectomy; fractures;
   myelitis; meningitis; polyradiculoneuritis)
Neuromuscular junction dysfunction (neuromuscular blocking agents; aminoglycoside antibiotics in
   conjunction with NM weakness; myasthaenia gravis; polyneuropathy; botulism)

Increased ventilatory efforts
Large airway obstruction (brachycephalic syndrome; pharyngeal masses; laryngeal oedema; recurrent
   laryngeal nerve paralysis; tracheal collapse; tracheal/peritracheal masses)
Small airway obstruction (bronchoconstriction)
Chest wall/diaphragmatic problems (open pneumothorax; loss of chest wall rigidity; abdominal enlargements)
Pleural space abnormalities (pneumothorax; hydrothorax; transudative; exudative; blood; chyle;
   diaphragmatic hernia)
Pulmonary parenchymal disease
   Elevated hydrostatic pressure (heart failure; hypervolaemia or high cardiac output; hypertension; neurogenic
     pulmonary oedema; mitral valvular stenosis)
   Increased capillary permeability (thoracic and non-thoracic trauma; haemorrhagic and septic shock; viral,
     bacterial, fungal or parasitic infections; thromboembolic; aspiration of acid gastric contents; inhalation of
     smoke and chemical fumes; inhalation of occupational mineral dusts; metabolic disorders such as
     haemorrhagic pancreatis, uraemia, hypercalcaemia; oxygen toxicity; ingestion of toxins such as paraquat;
     neoplasia; radiation pneumonitis; dermal thermal burns; immunologic disorders; drug reactions; DIC)
   Trauma
'Look-alike' disorders (hyperthermia; hypotension; hypovolaemia; pericardial tamponade; metabolic acidosis;
   anaemia; opioid drugs; fear, excitement, anxiety; stimulation of irritant respiratory receptors by inhalation of
   noxious gases or materials)
Pulmonary thromboembolism

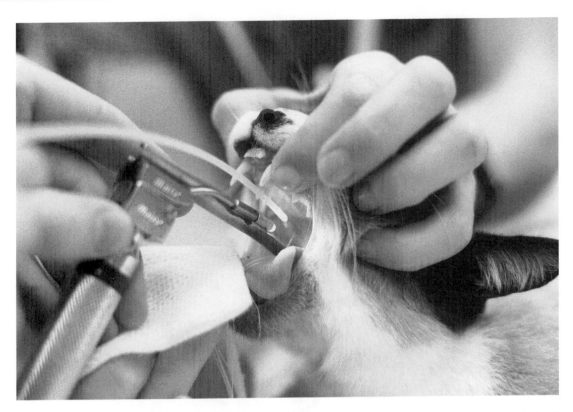

Fig. 13.5 A stiff urinary catheter can be placed into the larynx of an anesthetized cat and used as a stylet for blind intubation, for oxygen insufflation, or for high frequency jet ventilation.

wheezing. If widespread bronchoconstriction is life-threatening, a potent β_2-agonist such as terbutaline (1.25 mg/cat *per os* every 8–12 h) dopamine (0.2 mg/kg i/m) or adrenaline (0.02 mg/kg i/m) should be administered. If the bronchoconstriction is not life-threatening, aminophylline, which has minimal systemic effects, may be used. Glucocorticoids and antihistamines may also be beneficial. Anticholinergic agents such as atropine (0.04 mg/ kg) or glycopyrrolaate (0.02 mg/kg) may be useful if there is a parasympathetic component to the bronchoconstriction.

Pleural Space Abnormalities

Pleural space abnormalities are heralded by muffled heart or breathing sounds over large areas of the thorax, unilaterally or bilaterally. Good quality radiographs are often diagnostic if the patient can tolerate the stress and time necessary to take and develop them. Diagnostic thoracentesis will identify the nature of pleural space accumulation. A hypodermic needle or, better, an intravenous catheter, attached to a syringe, is introduced into the pleural space in a caudoventral or caudodorsal direction as close to the pleural surface as possible (Fig. 13.6). Thoracentesis may be repeated at several locations.

An indwelling chest drain is indicated whenever frequently repeated thoracentesis of fluid or air is necessary (Fig. 13.7). Indwelling chest tubes should be soft and non-irritating, and large enough to allow the passage of cellular debris and fibrin; usually a 10-Fr tube for a cat. The tube should have several large holes toward its tip to maximize the opportunity for fluid drainage. The chest tube must be inserted aseptically and must not allow air to leak into the chest (Paddleford & Harvey, 1989). The chest can be periodically drained using a large syringe, or the chest tube can be attached to a closed passive or active chest drainage system.

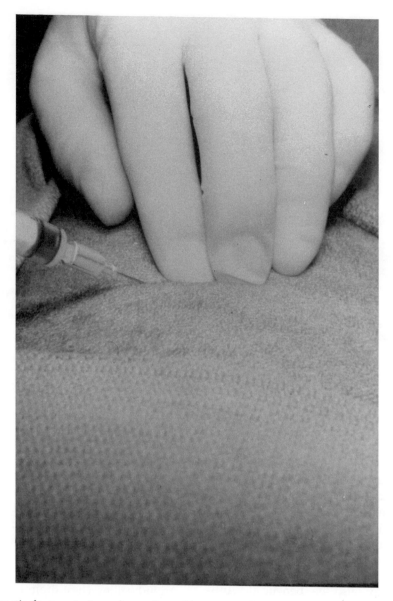

Fig. 13.6 A diagnostic thoracentesis can be performed by aseptically sliding a needle under the anterior edge of a rib, in a caudal direction, staying a flat as possible to the pleural surface.

Fluid and air will cease to drain if the pleural space is empty, or if the cannula is kinked or plugged with fibrin or mediastinal/lung tissue.

Pulmonary Parenchymal Disease

Pulmonary parenchymal disease may be heralded by abnormal lung sounds heard on auscultation: abnormally harsh breath sounds; crackling or crepitant ('popping') sounds at the beginning of inspiration or at the end of exhalation (may indicate the presence of some airway fluid); 'bubbling' fluid sounds during inspiration and expiration (airway fluid); localized areas of high-pitched wheezes, whistles or squeaks; or localized absence of vesicular sounds. Fluid sounds must be localized by their point of maximal intensity since referred upper airway fluid sounds can be heard over the chest. Because of the small volumes of air

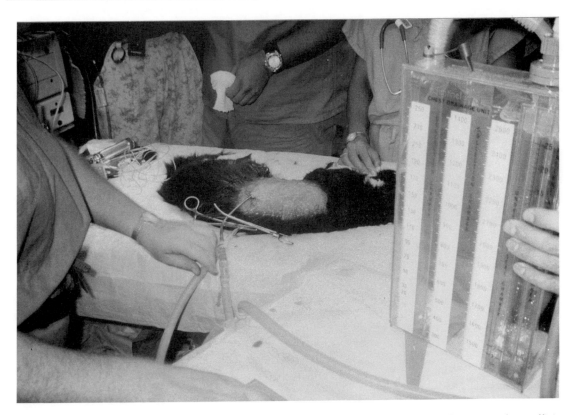

Fig. 13.7 An indwelling chest tube should be placed if the pleural space accumulation is of a sufficient magnitude that it would have to be drained several times daily.

moved during breathing, it is often impossible to rule out significant pulmonary parenchymal disease solely on the basis of normal thoracic auscultation.

Oxygen therapy
Oxygen therapy may be beneficial when the predominant cause of hypoxaemia is regional low ventilation to perfusion mismatching or diffusion impairment. Oxygen therapy cannot be expected to be particularly beneficial if the predominant cause of hypoxaemia is hypoventilation or small airway and alveolar collapse. The cat's response to oxygen therapy should be evaluated at periodic intervals.

Oxygen therapy may be achieved with an oxygen chamber or by insufflation through a nasal catheter inserted into the nasal cavity to the level of the medial canthus of the eye. Medical oxygen must be humidified by passing it through a water bath.

Intermittent positive pressure ventilation
Intermittent positive pressure ventilation (IPPV) is indicated whenever a cat cannot ventilate adequately or when pulmonary parenchymal disease is serious enough to make oxygen therapy alone unable to provide satisfactory oxygenation (Fig. 13.8). The general guidelines for IPPV are:

(1) a proximal airway pressure of 10–20 cmH$_2$O;
(2) an inspiratory time just long enough to achieve a full tidal volume;
(3) a tidal volume of 15–20 ml/kg;
(4) a ventilatory rate of 8–15 times per minute;
(5) a minute ventilation of 150–250 ml/kg/min; and
(6) a zero (atmospheric) end-expiratory pressure.

Diseased lungs are often less compliant than normal lungs, and therefore may be more difficult to ventilate. More aggressive ventilator settings may be necessary:

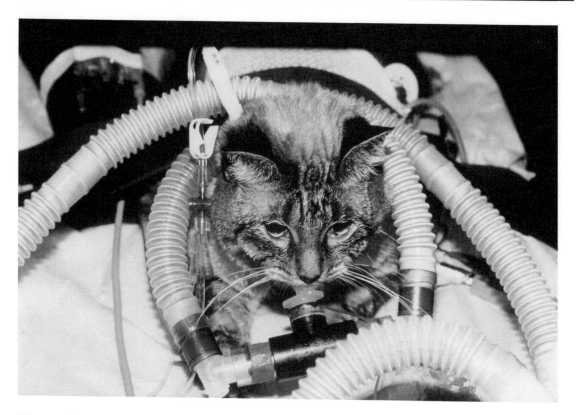

Fig. 13.8 Positive pressure ventilation is sometimes required for severe pulmonary parenchymal disease.

(1) a proximal airway pressure of up to 60 cmH$_2$O;
(2) an inspiratory time of up to 2 s;
(3) a tidal volume of up to 30 ml/kg;
(4) a ventilatory rate of up to 60/min;
(5) an inspired oxygen concentration of up to 100% for short periods of time; or
(6) an end-expired pressure of up to 15 cmH$_2$O. Positive end-expiratory pressure increases the transpulmonary pressure, functional residual capacity, and keeps small airways and alveoli open during the expiratory phase.

IPPV impedes venous return and diastolic ventricular filling. The degree of impairment of intrathoracic blood flow is proportional to the increase in pleural pressure, the inspiratory time, and the ventilation rate. Circulatory impairment is considered to be excessive if there is an associated diminution of pulse quality, arterial blood pressure, or cardiac output. Positive pressure ventilation may also

rupture pre-existing parenchymal bullae and could result in pneumomediastinum, pneumothorax, pulmonary haemorrhage, and air embolism.

Physical therapy

Cats with exudative pulmonary parenchymal disease (pneumonia) should be well hydrated; with transudative pulmonary disease (pulmonary oedema) they should be conservatively hydrated.

Secretions must be moved from the periphery of the airways to the central airways where they can be removed by cilia, coughing, or tracheal suctioning. Postural drainage (gravity) can facilitate this 'centralization' of secretions; recumbent cats should be repositioned at regular intervals. Mechanical chest vibration could be used for several minutes over the lung and should be repeated several times daily (Fig. 13.9).

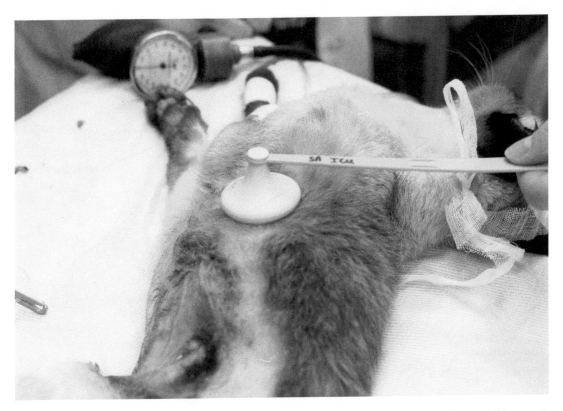

Fig. 13.9 Chest percussion with a paediatric bell-shaped percussion device can be used to mobilize exudates from the periphery of the airways in cats.

'Look-alikes'

There are several non-respiratory disorders which may cause tachypnoea or exaggerated ventilatory efforts and hyperventilation, but not hypoxaemia (Table 13.20).

Pulmonary Thromboembolism

Pulmonary thromboembolism may occur as a result of air, fat, or fibrin clot emboli to the lung. It has been associated with endocarditis, heartworm disease, cardiomyopathy, renal amyloidosis, Cushing's disease, hypovolaemic or septic shock, heat stroke, extensive neoplasia, visceral organ failure, and intravascular coagulation. Embolism is associated with severe dyspnoea and hypoxaemia. Effective treatment of the underlying disorder and heparinization are recommended as the first order of therapy.

Cardiovascular Complications

Adequate overall cardiovascular performance depends upon the appropriate interplay between multiple functions (Fig. 13.10). Arterial blood pressure is important as it influences cerebral and coronary circulation. Systemic vascular resistance is of particular importance in regulating peripheral (visceral) perfusion. Cardiac output is dependent upon an adequate preload (end-diastolic filling volume) and contractility. Central venous pressure (CVP) is commonly used as a measure of preload because CVP and end-diastolic right ventricular filling volume are related. Systemic oxygen delivery is the ultimate objective of the cardiopulmonary system. Specific diseases become significant when they impact on cardiovascular function to such an extent that oxygen delivery becomes insufficient.

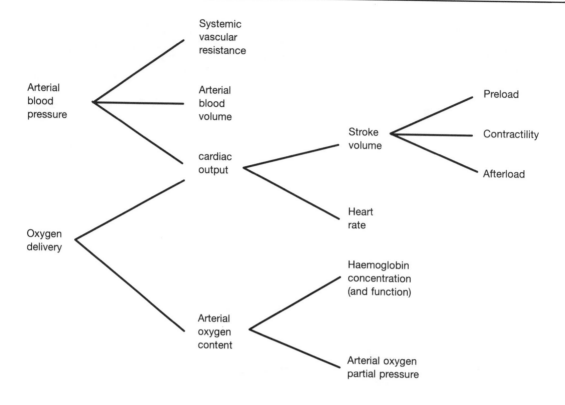

Fig. 13.10 Adequate oxygen delivery is dependent upon the efficient performance of several cardiopulmonary factors.

Bradycardia

Bradycardia in cats (Table 13.21) is generally defined as a heart rate below 50–60 beats per minute. If the underlying cause cannot be identified, a parasympatholytic should be administered. A non-responsive bradycardia may respond to a sympathomimetic with β_1-receptor activity such as dopamine (3–8 µg/kg/min or adrenaline (0.5 µg/kg/min).

Tachycardia

Sinus tachycardia (heart rate > 180 b.p.m) may be in compensation for poor venous return or contractility or may be a non-specific response to light depth of anaesthesia, the recovery phase of anaesthesia, hypoxaemia, hypercapnia, or hyperthermia. Specific treatment should be directed toward the underlying cause.

Premature Ventricular Contractions

Premature ventricular contractions (PVC, extra-systole) signify an underlying complication which may lead to more serious arrhythmias or cardiac arrest if unchecked (Table 13.22). Whenever PVCs are identified the following action should be taken: (1) eliminate obvious causes; (2) if intra-operative, evaluate the depth of anaesthesia and make appropriate adjustments; (3) maximize the inspired oxygen concentration; (4) provide ventilatory support to prevent or treat hypercapnia; (5) check proper function of the anaesthetic or other equipment; and (6) administer a bolus of fluids (Tilley, 1985).

Specific anti-arrhythmic therapy should be instituted: (1) when the rate exceeds (or would if the paroxysmal rhythm continued for an entire minute) 180–200 beats per minute; (2) when the arrhythmia is multiform in nature; (3) when the incidence or severity is becoming higher or more

Table 13.21 Causes of bradycardia

Anaesthetic drugs: many anaesthetics and some
muscle relaxants cause bradycardia by either
increasing vagal tone (narcotics, atropine,
anticholinesterase agents, such as neostigmine), or
by decreasing sympathetic tone (xylazine, β-
receptor blocking agents). Some agents directly
stimulate postganglionic cholinergic receptors
(succinylcholine) or affect myocardial
spontaneously depolarizing cells directly
(halothane, methoxyflurane, barbiturates,
lidocaine)
Excessive vagal tone which may be precipitated by
pharyngeal, laryngeal or tracheal stimulation by
foreign bodies; by pressure on the eyeball or rectus
muscles; by visceral inflammation or distention;
periosteal stimulation
Hypoxia – as a terminal event
Exogenous toxaemias (digitalis, organophosphates)
End-stage visceral organ failure or sepsis
Hyperkalaemia
Hypothermia – initially, indirectly, by decreasing
oxygen demands and, when severe, by direct
depression
Hypothyroidism
Sick sinus syndrome
Atrio–ventricular conduction disturbances

Table 13.22 Causes of premature ventricular
contractions

Endogenous release of catecholamines secondary to
any stress such as light levels of anaesthesia,
recovery from anaesthesia, pain, excitement,
hypoxia, hypercapnia, hypovolaemia, or
hypotension
Exogenous catecholamine therapy
Severe hypothermia
Digitalis toxicity (potentiated by hypokalaemia and
hypercalcaemia)
Hypokalaemia (potentiated by respiratory or
metabolic alkalosis, alkalinization therapy,
glucose/insulin therapy, β₂-agonist therapy,
calcium therapy)
Hyperkalaemia (potentiated by acidosis,
hypocalcaemia, suxamethonium or may be
iatrogenic)
Certain anaesthetics lower the threshold to
endogenous or exogenous catecholamines
(halothane, xylazine, thiamylal, thiopentone)
Myocardial inflammation, disease or stimulation
(intracardiac catheters, pleural tubes)
Thoracic and non-thoracic trauma
Congestive or hypertrophic heart failure
Visceral organ disease (gastric volvulus/torsion)
Intracranial disorders (increased pressure, hypoxia)

severe; (4) when the ectopic foci fires during the T wave of the preceding complex; and (5) when there is evidence of inadequate cardiac output (Bonagura, 1983; Kittleson, 1983).

Vasoconstriction

Vasoconstriction is sympathetic-mediated and may be a non-specific response to surgical stimulation, hypothermia, α-receptor agonist therapy, anaesthesia recovery or postoperative pain. Vasoconstriction may also be in compensation for hypovolaemia or poor cardiac output. The underlying cause should be corrected. Vasodilator therapy is not indicated until after blood volume restoration and unless arterial blood pressure is monitored.

Hypotension

Normal systolic, diastolic and mean blood pressures are approximately 100–160, 60–100

and 80–120 mmHg, respectively. Adequate cerebral and coronary perfusion is generally considered to require a mean systemic blood pressure of at least 50–60 mmHg. The causes of hypotension are listed in Table 13.23.

During general anaesthesia, the most effective treatment is to reduce the anaesthetic dose until the patient is just well enough anaesthetized to complete the surgical procedure. It may be necessary to change to anaesthetic agents which have less inherent cardiovascular depressant properties. If this is insufficient, and in non-anaesthetized cats, fluid therapy to restore an effective circulating volume is usually indicated. The CVP is commonly used to gauge the adequacy of the volume restoration. If forward-flow parameters are still low after the CVP has been increased by fluid therapy to about 10 cmH₂O, a sympathomimetic with β₁-agonist with minimal vasoconstriction effect is indicated (low-dose dopamine, dobutamine, see Table 13.24) (Shoemaker *et al.*, 1989; Lollgen &

Table 13.23 Causes of hypotension

Hypovolaemia
Extracellular fluid losses (dehydration)
Plasma/whole blood losses
    Vessel laceration
    Increased vascular permeability
    Low colloid oncotic pressure

Decreased cardiac output
Low preload
    Poor venous return
    Hypovolaemia
    Aggressive ventilator settings
    Intraoperative manipulation of heart and great
      veins
    Intraoperative manipulation of the liver
    Poor diastolic heart function
    Hypertrophic cardiomyopathy
    Pericardial tamponade
Poor contractility
    Intrinsic heart failure
    Anaesthetic drugs
    Toxaemia
    Severe electrolyte disturbances
Severe bradycardia/tachycardia
Severe arrhythmias

Vasodilatation
Anaesthetic drugs
    Acepromazine
    Bolus dosages of most anaesthetics
    Epidural or subarachnoid deposition of local
      anaesthetics
    Vasodilator drugs
Surface rewarming of hypothermic patients
Sepsis

Drexler, 1990). Occasionally it may be necessary to use drugs with more potent α-vasoconstrictor activity (noradrenaline, adrenaline) for a period of time to support arterial blood pressure (Hesselvik & Brodin, 1989; Schreuder *et al.*, 1989).

Oxygen delivery is the 'bottom line' of cardiovascular disease and therapeutic intervention (Fig. 13.10). It is the product of cardiac output and arterial blood oxygen content. Since cardiac output is seldom measured in the cat, the adequacy of oxygen delivery must be extrapolated from parameters such as pulse quality, capillary refill time, urine output, toe-web/core temperature gradient, base deficit, low venous PO_2, or high lactate.

Sepsis

Systemic infection is a common problem in critically ill cats. The clinical signs are due to the systemic inflammatory response to the infectious process, and include: lethargy; diminished appetite; hyperaemic mucous membranes; faster-than-normal capillary refill time; fever; leukocytosis with a left shift and possibly toxic neutrophils; tachycardia; low normal arterial and central venous blood pressures; a hyperkinetic pulse; hyperglycaemia; high venous oxygen; tachypnoea; respiratory alkalosis; and possibly a non-haemorrhagic diarrhoea. The systemic inflammatory response can lead to multiple organ failure: subnormal temperature; a decrease in leukocyte count, with a left shift and toxic neutrophilia; tachycardia with a weak pulse; vasoconstriction; low arterial and central venous blood pressures; hypoglycaemia; tachypnoea; high liver enzymes; haemoconcentration and hypoalbuminaemia; metabolic acidosis; coagulopathies; anuric renal failure, haemorrhagic diarrhoea, respiratory distress, and myocardial failure.

Haemodynamic Stabilization

Restoration of an effective circulating blood volume with crystalloid, colloid, and whole blood therapy is a first priority (Table 13.25). Sympathomimetic treatment is indicated when fluid therapy alone fails to restore acceptable arterial blood pressure and tissue perfusion.

Elimination of the Infection

The source of the infection should be removed or drained, if possible. The range of organisms potentially involved and their antibiotic susceptibilities is impossible to predict without blood culture. Antibiotic selections should be broad-spectrum and efficacious (Table 13.26). A combination of antibiotics is commonly selected to provide this broad coverage. Previous cultures and sensitivities help guide future antibiotic therapy. If the cat's condition does not appear to respond in 24 h, it may indicate

Table 13.24 Drugs used for cardiovascular support

Drug	Indication	Dosage
Dopamine	Increase renal (visceral) perfusion	$1\text{--}3\,\mu g/kg/min$
	Blood pressure and cardiac output support	$3\text{--}10\,\mu g/kg/min$
Dobutamine	Cardiac output and tissue blood flow support	$5\text{--}20\,\mu g/kg/min$
Norepinephrine	Blood pressure support	$0.1\text{--}1.0\,\mu g/kg/min$
Neosynephrine	Blood pressure support	$10\text{--}100\,\mu g/kg$
Ephedrine	Blood pressure and cardiac output support	$0.05\text{--}0.2\,mg/kg$
Nitroprusside	Vasodilation	$1\text{--}5\,\mu g/kg/min$
Hydralazine	Vasodilation	$0.2\text{--}0.5\,mg/kg$ PO
Acepromazine	Vasodilation and anxiolysis	$0.01\text{--}0.02\,mg/kg$ i/m

Table 13.25 Sepsis/septic shock checklist

Cardiovascular homeostasis
   Blood volume
   Sympathomimetics
Eliminate the infectious process
   Effective treatment of the underlying disease
   Remove or drain the source of infection
   Broad-spectrum, effective antibiotics
Support of organ function
   Renal failure
   Lung failure
   Gastrointestinal failure
   Coagulopathies
Support of abnormal biochemistries
   Hypoglycaemia
   Metabolic acidosis
Other
   Glucocorticosteroids
   Nutrition

infection with an organism resistant to the chosen antibiotic(s). A change of antibiotics is indicated.

Glucose

If the blood glucose concentration is very low, a bolus of glucose ($0.25\,g/kg$ i/v) should be administered. Blood glucose concentrations then can be maintained by an infusion of glucose ($2.5\text{--}10\%$ solution) titrated to the desired blood glucose concentration.

Anuria

Acute renal failure is a common consequence of sepsis. If restoration of an effective circulating volume does not generate an acceptable urine flow, diuretics (furosemide ($5\,mg/kg$), mannitol ($0.5\,g/kg$), or dopamine ($3\,\mu g/kg/min$)) should be administered. Diuresis therapy in an anuric patient should be monitored directly with a urinary catheter (see above).

Gastrointestinal Protection

The mainstay of gastrointestinal (GIT) protection is the restoration of an effective circulating blood volume. Misoprostol, a prostaglandin E_2 analogue, and superoxide dismutase and catalase, oxygen radical scavengers, have been reported to diminish gastric injury in septic shock. Methylprednisolone, however, was more effective in this regard than was a combination treatment of misoprostol, superoxide dismutase, and catalase (Arvidsson *et al.*, 1990). Drugs such as cimetidine ($4\text{--}10\,mg/kg$) and ranitidine ($2\text{--}4\,mg/kg$), which block histamine$_2$ receptors, decrease gastric acid secretion, as do some anticholinergic agents such as glycopyrrolate. Sucralfate ($5\text{--}30\,mg/kg$) acts to coat and protect existing ulcers.

Table 13.26 Categories of antibiotic effects (Brown, 1988; Dow, 1988; Donowitz & Mandell, 1988; Papich, 1988; Riviere, 1989; Karam, 1991; Olin *et al.*, 1991)

Antibiotic	Gram-negative	*Staph.* sp.	*Strep.* sp.	Anaerobes
Aminoglycosides (gentamicin, amikacin, netilmicin, tobramycin)	+	+	−	−
Quinolones (enrofloxacin, norfloxacin, and ciprofloxacin)	+	+	−	−
Penicillins Group 1 (penicillin G, ampicillin, amoxicillin)	−	±	+	+
B-lactam resistant (methicillin, nafcillin, oxacillin, cloxacillin)	−	+	+	−
Extended spectrum (ticarcillin, carbenicillin, azlocillin, piperacillin, mezlocillin)	+	+	+	+
Cephalosporins First generation (cephalothin, cefazolin, cephalexin, cephapirin, cephadrine, cefadroxil)	±	+	+	−
Second generation (cefoxitin, cefamandole, cefaclor, cefuroxime, cefonicid, ceforanide, cephotetan, cefmetazole)	+*	+	+	+
Third generation (cefotaxime, moxalactam, cefoperazone, ceftizoxime, ceftriaxone, ceftazidime, cefixime)	+	+	+	+
Imipenem/Cilastin	+	+	+	+
Aztreonam	+	−	−	−
Clindamycin	−	+	+	+
Metronidazole	−	−	−	+

* Except *Pseudomonas*

Hypoxaemia

A diffuse infiltrative pulmonary parenchymal disease is a common sequel to sepsis. This syndrome should be treated with oxygen and positive pressure ventilation in the same manner as outlined in the management of pulmonary parenchymal disease.

Coagulopathies

Acute disseminated intravascular coagulation (DIC) is a common consequence of sepsis. Effective treatment of the underlying disease process is the single most important aim of therapy. Hypercoagulation states should be treated with heparin (100 µg/kg, s/c, every 4–6 h). The objective of heparin therapy is to augment the effect of antithrombin III as an anticoagulant but not to prevent coagulation. Controlled clinical studies documenting the beneficial effects of heparin in treating DIC are lacking but the drug is commonly used in this disease. Low-dose heparin treatment is unlikely markedly to affect coagulation test results, and any marked changes in these values are most likely to be related to the septic process.

Hypocoagulation states may be due to fibrin degradation product inhibition of coagulation or to a depletion of coagulation precursors. Fresh plasma (if platelets are required) or fresh frozen plasma is indicated.

Corticosteroids

Pharmacological doses of corticosteroids have beneficial effects in various experiments in animals. The beneficial effects include: organelle- and cell-membrane stabilization, improved cellular metabolism and gluconeogenesis, improved microcirculation, decreased production of endogenous toxins such as myocardial depressant factor, decreased leukocyte activation and degranulation, and minimized reticuloendothelial depression and histological organ damage. The corticosteroids generally recommended are hydrocortisone (300 mg/kg), prednisolone (30 mg/kg), methylprednisolone (30 mg/kg), or dexamethasone (4 mg/kg). There is no clear evidence for greater beneficial effects of any one.

The efficacy of high dose corticosteroids in clinical septic shock is controversial. Some studies have demonstrated improved survival (White *et al.*, 1972; Schumer, 1976; Hoffman *et al.*, 1984) or reversal of the shock state (Sprung *et al.*, 1984). Others have reported no beneficial effects (Luce *et al.*, 1988) and no improvement in survival and an increased incidence of mortality associated with secondary infections (Hinshaw *et al.*, 1987; Bone *et al.*, 1987).

References

Arvidsson, S., Falt, K. & Haglund, U. (1990) Feline *E. coli* bacteremia – effects of misoprostol/scavengers or methylprednisolone on hemodynamic reactions and gastrointestinal mucosal injury. *Acta Chir. Scand.* **156**, 215–221.

Auer, L. (1982) Blood transfusion reactions in the cat. *J. Am. Vet. Med. Assoc.* **180**, 729–730.

Auer, L. & Bell, K. (1981). The AB blood group system of cats. *Anim. Blood Group Biochem. Genet.* **12**, 287–297.

Auer, L. & Bell, K. (1983) Transfusion reactions in cats due to AB blood group incompatibility. *Res. Vet. Sci.* **35**, 145–152.

Auer, L.A. & Bell, K. (1986) Feline blood transfusion reactions. *In: Current Veterinary Therapy* IX (ed. R.W. Kirk), pp. 515–521. WB Saunders, Philadelphia.

Authement, J.M. (1992) Blood transfusion therapy. *In: Fluid Therapy in Small Animal Practice* (ed. S.P. DiBartola), pp. 371–383. WB Saunders, Philadelphia.

Bonagura J. (1983) Therapy of cardiac arrhythmias. *In: Current Veterinary Therapy* VIII (ed. R.W. Kirk), pp. 360. WB Saunders, Philadelphia.

Bone, R.C., Fisher, C.J., Clemmer, T.P., *et. al.* (1987). A controlled clinical trial of high-dose methylprednisolone in the treatment of severe sepsis and septic shock. *New Eng. J. Med.* **317**, 653–658.

Bontempo F.A., (1993) General hematology and transfusion. *In: Pathophysiologic Foundations of Critical Care* (ed. M.R. Pinsky, & J.A. Dhainaur), p. 820. Williams & Wilkins, Baltimore.

Brooks, M. (1992) Transfusion medicine. *In: Veterinary Emergency and Critical Care Medicine* (ed. R.J.

Murtaugh & P.M. Kaplan), pp. 536–546. Mosby-Year Book, St. Louis.

Brown, S.A. (1988) Treatment of gram-negative infections. *In: Clinical Pharmacology; Veterinary Clinics of North America* (ed. M.G. Papich), pp. 1141–1165. WB Saunders, Philadelphia.

Concannon, K.T., Haskins, S.C. & Feldman, B.F. (1992) Hemostatic defects associated with two infusion rates of dextran 70 in dogs. *Am. J. Vet. Res.* **53**, 1369–1375.

Consensus Conference (1988) Red blood cell transfusion. *J. Am. Med. Assoc.* **260**, 2700–2703.

Dawidson, I., Gelin, L.E. & Haglund, E. (1980) Plasma volume, intravascular protein content, hemodynamic and oxygen transport changes during intestinal shock in dogs: Comparison of relative effectiveness of various plasma expanders. *Crit. Care Med.* **8**, 73–80.

DiBartola, S.P. (1992) *Fluid Therapy in Small Animal Practice*. WB Saunders, Philadelphia.

Donowitz, G.R. & Mandell, G.L. (1988) Beta-lactam antibiotics, *New Engl. J. Med.* **318**, 419–426; 490–500.

Dow, S.W. (1988) Management of anaerobic infections, *In: Clinical Pharmacology, Vet. Clin. North Am., Small Animal Practice* (ed. M.G. Papich), pp. 1167–1182. WB Saunders, Philadelphia.

Falk, J.L., Rackow, E.C. & Weil, M.H. (1989) Colloid and Crystalloid Fluid Resuscitation. *In: Textbook of Critical Care* (eds W.C. Shoemaker, *et. al.*), pp. 1055–1073. WB Saunders, Philadelphia.

Fulton, R.B. & Dennis, J.S. (1992) Blind percutaneous placement of a gastrostomy tube for nutritional support in dogs and cats. *J. Am. Vet. Med. Assoc.* **201**, 697–700.

Gandolfi, R.C. (1988) Feline neonatal isoerythrolysis: A case report. *Calif. Vet.* **42**, 9–10.

Giger, U. (1991) Feline neonatal isoerythrolysis: A major cause of the fading kitten syndrome. *Proc. Am. Coll. Vet Med.* pp. 347.

Giger, U. (1992) The feline AB blood group system and incompatibility reactions. *In: Current Veterinary Therapy* **XI** (eds R.D. Kirk, & J.D. Bonagura), pp 470–474. WB Saunders, Philadelphia.

Giger, U., Kilrain, C.G., Filippich, L.J. & Bell, K. (1989) Frequencies of feline blood groups in the United States. *J. Am. Vet. Med. Assoc.* **195**, 1230–1232.

Griffel, M.I. & Kaufman, B.S. (1992) Pharmacology of colloids and crystalloids. *In: Fluid Resuscitation of the Critically Ill; Critical Care Clinics* (ed. B.S. Kaufman), pp. 235–253. WB Saunders, Philadelphia.

Guyton, A.C. (1986) Physics of blood, blood flow, and pressure: hemodynamics. *In: Textbook of Medical Physiology* (ed. A.C. Guyton), pp. 206–217. WB Saunders, Philadelphia.

Hesselvik, J.F. & Brodin, B. (1989) Low dose norepinephrine in patients with septic shock and oliguria: Effects on afterload, urine flow, and oxygen transport. *Crit. Care Med.* **17**, 179–180.

Hinshaw, L., Peduzzi, P., Young, E., *et al.* (1987) Effect of high-dose glucocorticoid therapy on mortality in patients with clinical signs of systemic sepsis. *New Eng. J. Med.* **317**, 659–665.

Hoffman, S.L., Punjabi, N.H., Kumala, S., *et al.* (1984) Reduction of mortality in chloramphenicol-treated severe typhoid fever by high-dose dexamethasone, *N. Engl. J. Med.* **310**, 82–88.

Hubler, M., Kaelin, S., Hagen, A., *et al.* (1987) Feline neonatal isoerythrolysis in two litters. *J. Sm. Anim. Pract.* **28**, 833–838.

Hulse, J.D. & Yacobi, A. (1983) Hetastarch: an overview of the colloid and its metabolism. *Drug Intell. Clin. Pharmacy* **17**, 334–341.

Johnson, N.N. (1990) Neonatal isoerythrolysis in Himalayan kittens. *Aust. Vet. J.* **67**, 416–417.

Karam, G.H. (1991) New antibiotics in the critical care unit. *Critical Care Report* **2**, 128–135.

Kittleson, M. (1983) Drugs used in the therapy of cardiac arrhythmias. *In: Current Veterinary Therapy VIII* (ed. R.W. Kirk). pp. 297–301. WB Saunders, Philadelphia.

Klotz, U. (1987) Clinical pharmacokinetic considerations in the use of plasma expanders. *Clin. Pharmacokin.* **12**, 123–.

Kohn, C.W. & DiBartola, S.P. (1992) Composition and distribution of body fluids in dogs and cats. *In: Fluid Therapy in Small Animal Practice* (ed. S.P. DiBartola). pp. 1–34. WB Saunders, Philadelphia.

Lippert, A.C., Faulkner, J.E., Evans, T.E., Mullaney, T.P. (1989) Total parenteral nutrition in clinically normal cats. *J. Am. Vet. Med. Assoc.* **194**, 669–676.

Lollgen, H. & Drexler, H. (1990) Use of inotropes in the critical care setting. *Crit. Care Med.* **18**, S56–S60.

Luce, J.M., Montgomery, A.B., Marks, J.D., *et. al.* (1988) Ineffectiveness of high-dose methylprednisolone in preventing parenchymal lung injury and improving mortality in patients with septic shock. *Am. Rev. Respir. Dis.* **138**, 62–68.

Maxwell, M.H. & Kleeman, C.R. (1987) *In: Clinical Disorders of Fluid and Electrolyte Metabolism*, (ed. R.G. Narins) 4th edn. McGraw-Hill, New York.

Olin, B.R. (ed.) (1991) *Drug Facts and Comparisons*, pp. 1530–1710. JB Lippincott, St Louis.

Otto, C.M., McCall, Kaufman G. & Crowe D.T. (1989) Intraosseous infusion of fluids and therapeutics. *Comp. Cont. Ed.* **11**(4), 421–430.

Paddleford, R.R. & Harvey, R.C., (1989) Critical care

surgical techniques. *In: Critical Care, Veterinary Clinics of North America* (eds. R. Kirby & G.L. Stamp). pp. 1079–1094. WB Saunders, Philadelphia.

Papich, M.G. (1988) Therapy of gram-positive bacterial infections, *In: Clinical Pharmacology, Veterinary Clinics North America, Small Animal Practice*, (ed. M.G. Papich). pp. 1267–1285. WB Saunders, Philadelphia.

Pichler, M.E. & Turnwald, G.H. (1985) Blood Transfusion in the dog and cat. Part I. Physiology, collection, storage, and indications for whole blood therapy. *Compendium Continuing Education* **7**, 64–71.

Riviere, J.E. (1989) Cephalosporins. *In: Current Veterinary Therapy X* (ed. R.W. Kirk). pp. 74–77. WB Saunders, Philadelphia.

Rogers, Q.R., Baker, D.H., Hayes, K.C., *et al.* (1986) *Nutrient Requirements of Cats*. National Academy Press, Washington D.C.

Rose, D.B. (1989) *Clinical Physiology of Acid–Base and Electrolyte Disorders*, 3rd edn. McGraw-Hill, New York.

Schreuder, W.O., Schneider, A.J., Groeneveld, A.B.J. & Thijs, L.G. (1989) Effect of dopamine vs. norepinephrine on hemodynamics in septic shock. *Chest* **95**, 1282–1288.

Schumer, W. (1976) Steroids in the treatment of clinical septic shock. *Ann. Surg.* **184**, 333–341.

Shoemaker, W.C., Appel, P.L. & Kram, H.B., *et. al.* (1989) Comparison of hemodynamic and oxygen transport effects of dobutamine and dopamine in critically ill surgical patients. *Chest* **96**, 120–130.

Sprung, C.L., Caralis, P.V. & Marcial, E.H. (1984) The effects of high-dose corticosteroids in patients with septic shock. *New Eng. J. Med.* **311**, 1137–1143.

Stone, M.S. & Cotter, S.M. (1992) Practical guidelines for transfusion therapy. *In: Current Veterinary Therapy XI* (eds R.W. Kirk & J.D. Bonagura). pp. 475–479. WB Saunders, Philadelphia.

Stone, E., Badner, D. &Cotter, S.M. (1992) Trends in transfusion medicine in dogs at a veterinary school clinic: 315 cases (1986–1989). *J. Am. Vet. Med. Assoc.* **200**, 1000–1004.

Tilley, L.P. (1985) *Essentials of Canine and Feline Electrocardiography: Interpretation and Treatment*, 2nd edn. Lea & Febiger, Philadelphia.

Turnwald, G.H. & Pichler, M.E. (1985) Blood transfusion in dogs and cats, Part II: Administration, adverse effects, and component therapy. *Compend. Contin. Educ.* **7**, 115–122.

White, G.L., White, G.S., Kosanke, S.D., Archer, L.T. & Hinshaw, L.B. (1982). Therapeutic effects of prednisolone sodium succinate vs dexamethasone in dogs subjected to *E. coli* septic shock. *J. Am. Anim. Hosp. Assoc.* **18**, 639–648.

J.C.M. Lewis

14
Anaesthesia of Non-domestic Cats

Introduction

Although some non-domestic cat species and subspecies are well represented in captivity, many are not and some not at all. Furthermore, not all species in captivity breed readily. In the light of this and the increasing degree of specialization and professionalism adopted by some conservation centres, zoos, wild animal parks and private collections, there is a growing need for informed, specialist veterinary care. Similarly, projects designed to study rare and endangered non-domestic cats in the wild should demand ever-improving standards of veterinary expertise. Fundamental to the provision of such veterinary services is the ability to anaesthetize these animals competently.

A surprising amount of published information is available concerning anaesthesia of non-domestic cat species, although it has not previously been collated in depth. This chapter aims to summarize both the available literature and the author's experience in an attempt provide a comprehensive working guide to the subject. Where relevant, differences between animals in the wild and those in captivity are mentioned, although far more information is available concerning captive animals than their wild counterparts. Inevitably, therefore, the emphasis in this chapter is on anaesthesia of captive animals.

Indications for Anaesthesia

The practice of exotic animal medicine relies heavily on the use of immobilizing and anaesthetic drugs for even the most routine of procedures, and this is particularly true for the non-domestic cats. Nearly all manipulative procedures in the larger species and many in the smaller species require anaesthesia, although some simple procedures can be carried out under physical restraint. Thus anaesthesia is normally required for translocations, routine clinical examinations, blood and other tissue sampling, immobilization of trapped or marauding wild animals and the identification of free-living animals for ecological and ethological study. The indications for general anaesthesia in non-domestic cats are therefore far more likely to be related to handling fractious, aggressive or dangerous animals than rendering surgical patients insensible to pain. Consequently, the majority of non-domestic cats requiring anaesthesia are clinically normal. Anaesthesia is of course also required for the surgical, and in some cases medical, treatment of sick or injured animals.

Even in captive collections, the conditions available for the performance of anaesthesia are often far from ideal. Veterinary surgeons used to the more familiar surroundings of the comprehensively equipped veterinary clinic must adapt their technique to suit the crude conditions under which many captive and free-range non-domestic cats must be anaesthetized. With this in mind, anaesthesia in these species should never be undertaken lightly. Although modern drugs have a wide margin of safety in cats, there is still no absolutely risk-free anaesthetic technique and the anaesthetist must be prepared and equipped for the unexpected problem. All drugs and drug combinations have unique characteristics and it is helpful to use a technique with which the anaesthetist is familiar.

Whenever a cat is anaesthetized for whatever reason, it should be seen as an opportunity to examine it thoroughly as many problems go undetected in the conscious animal. Damaged teeth and overgrown claws are two common examples. It is also useful to take serum and other tissue samples for banking, as the opportunities for this rarely arise in the normal course of events.

Pre-anaesthetic Assessment and Preparation

Many of the problems that can arise during anaesthesia of non-domestic cats are avoidable by careful pre-anaesthetic assessment of the patient and consideration of the conditions under which the anaesthesia is to be performed. Owing to the difficulty in examination prior to anaesthesia, this is a more demanding task than with domestic cats. Consideration must be given to the species involved, the animal's medical condition, its weight, age, sex and temperament. Preparation of the area(s) to be used for induction and maintainence of anaesthesia must be carried out thoroughly. In the majority of cases conditions are far from ideal, and there is ample scope and need for improvization. After considering all the available information about a particular cat and its circumstances, the anaesthetist must be firmly convinced that the advantages of anaesthesia outweigh the disadvantages.

Physical Examination and History

The physical examination of a cat prior to anaesthesia is usually restricted to visual observation. This may be possible at close quarters in captive situations but binoculars will usually be required for free-living cats in their natural habitat unless trapped prior to anaesthesia. In the case of trained animals such as circus cats, a limited amount of 'hands on' examination may be tolerated, allowing, for example, auscultation of heart and lung. Under these circumstances, the anaesthetist needs to be very sensitive to the cat's behaviour and

have a high degree of trust in the owner's control.

A thorough history should be taken from the owner or keeper of captive animals concerning recent food and water intake, occurrence of coughing, breathlessness following exercise, diarrhoea, vomiting, excessive urine production, etc. Such information may provide the only clue to unrecognized problems that would influence the decision whether or not to anaesthetize. For example, it is not uncommon for cats with pneumonia to display few visual clues to their condition. If available, an animal's medical history can provide invaluable information about its general health status, existence of known disease conditions, current drugs in use and any previous unusual or idiosyncratic reactions to particular anaesthetics. Examination of previous haematology and serum biochemistry profiles and urinanalysis can also be rewarding. In addition, some idea of an animal's current weight can be gained from previous records.

Table 14.1 Approximate weights of adult non-domestic cats (Kitchener, 1991; Wallach & Boever, 1983; pers. experience)

Common name	Latin name	Adult weight range
Black-footed cat	(*Felis nigripes*)	1–3 kg
Bobcat	(*Lynx rufus*)	10–25 kg
Caracal	(*Felis caracal*)	7–20 kg
Cheetah	(*Acinonyx jubitus*)	30–70 kg
Clouded leopard	(*Neofelis nebulosa*)	15–30 kg
Eurasian lynx	(*Lynx lynx*)	15–30 kg
Fishing cat	(*Felis viverrina*)	5–15 kg
Jaguar	(*Panthera onca*)	40–100 kg
Jungle cat	(*Felis chaus*)	5–15 kg
Leopard	(*Panthera pardus*)	25–75 kg
Leopard cat	(*Felis bengalensis*)	2–5 kg
Lion	(*Panthera leo*)	120–250 kg
Margay	(*Felis wiedii*)	3–7 kg
Ocelot	(*Felis pardalis*)	7–15 kg
Puma	(*Felis concolor*)	25–75 kg
Rusty spotted cat	(*Felis rubiginosa*)	1–3 kg
Serval	(*Felis serval*)	8–18 kg
Snow leopard	(*Panthera uncia*)	25–60 kg
Tiger	(*Panthera tigris*)	75–300 kg
Wildcat	(*Felis silvestris*)	2.5–8 kg

Assessment of Weight

In order to calculate an appropriate anaesthetic dose, it is necessary to have some idea of the animal's weight. Given that under most circumstances it is not possible to weigh a cat whilst conscious, the anaesthetist must be able to estimate with accuracy. This can only be achieved with experience, especially when one considers the wide range involved from the smallest species at 2 kg or less (examples include the Black-footed cat, *Felis nigripes*, and the Rusty spotted cat, *Felis rubiginosa*) to the Siberian tiger (*Panthera tigris altaica*), which may weigh up to 300 kg or more. Approximate adult weight ranges for some of the more commonly seen non-domestic cat species are given in Table 14.1. It is important to record an animal's weight during anaesthesia in order to record the actual dose rates of induction agents, so that subsequent drugs doses are given accurately, and to gain data on the individual cat and the species. Small species can be weighed by conventional means used for any domestic animal. Medium-

sized cats may require nets or apparatus that can be suspended from suitable scales (Fig. 14.1). The large cats can be weighed on platform scales, or weights estimated from girth measurements and the application of regression equations (Seal *et al.*, 1976).

Temperament

Every cat has a different temperament, and often the differences between individuals within species are greater than those between species. Some lions, for example, are very phlegmatic, whilst others are always nervous and hence prone to overt aggression. Cats that are normally more aggressive and excitable will require higher anaesthetic doses than their calmer conspecifics. In some cases the difference in dose rate can be as much as two-fold. Free-living cats will usually require higher dose rates unless semi-tame. Even a calm, captive cat can become nervous and aggressive if disturbed sufficiently and thus it is important to minimize the amount of disturbance to which an animal is

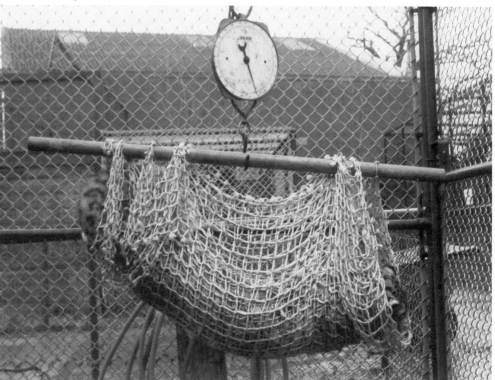

Fig. 14.1 Snow leopard: simple weighing technique using net, scaffold pole and meat scales.

exposed during pre-anaesthetic assessment or preparations. If at all possible, preparatory work for any cat anaesthetic should not be seen or heard by the animal. The delivery of induction agents should be carried out quickly, quietly and efficiently whichever method is used.

Intercurrent Disease

The possibility of intercurrent disease must be taken into account when deciding whether or not to carry out anaesthesia and which drugs to use. The significance of various conditions with respect to anaesthesia is described elsewhere (Hall & Clarke, 1991). However, it is important that the anaesthetist is aware of relevant conditions that have been described in non-domestic cats.

Anaemias are seen infrequently in non-domestic cats. Feline infectious anaemia (*Haemobartinella felis*) can affect any cat. Mild anaemia caused by chronic renal failure is far more common, especially in older animals, but rarely causes a significant problem unless the condition is advanced. Heavy flea infestations can cause anaemias in the smaller species and in cubs of medium-sized cats before they are weaned.

A history of diarrhoea and/or vomiting should be taken seriously as dehydration can be hard to determine prior to anaesthesia in many animals. Provision should be made for aggressive fluid therapy after induction of anaesthesia if there is any possibility of fluid deficits or electrolyte imbalances. Conscious non-domestic cats do not generally tolerate intravenous drips, thus deficits can often only be corrected during anaesthesia.

Liver disease is an important cause of morbidity and mortality. Clinical signs are similar to those seen in domestic cats. Hepatic tumours, diffuse necrotic hepatitis, hepatic fibrosis, active hepatitis and veno-occlusive disease have all been reported (Kelly *et al.*, 1980; Wallach & Boever, 1983; Munson & Worley, 1987; Gosselin *et al.*, 1988). The feline infectious peritonitis virus can cause hepatopathy in any species. Cheetah (*Acinonyx jubitus*) and snow leopard (*Panthera uncia*) seem especially prone to chronic liver disease, particularly

conditions involving widespread fibrosis (Dinnes & Henrickson, 1970; Ruedi *et al.*, 1980; Wahlberg, 1980; Munson & Worley, 1987, 1991; Gosselin *et al.*, 1988). Although severe liver failure must be present before the metabolism of many drugs is noticeably distorted, prolonged recoveries from ketamine-based anaesthetics are possible in affected cats and the use of halothane in such animals should be avoided.

Renal disease is also a common cause of morbidity and mortality. Glomerulonephritis, congenital malformations, toxic nephroses, renal lymphosarcoma, feline infectious peritonitis, diabetes mellitus, leptospirosis, urolithiasis and chronic interstitial nephritis have all been reported (Benirschke *et al.*, 1976; Bush *et al.*, 1987; Fowler, 1986). For example, renal disease is recognized as a problem in all ages of tiger, with chronic interstitial nephritis being the most common lesion (Benirschke *et al.*, 1976). The authors suggested that Siberian tigers may be particularly susceptible. Captive black-footed cats are very prone to renal failure resulting from tubular necrosis and interstitial nephritis, although the cause is unknown. The symptoms of renal failure are polydypsia, polyuria, anorexia, depression, vomiting, decreased gut transit time and sometimes convulsions. Although pre-anaesthetic urinalysis can be valuable in assessing anaesthetic risk in older cats, caution should be excercised in extrapolation from the domestic cat. For example, normal tiger urine occasionally contains fat droplets and a trace of protein (Hewer *et al.*, 1948). Given that a large part of ketamine is excreted unchanged by the kidney in domestic cats (Wright, 1982), care should be excercised when using cyclohexylamines in cats with renal insufficiency. Recoveries are likely to be prolonged in affected animals.

Respiratory disease is a common cause of death (Schmidt *et al.*, 1986). Given that they tend to take little excercise, captive animals often show little more evidence of long-standing respiratory infection than a chronic nasal discharge (Haigh *et al.*, 1978). Bacterial pneumonias are probably the most common condition encountered, and the possibility of pulmonary tuberculosis should always be considered.

Preparation of Animal and Area

Once a careful assessment of an animal has been carried out and anaesthetic drugs and doses chosen, it is necessary to prepare both the cat and the area to be used. In the case of wild animals many of these steps will not be possible.

To ensure an empty stomach and thereby reduce the risk of vomiting, large cats like lion and tiger should be starved for at least 24–48 h, and water witheld for 12 h unless dehydration is suspected. Twenty four hours starvation is usually sufficient for medium-sized species such as the leopard (*Panthera pardus*), and 12 h for the smaller species. Water should be witheld for 2 h prior to anaesthesia in small species. The cat should be moved to a suitable indoor den or squeeze facility and, if excited, allowed to calm down prior to injection of anaesthetic drugs or any other procedure. A cat should never be anaesthetized when another is present in the same area.

The site chosen for anaesthesia should be quiet, warm and safe. This is easier to achieve in indoor dens than in outside enclosures. Feed trays, water bowls and any movable items should be removed before allowing the cat access. If anaesthesia has to be induced outside, the weather should be considered, pools drained, the risk of falling from platforms or trees after induction considered and the possibility of the animal hiding out of range of a dart in rock-work, etc. eliminated. The public should be excluded from any area that is to be used. Wherever the procedure is to carried out, access to emergency equipment and exits should be assured. Where necessary, the means of transporting the cat from the site of induction has to be prepared. A robust stretcher is the most convenient way to move large cats although strong nets can be used. If the distance involved is great, it is safer to carry the cat in a secure box or crate.

Methods of Drug Administration

Whilst it may be desirable to administer anaesthetic induction agents intravenously

(i/v), this is rarely practical in non-domestic species. Even small species can be very difficult to hold sufficiently still. To attempt i/v administration in the conscious animal is not only stressful for the cat and difficult for the handler, but is also accompanied by the risk of injury to both. In the smaller cats, or young of larger species, anaesthetic gases can be delivered by mask to achieve induction. This does not eliminate the difficulty of handling, although the animal does not have to be held as still as for intravenous injections. By far the majority of anaesthetic induction agents are therefore given by the intramuscular (i/m) route, either by physically restraining the animal for injection by hand or by using remote injection systems.

Physical Restraint

Small animals can often be handled for minor examinations and injections, but the extent to which this is tolerated varies widely. Thick leather gloves are favoured by some, but many species will bite through gloves and the handler's sensitivity is markedly reduced so that escapes are common. An alternative approach is to envelop the cat in a blanket from which it has great difficulty in escaping. Where space allows, a better option is the hand-held hoop net which can cope with animals up to 15 kg or so. These should be deep enough to allow the hoop to be turned over on itself after capture in order to prevent escapes through the net entrance. Padded hoop rims will help prevent damage to teeth if the cat bites into the rim during capture. Commercially available, portable, small animal squeeze cages are rarely practical for small cats as the animal has to handled to be transferred into them. The occasional animal will allow itself to be harried into a suitably designed crush cage that is positioned against a den exit, but most cats will be suspicious of this arrangement unless it is part of their usual routine. When designing new cat facilities, a crush can be built into runs that animals use to reach outside enclosures. Therefore, each cat will pass through the open crush every day and will be easier to trap for injections when required.

Medium-sized cats can be caught and held

with pole-mounted quick-release snares, but this is difficult and potentially dangerous for cat and handler. The snare is placed around the neck and one fore leg and tightened so that the front of the animal is controlled. As soon as the snare is in place the tail is grasped to straighten the cat, thus allowing a second operator to inject into hind leg muscles. Some species such as cheetah may tolerate this, whereas others such as leopard will thrash until exhausted. Accidental strangulation and musculoskeletal damage is not uncommon, and the extreme agility of many cats limits the use of the method. An inbuilt crush facility is a far more practical and humane system where the arrangement of dens and enclosures allows, and permits a considerably greater degree of safety for handler and cat.

Physical restraint of larger species such as lion and tiger is limited to the use of crush (or squeeze) facilities. Ideally the crush should be built into an access corridor between inside dens or between inside dens and outside enclosures (Fig. 14.2). As the animal will be familiar with the apparatus, it is a relatively easy matter to trap it in the crush for injections. The best crushes are those with a low roof to limit the animal's vertical travel when squeezed, no gaps between crush and surrounding structures, and a quick release mechanism should the cat develop respiratory distress or collapse whilst being crushed. Some collections have preferred to make crush or squeeze dens, particularly in zoo hospitals (Fig. 14.3). These are modified, usually full size, dens with a sliding metalwork wall that can squeeze the cat against the back of the den. The den can then be used both as sleeping/living quarters or a crush, with animal access provided from adjacent dens into the back of the crush den by standard sliding doors. These are more cumbersome to use as the crush wall has further to travel, and the animal usually has more ability to move up or along when crushed. However, they are extremely useful when repeated injections or anaesthetics are necessary for a cat under intensive care. Details of mobile restraint boxes for the larger

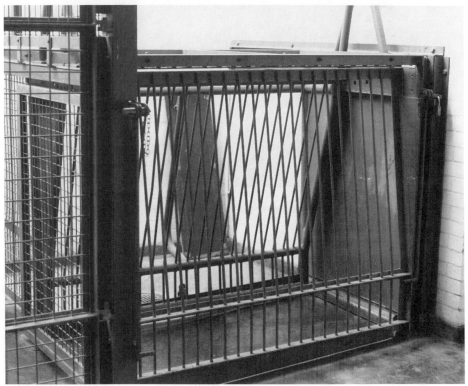

Fig. 14.2 Inbuilt crush cage for large cats sited between indoor dens (left) and door to outside enclosure (right). (Courtesy of Zoological Society of London.)

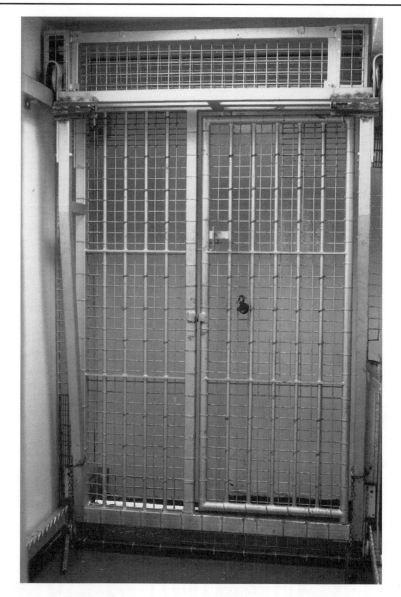

Fig. 14.3 Front of crush den. Note floor level ratchet. (Courtesy of Zoological Society of London.)

species were described by Graham-Jones (1964).

Most cat species can be trapped or snared in the wild when necessary, although this is far from easy and should not be undertaken by the inexperienced. Detailed descriptions of trap and snare designs suitable for wild cats are given in the 'Wildlife Restraint Series' (1991) and McKenzie (1993). With regard to the smaller species and feral domestic cats, the Universities Federation for Animal Welfare has also published designs of a suitable trap and crush cage (UFAW, 1981).

Whatever method of physical restraint is used to allow administration of i/m anaesthetic agents, the anaesthetist must be quick. Non-domestic cats of all sizes are remarkably strong and will wriggle however restrained. Consequently, it is important to have all injections prepared in advance and to use sufficiently robust needles. For very small species, a short 23-gauge needle is advised, for small- to medium-sized animals a 21-gauge needle is appropriate, and for the larger species a 19- or 18-gauge needle is required. Using needles of lesser diameters will prolong the injection unnecessarily with the risk that the cat may move during the procedure leading to bent needles and incomplete injections.

Remote Injection

Remote injection techniques fall into two categories—the pole syringe and the dart. A pole syringe is essentially a syringe mounted on a pole which extends the arm by 1–1.5 m. Thus an animal can be injected in a relatively confined space such as a small cage without physical restraint. However, as cats are extremely quick to respond to painful stimuli, the operator must be equally fast. It also follows that only very high gauge needles are appropriate to avoid slow injection. In the author's opinion, pole syringes are of limited use and must never be used on small cats.

In a very high percentage of cases involving the medium-sized and larger cats, using a dart to deliver anaesthetics is the easiest method of administration. If an appropriate dart is chosen and the procedure carried out quickly, quietly and with accuracy, it is usually far simpler and safer than hand injection in physically restrained animals, and produces far less stress and excitement prior to induction. Darting techniques are suitable not only for the delivery of anaesthetics to caged or trapped animals, but also to animals in outside enclosures and to untrapped, free-living larger cats such as lions. Many types of dart are available, although not all are suitable for cats. These are reviewed in detail elsewhere (Kock, 1987; Wildlife Restraint Series, 1991; McKenzie, 1993). Licences are required in the UK for the use of dart systems and relevant legislation is detailed in Kock (1987). Whichever system is chosen, it is essential that the operator familiarizes him/herself with it well in advance of using it on an animal as all systems have their own individual characteristics.

The dart and needle type selected depends on the individual animal involved and the conditions under which darting is carried out. Bearing in mind that the majority of drugs are best given i/m, allowances must be made in selecting the length of needle required for obese

animals. Subcutaneous (s/c) delivery of most anaesthetic agents will result in slow and sometimes incomplete inductions. Darts should be prepared well away from the cat to minimize excitement prior to induction and care must be taken not to contaminate the outside of any dart or blowpipe mouthpiece with anaesthetic drugs. Each dart should be fired from the *minimum* safe range to ensure accuracy. Suitable target areas are the muscle masses of the upper limbs and, in larger species, the neck. Many cats will chew a dart if they can get to it, but they rarely swallow component parts. It is more difficult for a cat to reach a dart if it has been placed in neck muscles. However, in male lions the mane will often prevent a dart penetrating fully. If possible, cats should be darted when standing still. The loose skin folds present when sitting or lying down will often absorb much of a darts' impact energy, resulting in s/c delivery or even failure to penetrate the skin at all. If the cat is moving when darted, there is a high risk of dart deflection and inaccurate placement. In the event of a suspected dart failure or partial drug delivery, it is wise to wait a full 20 min before giving additional drugs.

Small cats < 10 kg are best darted with lightweight plastic darts of 1–2 ml capacity used in conventional blowpipes, for example those made by Telinject (UK) (Fig. 14.4). In experienced hands, these are accurate up to 10 metres, although are suitable for any lower distance. Used with fine needles, such darts easily penetrate the skin and inflict negligible impact trauma. It is possible to see whether a drug has been completely injected as the darts are translucent. To minimize damage caused by innaccurately placed darts, small cats should not be darted at a greater range than 10 m.

Although lightweight plastic darts fired through a conventional blowpipe can be used on larger animals with thicker skins and coats, it is not generally advised as s/c injections often result from incomplete penetration of the needle. The medium-sized and large cats usually require an injection volume of < 3–3.5 ml, thus the larger, more robust, nylon darts such as the Telinject 'Vario' range are more appropriate (Fig. 14.4). These are fired through a blowpipe assisted by a charge of compressed CO_2, and

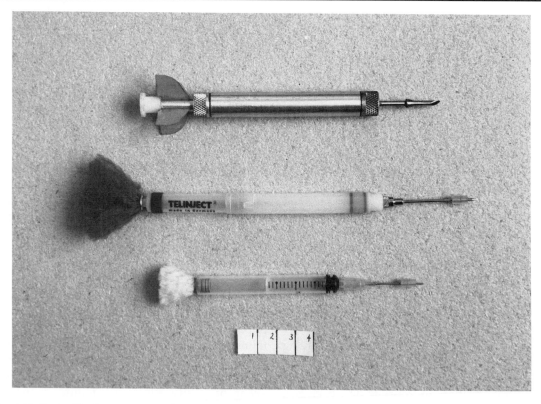

Fig. 14.4 Projectile darts: Top, 4-ml metal type dart (D. Lowndes); middle, Telinject 3.5-ml 'Vario' blowpipe dart; bottom, Telinject 1.5-ml blowpipe dart. Scale in centimetres.

hence have a greater impact energy. Fitted with sturdier needles, they penetrate thick skin well, discharge their contents quickly, yet create very little soft tissue damage. Different lengths of needle are available to suit the different species of cat. An effective range of 15–20 m can be achieved using a 1-m blowpipe and a hand-held pistol adaptor supplying the CO_2. The range can be increased to 30–40 m by using the same darts in a rifle. For captive cats at limited range (< 20 m) the 'Vario' type system is hard to better for reliable drug delivery. This system should not be used on the smallest species.

More traditionally, metal darts (Fig. 14.4) fired from gas or blank cartridge powered pistols or rifles such as the 'Capchur' system were used on the medium and large cats, but for the majority of captive situations they are unnecessarily traumatic. On impact the drug is delivered by the detonation of a small charge behind a plunger within the dart, whereas with most blowpipe systems the drug delivery relies on air or butane gas pressure behind the plunger.

Given this detonation system, the larger bore needles used and the more powerful delivery system, not only does the dart hit the animal with greater energy, but drugs delivered by the darts are pushed into the animal with greater force. As a result they inevitably inflict more trauma. If used on smaller species it is possible to fracture bones and inflict wounds requiring treatment. However, the metal darts may have significant advantages over their plastic counterparts when darting medium and large cats out-of-doors at long range, particularly in windy conditions.

Darting animals is not without hazards. In captivity these are usually restricted to problems arising from inaccurate placement of the dart. Damage to major nerve trunks, blood vessels and bones is only likely in the smaller cats where the dart type, velocity or weight is inappropriate. In animals of the size of a leopard or cheetah, the Telinject type of dart rarely causes any significant damage even if placed on the chest or abdominal wall. This is not true of the heavier metal darts. Whatever dart is chosen, the possibility of damage to vulnerable structures such as eyes resulting from a poorly judged shot cannot be completely eliminated. Dart richochets are fortunately rare, but the operator must always ensure that no people are within range when firing.

When darting animals out-of-doors and particularly in the wild, the potential for problems is far greater and almost entirely beyond the operator's control. No anaesthetic agent works immediately, and during the time between darting and induction many things can happen. Animals can be lost in heavy undergrowth during the partially anaesthetized stage or they may fall into water, down steep inclines or out of trees in which they have sought refuge. Reassuringly, in one study of wild African lion and leopard (King *et al.*, 1977) darted animals only ran 10–30 m before sitting down. The possibility of other predators attacking an anaesthetized cat should also be borne in mind.

Premedication and Sedation

There are several reasons why premedication can be unnecessary, undesirable or even counterproductive in non-domestic cats. Premedicant drugs only produce predictable and reliable effects when injected, as the uptake of many following ingestion is highly variable. Therefore to administer premedicants to most captive or free-living non-domestic cats, the animal must be handled or darted twice to achieve anaesthesia. This can result in an excited animal at exactly the wrong time, negating any potential benefit from a sedative. Where cats have to be darted in free-ranging situations, there may only be one chance to do so successfully. The valuable anaesthetic sparing effect of some sedatives is retained by incorporating them with anaesthetic drugs, the two given simultaneously for induction (see later). Furthermore, although premedicant sedatives may reduce the amount of general anaesthetic necessary, they also increase the total recovery time, which is often undesirable.

Most gaseous general anaesthetics now recommended for use in non-domestic cats do not irritate the tracheobronchial tree to a significant extent which reduces the need for pre-anaesthetic anticholinergics. Pre-induction mydriasis produced by anticholinergics is undesirable in any cat. Many will be anxious prior to induction and visual disturbances will only make matters worse. In free-living or extensive captive situations the effects could be disasterous. Furthermore, the use of anticholinergics prior to anaesthetic combinations including certain α_2-agonists is controversial. α_2-Agonists are used widely in the anaesthesia of non-domestic species.

Thus, although exceptions will always arise, the use of pre-anaesthetic medication with sedatives and anticholinergics is not generally recommended in non-domestic species. There may be some value in premedicating hand-tame captive animals, but this is rarely necessary. Situations do arise where the use of anticholinergics during an anaesthetic is desirable, or when mild sedation alone is required without subsequent anaesthesia.

Anticholinergics

Atropine given at 0.01–0.02 mg/kg has been recommended for use in non-domestic cat species for the control of ketamine-induced salivation and the prevention of xylazine-induced bradycardia (Wildt *et al.*, 1992). In domestic cats i/m or s/c atropine up to 0.1 mg/kg is safe and effective (Hall & Clarke, 1991), and there is no reason to suppose that the same may not be true in the smaller species of non-domestic cat.

The cyclohexamine anaesthetics phencylidine, ketamine and tiletamine all cause a degree of hypersalivation, and the use of atropine is recommended as necessary when these drugs are used. Atropine can be given in the immobilizing mixture or immediately after induction. In the majority of species, it is rarely necessary to give an anticholinergic to control tracheobronchial secretions during gaseous anaesthesia using halothane or isoflurane as these gases are not very irritant. However, it is a wise precaution for cats of less than 5 kg in which even relatively minor amounts of secretion can cause significant obstructions in the small airways.

The use of anticholinergics to block bradycardia produced by α_2-agonists remains controversial and is only recommended in cases of overdose. Atropine is not reliable in blocking xylazine-induced bradycardia in domestic cats (Klide *et al.*, 1975). Cardiac output may actually be decreased in domestic cats, presumably due to the resulting tachycardia preventing adequate filling of the heart during diastole (Dunkle *et al.*, 1986). However, this would not necessarily apply to larger species. Furthermore, A–V blockade may be produced by the use of anticholinergics following medetomidine in cats (Jalanka, pers. commun.)

Glycopyrrolate is probably a better anticholinergic for cats (Hall & Clarke, 1991). As it does not cross the blood–brain barrier readily, central effects such as mydriasis and marked tachycardia are not so much of a problem as with atropine. Furthermore, in domestic cats it does not cause as marked an increase in heart rate. Unfortunately, there are no studies of its use in non-domestic cats.

Sedatives

In some circumstances mild sedation or tranquillization may be desirable. Introducing or transporting nervous cats and bringing animals into unfamiliar surroundings such as hospital dens are two examples. However, sedatives alone should not generally be used to facilitate examination or treatment.

Phenothiazines

Phenothiazine derivatives were widely used to sedate or tranquillize nervous cats in the past, but have largely been superseded. All phenothiazine derivatives are α_1-adrenoceptor blockers and as such produce hypotension due to peripheral vasodilation in addition to any anti-adrenaline effect. All drugs in this class impair thermoregulation. The degree of sedation achieved in each cat is variable, especially when given orally, and in certain individuals a paradoxical excitement may occur. Acepromazine may be given orally at 0.5–2 mg/kg and

promazine at 2–6 mg/kg (Wallach & Boever, 1983).

Benzodiazepines

Benzodiazepines can produce mild tranquillization in non-domestic cats with far fewer side-effects. In addition these drugs possess anxiolytic, amnesic, anticonvulsant and muscle-relaxing properties. Although vasodilation and a moderate decrease in cardiac contractility may occur, sympathetic nervous system reflexes are not impaired. Hence cardiac output and blood pressure will return to normal after administration of benzodiazepines as a result of catecholamine release (Klein & Klide, 1989).

Diazepam is not water soluble and is less well absorbed following i/m administration than when given orally. Diazepam solutions may also cause pain on i/m injection. Suggested initial oral doses in non-domestic cats are 0.25–1.0 mg/kg, although there is a great deal of individual variation in response. In small cats this can be repeated at 8-h intervals if necessary, less frequently in larger species. Given i/v as an anticonvulsant, doses of 0.3–0.5 mg/kg are appropriate (Dinnes, 1980). In domestic cats short courses of oral diazepam at 0.25–0.5 mg/kg have been recommended as an appetite stimulant (Bedford & Godsall, 1988; Davies, 1988). There may be benefit in trying a similar approach in non-domestic cats newly arrived in a collection where mild tranquillization and appetite stimulation is appropriate, although there have been no relevant studies published to date. Where an i/m benzodiazepine is required, midazolam is the preferred drug. Midazolam is water soluble, is rapidly absorbed from muscle, and does not cause pain on injection. Doses of < 0.2 mg/kg will provide mild tranquillization. Midazolam (approximately 0.1 mg/kg) has been administered orally in baits to free-living lions to calm nervous or very cautious animals prior to darting (McKenzie, 1993, p. 254).

α_2-Adrenoceptor agonists

Despite a wide range of undesirable physiological effects, parenteral α_2-agonists can produce the most effective sedation of any class of sedative drug in the cat. In addition, their effects are reversible by the use of α_2-adrenoceptor antagonists such as idazoxan or atipamezole (see 'Recovery from anaesthesia'). However, α_2-agonists should not be used alone to handle the larger species. In all species, high doses will produce a sleep-like state with marked muscular relaxation. When stimulated, cats will arouse from this condition and are capable of reacting aggressively. Many α_2-agonists cause significant uterine muscle stimulation and are therefore contraindicated in early or late pregnancy.

Doses of between 1 and 5 mg/kg xylazine have been recommended to facilitate handling a variety of non-domestic cat species (York & Huggins, 1972; Dinnes, 1980) but the author's experience is that these doses will not provide sufficiently reliable immobilization in larger species unless hand-tame. Where large enough doses have been given to tiger to allow handling, severe respiratory depression occurs representing overdose (Bush *et al.*, 1987).

Medetomidine is a very potent, selective and specific full agonist at pre- and postsynaptic α_2-adrenoceptors, with far greater affinity and selectivity than xylazine (Virtanen *et al.*, 1988; Virtanen, 1989). Used alone, medetomidine at 100–150 µg/kg i/m or s/c can provide profound sedation in smaller species sufficient for superficial examination and simple procedures such as blood sampling, without apparently causing dangerous respiratory or cardiovascular depression. Although peak plasma levels are achieved in domestic cats 30 min after i/m injection (Salonen, 1989), most small cats are safe to handle after 5–10 min. As in the domestic cat the depth of sedation does not increase at higher than recommended doses, only the duration of effect (Salonen, 1989; Vaino, 1989). Doses of up to 200 µg/kg have been tolerated in the Black-footed cat (pers. experience). In juveniles of the larger species sufficient sedation may be achieved for superficial examination, but this is a dangerous practice in adults due to insufficient restraint and the ability of an animal to respond to stimulation by arousal. For example, in adult snow leopards 60–107 µg/kg medetomidine provides moderate to deep sedation, but with insufficient immobilization to allow safe handling (Jalanka, 1987, 1989a).

Other α_2-agonists such as detomidine and romifidine have not been sufficiently tested in the non-domestic cat species and therefore cannot be recommended for use at present.

Long-acting Sedatives

For many years, wildlife veterinarians in South Africa have used long-acting sedatives or tranquillizers to provide prolonged periods of calming in wild hoofstock confined to temporary captivity, during transportation or immediately after relocation (Ebedes & Burroughs, 1989). Such drugs are slow-release sedative depots and produce sedation of up to 4 weeks depending on the drug and dose chosen. Unfortunately, there has been no published accounts of their use in carnivora. On occasions, long-acting sedation following a single injection may be desirable in non-domestic cats, such as the introduction of animals or the confinement in unfamiliar surroundings, particularly given that orally administered sedatives are unreliable in their effect. The author has used pipothiazine palmitate ('Piportil depot'— May & Baker) in adult male lion at 1–2 mg/kg i/m with some success. Mild tranquillization for up to 2 weeks was achieved both in the animals' dens and outside enclosures, but without any reduction in intraspecific aggression between males. The more rapidly effective but shorter acting zuclopenthixol acetate, a neuroleptic of the thioxanthone series with apparent dopamine antagonist activity (Clopixol-Acuphase; Lundbeck) shows great promise in many species, but has yet not been assessed in cats.

Induction of General Anaesthesia

The choice of induction agent(s) should be based on a knowledge of available drugs, consideration of what is required of the anaesthetic and a careful appraisal of the species and particular animal concerned. Each drug or drug combination has its own individual characteristics, and it is always helpful to use an anaesthetic agent with which the anaesthetist is familiar. This is particularly important when large cats are anaesthetized by veterinary surgeons who do not regularly deal with the more dangerous species. Equally important is the principle of administering sufficient anaesthetic for reliable induction. Underdosing any cat can create difficulties as some agents will cause excitement in low doses whilst others will produce profound ataxia. The safety of personnel must be a high priority when anaesthetizing any of the larger, more dangerous species and it is the responsibility of the anaesthetist to ensure effective and safe immobilization.

Wild animals often require higher doses of anaesthetic induction agents than their captive counterparts. However, direct comparisons between published data for wild and captive animals are difficult to make as no standards of anaesthetic depth or pre-anaesthetic excitement are applied. Wild cats are often anaesthetized for simple, relatively non-invasive procedures—radiocollaring, translocation, blood sampling, etc.—during which the main requirement is for safe immobilization. Whilst this is also the case with many captive cat anaesthetics it is not invariably so. Conditions under which general anaesthesia is conducted on wild animals are often far from ideal, a fact which will also lead field operators to accept and even require a lighter plane of anaesthesia than would be acceptable in the captive situation. Reference will be made to differences between doses required for wild and captive animals later in this section.

Even today, no anaesthetic agent or combination of agents possesses all the desired properties for non-domestic cat anaesthesia. The ideal drug would have high solubility and potency to allow small injection volumes; be effective via the i/m route and rapidly produce immobilization; provide adequate anaesthesia, analgesia and muscle relaxation of suitable duration; be free from adverse cardiovascular, respiratory and thermoregulatory effects; be harmless to the operator; and be capable of complete and permanent reversal. Up until the mid 1960s i/v barbiturates were commonly used in captive cats (Klos & Lang, 1976), but this was practically difficult and of little use in wild animals. Suxamethonium immobilization has been used for field studies of wild cats (e.g. Hornocker *et al.*, 1965), but this cannot be described as anaesthesia and is ethically unacceptable. The

first relatively safe i/m agent that found widespread use in both captive and wild cats was phencylidine, one of the cyclohexamine derivatives. Effective in very low volumes, phencylidine came into use in the late 1960s and early 1970s. However, even with the concurrent use of sedatives, major adverse side-effects occurred commonly and the drug was quickly superceded by other cyclohexamines, ketamine and tiletamine, either alone or in combination with sedatives or tranquillizers. Most modern anaesthetic regimes in use today for the non-domestic cats involve drug combinations including either ketamine or tiletamine.

Barbiturates

With small, handlable or tame animals, short-acting barbiturates can be given i/v to induce anaesthesia. Methohexitone sodium (0.5%) is effective at 3–5 mg/kg, or thiamylal sodium or sodium pentothal can be given to effect (Dinnes, 1980). In such cases the cephalic vein is probably the most convenient.

Barbiturates are more commonly encountered as poisons when contaminated meat is fed to non-domestic cats (Bush & Teeple, 1975; Martin & Mallock, 1987). Horse meat is usually implicated in accidental poisonings when neck muscle has been contaminated with pentobarbitone sodium during perivascular administration for destruction. Cases of malicious barbiturate poisoning also occur. The particular drug involved is usually other than pentobarbitone sodium, and can be readily identified by serum analysis. Affected cats often recover, sometimes after days of sedation or even anaesthesia. However, complications such as respiratory depression and arrest, hypothermia, renal failure and aspiration pneumonia can occur during the extended period of immobilization. Treatment of barbiturate poisoning is by aggressive diuresis and supportive care until the effects wear off (Fowler, 1986; Martin & Mallock, 1987).

Etorphine

Cats should never be anaesthetized with etorphine or etorphine combinations. In a series of 11 anaesthetics using etorphine in zoo cats,

Robinson (1976) reported severe side-effects including respiratory depression, cyanosis, tremors, muscle rigidity and convulsions. The concurrent use of acetylpromazine did not prevent convulsions. Euthanasia of very large cats can be carried out with etorphine after induction of general anaesthesia, but extreme care must be taken to handle and dispose of the carcases safely.

Phencyclidine

The cyclohexamines phencyclidine, tiletamine and ketamine have been used extensively in Felidae. Phencyclidine hydrochloride was the first member of the group to become widely available. Owing to its high potency, low injection volumes were required even for adult lion and tiger. Thus phencyclidine became the first practical anaesthetic agent for field immobilization of larger species where the necessity for remote injection limited the volume of drug that could be given with accuracy. Although phencyclidine has long been superceded by drugs and drug combinations with more favourable characteristics, a considerable amount of data were published on its use in cats and these will be summarized here.

Phencyclidine at 0.5–1.5 mg/kg i/m produces restraint accompanied by a dissociative-type anaesthesia in most species (Mayo, 1967; Theobald, 1970; Ebedes, 1973; Reed & Tennant, 1975; Klos & Lang, 1976; Wallach & Boever, 1983) although smaller cats may require < 2 mg/kg (Klos & Lang, 1976). Once anaesthetized, animals remain with their eyes open and have at least partially intact laryngeal and pharyngeal reflexes. Analgesia is adequate. However, induction and recovery times are long and may be accompanied by excitement, excessive salivation is common, and thermoregulation is impaired. Total recovery time of wild lions given phencyclidine at 1.7 mg/kg was found in one study to be <15 h (Smuts et al., 1973). Most seriously, relaxation is poor with a tendency towards spontaneous involuntary muscle movement and convulsions. Cheetah and tiger seem particularly prone to convulsions under phencyclidine (Seal & Erickson, 1969; Jones, 1972; Ebedes, 1973). Cheetah should not be given

more than 0.8 mg/kg (Jones, 1972; Ebedes, 1973), higher doses resulting in a greater incidence of convulsions, hyperthermia and recoveries lasting < 72 h. Conversely, jaguars (Panthera uncia) may require higher doses than other members of the Panthera genus to achieve comparable immobilization (Seal et al., 1970). Higher doses are also necessary for wild versus captive animals (Ebedes, 1973). Some authors believe that hallucinations characterized by continuous roaring may follow the use of phencyclidine in lions. A few sex differences have also been observed. In one study, male bobcats (Lynx rufus) were found to be more sensitive to phencyclidine than females (Baily, 1971) and in another, male Canadian lynx (Lynx canadensis) were anaesthetized for twice as long as females given the same dose (Berrie, 1972).

Some of the major side-effects seen with phencyclidine in cats can be at least partially prevented by the concurrent use of other drugs. Atropine is usually sufficient to control the excessive salivation (Jones, 1972; Ebedes, 1973). Many authors reported a decrease in induction times and incidence of convulsions plus an improvement in relaxation when phenothiazines such as promazine or acepromazine were used in combination with phencyclidine (Seal et al., 1970; Ebedes, 1973; Bush et al., 1978; Wallach & Boever, 1983). Acepromazine is included at < 0.34 mg/kg (Ebedes, 1973; Bertram, 1976; Sitton & Weaver, 1976) and promazine at < 1 mg/kg (Seal et al., 1970). Alternative tranquillizers such as xylazine at 0.5–0.75 mg/kg or azaperone at 0.4–0.6 mg/kg (Ebedes, 1973) produce a similar improvement in relaxation and induction times. However, convulsions are still seen even with the use of phenothiazines (Baily, 1971; Hornocker & Wiles, 1972; Bertram, 1976; Bush et al., 1978; Dinnes, 1980), xylazine or azaperone (Ebedes, 1973; Greenwood, pers. commun.), and most of these drugs further impair thermoregulation.

An alternative approach to prevent convulsions is to give sufficient phencylidine with or without a phenothiazine tranquillizer to safely immobilize an animal, followed by i/v barbiturates to induce anaesthesia or permit intubation, etc. (Jones, 1972; Klos & Lang, 1976). However, recoveries are even more prolonged. Given that phencyclidine has now been superceded by other drugs, further investigations into alternative tranquillizers and shorter acting intravenous agents to be used in combination have not been necessary.

For the capture of wild lion and leopard, oral phencyclidine is still found to be useful by some owing to its high potency (McKenzie, 1993, pp. 251–254). Although this technique should be considered only as a last resort, it may be necessary for animals too wary of traps or situations in which they may be darted. Doses of 2.5–3.5 mg/kg will usually achieve immobilization, but induction times may be as long as 4 h and a long period of incapacity is usual.

Ketamine

Ketamine hydrochloride is a shorter acting analogue of phencyclidine, possessing < 20% of the activity of the parent compound (Beck, 1972). It is soluble in water producing irritant solutions of low pH. Ten per cent solutions are commercially available (e.g. 'Vetalar'—Parke-Davis) but where higher concentrations are required it is possible to obtain ketamine powder (Parke-Davis) which can be made up to 20% solutions at normal ambient temperatures or even 25% at 25°C. Used alone in clinically normal cats, ketamine rapidly induces dissociative or cateleptoid anaesthesia accompanied by analgesia, an increase in heart rate, cardiac output and blood pressure, and minimal respiratory depression. However, there are some doubts over its effectiveness as a deep visceral analgesic (Sawyer *et al.*, 1991a). Salivation is increased (although less than with phencyclidine) and can obstruct the airway of smaller cats despite partial preservation of laryngeal and pharyngeal reflexes. However, intubation is usually accomplished easily under ketamine (Klein, 1980), and atropine is effective in preventing salivation.

Muscle tone is maintained under ketamine and tremors, limb muscle spasms and muscular rigidity are often seen even without further stimulation. Furthermore, like phencyclidine, ketamine can induce convulsions in cats when given alone. This is not a dose-dependant effect (Beck, 1972), and all species can be affected.

Some species such as tiger and cheetah appear particularly susceptible (Klos & Lang, 1976; Bush *et al.*, 1987). Estimates of the incidence of ketamine-induced convulsions in non-domestic cat are in the order of 5% (Klos & Lang, 1976; Beck, 1976). Such convulsions are usually controllable with i/v benzodiazepines (Beck, 1976; Bush *et al.*, 1987), although they are often self-limiting. Phenothiazines do not prevent convulsions (Dinnes, 1980). Other occasional side-effects that occur with the sole use of ketamine in cats include occasional prolonged and ataxic recoveries, excitement during induction if underdosed, and mania in kittens. The latter condition is characterized by vocalization, wall climbing and the kitten throwing itself on its back (Fowler, 1986). Such mania is not responsive to diazepam. Ketamine is detoxified in the liver, but the majority is excreted unchanged in urine. Prolonged recoveries can therefore be expected in animals with compromised hepatic or renal function. Ketamine rapidly crosses the placenta (Hall & Clarke, 1991).

Despite its many undesirable side-effects, ketamine has a wide safety margin in non-domestic cats (Dolensek, 1971; Klos & Lang, 1976), and i/m ketamine alone can be used to anaesthetize all species of non-domestic cat. In captivity, small species require 15–30 mg/kg (Beck, 1976; Klos & Lang, 1976; Wallach & Boever, 1983); medium-sized cats require 10–15 mg/kg (e.g. Wildt *et al.*, 1985); and the large species such as lion and tiger can be anaesthetized with < 10 mg/kg. Studies on wild lion suggest doses of at least 12 mg/kg are necessary before immobilization is safely acheived (Ebedes, 1973; Smuts *et al.*, 1973). Cheetah should not be given more than 6–10 mg/kg (Smuts *et al.*, 1973; Beck, 1976). Additional ketamine given to deepen or extend anaesthesia should be given i/v at 0.5–2 mg/kg to avoid the prolonged recoveries that result from supplementary i/m doses and minimizing the total dose given (Fowler, 1986; Wildt *et al.*, 1992). Smaller species tend to recover consciousness within 30–45 min following a single i/m dose (Klos & Lang, 1976), and large species such as lion take about an hour (Smuts *et al.*, 1973). However, the return of consciousness is usually followed by a period of ataxia and limited mobility lasting several hours. During recovery, the hind quarters remain paretic long after the fore quarters have regained co-ordination (Smuts *et al.*, 1973).

The adverse side-effects of induction excitement, salivation, poor muscle relaxation and convulsions seen when ketamine is used alone are unacceptable to most anaesthetists today. In addition, large delivery volumes are required for medium and large species, making remote injection difficult. Therefore ketamine is now usually combined with sedatives and anticonvulsants, particularly benzodiazepines and α_2-agonists.

Ketamine plus Benzodiazepines

Benzodiazepines improve muscle relaxation and reduce the incidence of convulsions caused by ketamine (Klein, 1980). Unlike α_2-agonists, they do not significantly reduce the requirement for cyclohexamines, and hence are used with ketamine at the standard doses given above. Midazolam (0.2 mg/kg) is a better choice than diazepam where the induction agents are given together in one dart or injection as it is water soluble and absorbed more rapidly. Diazepam at 0.1–0.5 mg/kg can be given with ketamine in all species (Fowler, 1986). As benzodiazepines produce minimal cardiovascular or respiratory depression in cats (Klein & Klide, 1989), ketamine/benzodiazepine combinations may be preferred to those containing α_2-agonists for the induction of anaesthesia in severely debilitated or shocked animals.

Ketamine plus Xylazine

Concurrent use of xylazine markedly reduces induction excitement, muscle tone and spontaneous movements due to ketamine in non-domestic cats. The incidence of convulsions is reduced, although not eliminated. Furthermore, xylazine doses as low as 0.5–1 mg/kg significantly lower the amount of ketamine required for induction of anaesthesia (Klein, 1980). In domestic cats, the plasma half-life of ketamine is nearly doubled by xylazine premedication (Waterman, 1983). Thus, in captive situations

where injection volumes are not critical, large cats and cheetah can be satisfactorily induced with 7–8 mg/kg ketamine plus 0.5–1 mg/kg xylazine, all other medium-sized species with 8–10 mg/kg ketamine plus 0.5–1 mg/kg xylazine, and the smaller species with 10–20 mg/kg ketamine plus 1–2 mg/kg xylazine. With these doses, animals are usually immobilized within 5–10 min and remain usefully anaesthetized for longer periods than with ketamine alone. Convulsions may occasionally occur in the larger species, usually precipitated by handling, disturbance or overdose. As a precautionary measure it is advised that all medium and large cats are given 5–10 mg diazepam i/v as soon as they are safely immobilized. Recoveries are generally smooth, although ataxia may be noted for a couple of hours. Excessive salivation is not usually a problem, and atropine is effective where necessary. Atropine is recommended with smaller species due to the small diameter airways.

Very few reports are available describing the haematological and biochemical effects of ketamine/xylazine in non-domestic cats, possibly due to a lack of baseline data in conscious animals. Seal *et al.* (1987) described a 10% rise in haematocrit and minor increases in serum potassium, glucose and bilirubin in tigers lightly anaesthetized with 3.5 mg/kg ketamine plus 1 mg/kg xylazine as compared with 5 mg/kg ketamine plus 0.3 mg/kg xylazine. A decrease in serum chloride was also noted. It is not clear from this report whether the differences are due to higher xylazine or lower ketamine doses.

One major disadvantage using ketamine and xylazine as above in large cats is the high volume required for remote injection even when ketamine is available at 200 mg/ml. However, a practical alternative to phencyclidine for field anaesthesia can be made by increasing the proportion of xylazine and reducing that of ketamine. With this approach not only can low volume darts be used, but partial reversal of anaesthesia also becomes possible. No reversal agent is available for ketamine, but there are several drugs described below (see 'Recovery from anaesthesia) that will antagonize the effects of α_2-agonists. As higher xylazine doses significantly increase immobilization and recovery times (Bush *et al.*, 1987) reversal is often desirable.

Medium and large cats including cheetah can be anaesthetized with 2–4 mg/kg ketamine plus 2–3 mg/kg xylazine (Wiesner, 1977; Wiesner & von Hegel, 1985; Gonzales & McDonnel, 1986; Bush *et al.*, 1987; Goltenboth & Klos, 1987). Wiesner (1977) described a simple method of dissolving 500 mg lyophilized xylazine ('Rompun dry substance'—Bayer) in 4 ml of 10% ketamine solution to produce approximately 4 ml of 'Hellabrunner mixture' containing 125 mg xylazine plus 100 mg ketamine per millilitre. Even with large cats, very low volumes are required. Adult tigers, for example, can be immobilized with 3.0 ml 'Hellabrunner mixture' (Wiesner & von Hegel, 1985) or 3.0 ml 'Hellabrunner mixture' plus 100 mg ketamine for larger specimens (Bush *et al.*, 1987).

Studies on free-living cats suggest that higher doses of ketamine and xylazine are generally required for immobilization and anaesthetic induction. Logan *et al.* (1986) found that wild puma (*Felis concolor*) required approximately 11 mg/kg ketamine plus 1.8 mg/kg xylazine to achieve light to moderate general anaesthesia. Even at these dose rates, the period of useful immobilization and time to recovery was extremely variable. Differing levels of pre-induction excitement may have affected the results, although this was not assessed. At 20 mg/kg ketamine plus 3.3 mg/kg xylazine approximately 2 h immobilization was achieved, and recoveries took 4 h. No fatalities were recorded. Van Wyk & Berry (1986) were able to effect immobilization of free-ranging African lion for up to 4 h with ketamine at 8 mg/kg plus 3.2 mg/kg xylazine. Similar doses of ketamine and xylazine are advised by McKenzie (1993, p. 227) for safe immobilization of wild African lions.

The use of xylazine in non-domestic cat anaesthesia does produce a few problems. Vomiting or retching may occur prior to immobilization in some animals (Klos & Lang, 1976; Logan *et al.*, 1986; Bush *et al.*, 1987), much as it does in domestic cats (Cullen & Jones, 1977). In the tiger, xylazine inhibits gastrointestinal motility, delaying the passage of barium from stomach to duodenum (Cook & Kane, 1980). Thus anaesthetic combinations including xylazine would be contraindicated for studies of gastric emptying. It is likely that this would apply to other cat species and other α_2-agonists. Xylazine induced bradycardia is rarely a significant problem where doses are low. However, in combinations using high xylazine doses it may be wise to give an anticholinergic soon after immobilization, despite the controversy over the use of atropine to control α_2-agonist mediated bradycardia. Respiratory depression has been noted by a number of authors, particularly where high xylazine doses are used (Logan *et al.*, 1986; Bush *et al.*, 1987). Particular attention should be paid to the monitoring of blood gases in these cases, most practically in field situations by the use of pulse oximetry.

Medetomidine plus Ketamine

In recent years, combinations of medetomidine with ketamine have become very popular in Europe for the safe and reliable anaesthetic induction of non-domestic cats. α_2-Agonists markedly reduce ketamine requirements both by direct CNS effects and by increasing the bioavailability of ketamine (Klein & Klide, 1989). This is particularly so in the case of the highly specific α_2-agonist medetomidine (Jalanka, 1987; Roeken, 1987), allowing the use of very low ketamine doses and effective reversal of anaesthesia with α_2-antagonists. To an extent, the disadvantages of medetomidine and ketamine are counterbalanced when used in combination (Verstegen *et al.*, 1991). Medetomidine compensates for the poor muscle relaxing and analgesic effects of ketamine, whilst the cardiac stimulating properties of ketamine partially compensate the medetomidine-induced bradycardia. Ketamine causes peripheral vasodilation, whereas medetomidine causes peripheral vasoconstriction.

Suitable doses for the induction of anaesthesia in different species are given in Table 14.2. Medetomidine is available in two strengths: 1 mg/ml ('Domitor'—Norden Laboratories) and 10 mg/ml ('Zalopine'—Farmos). Using 10 mg/ml medetomidine and 200 mg/ml ketamine any

Table 14.2 Intramuscular doses of medetomidine and ketamine suitable for anaesthetic induction of adult non-domestic cats (i.e. doses required to achieve complete immobilization, good muscle relaxation and no arousal after stimulation. Intubation should be possible at higher end of ranges quoted.) (Lewis, pers. exp.; Jalanka, 1987; 1989a,b; Barnett & Lewis, 1990; Jalanka & Roeken, 1990; Lewis, 1991)

Species	Medetomidine (per kg)	Ketamine (per kg)
Small cats		
Black-footed cat		
Caracal		
Fishing cat		
Jungle cat	80–100 µg	3–5 mg
Lynx		
Ocelot		
Serval		
Medium cats		
Cheetah		
Clouded leopard		
Jaguar	60–80 µg	2.5–3 mg
Leopard		
Puma		
Snow leopard		
Large cats		
Lion		
Tiger	30–40 µg	1–2 mg

cat can be anaesthetized with less than 3.5 ml total drug volume. Lower doses than those given can be used in exceptionally calm or tame cats, but this is not wise in the larger species. With excited or aggressive animals, the dose of both medetomidine and ketamine should be increased to ensure safe immobilization and relaxed anaesthesia. For example, in excited lion or tiger, 50 µg/kg medetomidine plus 2–3 mg/kg ketamine are more appropriate than the 30–40 µg/kg medetomidine plus 1–2 mg/kg ketamine quoted in Table 14.2. Where rapid immobilization is required (for the recapture of escaped animals for example) a similar increase in dose is appropriate (Jalanka, pers. commun.). Young of any species should be dosed according to size. For example, a 40-kg lion should be given 60–80 µg/kg medetomidine plus 2–3 mg ketamine as for the medium-sized cats.

Few studies of medetomidine and ketamine combinations in wild cats have yet been published. However, where such animals are more than usually excited prior to anaesthesia, it is likely that the doses of both compounds required would be higher than those quoted for their captive counterparts. Wild bear chased prior to darting have required up to twice the medetomidine and ketamine doses found reliable in captive animals (Roeken, 1987). Not all free-living cats are excited prior to anaesthesia, and doses may have to be selected according to the mental state of any particular animal. This principle is probably true for other anaesthetic drugs, but little attention has been paid to the point in published accounts of wild animal anaesthesia.

Induction of anaesthesia with medetomidine/ketamine is extremely smooth, animals generally lying down and appearing to be asleep within 5–10 min. Although it is generally safe to handle a cat at this point, 15–20 min should be allowed for the full effect. Although difficult to explain, the tail is the last area to lose sensation with medetomidine/ketamine. In large cats it is essential to check the response to applying pressure to the tail before assuming an animal is satisfactorily immobilized and therefore safe to handle. Vomiting or retching is occasionally seen on induction, and less commonly during the recovery period. This is minimized by pre-anaesthetic starvation. Fasciculation or twitching of leg muscles is sometimes seen in the late induction period although this is generally self-limiting.

The relaxation of skeletal muscle produced by medetomidine/ketamine is excellent, laryngeal and pharynegeal reflexes are partially preserved, and excessive salivation is not seen—presumably due to the low doses of ketamine employed. Ketamine-induced convulsions are very rare with this combination, but mild fitting has been observed in two lions on two occasions soon after induction (pers. observation). In large species, 1–1.5 h of useful anaesthesia will be provided by a single i/m dose of medetomidine/ketamine, although undisturbed the animals will often stay down for 2–3 h. In medium-sized species, relaxed anaesthesia tends to persist for 45–60 min. If no antagonist is given, these cats usually start to observe their surroundings 1.5–2 h after darting (Jalanka, 1989a). Smaller species tend to be anaesthetized for shorter periods. In domestic cats the duration of anaesthesia is related to the amount of ketamine given (Verstegen *et al.*, 1991) and this is probably the case in non-domestic species. Jalanka (1989b) found that induction times with medetomidine/ketamine in snow leopards were shorter than with ketamine/xylazine, and that medetomidine/ketamine treated animals showed superior muscle relaxation, a longer duration of useful immobilization and shorter total recovery times. Haematology, serum biochemistry and arterial blood gas values were comparable.

A limited amount of information is available about the physiological effects of medetomidine/ketamine combinations in non-domestic species. In his studies with snow leopards, Jalanka (1989a) reported stable heart and respiratory rates. However, it is the author's experience that both respiratory rate and oxygen saturation was usually depressed for a short period immediately following induction. This is consistent with an early depression in PO_2 with subsequent compensation observed in snow leopards (Jalanka, 1989a), although the Jalanka did not refer to changes in respiratory rate. Mucous membrane colour may appear cyanosed shortly after induction, although it usually rapidly returns to normal thereafter. In domestic cats, a 30% fall in heart rate was recorded by Young and Jones (1990) within 10 min of induction without causing a problem. This may occur in non-domestic species, but baseline values in conscious animals are not available. A slowing of the heart rate after a period of stable anaesthesia may indicate the onset of recovery, presumably due to the effects of ketamine wearing off in the presence of continued medetomidine-induced bradycardia. Changes in heart rate should therefore be interpreted carefully. No arrythmias or A–V blocks were seen with electrocardiography in the snow leopards studied by Jalanka (1987, 1989a). However, in a recent study of medetomidine and ketamine in African lions sinus arrhythmia, sinoatrial blocks and second degree A–V blocks were recorded in some animals

(Quandt, 1993). Thermoregulation is impaired, and although rectal temperatures remain stable when an animal is maintained at room temperature (Jalanka, 1989a) core temperatures should be monitored during long anaesthetics whenever medetomidine/ketamine has been used. Packed cell volumes decrease and blood glucose levels increase during medetomidine/ketamine induced anaesthesia (Jalanka, 1989a). Therefore it is important to standardize the time after darting at which blood samples are taken if samples are to be compared.

Medetomidine and ketamine provides safe, reliable anaesthesia for non-domestic cats, with few adverse side-effects even in animals of compromised health status (Jalanka & Roeken, 1990). In a series of 156 non-domestic cat immobilizations carried out at Helsinki and Kolmarden zoos Jalanka and Roeken (1990) reported only minor side-effects and no fatalities. Similarly, the author has used medetomidine/ketamine combinations on over 300 non-domestic cats without fatality. The safety margin thus appears to be extremely high, particularly given that both series quoted included a number of seriously ill animals. No adverse effect was seen in a late pregnant snow leopard in Jalanka and Roeken's series, but insufficient data are available to draw firm conclusions about the safety of this drug combination in pregnant animals generally. Jalanka reported administration of medetomidine at 625 µg/kg plus ketamine at 9.4 mg/kg to a lynx without complication (Jalanka, 1989a). Medetomidine at 325 µg/kg with 4 mg/kg ketamine was tolerated in an adult cheetah anaesthetized by the author. Lions and tigers given an additional 120 µg/kg medetomidine i/v following induction at standard doses suffered no ill effects (Barnett & Lewis, 1990). Thus, in dangerous species, it is preferable to over estimate than underestimate an animal's weight for calculation of medetomidine dose to avoid the risk of incomplete immobilization. However, caution should be excercised in calculating the amount of ketamine used due to the potentiation of its effect by the α_2-agonist.

Tiletamine plus Zolazepam

The cyclohexamine tiletamine hydrochloride has at least twice the potency of phencyclidine, but characteristically produces poor muscle relaxation and convulsions when used alone in non-domestic cats (Beck, 1972; Boever *et al.*, 1977; Wallach & Boever, 1983). When combined with the benzodiazepine zolazepam hydrochloride these effects are significantly reduced and the combination provides dose related anaesthesia ranging from chemical immobilization to cateleptoid or dissociative anaesthesia (Schobert, 1987). A 1:1 lyophilized mixture of the two compounds is available in the USA as 'Telazol' (A.H. Robbins) and in Europe as 'Zoletil' (Reading Laboratories). It is not yet available in the UK. The dry powder has a very long shelf-life and can be made up to highly concentrated solutions containing < 500 mg/ml.

Intramuscular tiletamine/zolazepam produces extremely rapid immobilization with onset of effects being seen in as little as 2–3 min (Smeller & Bush, 1976; Bush *et al.*, 1987; Wildt *et al.*, 1992). Induction of anaesthesia is frequently completed within 10 min, and the speed of induction is not apparently related to dose rate (King *et al.*, 1977). The ability to produce very rapid induction combined with high solubility and hence low delivery volume makes tiletamine/zolazepam particularly suitable for the recapture of escaped animals and the capture of free-living animals that are likely to run after being darted. Where available, it is the combination of choice for these purposes. Low doses are used for simple restraint, minor procedures and endotracheal intubation (Gray *et al.*, 1974). Higher doses can be used for surgical procedures as tiletamine does provide reasonable levels of analgesia (Schobert, 1987; Verstegen *et al.*, 1991). However, this is not recommended because of the limited degree of muscle relaxation produced (Smeller & Bush, 1976; Verstegen *et al.*, 1991) presumably due to preservation of spinal reflexes (Schobert, 1987). A greater degree of muscle relaxation is achieved in medium and large species, although this is dose dependent to an extent.

Tiletamine/zolazepam combinations are considered by many to have very wide safety margins. Respiratory depression is minimal, and cardiovascular integrity is maintained (Bush *et al.*, 1987; Wildt *et al.*, 1992). In domestic cats tiletamine/zolazepam causes tachycardia with a slight rise in blood pressure and cardiac output coupled with initial respiratory stimulation followed by mild depression of breathing (Hall & Clarke, 1991). Respiratory depression has been recorded in debilitated animals given high doses (Schobert, 1987). Insignificant alterations to acid–base balance have been recorded in cheetah and lion (Smeller & Bush, 1976; Bush *et al.*, 1978). Excessive salivation is recorded in some cats (Boever *et al.*, 1977), but did not occur in every case (Bush *et al.*, 1987; Wildt, 1992). Pharyngeal and laryngeal reflexes are at least partially preserved, and anticholinergics are effective in reducing salivation (Schobert, 1987).

Mild tremors and convulsions are occasionally seen during anaesthesia (Seidensticker *et al.*, 1974; Bush *et al.*, 1987; Wildlife Restraint Series, 1991; Wildt *et al.*, 1992), but these are generally not a significant problem. In common with many other anaesthetics, tiletamine/zolazepam appears to impair thermoregulation (King *et al.*, 1977). The main drawbacks of tiletamine/zolazepam combinations are seen in the recovery or post-recovery periods. Recoveries are generally smooth and usually occur within 4 h. Although the period and depth of anaesthesia is related to dose, the time required for recovery of the ability to walk is not necessarily so (Seidensticker *et al.*, 1974). A small percentage of cats show a dramatically prolonged recovery often characterized by disorientation (Boever *et al.*, 1977; Wildlife Restraint Series, 1991; R. Cooper, pers. commun.) and in some cases the recovery is stormy (King *et al.*, 1977; Verstegen *et al.*, 1991). Tigers are frequently dull for a couple of days following tiletamine/zolazepam (L.Gage, pers. commun.) and there are many reports of resedation occurring in this species (particularly white tigers and the Siberian subspecies) between 1 and 5 days after anaesthesia. Following an apparently complete recovery, these episodes usually take the form of mild sedation with ataxia. In some cases supportive care is required for a variable period (Bush *et al.*, 1987; Cooper, 1989; Wildt *et al.*, 1992; L.Gage, pers.commun.). In exceptional cases, complete recoveries may take up to 3 weeks (Cooper, 1989). Post-recovery resedation has also been observed in lion, cheetah and fishing cat (Wildt *et al.*, 1992; R. Cooper, pers. commun.). More seriously, convulsive episodes have been observed during the post-recovery period in Siberian and white tigers (Cooper, 1989; L. Gage, pers. commun.), serval (R. Cooper, pers. commun.), and cheetah (E. Blumer, pers. commun.). Diazepam is usually effective in controlling such fits. In one case, a tiger fitted intermittently for 48 h 3 days following anaesthesia (L. Gage, pers. commun.). The majority of animals showing post-recovery neurological problems have been clinically normal and there appears to be no age or sex predisposition. However, in a proportion of cases there is a history of multiple tiletamine/zolazepam anaesthetics. These complications are almost certainly due to the tiletamine (Klein, 1980). When selecting an anaesthetic protocol for a cat it should be borne in mind that tiger and cheetah seem to be particularly susceptible to cyclohexamine-induced convulsions irrespective of which analogue is given.

Suggested combined doses of tiletamine and zolazepam for non-domestic cat species are given in Table 14.3. The wide ranges given reflect the large variation quoted in the literature, the dose dependancy of anaesthetic depth and the wide safety margin of the compounds. Furthermore, when reviewing the literature it is apparent that different authors are using tiletamine/zolazepam for widely varying purposes which makes their recomendations very difficult to compare without standardized measures of anaesthetic depth. Table 14.3 should therefore be considered as a guideline only. Very calm animals can be immobilized with lower doses than the minimums quoted (Bush *et al.*, 1987). There is some evidence that wild cats require doses at the upper end of or slightly above the ranges in Table 14.3 (Seidensticker *et al.*, 1974; Bertram & King, 1976; King *et al.*, 1977). Interestingly, wild male lions and leopards have been found to require lower doses of tiletamine/zolazepam than females to achieve the same effect (Bertram & King, 1976; King *et al.*, 1977, McKenzie, 1993, p. 227).

Tiletamine/zolazepam anaesthesia is not effectively reversible, although short-term reversal of the effects of benzodiazepines can be achieved with flumazenil. Despite this limitation and the occasional post-recovery neurological complications, the combination offers a rapidly acting, high potency/low volume immobilizing and anaesthetic agent with a wide safety margin. It is particularly convenient for the anaesthesia of large, free-living cats in the field or in animals where it is only possible to administer very low volumes for induction.

Saffan

The steroid combination of 9 mg/ml alphaxalone and 3 mg/ml alphadolone known as 'Saffan' (Glaxo) has not found wide use in non-domestic cat anaesthesia. Green (1979) reported its use at 12–18 mg/kg i/m in zoo felids held in restraining cages, but commented on the large volume needed which restricts the possibility of remote injection techniques. Saffan has been used at 3 mg/kg intravenously to induce light anaesthesia suitable for minor procedures in captive cheetah (Button *et al.*, 1981). Left alone, these animals remained recumbant for 1–3 h, but showed evidence of impaired thermoregulation. Greenwood (pers. commun.) was able to achieve restraint in cheetah by using Saffan at 5 mg/kg i/m. Subsequent doses were given i/v. Intravenous Saffan (approximately 2.4 mg/kg) is considered

Table 14.3 Intramuscular doses of tiletamine and zolazepam suitable for immobilization and anaesthetic induction of adult non-domestic cats (Gray *et al.*, 1974; Boever *et al.*, 1977; Schobert, 1987; Smeller & Bush, 1976; Wildlife Restraint Series, 1991; McKenzie, 1993)

Species	Total combined dose (mg/kg)	
	Light anaesthesia immobilization	Anaesthesia of moderate depth
Small cats	3–5	10–15
Medium cats	2.5–5	10
Large cats	2–4	8–10

the drug of choice by McKenzie (1993, p. 236) for immobilization of wild cheetah in traps.

Saffan does not offer any advantages over other anaesthetics available for non-domestic cats and is impractical for most situations. In domestic cats, the use of Saffan may be associated with hyperaemia and swelling of paws, ears and noses, with occasional cases of laryngeal and pulmonary oedema, presumably due to histamine release (Hall & Clarke, 1991). Although none of these side effects has yet been reported in non-domestic cats, there would seem little justification in testing the product further in these species.

Inhalation Agents

As with most other mammals, induction using gaseous anaesthetics is possible with non-domestic cats. In the 1960s Graham-Jones (1964) used ether and chloroform mixtures to induce anaesthesia in large- and medium-sized species by pumping the gases into specially constructed cages. The enormous practical difficulties were perhaps warranted at that time owing to the lack of safe alternative injectable anaesthetics, but fortunately this is no longer the case. If small or very young cats can be suitably restrained, induction can be achieved with halothane (Robinson & Benirschke, 1981), methoxyflurane or isoflurane administered via a face mask. However, this may require forcible restraint for long periods, involving a significant degree of stress and resultant catecholamine release with possible adverse cardiovascular consequences (Jones, 1983). Therefore, in most cases, induction with injectable anaesthetics is preferable. When mask induction is unavoidable, isoflurane is probably the best tolerated as it is less unpleasant than other agents.

Maintenance of Anaesthesia

When it is necessary to prolong anaesthesia beyond the useful and safe period allowed by a single dose of the induction agent(s), maintenance with inhalation agents administered via an endotracheal tube is the best option. Gaseous anaesthesia allows complete control of the airway, accurate control of the depth of anaesthesia and more rapid recoveries than with incremental parenteral drugs. The equipment necessary for inhalation anaesthesia can be portable and is practical in all but the most extreme field conditions. If it is necessary to transport such equipment by air to more remote locations, oxygen cylinders can be replaced by oxygen concentrators as used by army medical corps. However, circumstances will inevitably arise when inhalation anaesthesia is not available or the need for it was not predicted. In these cases the use of incremental i/v agents will be necessary. Even if not ideal, with care this approach can be used successfully in all but the most critically ill patients.

However maintenance of anaesthesia is achieved, it is possible during selected surgical procedures to use local anaesthesia as an adjunct to general anaesthesia. For example, local nerve blocks applied during invasive dental procedures can avoid the need to deepen an anaesthetic simply to provide a high degree of local analgesia. Neuromuscular blocking agents can be used in non-domestic cats to provide a greater degree of relaxation during balanced anaesthesia as they can in the domestic cat. Although these agents allow a lower level of general anaesthesia to be employed, it must be remembered that they provide no analgesia or anaesthesia in their own right and require the provision of intermittent positive pressure ventilation. Furthermore, assessment of the depth of anaesthesia becomes difficult with their use (Hall & Clarke, 1991). Therefore the use of neuromuscular blockade should only be undertaken by the most experienced anaesthetists.

Intubation and Anaesthetic Circuits

To ensure operator safety, a mouth gag should be applied to all medium- and large-sized non-domestic species before intubation or examination of the mouth is attempted. The simplest design is a section of thick-walled plastic tubing of appropriate length placed between the upper and lower canine teeth of one side, with the tooth crowns positioned within the tube lumen. Polyethylene water pipe with an external diameter of 20 mm and wall thickness of 2 mm has proved useful in a wide range of species.

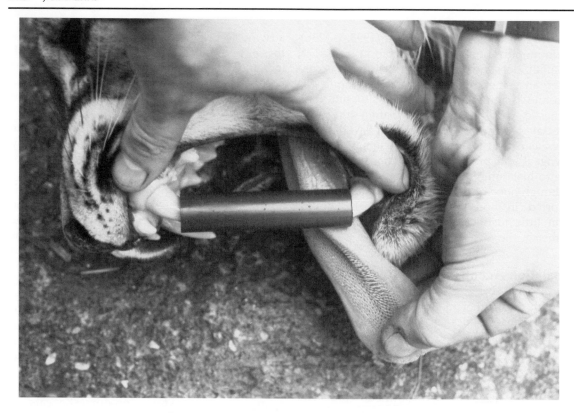

Fig. 14.5 Snow leopard: correctly fitted tube gag.

The canines of the larger species are sufficiently curved to allow the ends of the tube to rest upon the proximal tooth crown and not the gums where they may cause trauma (Fig. 14.5). Such tube gags are only intended for use in fully anaesthetized cats. They may be crushed or split by a semiconscious animal.

In most species, intubation is easily achieved during inspiration and does not require topical anaesthesia of the larynx. In all species except the leopard (*Panthera pardus*), intubation is performed under direct vision using an appropriately sized laryngoscope blade having extended the head on the neck and the tongue as far forward as possible. The larynx of the leopard is situated relatively further down the neck towards the thoracic inlet than in other cats and intubation is made easier by the use of a rigid endoscope. Cuffed endotracheal tubes of various designs can be used, but in medium and large species the thick walls of the traditional Magill curved tubes prevent accurate alignment with the shape of the trachea and may restrict gas flow at the point of delivery within the

trachea. A more suitable design for these animals is the straighter, flexible, silicone tube ('Aire-cuff') made by Bivona Inc., USA and currently imported to the UK by Bowring Medical Engineering of Oxfordshire (Fig. 14.6). These tubes are also available with wire reinforcement to prevent kinking. Introduction of the endotracheal tube in the larger species may be aided by the use of a tube stiffener. Most tubes of high diameter are too long for cats leading to the risk of endobronchial intubation. This can be avoided by reducing their length to match the distance between the nostrils and the point of the shoulder (Hall & Clarke, 1991). Even the largest of cats can be intubated with tubes of less than 70 cm in length. Tubes of internal diameters between 12 and 18 mm are generally suitable for adult medium-sized cats, with adult lion and tiger accepting tubes of up to 26 mm internal diameter.

The choice of anaesthetic circuit will be determined largely by the size of the cat according to standard principles that apply to any domestic species. Circuits with limited dead

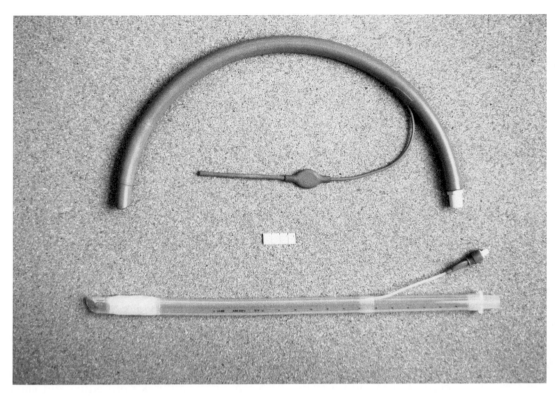

Fig. 14.6 Curved 14-mm Magill type endotracheal tube (top) and straight, flexible 14-mm silicone 'Aire-cuff' endotracheal tube (Bivona).

space such as the Ayres T piece and co-axial Baines are suitable for smaller species. The medium- and large-sized cats can be maintained on non-rebreathing circuits, but this is wasteful of gas and unnecessarily expensive. Thus circle or to-and-fro circuits are more usually employed with such animals. Assisted ventilation is rarely required, but the ability to apply positive pressure ventilation should be available in the event of respiratory failure.

Inhalation Agents

Currently, isoflurane is considered to be the inhalant anaesthetic agent of choice in non-domestic cats, and has been used widely in many species without adverse effects (Personal experience; Bush *et al.*, 1987; Wildt *et al.*, 1992). The use of halothane has also been widely documented (Dinnes, 1980; Robinson & Benirschke, 1981; Wallach & Boever, 1983; Bush *et al.*, 1987). However, there is some evidence that prolonged maintenance with

halothane may produce hepatotoxicity, at least in snow leopard (Fanton *et al.*, 1984). Cardiac arrythmias frequently occur in domestic cats receiving halothane (Hall & Clarke, 1991), and the hypotensive effects of halothane are well recognized. Therefore, isoflurane should be used in preference to halothane in cats with cardiac or hepatic disease. Methoxyflurane can also be used (Krahwinkel, 1970; Dinnes, 1980; Wallach & Boever, 1983; Bush *et al.*, 1987) and is less likely to vaporize to lethal concentrations than halothane. Recoveries after methoxyflurane anaesthesia may take up to 1.5 h (Wallach & Boever, 1983). Nitrous oxide can be used as part of balanced gaseous anaesthesia, although there is no specific documentation of its use in non-domestic species.

Special care should be exercised with the use of inhalation agents following induction with α_2-agonists, particularly medetomidine. The dose requirements for halothane are markedly reduced by medetomidine in the dog (Vickery & Maze, 1989; Raiha *et al.*, 1989) and rat (Segal *et al.*, 1989) and this is apparently true in non-domestic cats maintained on isoflurane. Overdose with a gaseous agent is therefore easier to achieve following induction with medetomidine combinations than when using the same agents following induction regimes that do not include α_2-agonists.

Intravenous Agents

Induction of anaesthesia in most non-domestic cats involves the use of a cyclohexamine, particularly ketamine or tiletamine, and it is possible to use incremental i/v ketamine to prolong or deepen anaesthesia. Ketamine should be given slowly to effect and in decreasing doses. Diazepam should always be available to control ketamine-induced fits if these occur. Although such an approach will inevitably increase recovery periods, it will do so to a far lesser extent than with the use of incremental i/m ketamine.

Theroretically, where tiletamine/zolazepam combinations have been used to induce anaesthesia, i/v maintenance should be with ketamine rather than with more of the induction mixture. The half-lives of tiletamine and zolazepam are different in the cat and thus the ratio of drugs will vary with each incremental dose. However, practical experience suggests that few problems arise from the use of further tiletamine/zolazepam to provide maintenance if absolutely necessary (L.Gage, pers. commun.).

Although the short-acting, substituted phenol derivative propofol ('Rapinovet'—Pitman-Moore) is impractical as an induction agent due to the necessity for i/v administration, it may have potential for i/v maintenance or short-term prolongation of anaesthesia in non-domestic cats. In domestic cats i/v maintenance doses of 0.5 mg/kg per minute have been suggested (Brearley *et al.*, 1988). No evidence of cumulative effects were found by Morgan and Legge (1989) in domestic cats given incremental doses, and heart rate and blood pressure are maintained (Hall & Clarke, 1991). However, propofol does cause respiratory depression (Brearley *et al.*, 1988) and longer recoveries than in domestic dogs as cats do not metabolize phenols as rapidly (Hall & Clarke,

1991). In the author's limited experience, intravenous propofol given to tigers and lions at 1 mg/kg following induction with medetomidine and ketamine can result in temporary apnoea and a shallow respiratory pattern if given too rapidly. Maintenance of large cats with propofol for any length of time would be extremely expensive, thus in practice its use would probably be restricted to smaller species.

Anaesthesia for Transport

Captive cats and the smaller, free-living species usually remain calm for transportation in crates provided they are left relatively undisturbed and in reduced light. However, free-living lion, leopard and occasionally cheetah are very excitable and may inflict serious injury to themselves in their violent attempts to escape from transport crates. Consequently it is common practice for such animals to be heavily sedated or even anaesthetized during transport, particularly where journey times are kept below 8 h. This is a very risky procedure and should only be attempted by the most experienced veterinarians. A detailed account of the techniques and risks is given in McKenzie (1993, p. 286–292).

Anaesthesia and Reproduction

As certain species of non-domestic cat become increasingly rare and in some cases difficult to breed, more and more attempts are being made to apply artificial reproductive techniques, such as artificial insemination (AI), *in vitro* fertilization (IVF) and embryo transfer (ET) to captive breeding programmes. Recent experience suggests that the anaesthetics used during some procedures may adversely influence reproductive function. For example, during electroejaculation attempts to collect semen, relaxation of the bladder neck may lead to contamination of the semen with urine which is potentially spermicidal. Many anaesthetic drugs produce this effect including diazepam, phenothiazines and the volatile agents halothane and isoflurane (Howard, 1993). A combination of ketamine, acepromazine and halothane given during the follicular phase of the ovarian cycle was thought to be responsible for inhibition of ovulation in domestic cats (Howard, 1992). It is clear that great care must be taken to select and assess appropriate anaesthetic agents during reproductive procedures.

Anaesthetic Monitoring and Fluid Therapy

The principles of anaesthetic monitoring in non-domestic cats are no different to those applied to domestic species, and have been discussed at length elsewhere (Chapter 10). To be able to appreciate deterioration of a patient's condition during an anaesthetic allows remedial action to be taken and disaster avoided. However crude the conditions under which a cat is anaesthetized, the need for monitoring remains the same. It is rarely the case that hospital facilities are available for non-domestic cats and therefore monitoring equipment should generally be portable and independently powered. Fortunately, there is a wide range of simple and battery operated equipment now available and thus no excuse exists for failing to monitor a patient during anaesthesia irrespective of the conditions under which it is performed.

Initial Assessment after Induction

Once a cat has been apparently immobilized following administration of the induction agent(s) it is necessary to assess the depth and effectiveness of anaesthesia carefully before any procedures are carried out. This is especially important with dangerous species. An animal's response to stimuli (prodding with a pole from safe position, pinching between toes, palpebral reflex, light touch on inner aspect of ears), its respiration rate, mucous membrane colour, pulse rate and quality and muscle tone (limb and jaw) should all be assessed without delay and at intervals thereafter. In medium and large cats it is wise to secure the head by placing a fork (Fig. 14.7) over the neck or applying pressure with a broom on the neck (Fig. 14.8) whilst initial observations are made. In danger-

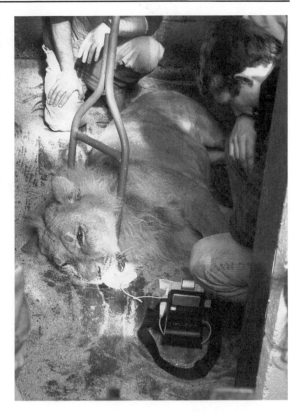

Fig. 14.7 Lioness secured immediately after induction with metal fork whilst initial assessment is made.

ous species following induction with medetomidine and ketamine it is *essential* to check the response to pressing or pinching the tail and hind feet before assuming the animal is safe to handle (Lewis, 1991). Personal experience with lion and tiger suggests that these areas are the last to lose sensation, and stimuli applied here early in induction may arouse an apparently immobilized animal. With most induction agents, immobilization occurs well in advance of anaesthesia. Therefore it is important with dangerous species to allow sufficient time for induction before disturbing the animal. This may be < 20 min following i/m administration and longer if induction agents have been delivered s/c. Indications of light anaesthesia include reflex limb movements, lacrimation, pupillary dilatation and movement of the eyes. Opening the jaw wide may produce short periods of apnoea in lightly anaesthetized cats. Should initial observations reveal that a cat is too lightly anaesthetized to handle safely,

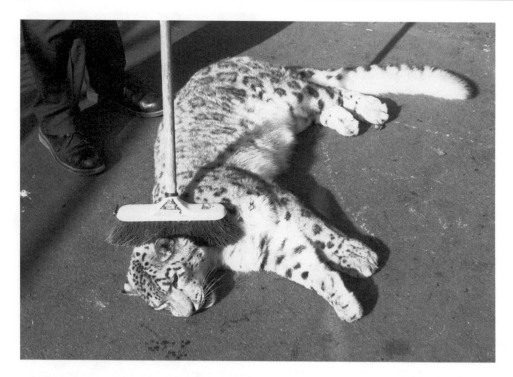

Fig. 14.8 Snow leopard: restraint with broom for initial post-induction assessment.

placing a blindfold over the eyes will reduce the risk of arousal. Given that the last sense to be abolished by general anaesthesia is usually hearing, it is good practice to insist on quiet around any anaesthetized cat. Immediately following initial examination, a plain eye cream should be applied to each cornea to prevent drying and the eyes covered to protect them from strong sunlight where appropriate. Cyclohexamines cause marked pupillary dilation and retinal damage may result from direct sunlight.

Monitoring During Anaesthesia

Basic, clinical cardiopulmonary monitoring is usually sufficient during short procedures without resorting to the use of sophisticated equipment. One exception to this is the use of pulse oximeters which take only seconds to set up if the user is familiar with sensor placement. Attention should be paid to respiratory rate, depth and pattern; colour of the mucous membranes and capillary refill time; and pulse rate, strength and rhythm. A peripheral pulse can be appreciated in most individuals in the lingual artery or the dorsal metatarsal artery. The femoral pulse is not a good indicator of peripheral circulation. Large cats have heart rates of approximately 40–50 b.p.m., with respiratory rates of around 10 per minute. Heart rate will tend to increase as anaesthetic depth decreases, providing one of the early indications of arousal. However, with medetomidine/ketamine combinations the reverse is true as the effects of medetomidine persist longer than those of ketamine. Although there are many other causes of heart rate slowing, one must always be aware that it may indicate impending arousal following medetomidine/ketamine induction and should carefully check the observation against other signs. In medium and large species, this effect will usually be seen at 30–60 min following induction.

Capillary refill times of between 2 and 3 s are usual. Cyanosis of mucous membranes can only usually be seen where there is adequate blood flow to carry deoxygenated haemoglobin to the periphery. In practice, except where an α_2-agonist has been used, it is rarely observed during anaesthesia unless there is profound oxygen lack due to severe lung disease or failure of oxygen supply (Hall & Clarke, 1991).

Prolonged Anaesthetics

A more comprehensive approach to monitoring should be adopted during prolonged anaesthetics and with any anaesthesia carried out in poor risk subjects. However, sophisticated monitoring equipment should only be used to augment and not replace clinical observation. It is tempting to place too much reliance on technological gadgets, the servicing of which during anaesthesia can distract one's attention from direct observation of the patient. Oesophageal stethoscopes, respiratory rate monitors, apnoea alarms, tidal and minute volume monitors, the measurement of arterial blood gas values and capnography can all be applied to the assessment of respiratory function in non-domestic cats as they can in domestic animals. Similarly, oesophageal stethoscopes, heart rate monitors, electrocardiography and pulse monitors can provide valuable information about the state of the circulation during anaesthesia.

Although detailed discussion of the use of monitoring devices can be found elsewhere (Chapter 10) it is worth emphasizing that heart rate monitors without an ECG facility are of limited use. These devices may be triggered by electrical noise or both R and T waves when electrodes are incorrectly placed. They may also double count when receiving high amplitude signals. Electrocardiography not only provides more accurate information about the heart rate, but also about disturbances of cardiac rhythm, myocardial ischaemia and differential diagnosis of cardiac arrest should this occur. More relevant information concerning the effectiveness of the heart as a pump and the adequacy of circulatory volume can be derived from measurement of arterial blood pressure.

Direct measurement of arterial blood pressure requires the placement of intra-arterial cannulae or transducers. In medium and large species, the dorsal metatarsal artery can be used (Fig. 14.9), but in smaller species it may be necessary to use the femoral artery (see Chapter 10). In the latter case, particular care should be taken to avoid post-withdrawal haematoma formation. Although not as accurate, indirect measurement of arterial blood pressure by sphygmomanometry is easier for the operator, less invasive and yet can still detect trends in systolic and

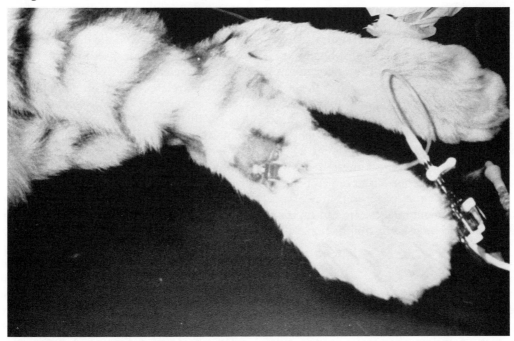

Fig. 14.9 Tiger: intra-arterial cannula in dorsal pedal artery for direct measurement of arterial blood pressure.

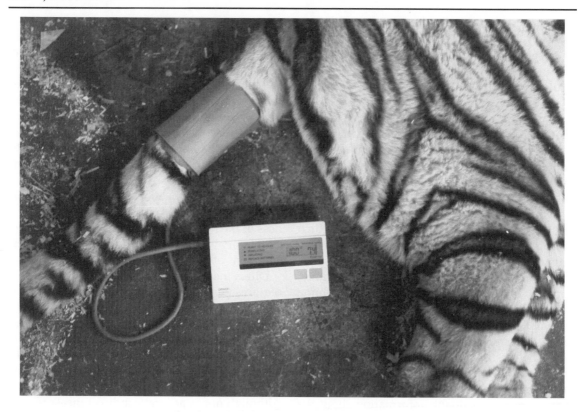

Fig. 14.10 Tiger: Omron portable sphygmomanometer with cuff placed around base of tail.

diastolic pressures. In medium and large species suitably sized sphygmomanometry cuffs can be placed around the distal fore leg or hind leg (medial aspect), or proximal tail (ventral aspect). A simple, cheap and effective sphygmomanometer (Automatic digital BP monitor, Omron Corporation, Japan) suitable for use in the larger species under field conditions is illustrated in Fig. 14.10. For a detailed comparison of direct and indirect blood pressure measurement and methods see Hall and Clarke (1991, pp. 24–31). With either direct or indirect measurement of blood pressure it is important to remember that pressure does not equal perfusion, thus assessment of mucous membrane colour and capillary refill time should be used in conjunction.

Pulse Oximetry

The application of pulse oximetry in non-domestic cats deserves special mention. Given the difficult and crude circumstances under which many non-domestic species are anaesthetized, there is always need for simple, portable,

non-invasive monitors that are quick to apply yet yield useful information in addition to clinical observation. Pulse oximeters provide one such technique and are described in Chapter 10. Although in man, pulse oximetry measurements of haemoglobin oxygen saturation (SpO_2 values) correlate well with *in vitro* measurements of arterial blood oxygen saturation (SaO_2), this has yet to be established in non-domestic animals. However, pulse oximeters are thought to be sufficiently accurate to monitor trends in haemoglobin oxygen saturation in a wide variety of non-domestic species (Allen, 1990, Zuba & Allen, 1992) even if the absolute oxygen saturation is more difficult to interpret. To be able to monitor blood oxygenation without the need for animal-side laboratory facilities necessary for direct blood gas analysis is extremely valuable, especially given that pulse oximeters are now available as battery-operated, portable units. One such is shown in Fig. 14.11.

The choice of sensor used with any pulse oximeter and the site of placement is crucial to

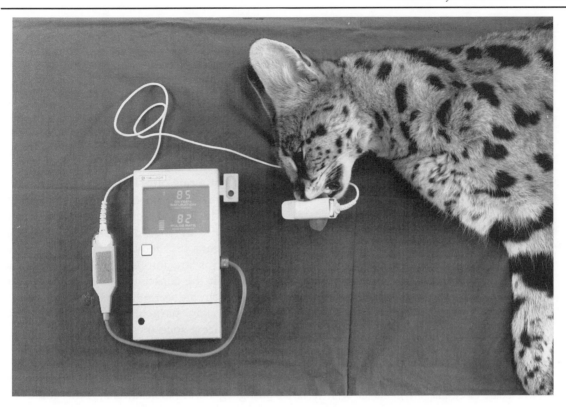

Fig. 14.11 Serval: portable, battery operated pulse oximeter (Nellcor) in use. Note finger-sensor on tongue.

ensure accurate results. Human finger sensors work adequately on the tongues of medium and large cats. Veterinary 'clamp' type sensors (Nellcor Inc. USA) can be applied to the tongue of any cat although they are easily dislodged. In theory, the clamp type sensors can be applied to any non-pigmented area but hair must be removed first to allow light transmission. In some cats the ears and even the lips can be used. Reflectance sensors applied to skin overlying bone may be applicable in some circumstances. Further development of this type may allow reliable rectal or oesophageal probe sensors to be designed in the future (Allen 1992).

Temperature Monitoring

Core temperature should be monitored during prolonged anaesthesia as most anaesthetic agents used in non-domestic species impair thermoregulation. When working in extremely high or low ambient temperatures, it is necessary to monitor core temperatures for all anaesthetics. Normal rectal temperatures of non-domestic cats range from 37.7 to 39°C. Simple, inexpensive, battery-operated, electronic thermometers with thermistor probes are now widely available allowing continuous monitoring of rectal or oesophageal temperature (Fig. 14.12).

Hypothermia can occur in any species during prolonged anaesthesia, but affects smaller species and critically ill animals to a greater extent. Although hypothermia can be corrected, it is far better to prevent its occurrence by attention to environmental conditions during anaesthesia.

Hyperthermia can result from pre-anaesthetic excitement, convulsions, high environmental temperatures and exposure to direct sunlight. Untreated, hyperthermia will lead to brain damage and death from pulmonary oedema. Even in less extreme cases a prolonged recovery from anaesthesia can be expected. As little as 10 min excitement in puma has been known to increase the body temperature to 42.2°C (A. Greenwood, pers. commun.). In tigers, core temperatures above 39.4°C are considered to

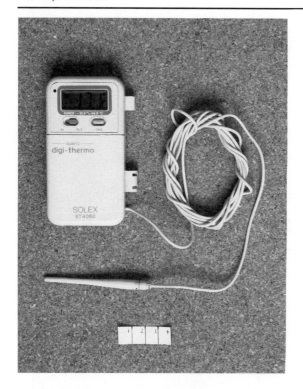

Fig. 14.12 Solex electronic thermometer with rectal probe.

require reduction by externally applied water and increased air cooling. Core temperatures rising above 40.6°C demand more aggressive therapy including water immersion, cold water enemas, intravenous fluids, corticosteroids and antibiotics (Bush *et al.*, 1987). To avoid further increases in body temperature, overheated cats should never be enclosed in a box. Prevention of hyperthermia is particularly important when anaesthetizing free-ranging species in high ambient temperatures. Conscious cats lose heat in these conditions primarily by panting. Panting rates of between 120 and 150 per minute have been observed in lions in ambient temperatures of 40°C (van Wyk & Berry, 1986). Under field conditions, being unable to lose heat in this manner during anaesthesia can rapidly lead to hyperthermia.

Fluid Therapy

The principles of fluid therapy in non-domestic cats are the same as for domestic animals. Colloidal and crystalloid fluids used in domes-

tic animal medicine are suitable for all cat species, with no adverse reactions being reported in the literature or experienced by the author. Apart from the correction of specific deficits, fluids are given during prolonged anaesthetics to maintain intravenous access and extracellular fluid volume. Michell *et al.* (1989) recommended that such prophylactic use of fluids should be restricted to lactated Ringer's solutions at a rate of 5–10 ml/kg/h.

In severely dehydrated animals, it is desirable to replace the fluid and electrolyte losses prior to anaesthesia. In non-domestic species this usually means oral rehydration fluids as intravenous drips are impossible to establish and maintain in the conscious subject. Not all cats take oral rehydration solutions which can create the need for particularly aggressive fluid therapy during anaesthesia. Under such circumstances the monitoring of central venous pressure is advisable where possible. Urine output and quality are not usually monitored during general anaesthesia, but could be considered in cases such as these and where there is severe renal impairment.

Suitable sites and techniques of intravenous cannula placement in smaller species are as for domestic cats. For the smallest of species the jugular vein is the most practical vessel and is very superficial in tiny cats. The jugular can be employed in medium and large species, and should be used if large volumes are to be given. The cephalic vein on the dorsal aspect of the foreleg can be used in small, medium and young of the larger species, but can be hard to locate in adult lion and tiger. The medial saphenous vein which crosses the medial tibial region (Chapter 1) is convenient in all medium and large cats (Fig. 14.13), and is easily immobilized for cannulation. The lateral saphenous vein or recurrent tarsal vein (Fig. 14.14) can also be used, but is far more mobile in many species making placement awkward. Lateral tail veins can be used in larger species, but many captive specimens will have substantial deposits of fat overlying the veins. A cut down approach to the veins of medium and large cats greatly assists cannula placement, especially with over-the-needle cannulae. The skin is surprisingly

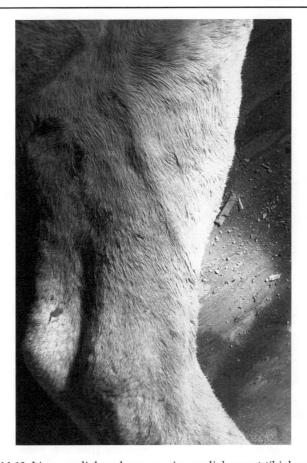

Fig. 14.13 Lion: medial saphenous vein, medial aspect tibial region.

thick in these species and will damage a cannula tip if percutaneous placement is attempted.

Recovery from Anaesthesia

General Considerations

Clarke and Hall (1990) calculated that 40% of the fatalities in healthy domestic cats undergoing general anaesthesia occur during the recovery period. No comparable figures are available for non-domestic species, but it is clear from these figures that the recovery period is a critical phase and that considerable attention should be directed towards ensuring the safety of a cat during recovery. Consideration must be given to both the monitoring of cats during recovery and the conditions under which they are expected to recover. When α_2-agonists have been used, recovery can be accelerated by the use of α_2-antagonist drugs.

All animals should be allowed to recover undisturbed in quiet, dimly lit conditions within a secure area free from physical hazards. Provision must be made to prevent the development of either hypothermia or hyperthermia. In captivity, access to platforms or other structures from which the cat may fall before recovery is complete must be restricted. In practice an unfurnished indoor den will usually suffice. Under free-ranging conditions access to other natural hazards such as free-standing water and substantial drops must be limited, although this may tax the imagination. Where possible cats destined to be released directly into the wild are better recovering in a large box or restricted area before they are freed. Food and water should be withheld in all cases until recovery is complete.

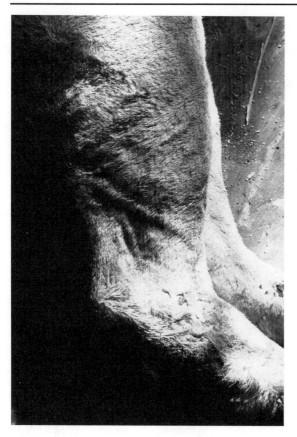

Fig. 14.14 Lion: recurrent tarsal vein, lateral aspect distal tibial region.

Cats should be placed in lateral recumbancy for recovery, preferably with the nose positioned below the level of the pharynx so that any secretions or regurgitated ingesta can drain. If the animal allows, the tongue should be extended. The animal should be made comfortable with appropriate bedding material and consideration given to postoperative analgesia where applicable. In smaller species endotracheal tubes should be removed whilst the animal is still relatively deep to avoid laryngeal spasm that may arise from extubation during light anaesthesia. In the larger species, laryngeal spasm does not appear to be a problem and extubation can be delayed until cough reflexes are present. It has been common practice to turn cats periodically during prolonged recoveries to prevent partial airway collapse and congestion of the lower lung. However, studies by Taylor (pers. commun.) in the horse suggest that this is unnecessary and may be counterproductive in heavy animals. No direct evidence is available for non-domestic cats in this regard, but certainly caution should be exercised in repeated turning of large lion and tiger. Reversible anaesthetics are now used widely in non-domestic species reducing the need to consider turning, but where it is practised during prolonged recoveries it is advisable to assess respiratory function using pulse oximetry until this becomes unsafe for the operator and equipment. During recovery from any anaesthetic, cats should be frequently monitored and attended at least until they are capable of maintaining sternal recumbency.

Reversal of Anaesthetic Drugs

Chemical reversal of anaesthesia is more commonly practised and desirable in the non-domestic species than in the domestic cat. Ideal circumstances for recovery rarely exist either in captive or free-ranging conditions. The elimination of physical hazards including inappropriate ambient temperatures is virtually impossible, particularly in the field. Postanaesthetic monitoring is particularly difficult to provide with species that are potentially dangerous and all non-domestic cats resent human interference during recovery unless exceptionally tame. In the domestic animal such intervention may be reassuring whereas in non-domestic animals it will represent additional stress causing unnecessary excitement. Adequately trained staff are usually unavailable for observation of non-domestic cat recoveries requiring that the veterinarian is present at all times until the cat is sufficiently aroused. This is often impractical. For wild animals there is considerable advantage in being able to return the cat to its normal surroundings as soon as possible, and ideally this should only be done when full recovery has been achieved.

α_2-Antagonists

In recent years several α_2-antagonist drugs have been used to reverse anaesthesia in non-domestic cats where induction combinations include α_2-agonists. Most such combinations are based on ketamine plus xylazine or medetomidine, and residual impairment of motor and mental functions can occur for several hours if the α_2-agonist is not reversed. Conversely, where α_2-antagonists are given before the effects of ketamine have worn off, residual ataxia and excitement may occur as the cat is exposed to the effects of the cyclohexamine. In this regard the development of medetomidine/ketamine combinations has improved matters as very low doses of ketamine can be used with safety, particularly in the larger species. Nevertheless, at least 30 min should be allowed before an α_2-agonist is antagonized when it has been used in combination with ketamine.

α_2-Antagonists have intrinsic central nervous and cardiovascular effects and must be used with care (Klein & Klide, 1989). In theory, the amount of antagonist given at any point in time should be related to the amount of agonist activity remaining. This calculation requires knowledge not only of the administered dose and the time of administration, but also of the elimination rates of α_2-agonists in different species. Unfortunately, this information is not available. Dose rates of reversal agents in non-domestic species are therefore based on the practical experience of investigators and extrapolation from the situation in domestic cats. α_2-Antagonists work by blocking central and peripheral α_2- and α_1-adrenoceptors. However, the degree of specificity varies widely between different compounds due to varying α_2/α_1 selectivity ratios (Virtanen & MacDonald, 1987).

The unselective alpha blocker tolazoline ('Priscoline'—CIBA) was used in early work, but has now been largely superseded. Van Wyk and Berry (1986) demonstrated that wild lions anaesthetized with ketamine (8 mg/kg) plus xylazine (3.2 mg/kg) recovered far more rapidly following i/m or i/v tolazoline at 4 mg/kg than without reversal. After i/m tolazoline recoveries were noted within 1 h and after i/v tolazoline recoveries were seen within 20 min. Residual ataxia was present in all animals. Tolazoline at 5 mg/kg produced convulsions. Tolazoline has direct peripheral vasodilatory effects (Martindale, 1982) and i/v administration cannot therefore be recommended.

Yohimbine ('Antagonil'—Wildlife Laboratories) is one of a group of indole alkaloids possessing α-adrenergic blocking properties. It has low α_2/α_1 selectivity and also causes excitation if used in excess. It has been extensively used in the USA to reverse the effects of α_2-agonists in non-domestic species including cats. Intravenous doses of approximately 0.1 mg/kg are reported by several authors as effective in hastening recovery in a wide variety of medium and large cats, including tiger, leopard, jaguar and puma, that have been anaesthetized with the 'Hellabruner mixture' of ketamine and xylazine (Gonzales & McDonnel, 1986; Bush *et al.*, 1987; Goltenboth & Klos, 1987). However, direct comparisons between studies are very difficult to make as no universal standards of what constitutes a recovery were used and reversal agents were given at varying times after the α_2-agonists. Arousal times of 5–15 min were reported by Gonzales & McDonnel (1986) following i/v administration, with 'walk times' of 15–30 min. Higher doses are advocated for i/m administration (Goltenboth & Klos, 1987; Wildlife Restraint Series, 1991). In only one study was the amount of yohimbine related to the amount of xylazine given. Seal *et al.* (1987) recommended that in tigers i/v yohimbine should be used at 10% of the xylazine dose to achieve recovery times of less than 10 min. In the experience of the International Zoo Veterinary Group i/m doses of up to 0.15 mg/kg are effective in large cats and up to 0.5 mg/kg is appropriate in small species.

Idazoxan (Reckitt & Colman) is another imidazoline derivative, but with far greater α_2 selectivity and potency than yohimbine. In the UK it is not available commercially. Intramuscular doses of approximately 0.05–0.1 mg/kg are effective in reversing the sedative and cardiovascular effects of xylazine (Crawshaw *et al.*, 1986). Although doses of 0.1 mg/kg i/m have been used to reverse the effects of medetomidine in some tigers and lions by the author, not all animals respond equally and some not at all.

The idazoxan analogue, 2-methoxy-idazoxan (RX821002A—Reckitt & Colman) has shown great potential as a specific α_2-antagonist in cats, although insufficient data are available to make firm recommendations about dose rates.

Unfortunately, this drug is also not commercially available as yet. Its potency and specificity is claimed to be far greater than idazoxan (Reckitt & Coleman, pers. commun.) and preliminary experience with the compound would appear to bear this out. Kock *et al.* (1989) achieved reversal of the effects of xylazine in tiger, cheetah, jaguar and lion with 2-methoxy-idazoxan (2-MI) at 5–40 µg/kg i/m, although residual depression and ataxia were noted. The author has observed satisfactory reversal of medetomidine within 20 min in captive lions, tiger and snow leopard using 2-MI at 10–33 µg/kg i/m at 30–45 min after induction. Residual depression was noted in 2 out of 15 lions. These doses represent 25–50% of the dose of medetomidine used. One jaguar given 12 µg/kg 2-MI i/m to reverse medetomidine (equivalent to 33% of medetomidine dose) became overexcited during recovery. Although the drug can be given i/v to hasten recovery (personal observation), Kock *et al.* (1989) reported convulsions in a lion and a tiger given i/v 2-MI at 5 µg/kg and 20 µg/kg respectively. It is not clear whether this was a direct effect of the 2-MI or as a result of exposure to residual effects of ketamine.

Another idazoxan analogue, atipamezole, ('Antisedan' Norden) has been widely used in non-domestic cats to reverse the effects of medetomidine. Atipamezole is a highly potent, specific α_2-adrenoceptor competitive antagonist with considerably greater α_2 receptor specificity than idazoxan (Virtanen, 1989). Following anaesthesia with medetomidine/ketamine as described earlier, i/m doses of atipamezole at 2.5–3 times the dose of medetomidine will lead to smooth arousal within 10–20 min. The first signs of reversal are usually pupillary dilatation followed by raising of the head. Soon thereafter animals are able to sit on their brisket and walk. Control of the hind legs is generally achieved after that of the fore legs and hind leg ataxia may persist for a while. The amount of atipamezole given should be reduced where anaesthesia is prolonged. Atipamezole given at 4–5 times the medetomidine dose is tolerated by many species but may cause post-recovery restlessness, excitement, hyperaesthesia and hyperextension of claws in the jaguar, puma

and ocelot. It is interesting to note that these are all New World species. If absolutely necessary, recovery can be further hastened by dividing the atipamezole dose between the i/v and i/m routes. In this case reversal will be achieved within 5–10 min but often with some degree of post-recovery overalertness or excitement (Jalanka & Roeken, 1990; personal observation). The i/v route is not recommended for New World species and is usually unnecessary in any cat. Cats occasionally vomit on recovery following atipamezole. Some individuals show a tendency apparently to sleep after a complete recovery, but are aroused by the slightest stimulus.

Miscellaneous Drugs

The short-acting analeptic doxapram has been shown to be ineffective at reversing xylazine in domestic cats although there is a temporary initial stimulation (Hartsfield *et al.*, 1991). However, doxapram is an effective respiratory stimulant in non-domestic cats, but its effects are short-lived.

Although overdose is unlikely in non-domestic cats, benzodiazepine-induced sedation, muscle relaxation and apnoea can be temporarily reversed with the short-acting compound flumazenil ('Anexate'—Roche). This drug has virtually no pharmacological effect when given alone (Klein & Klide, 1989).

Analgesia

The control of postoperative and other kinds of pain in non-domestic cats has received virtually no attention and is often completely neglected even today. This is due, at least in part, to the low proportion of general anaesthetics administered to facilitate surgery. Although all cats show minimal overt signs of pain, there is little reason to suppose that invasive surgery, trauma and various severe medical conditions do not produce pain. Therefore the anaesthetist must at least consider the need for analgesia, both on welfare grounds and in consideration of the fact that postoperative pain may well delay healing and prevent adequate feeding.

Guidelines for analgesia in the domestic cat have been produced by Taylor (1985), and what little advice that can be given for non-domestic species must be largely based on such information in addition to the author's practical experience. In general, opiates are considered necessary for the control of acute and severe pain, with non-steroidal anti-inflammatory drugs (NSAIDs) being used to alleviate chronic and low-grade pain (Taylor, 1985).

Opiates

Various opioids can be used to control pain in cats, but all have the disadvantage of a limited period of activity. Butorphanol at doses of between 0.05 and 0.1 mg/kg s/c, i/m or i/v have been found to provide effective visceral analgesia in domestic cats for between 4 and 6 h (Sawyer *et al.*, 1991a). It is effective via the oral route at 5–10 times the parenteral dose rate (Hall & Clarke, 1991, p. 69). Pethidine can be effective i/m at 2–4 mg/kg in domestic cats every 3–4 h postoperatively (Hall & Clarke, 1991). Although 0.1 mg/kg morphine i/m will provide a similar period of analgesia, its use should be restricted to once daily (Taylor, 1985; Hall & Clarke, 1991). Buprenorphine ('Temgesic'—Reckitt & Colman) has also been used in domestic cats at 6–10 μg/kg to good effect, but is found to significantly delay recovery from general anaesthesia. For practical reasons, the use of these opiate analgesics in non-domestic cats will usually be restricted to the immediate postoperative period.

Non-steroidal Anti-inflammatory Drugs

Despite their potential toxicity, NSAIDs can be used with care in cats. Excretion follows conjugation with glucuronic acid in the liver, a process that requires glucuronyl transferase. The feline liver has a relative deficiency of this enzyme compared to other species, and the resulting longer half-life of NSAIDs increases the risk of toxicity. Although all drugs in this class have the potential to cause gastric ulceration after long-term use, this has not been seen

by the author in the larger species medicated for periods not exceeding 7 days.

Aspirin has been used by the author in cheetah and lion with no apparent ill effect at oral doses of < 25 mg/kg once daily or once every other day for periods up to 7 days. Taylor (1985) commented on the development of aplastic anaemia and thrombocytopaenia in domestic cats following prolonged use of aspirin, although there is no information on this point in respect of non-domestic species.

Flunixin meglumine is a potent analgesic and anti-inflammatory in many species. Preliminary studies by Taylor *et al.* (1991) in domestic cats suggested that 1 mg/kg given every 12–24 h would not lead to drug accumulation. Furthermore, empirical observations by the author in lion, serval and jaguar suggest that the short-term (< 7 days) use of flunixin at 1 mg/kg once daily provides analgesia and anti-inflammatory activity without producing overt toxicity. Flunixin can cause renal papillary necrosis and therefore caution should be exercised with the use of this drug in dehydrated cats or those suffering any degree of renal impairment (Bush *et al.*, 1987).

Other NSAIDs that may have application in the non-domestic species include phenylbutazone and ketoprofen. Phenylbutazone has been used by the author on a few occasions in the larger species at ~ 10 mg/kg daily in divided oral doses for periods of up to 7 days with no apparent adverse side-effects. Ketoprofen ('Ketofen'—Rhone-Merieux) has recently been introduced for use in domestic cats and is claimed to be a potent analgesic and anti-inflammatory agent. Recommended dose rates are 2 mg/kg s/c once daily for 3 days or 1 mg/kg *per os* once daily for 5 days. Due to the low toxicity in the domestic cat, ketoprofen should be seriously considered for further investigation in non-domestic species.

α₂-Agonists

Medetomidine and other α_2-agonists possess analgesic properties at relatively low doses. Where these drugs have been included in the induction regime and their action not subsequently reversed, a degree of analgesia will persist beyond the period of anaesthesia. Therefore, by appropriate choice of induction agents such residual analgesia can be exploited following minor procedures that may be mildly painful for short periods. Furthermore, α_2-agonists augment the visceral analgesia provided by butorphanol in domestic cats (Sawyer *et al.*, 1991b). Thus, one of many factors in the decision to antagonize α_2-agonists or not should be consideration of postoperative analgesia.

References

Allen, J.L. (1990) Pulse oximetry: Clinical applications in zoological medicine. *Proc. Ann. Conf. AAZV*, pp. 163–164.

Allen, J.L. (1992) Pulse oximetry: everyday uses in a zoological practice. *Vet. Rec.* **130**, 354–355.

Baily, T.N. (1971) Immobilization of bobcats, coyotes and badgers with phencyclidine hydrochloride. *J. Wildl. Manage.* **35**, 847–849.

Barnett, J.E.F. & Lewis, J.C.M. (1990) Medetomidine and ketamine anaesthesia in zoo animals and its reversal with atipamezole. A review and update with specific reference to work in British zoos. *Proc. Ann. Conf. AAZV*, pp. 207–214.

Beck, C.C. (1972) Chemical restraint of exotic species. *J. Zoo Anim. Med.* **3**, 3–66.

Beck, C.C. (1976) VETALAR (ketamine hydrochloride). A unique cataleptoid anesthetic agent for multispecies usage. *J. Zoo Anim. Med.* **7**, 11–38.

Bedford, S.W. & Godsall, S.A. (1988) Letter to *Veterinary Rec.* 11.6.88, pp. 590–591.

Benirschke, K., Griner, L.A. & Saltzstein, S.L. (1976) Pathological findings in Siberian tigers. *Erkrankungen der Zootiere* **18**, 263–274.

Berrie, P.M. (1972) Sex differences in response to phencyclidine hydrochloride in lynx. *J. Wildl. Manage.* **36**, 994–996.

Bertram, B.C.R. (1976) Lion immobilization using phencyclidine (Sernylan). *E. Afr. Wildl. J.* **14**, 233–235.

Bertram, B.C.R. & King, J.M. (1976) Lion and leopard immobilization using CI-744. *E. Afr. Wildl. J.* **14**, 237–239.

Boever, W.J., Holden, J. & Kane, K.K. (1977) Use of Telazol (CI-744) for chemical restraint and anesthesia in wild and exotic carnivores. *Vet. Medicine/Small Anim. Clinician* **72**, 1722-1725.

Brearley, J.C., Kellagher, R.E.B. & Hall, L.W. (1988) Propofol anaesthesia in cats. *J.S.A.P.* **29**, 315–322.

Bush, M. & Teeple, E. (1975) Barbiturate toxicity in lions. *J. Zoo Anim. Med.* **6**, 25–26.

Bush, M., Custer, R., Smeller, J., Bush, L.M., Seal, U.S. & Barton, R. (1978) The acid–base status of lions, *Panthera leo*, immobilized with four drug combinations. *J. Wildlife Dis.* **14**, 102–109.

Bush, M., Phillips, L.G. & Montali, R.J. (1987) Clinical management of captive tigers. *In: Tigers of the World* (ed. R.L. Tilson & U.S. Seal), pp. 171–204. Noyes Publications, New Jersey.

Button, C., Meltzer, D.G.A. & Mulders, M.S.G. (1981) Saffan induced poikilothermia in cheetah (*Acinonyx jubitus*). *J. S. Afri. Vet. Assoc.* **52**, 237–238.

Clarke, K.W. & Hall, L.W. (1990) A survey of anaesthesia in small animal practice: AVA/BSAVA report. *J. Assoc. Vet. Anaesth.* **17**, 4–10.

Cook, C.S. & Kane, K.K. (1980) Apparent suppression of gastrointestinal motility due to xylazine—A comparative study. *J. Zoo Anim. Med.* **11**, 46–47.

Cooper, R. (1989) A precautionary note concerning the use of Telazol in the Siberian tiger. *Amer. Assoc. Zoo Vet. Newsletter* **5**, 3.

Crawshaw, G.J., Mehran, K.G. & Black, S. (1986) Antagonism of xylazine and ketamine/xylazine combinations in exotic species by idazoxan and RX821002. *Proc. Ann. Conf. AAZV*, pp. 1–2.

Cullen, L.K. & Jones, R.S. (1977) Clinical observations on xylazine/ketamine anaesthesia in the cat. *Vet. Rec.* **101**, 115–116.

Davies, M. (1988) Letter to *Vet. Rec.* 25.6.88, p. 640.

Dinnes, M.R. & Henrickson, R. (1970) Liver disease in cheetahs. A preliminary report. *Proc. Ann. Conf. AAZV*, 110 – 114.

Dinnes, M.R. (1980) Medical care of non-domestic carnivores. *In: Current Veterinary Therapy* **VII**, pp. 710–753. W.B. Saunders.

Dolensek, E.P. (1971) Anesthesia of exotic felines with ketamine HCL. *J. Zoo Anim. Med.* **2**, 16–19.

Dunkle, N. Moise, N.J., Scarlettg-Kranz, J. & Short, C.E. (1986) Cardiac performance in cats after administration of xylazine or xylazine and glycopyrrolate: echocardiographic evaluations. *Amer. J. Vet. Res.* **47**, 2212–2216.

Ebedes, H. (1973 The drug immobilization of carnivorous animals. *In: The Capture and Care of Wild Animals* (ed. E. Young), pp. 62–68. Human & Rousseau Publishers, Cape Town.

Ebedes, H. & Burroughs, R. (1989) Long-acting neuroleptics in wildlife. Ms Paper presented at the Tranquilizer Symposium held at the National

Zoological Gardens, 17th March, 1989. Pretoria, South Africa.

Fanton, J.W., Hubbard, G.B. & Fletcher, K.C. (1984) Halothane induced hepatic necrosis in a snow leopard. *J. Zoo Anim. Med.* **15**, 108–111.

Fowler, M.E. (1986) *Zoo and Wild Animal Medicine*, 2nd edn. W.B. Saunders, Philadelphia.

Goltenboth, von R. & Klos, H-G. (1987) Versuche mit yohimbin als antidot bei durch xylazin immobilisierten zootieren im Zoo Berlin. *In: Proc. 29th Int. Symp. uber die Erkrankungen der Zootiere*, 20.5.87, Cardiff.

Gonzales, B.J. & McDonnel, T. (1986) The effects of yohimbine on xylazine–ketamine anesthesia in exotic felidae. *Proc. Ann. Conf. AAZV*, pp. 142–143.

Gosselin, S.J., Loudy, D.L., Tarr, M.J., Balistreri, W.F., Setchell, K.D.R., Johnston, J.O., Kramer, L.W. & Dresser, B.B. (1988) Veno-occlusive disease of the liver in captive cheetah. *Vet. Pathol.* **25**, 48–57.

Graham-Jones, O. (1964) Restraint and anaesthesia of some captive wild mammals. *Vet. Rec.* **76**, 1216–1248.

Gray, C.W., Bush, M. & Beck, C.C. (1974) Clinical experience using CI-744 in chemical restraint and anesthesia of exotic specimens. *J. Zoo Anim. Med.* **5**, 12–21.

Green, C.J. (1979) *Animal Anaesthesia*. Laboratory Animals, London.

Hall, L.W. & Clarke, K.W. (1991) *Veterinary Anaesthesia*, 9th edn. Baillière Tindall, London.

Haigh, J.C., Pharr, J.W. & Daoust, P.Y. (1978) Pleuropericarditis and pneumonia due to listeria monocytogenes in an African lion. *J. Zoo Anim. Med.* **9**, 38–42.

Hartsfield, S.M., Matthews, N.S., Miller, S., Cornick, J. & Jacobson, J.D. (1991) Comparison of the effects of tolazoline, yohimbine, and doxapram in cats medicated with xylazine. *Proc. 4th Int. Congress of Vet. Anaesth.* pp. 71–73.

Hewer, T.F., Harrison, L. & Malkin, T. (1948) Lipuria in tigers. *Proc. Zool. Soc. London* **118**, 924–928.

Hornocker, M.G., Craighead, J.J. & Pfeiffer, E.W. (1965) Immobilizing mountain lions with succinylcholine chloride and pentobarbital sodium. *J. Wildl. Manage.* **29**, 880–883.

Hornocker, M.G. & Wiles, W.V. (1972) Immobilizing pumas (*Felis concolor*) with phencyclidine hydrochloride. *Int. Zoo Yearb.* **12**, 220–223. Zoological Society of London.

Jalanka, H. (1987) Clinical-pharmacological properties of a new sedative—Medetomidine—and its antagonist, MPV-1248. *Proc. 1st Int. Conf. Zoo & Avian Med.* pp. 530–534.

Jalanka, H.H. (1989a) Medetomidine- and ketamine-induced immobilization of snow leopards (*Panthera uncia*): Doses, evaluation, and reversal by atipamezole. *J. Zoo & Wildl. Med.* **20**, 154–162.

Jalanka, H.H. (1989b) Evaluation and comparison of two ketamine-based immobilization techniques in snow leopards (*Panthera uncia*). *J. Zoo & Wildl. Med.* **20**, 163–169.

Jalanka, H.H. & Roeken, B.O. (1990) The use of medetomidine, medetomidine–ketamine combinations, and atipamezole in non-domestic mammals: A review. *J. Zoo & Wildl. Med.* **21**, 259–282.

Jones, D.M. (1972) The use of drugs for immobilization, capture, and translocation of non-domestic animals. *Veterinary Annual*, pp. 320–352.

Jones, R.S. (1983) Intravenous anaesthesia in cats. *In: The Veterinary Annual*, 23rd issue, pp. 276–280. Scientechnica, Bristol.

Kelly, D.F., Pearson, H., Wright, A.I. & Greenham, L.W. (1980) Morbidity in captive white tigers. *In: The Comparative Pathology of Zoo Animals* (ed. R.J. Montali, & G. Migaki), pp. 183–188. Smithsonian Institution Press, Washington DC.

King, J.M., Bertram, B.C.R. & Hamilton, P.H. (1977) Tiletamine and zolazepam for immobilization of wild lions and leopards. *J.A.V.M.A.* **171**, 894–898.

Kitchener, A. (1991) *The Natural History of the Wild Cats*. Christopher Helm, London.

Klein, L. (1980) Clinical pharmacology of agents used in the restraint of felidae and hoofed stock. *Proc. Ann. Conf. AAZV*, pp. 7–12.

Klein, L.V. & Klide, A.M. (1989) Central α_2 adrenergic and benzodiazepine agonists and their antagonists. Review article. *J. Zoo & Wildlife Med.* **20**, 138–153.

Klide, A.M., Calderwood, H.W. & Soma, L.R. (1975) Cardiopulmonary effects of xylazine in dogs. *Am. J. Vet. Res.* **36**, 931–935.

Klos, H-G & Lang, E.M. (eds) (1976) *Handbook of Zoo Animal Medicine*. Van Nostrand Reinhold, New York.

Kock, R.A. (1987) Remote injection systems: Science and art. *Vet. Rec.* **121**, 76–80.

Kock, R.A., Jago, M., Gulland, F.M.D. & Lewis, J.C.M. (1989) The use of two novel alpha 2 adrenoceptor antagonists, idazoxan and its analogue RX821002A in zoo and wild animals. *J. Ass. Vet. Anaesth.* **16**, 4–10.

Krahwinkel, D.J. (1970) The use of tiletamine hydrochloride as an incapacitating agent for a lion. *J.A.V.M.A.* **157**, 622–623.

Lewis, J.C.M. (1991) Veterinary considerations. *In: Management Guidelines for Exotic Cats* (ed. J.

Partridge), pp. 126–130. Association of British Wild Animal Keepers, Bristol, UK.

Logan, K.A., Thorne, E.T., Irwin, L.L. & Skinner, R. (1986) Immobilizing wild mountain lions (*Felis concolor*) with ketamine hydrochloride and xylazine hydrochloride. *J. Wildl. Dis.* **22**, 97–103.

Martin, H.D. & Mallock, A. (1987) Management of barbiturate intoxication in cougars (*Felis concolor*). *J. Zoo Anim. Med.* **18**, 100–103.

Martindale, W. (1982) Tolazoline hydrochloride. *In: The Extra Pharmacopoeia*, 28th edn (ed. J.E.F. Reynolds), pp. 1633–1634. The Pharmaceutical Press, London.

Mayo, J.G. (1967) Report on the tranquillisation of a male snow leopard (*Panthera uncia*) for semen extraction. *Int. Zoo Yearb.* **7**, 148–150.

McKenzie, A.A. (1993) (ed.) *The Capture and Care Manual: Capture, Care, Accommodation and Transportation of Wild African Animals.* Wildlife Decision Support Services and The South African Veterinary Foundation, Pretoria.

Michell, A.R., Bywater, R.J., Clarke, K.W., Hall, L.W. & Waterman, A.E. (1989) Anaesthesia, surgery and fluid therapy: *In: Veterinary Fluid Therapy* (ed. A.R. Michell *et al.*), pp. 215–221. Blackwell Scientific Publications, Oxford.

Morgan, D.W.T. & Legge, K. (1989) Clinical evaluation of propofol as an intravenous anaesthetic agent in cats and dogs. *Vet. Rec.* **124**, 31–33.

Munson, L. & Worley, M.B. (1987) The prevalence and morphology of liver disease in captive large cats: A comparison between snow leopards and cheetahs. *Proc. 1st Int. Conf. Zoo & Avian Med., AAZV*, p. 492.

Munson, L. & Worley, M.B. (1991) Veno-occlusive disease in snow leopards (*Panthera uncia*) from Zoological Parks. *Vet. Pathol.* **28**, 37–45.

Quandt, S. (1993) The immobilization of African lions (*Panthera leo*) with medetomidine/ketamine in comparison with tiletamine/zolazepam and phencyclidine (abstract). *Proceedings of International Symposium: Capture, Care and Management of Threatened Mammals.* Wildlife Group of South African Veterinary Association and W.A.W.V., Skukuza, South Africa, Sept. 1993.

Raiha, M.P., Raiha, J.E. & Short, C.E. (1989) A comparison of xylazine, acepromazine, meperidine and medetomidine as preanaesthetics to halothane anaesthesia in dogs. *Acta Vet. Scand.* **85**, 97–102.

Reed, G.T. & Tennant, M.B. (1975) Vasectomy procedure for African lions. *J. Zoo Anim. Med.* **6**, 15.

Robinson, P.T. (1976) Immobilization of felidae with M99. *J. Zoo Anim. Med.* **7**, 31.

Robinson, P.T. & Benirschke, K. (1981) Removal of a conjunctival dermoid in an African lion (*Panthera leo*). *J. Zoo Anim. Med.* **12**, 85–88.

Roeken, B.O. (1987) Medetomidine in zoo animal anaesthesia. *Proc 1st Int. Conf. Avian & Zoo Med., AAZV*, pp. 535–538.

Ruedi, D., Helstab, A & van den Ingh, T. (1980) Liver cirrhosis in snow leopards—further results. *Int. Ped. Book of Snow Leopards* **11**, 195–204.

Saint John, B.E. (1992) Pulse oximetry: Theory, technology and clinical considerations. *Proc. Ann. Conf., AAZV*, pp. 223–229.

Salonen, J. (1989) Pharmacokinetics of medetomidine. *Acta Vet. Scand.* Suppl. **85**, 49–54.

Sawyer, D.C., Rech, R.H. & Durham, R.A. (1991a) Does ketamine provide adequate visceral analgesia when used alone or in combination with acepromazine, diazepam, or butorphanol in cats? *Proc. 4th Int. Congr. Vet. Anaesth.* p. 381.

Sawyer, D.C., Rech, R.H., Durham, R.A., Jandron, S.R., Richter, M.A. & Striler, E.L. (1991b) Does butorphanol provide adequate surgical analgesia in the dog and cat? *Proc. 4th Int. Congr. Vet. Anaesth.* pp. 383–384.

Schmidt, R.E., Hubbard, G.B. & Fletcher, K.C. (1986) Systematic survey of lesions from animals in a zoologic collection: III. Respiratory system. *J. Zoo Anim. Med.* **17**, 17–23.

Schobert, E. (1987) Telazol use in wild and exotic animals—clinical experience and a review of the literature. *Vet. Med.* Oct 1987, pp. 1080–1088.

Seal, U. S. & Erickson, A.W. (1969) Immobilization of carnivora and other mammals with phencyclidine and promazine. *Fed. Proc.* **28**, 1410–1416.

Seal, U.S., Erickson, A.W. & Mayo, J.G. (1970) Drug immobilisation of the carnivora. *Int. Zoo Yearb.* **10**, 157–170. Zoological Society of London.

Seal, U.S., Barton, R., Mether, L., Olberding, K., Plotka, E.D. & Gray, C.W. (1976) Hormonal contraception in captive female lions (*Panthera leo*). *J. Zoo Anim. Med.* **7**, 12–20.

Seal, U.S., Armstrong, D.L. & Simmonds, L.G. (1987) Yohimbine hydrochloride reversal of ketamine hydrochloride and xylazine hydrochloride immobilization of Bengal tigers and effects on haematology and serum chemistries. *J. Wildl. Dis.* **23**, 296–300.

Segal, I.S., Vickery, R.G. & Maze, M. (1989) Dexmedetomidine decreases halothane anesthetic requirements in rats. *Acta Vet. Scand.* **85**, 55–59.

Seidensticker, J., Tamang, K.M. & Gray, C.W. (1974) The use of CI-744 to immobilize free ranging tigers and leopards. *J. Zoo Anim. Med.* **5**, 22–25.

Sitton, L. & Weaver, D. (1976) *A Study of California*

Mountain Lions. Calif. Dept. of Fish & Game, Pittman-Robertson report.

Smeller, J. & Bush, M. (1976) A physiological study of immobilized cheetahs. *J. Zoo Anim. Med.* **7**, 5–7.

Smuts, G.L., Bryden, B.R., de Vos, V. & Young, E. (1973) Some practical advantages of CI-581 (ketamine) for the field immobilization of larger wild felines, with comparative notes on baboons and impala. *Lammergeyer*, **18**, 1–14.

Taylor, P. (1985) Analgesia in the dog and cat. *In Practice*, **7**, 5–13.

Taylor, P.M., Lees, P., Reynoldson, J., Stodulski, G. & Jefferies, R. (1991) Pharmacodynamics and pharmacokinetics of flunixin in the cat: a preliminary study. *Vet. Rec.* **128**, 258.

Theobald, J. (1970) Experience in maintaining an exotic cat collection at the Cincinnatti Zoo. *J. Zoo Anim. Med.* **1**, 4–9.

Universities Federation for Animal Welfare (1981) Feral cats: Notes for veterinary surgeons. *Vet. Rec.* **108**, 301–303.

Vaino, O. (1989) Introduction to the clinical pharmacology of medetomidine. *Acta. Vet. Scand.* **85**, 85–88.

Van Wyk, T.C. & Berry, H.H. (1986) Tolazoline as an antagonist in free-living lions immobilised with a ketamine–xylazine combination. *J. Sth Afr. Vet. Assoc.* **57**, 221–224.

Verstegen, J., Fargetton, X., Donnay, I. & Ectors, F. (1991) An evaluation of medetomidine/ketamine and other drug combinations for anaesthesia in cats. *Vet. Rec.* **128**, 32–35.

Vickery, R.G. & Maze, M. (1989) Action of the stereoisomers of medetomidine in halothane-anaesthetised dogs. *Acta Vet. Scand.* **85**, 71–76.

Virtanen, R. (1989) Pharmacological profiles of medetomidine and its antagonist, atipamezole. *Acta Vet. Scand.* **85**, 29–37.

Virtanen, R. & MacDonald, E. (1987) Reversal of the sedative/analgesic and other effects of detomidine and medetomidine by MPV-1248, a novel α_2-antagonist. *Pharmacol. Toxicol.* **60** (Suppl.), 73.

Virtanen, R., Savola, J., Saano, V. & Nyman, L. (1988) Characterization of the selectivity, specificity, and potency of medetomidine as an α-2-adrenoceptor agonist. *Eur. J. Pharmacol.* **150**, 9–14.

Wahlberg, C. (1980) Autopsy findings and causes of death in captive snow leopards (*Panthera uncia*): A preliminary report. *Int. Ped. Book of Snow Leopards*, **2**, 205–217.

Wallach, J.D. & Boever, W.J. (1983) *Disease of Exotic Animals. Medical and Surgical Management.* W.B. Saunders, Philadelphia.

Waterman, A.E. (1983) Influence of premedication with xylazine on the distribution and metabolism of intramuscularly administered ketamine in cats. *Res. Vet. Sci.* **35**, 285–290.

Wiesner, H. (1977) Tranquilization by the 'blowgun rifle' method. *Kleintierpraxis*, **22**, 327–330.

Wiesner, H. & von Hegel, G. (1985) Praktische hinweise zur immobilisation von wild- und zootieren. *Tierarztl. Prax.* **13**, 113–127.

Wildlife Restraint Series (1991) International Wildlife Veterinary Services Inc., 1850 North Main Street, Salinas, California, 93906, USA.

Wildt, D.E., Howard, J. & Bush, M. (1985) Ejaculate characteristics and adrenal–pituitary–gonadal relationships in clouded leopards evaluated throughout the year. *Proc. Ann. Conf. AAZV*, pp. 33–36.

Wildt, D.E., Mellen, J.D. & Seal, U.S. (1992) *In: Felid Action Plan, 1991 and 1992: AAZPA Felid Taxon Advisory Group Regional Collection Plan and IUCN Captive Breeding Specialist Group Global Felid Plan*, pp. 150–152. Conservation and Research Center, Smithsonian Institution, Virginia.

Wright, M. (1982) Pharmacological effects of ketamine and its use in veterinary medicine. *J.A.V.M.A.* **180**, 1462–1471.

York, W. & Huggins, K. (1972) Rompun (Bay Va 1470). *J. Zoo Anim. Med.* **3**, 15–17.

Young, L.E. & Jones, R.S. (1990) Clinical observations on medetomidine/ketamine anaesthesia and its antagonism by atipamezole in the cat. *J.S.A.P.* **31**, 221–224.

Zuba, J.R. & Allen, J.L. (1992) Affordable, portable, noninvasive monitoring equipment and its place in zoo and wildlife medicine. *Proc. Ann. Conf. AAZV*, pp. 230–234.

Index